# Therapeutic Use of Plant Secondary Metabolites

Edited by

## Saheed Sabiu

*Department of Biotechnology and Food Science*
*Faculty of Applied Sciences*
*Durban University of Technology*
*Durban 4000*
*South Africa*

# Therapeutic Use of Plant Secondary Metabolites

Editor: Saheed Sabiu

ISBN (Online): 978-981-5050-62-2

ISBN (Print): 978-981-5050-63-9

ISBN (Paperback): 978-981-5050-64-6

© 2022, Bentham Books imprint.

Published by Bentham Science Publishers Pte. Ltd. Singapore. All Rights Reserved.

First published in 2022.

need for a court order if at any point you breach any terms of this License Agreement. In no event will any delay or failure by Bentham Science Publishers in enforcing your compliance with this License Agreement constitute a waiver of any of its rights.

3. You acknowledge that you have read this License Agreement, and agree to be bound by its terms and conditions. To the extent that any other terms and conditions presented on any website of Bentham Science Publishers conflict with, or are inconsistent with, the terms and conditions set out in this License Agreement, you acknowledge that the terms and conditions set out in this License Agreement shall prevail.

**Bentham Science Publishers Pte. Ltd.**
80 Robinson Road #02-00
Singapore 068898
Singapore
Email: subscriptions@benthamscience.net

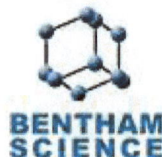

# CONTENTS

# FOREWORD

For centuries, plants have played vital roles in biological beings' economic, social, spiritual, cultural and health wellbeing. Interestingly, through knowledge and advances in research and technology, human beingare gaining a deeper understanding of the significant contributions of plants to human and animal health and development. There is abundant evidence showing that medicinal plants and their secondary metabolites are useful in preventing, ameliorating and in the treatment of various disease conditions such as diabetes, cancer, bacterial, fungal and viral infections. I am aware that many books on medicinal plants and secondary metabolites are in the market and university libraries. However, the current book on "Therapeutic use of plant secondary metabolites" is unique in its content, diversity, and originality of materials. Its depth and expertise of various national and international contributors make it a must-have and a must-read for scientists in the field of medicinal plants, agriculture, food science, postgraduate students, health professionals, and traditional healers. The book covers important topics such as drug discovery and their metabolites in health management, plant secondary metabolites as therapeutic agents in degenerative and microbial infections, etc. The topics are well-structured, covering 15 chapters (chapters 1-15). These topics/chapters provide a framework and stimuli for further in-depth research in the field.

I strongly endorse the book.

**Oluwafemi Omoniyi Oguntibeju**
Department of Biomedical Sciences
Faculty of Health & Wellness Sciences
Cape Peninsula University of Technology
Bellville, South Africa

# PREFACE

The concept of phytotherapy is as old as mankind. During the last decades, it has become evident that there exist several plants with therapeutic potential, and it is increasingly being accepted that phytotherapy could offer potential lead compounds in the drug discovery/development process. The interest in phytotherapy could be associated with secondary metabolites that could act individually, additively, or in synergy to improve health and wellbeing. Indeed, medicinal plants, unlike conventional drugs, commonly have bioactive constituents working together catalytically and synergistically to produce a combined effect that may surpass the total activity of the individual constituents. The combined actions of these metabolites tend to increase the activity of the main constituent by speeding up or slowing down its metabolism in the body. Also, the secondary metabolites might minimize the rate of undesired adverse effects, and have an additive, potentiating, or antagonistic effect.

The book offers evidence-based mechanistic views on complementary and alternative medicine with a focus on biological mechanisms of action of plant secondary metabolites in degenerative and microbial diseases such as diabetes, cancer, neurodegenerative disorders, antimicrobial resistance, etc., while reporting health benefits. The chapters are written by enviable scholars, lecturers, and experts in indigenous knowledge systems (IKS), industrial and medicinal plants, phytotherapeutics, and phytoinformatics. **Therapeutic Uses of Plant Secondary Metabolites** is timely and highly valuable for both undergraduate and postgraduate students, as well as researchers and professionals in IKS, phytomedicine, ethnopharmacology, phytopharmacology, plant biotechnology, drug discovery and development, and phytotherapeutics.

**Saheed Sabiu**

Department of Biotechnology and Food Science
Faculty of Applied Sciences
Durban University of Technology
Durban 4000
South Africa

# List of Contributors

**A.K. Oyebamiji**
Computational Chemistry Research Laboratory, Department of Pure and Applied Chemistry, Ladoke Akintola University of Technology, Ogbomoso, Oyo State, Nigeria

**Adeyemi O. Aremu**
Indigenous Knowledge Systems (IKS) Centre, North-West University, Faculty of Natural and Agricultural Sciences, Private Bag X2046, Mmabatho 2790, South Africa
School of Life Sciences, Scottsville 3209, University of KwaZulu-Natal Pietermaritzburg, Private Bag X01, Scottsville 3209, South Africa

**Aderonke F. Ajayi-Smith**
International Centre for Genetic Engineering and Biotechnology (ICGEB), Cape Town, South Africa

**Adeniyi C. Adeola**
State Key Laboratory of Genetic Resources and Evolution, Yunnan Laboratory of Molecular Biology of Domestic Animals, Kunming Institute of Zoology, Chinese Academy of Sciences, China

**Abdulwakeel A. Ajao**
Department of Botany and Plant Biotechnology, University of Johannesburg, PO Box 524, Auckland Park 2006, Johannesburg, South Africa

**Babatunji E. Oyinloye**
Wits Advanced Drug Delivery Platform Research Unit, Department of Pharmacy and Pharmacology, School of Therapeutic Science, Faculty of Health Sciences, University of the Witwatersrand, Johannesburg, York Road, Parktown, South Africa
Phytomedicine, Biochemical Toxicology and Biotechnology Research Laboratories, Department of Biochemistry, Faculty of Sciences, Afe Babalola University, Ado Ekiti, Nigeria

**Bulama I.**
Department of Veterinary Physiology and Biochemistry, University of Maiduguri, Maiduguri, Nigeria

**Bilbis L.S.**
Department of Biochemistry, Usmanu Danfodiyo University Sokoto, Nigeria

**Chinedu E. Udekwu**
Department of Biochemistry, College of Natural Sciences, Michael Okpara University of Agriculture, Umudike, Abia State, Nigeria

**Christiana E. Aruwa**
Department of Biotechnology and Food Science, Durban University of Technology, P.O.Box 1334, Durban 4000, South Africa

**Depika Dwarka**
Durban University of Science, Department of Biotechnology and Food Science, Durban, KwaZulu-Natal, South Africa

**Emmanuel O. Ajani**
Department of Medical Biochemistry and Pharmacology, Kwara State University, Malete, P.M.B. 1530, Ilorin, Nigeria

**Fatai O. Balogun**
Department of Biotechnology and Food Science, Durban University of Technology, P.O.Box 1334, Durban 4000, South Africa

**Fikisiwe C. Gebashe**
Agricultural Research Council – Vegetables, Industrial and Medicinal Plants, Pretoria, Private Bag X293, Pretoria 0001, South Africa

| | |
|---|---|
| **Henry A. Adeola** | Department of Oral and Maxillofacial Pathology, Faculty of Dentistry, University of the Western Cape and Tygerberg Hospital, Cape Town, South Africa<br>Division of Dermatology, Department of Medicine, Faculty of Health Sciences and Groote Schuur Hospital, University of Cape Town, Cape Town, South Africa |
| **Himansu Baijnath** | University of KwaZulu-Natal, School of Biological Sciences, Durban, South Africa |
| **Ismaila O. Nurain** | Department of Pharmacology, The University of Minnesota Medical School, Minneapolis, USA |
| **J.O. Aribisala** | Department of Biotechnology and Food Science, Faculty of Applied Sciences, Durban University of Technology, South Africa |
| **John Jason Mellem** | Durban University of Technology, Department of Biotechnology and Food Science, Durban, KwaZulu-Natal, South Africa |
| **Karishma Singh** | Department of Biotechnology and Food Science, Durban University of Technology, P.O.Box 1334, Durban 4000, South Africa |
| **Kazeem A. Alayande** | Antibiotic Resistance and Phage Biocontrol Research Group, Department of Microbiology, North-West University, Mmabatho 2745, South Africa<br>Unit for Environmental Sciences and Managements, North-West University, Potchefstroom, South Africa |
| **M.O. Kaka** | Department of Microbiology, Adeleke University, Ede, Osun State, Nigeria |
| **Michael C. Ojo** | Department of Biochemistry and Microbiology, University of Zululand, KwaDlangezwa, South Africa |
| **Mariam O. Oyedeji-Amusa** | Department of Botany and Plant Biotechnology, University of Johannesburg, PO Box 524, Auckland Park 2006, Johannesburg, South Africa |
| **Ohanaka N.J.** | Department of Biochemistry, Nile University of Nigeria, Abuja, Nigeria |
| **Pillay Charlene** | Department of Biotechnology and Food Science, Durban University of Science, Durban, South Africa |
| **Ramdhani Nishani** | Council for Scientific and Industrial Research, Durban, South Africa |
| **Raphael T. Aruleba** | Department of Molecular and Cell Biology, Faculty of Science, University of Cape Town, Cape Town, South Africa |
| **Rashmi Bhardwaj** | Centre for Medical Biotechnology, Maharshi Dayanand University, Rohtak, Haryana, India |
| **Saheed Sabiu** | Department of Biotechnology and Food Science, Durban University of Technology, P.O.Box 1334, Durban 4000, South Africa |
| **Singh Seema** | Subinite (Pty) Ltd, Godrej Consumer Products South Africa, Durban, South Africa |

**Stephen O. Amoo**  Agricultural Research Council – Vegetables, Industrial and Medicinal Plants, Pretoria, Private Bag X293, Pretoria 0001, South Africa
Indigenous Knowledge Systems (IKS) Centre, North-West University, Faculty of Natural and Agricultural Sciences, Private Bag X2046, Mmabatho 2790, South Africa
Department of Botany and Plant Biotechnology, Faculty of Science, University of Johannesburg, P.O. Box 524, Auckland Park 2006, South Africa

**Suleiman N.**  Department of Veterinary Physiology and Biochemistry, Faculty of Veterinary Medicine, Usmanu Danfodiyo University Sokoto, Sokoto, Nigeria

**T.A. Ajayeoba**  Department of Microbiology, Adeleke University, Ede, Osun State, Nigeria

**Taofik Olatunde Uthman**  School of Medicine and Department of Biological Sciences, University of Limerick, Limerick, Ireland

**Tayo A. Adekiya**  Wits Advanced Drug Delivery Platform Research Unit, Department of Pharmacy and Pharmacology, School of Therapeutic Science, Faculty of Health Sciences, University of the Witwatersrand, Johannesburg, York Road, Parktown, South Africa

**Uwazie C. Kenneth**  Department of Biochemistry, Nigeria, Ladoke Akintola University of Nigeria, Ogbomoso, Oyo State, Nigeria

**CHAPTER 1**

# The Role of Plant Secondary Metabolites in Health Management

**Taofik Olatunde Uthman[1,*]**

*[1] School of Medicine and Department of Biological Sciences, University of Limerick, Limerick, Ireland*

**Abstract:** Plant secondary metabolites (PSM) are bioactive compounds produced by plants for protection against predatory organisms and to attract insects for pollination. Recently, greater attention is being focused on PSM due to their perceived ability to elicit pharmacological activities, including antihypertensive, antiarrhythmic, antimalarial, anticancer, analgesic, antispasmodic, antidiabetic, and antimicrobial effects. Therefore, many plant species are continually screened for PSM, such as alkaloids, flavonoids, terpenes, saponins, cardiac glycosides, fatty acids, steroids, and tannins with a view to exploiting them in the manufacture of drugs and pharmaceuticals. In this review, the pharmacological activities and possible mechanisms of action of selected PSM are discussed.

**Keywords:** Alkaloids, Biological activity, Flavonoids, Polyphenols, Secondary metabolites, Saponins, Terpenes.

## 1. INTRODUCTION

The term 'metabolites' refers to intermediates and products of metabolism. They are usually small molecules with diverse functions, including structural, signaling, stimulatory, inhibitory, catalytic and defensive roles as well as providing fuel. Metabolites in plants can be of two types namely primary and secondary metabolites. Primary metabolites in plants are essential for life processes such as growth and development of cells. They are produced continuously during growth phase of plants where they are involved in important metabolic processes such as photosynthesis and respiration. Primary metabolites are generally heavy molecular weight compounds with diverse structures, including DNA, proteins, carbohydrates, and lipids.

* **Corresponding author Taofik Olatunde Uthman:** School of Medicine and Department of Biological Sciences, University of Limerick, Limerick, Ireland; E-mail: taofik.uthman@ul.ie

Unlike primary metabolites, secondary metabolites refer to a vast and diverse group of active organic compounds produced by plants for the purpose of increasing the likelihood of their survival by repelling or attracting other organisms. This implies that secondary metabolites play a defensive role against herbivory and other interspecies protection. They are not essential for the growth and development of the producing plants and are often differentially distributed among limited taxonomic groups within the plant kingdom. Their absence does not result in plant death but can impair survivability, fecundity, and aesthetics of plants. Apart from the protective role, some secondary metabolites are involved in the pigmentation of flower and seed, which attract pollinators, thereby enhancing seed dispersal and plant reproduction. More importantly, plant secondary metabolites have been reported to possess a myriad of pharmaceutical properties which can be exploited for human health [1]. Secondary metabolites are biosynthesized from primary metabolites by specialized cell types at distinct developmental stages. They are generally low molecular weight compounds, varying in quality and quantity for a specific plant species depending on location.

The main biotic factor that affects plants is a pathogenic infection caused by bacteria, viruses, fungi, and nematodes. Other biotic antagonists include attacks by mites, insects, mammals, and other herbivorous animals and competition from other plants arising from parasitism and allelopathy. The most significant abiotic environmental stresses faced by plants are excessive temperature and water as well as exposure to radiation and chemicals. To combat these stress factors, plants have evolved a defensive system involving the production of secondary metabolites, which serve to protect against predators and microbial pathogens [2]. These natural products are able to perform a defensive role due to their toxic nature, which allows them to repel herbivores and microbes as well as dominate other plants within the same locality [3]. One of the mechanisms employed by secondary metabolites is acting as antimicrobial agents, which may be pre-formed or induced by infection. Other modes of defense include formation of polymeric barriers to prevent penetration of pathogens, and synthesis of enzymes capable of degrading pathogenic cell wall. It is also possible for plants to employ secondary metabolites as specific recognition and signaling systems, which allows rapid detection of pathogenic invasion and triggering of defensive responses.

Plants can also efficiently respond to environmental stresses through sensors regulated by feedback mechanisms. To achieve this, plants use secondary metabolites as messengers under sub-optimal conditions to trigger their defense mechanism, which involves the production of phytochemicals, hormones and a variety of proteins necessary to protect the ultra-structure of plants from such hazards [4]. Elevated synthesis of secondary metabolites has also been observed under abiotic stresses like salinity and drought. These are utilized efficiently in defense mechanisms and biochemical pathways facilitating water and nutrient acquisition, chloroplast function, ion uptake and balance, synthesis of osmotically active metabolites and specific proteins, production of metabolites acting as osmo-protectants and detoxifying radicals [5].

## 2. CLASSIFICATION OF PLANT SECONDARY METABOLITES

It has been estimated that well over 300,000 secondary metabolites exist in nature [6]. There is no rigid scheme for classifying these secondary metabolites due to their immense diversity with respect to structure, function, and biosynthesis. Hence, it is difficult for them to fit perfectly into a few simple categories. For ease of reference, PSM may be grouped based on the presence of a recurring structural feature. For example, flavonoid compounds are oxygenated derivatives of aromatic ring structure, while alkaloids having an indole ring are called indole alkaloids. Terpenes consist of five carbon isoprene units, which are assembled in different ways.

PSM may also be classified according to the genus to which the plant source belongs. For example, morphine and codeine are examples of opium alkaloids. Grouping is also possible according to biological activities and physiological effects they elicit, such as antimicrobials, antibiotics, analgesics, *etc*. PSM can also be classified based on similarities in biosynthetic pathways. Generally, classifications based on structure and biosynthesis are more realistic and make the most sense.

## 3. POLYPHENOLS – A MAJOR CLASS OF PLANT SECONDARY METABOLITES

Polyphenols are secondary metabolites essential for the protection and survival of plants. They represent one of the most widespread groups of secondary metabolites in plants, with more than 8,000 identified phenolic structures [7]. These compounds can be found in almost all organs of plants, where they perform a myriad of functions, including skeletal constituents of different tissues and pigmentation of several plant organs [8], defense against various pathogens [9] and signaling molecules in plant cells [10]. The main sources of phenolic compounds are woody vascular plants, especially bark.

### 3.1. Classes of Polyphenols

Fig. (**1**) depicts the sub-divisions of polyphenols into different classes based on their chemical structures, namely phenolic acids, flavonoids, stilbenes and lignans [11, 12].

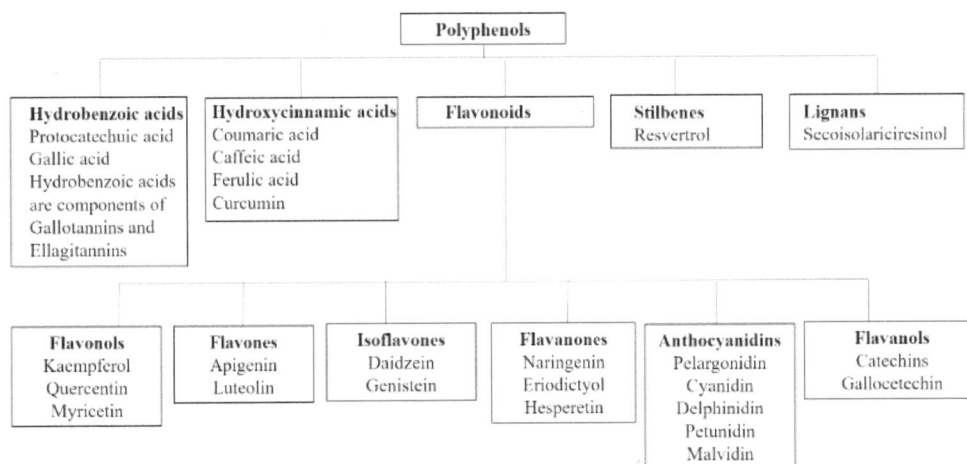

Fig. (1). Sub-divisions of polyphenols [13].

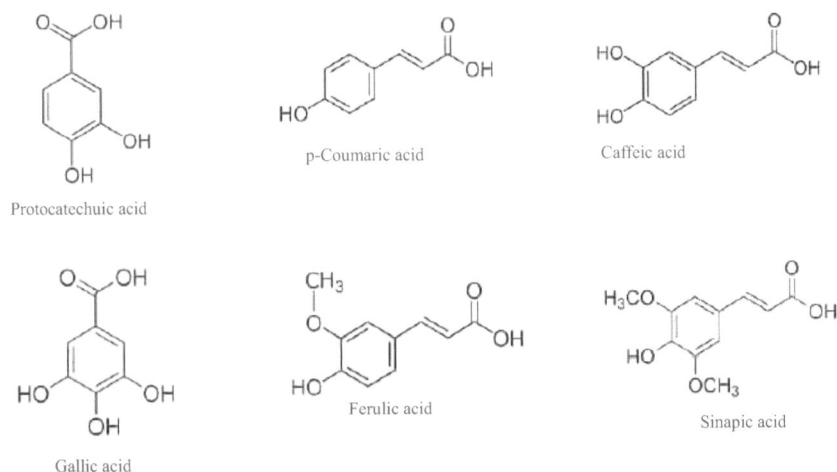

Fig. (2). Chemical structure of phenolic acids [7].

## 3.1.1. Phenolic Acids

Phenolic acids constitute one of the main classes of polyphenolic compounds found in plants where they rarely occur in free form but as esters, glycosides, or amides [14]. The structural variation of phenolic acids depends on the number and position of hydroxyl groups on the aromatic ring. Phenolic acids have two distinctive structures, namely benzoic acid and cinnamic acid derivatives (Fig. 2). The most common benzoic acid derivatives found in the bark of woody plants are vanillic, gallic, syringic and protocatechuic acid [15 - 17], while p-coumaric, caffeic, ferulic and synaptic acids represent the most common cinnamic acid derivatives [18]. Phenolic acids often occur in bound form and can only be hydrolyzed by acid, alkaline or enzymatic hydrolysis [19, 20].

### 3.1.2. Flavonoids

Flavonoids are composed of two aromatic rings joined by a unit of three carbon atoms. The unique arrangement of carbon skeleton explains the chemical diversity of this family of compounds [21]. (Fig. **3**) presents the six different sub-groups into which flavonoids can be further divided based on the type of heterocycle involved namely flavonols, flavones, isoflavones, flavanones, anthocyanidins, and flavanols [22]. Over 4,000 flavonoids have been identified in plants, with the possibility of many more to be identified [23].

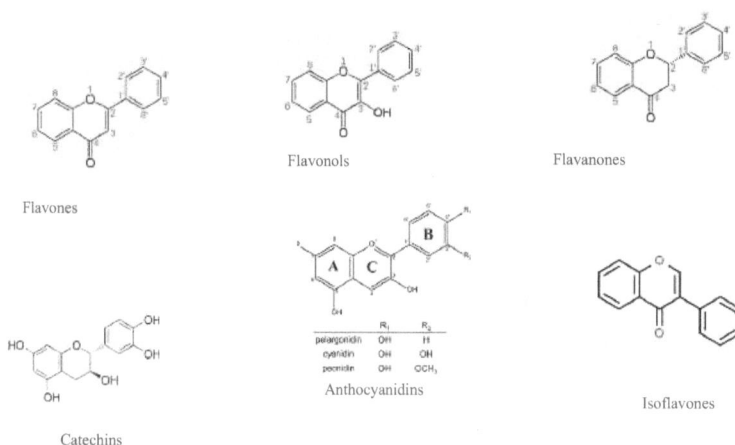

Flavones

Flavonols

Flavanones

Catechins

Anthocyanidins

Isoflavones

**Fig. (3).** Subclasses of flavonoids [22].

Flavonols constitute the most common sub-group of flavonoids and they include such compounds as quercetin, kaempferol and myricetin [24 - 26], followed by flavones (such as apigenin, luteolin) and flavanols (such as catechin, epicatechin) [27]. Flavanols exist in both monomeric and polymeric forms. The monomeric forms of flavanols include catechin and epicatechin as well as their derivatives such as gallocatechins, which represent the major flavanols found in tea leaves and cacao beans [28]. Catechin and epicatechin form polymeric flavanols, which are often referred to as proanthocyanidins whose polymeric chains can be cleaved by acid catalysis to produce anthocyanidins [7]. Proanthocyanidins are traditionally considered to be condensed tannins dimers, oligomers, and polymers of catechins [29]. Depending on inter-flavanic linkages, oligomeric proanthocyanidins can be A-type structure in which monomers are linked through C2–O–C7 or C2–O–C5 bonding, or B-type in which C4–C6 or C4–C8 are common.

### 3.1.3. Lignans and Stilbenes

Lignans and stilbenes constitute the last two groups in the polyphenol family. They are closely related and widely distributed in different parts of plants, including roots, rhizomes, stems, bark, leaves, and fruits. Lignans are synthesized by oxidative dimerization of two phenylpropane units forming diverse structures of different linkage patterns. Several lignans, such as secoisolariciresinol, are considered to be phytoestrogens [30]. They are majorly found in linseed, which contains secoisolariciresinol and relatively low quantities of matairesinol. Stilbenes are also biosynthesized from phenylpropanoids which can be further oxidized to form oligomers *via* two-carbon methylene bridge. Most stilbenes in plants have been reported to act as antifungal phytoalexins, which are synthesized only in response to infection or injury.

Resveratrol is one of the most studied stilbenes, and it is found predominantly in grapes [31].

It exhibits neuroprotective activity against Parkinson's and Alzheimer's diseases by virtue of its ability to influence and modulate cellular processes such as signaling, proliferation, apoptosis, redox balance and differentiation [32, 33]. It also plays neuroprotective role through inhibition of nuclear factor κB signaling in the progression of Alzheimer's disease [34]. Resveratrol also inhibits development of cancers of the lung, skin, breast, prostate, gastric and colon through suppression of angiogenesis and metastasis. The anti-carcinogenic activity of resveratrol is closely linked with its antioxidant activity which involves inhibition of cell cycle enzymes and regulators [35]. Resveratrol functions as an anti-diabetic agent by modulating Sirtuin 1 (SIRT1). A protein which improves glucose homeostasis and insulin sensitivity in humans [36, 37]. The compound also inhibits diabetes-induced nephropathy and ameliorates renal dysfunction through inhibition of $K^+$ ATP and $K^+$ V channel in beta cells [38]. Resveratrol also acts as an anti-aging agent and plays a prominent role in prolonging life span [36].

## 4. MEDICINAL PLANTS

Medicinal plants refer to plants whose parts including leaves, root, stem bark, fruits and seeds can be used for treatment and/or management of diseases affecting humans and animals. According to World Health Organization, plants that are rich in substances which can be used for therapeutic purposes or serve as precursors for producing synthetic drugs are referred to as medicinal plants [1]. In most parts of the world, particularly in developing countries, plants are used to treat many ailments affecting humans including diabetes, diarrhea, constipation, ulcer, fever, cold and dental infection. This explains why majority of medications used in traditional healthcare system are derived from plants. Despite advancements in the production of synthetic drugs and antibiotics, plants still remain a major source of therapy in many parts of the world.

The widespread use of herbal remedies and preparations have been traced to the presence of specific natural products with medicinal properties [39]. The biological activities exhibited by plants are mainly attributed to the presence of secondary metabolites which are usually expressed in certain parts of the plants [40, 41]. Therefore, medicinal plants are rich sources of secondary metabolites that have been extensively used in the manufacture of drugs and pharmaceuticals [42]. Many of the plant secondary metabolites are produced constitutively in healthy plants in their biologically active forms while others occur as inactive precursors but become activated when there is tissue damage or pathogenic attack.

## 5. PLANTS SECONDARY METABOLITES IN HEALTH MANAGEMENT

It is noteworthy that the traditional use of plant extracts for the formulation of herbal remedies provides the foundation for the establishment of modern system of medicine. The therapeutic effect of plant materials can be attributed to the combinations of secondary metabolites present in the plant such as alkaloids, flavonoids, terpenes, saponins, cardiac glycosides, fatty acids, steroids, and tannins. To date, several plant species are continually screened for these secondary metabolites with a view to isolating them for drug manufacture. This section explores secondary metabolites from plants that have been exploited in health management due to their biological activities.

### 5.1. Alkaloids

Alkaloids are a group of naturally occurring chemical compounds that contain mostly basic nitrogen atoms. They are extremely toxic and bitter but show marked therapeutic effects in small quantities [43]. Therefore, plant alkaloids and their synthetic derivatives are used as medicinal agents in many parts of the world [44]. According to reports, about 12,000 known alkaloids have been exploited as pharmaceuticals due to their potent biological activities [1]. The pharmacological activities of alkaloids include antihypertensive, antiarrhythmic, antimalarial, anticancer, analgesic, antispasmodic, antidiabetic, and antimicrobial effects [45].

For instance, benzylisoquinoline and indoquinoline alkaloids have been shown to have antiviral and antibacterial activities respectively while quinine alkaloid is widely known for its antimalarial activity against the plasmodium parasite [46]. Alkaloids extracted from different plants also exhibited antidiabetic property through inhibition of alpha amylase activity [47 - 49]. Morphine and its methyl ether derivative codeine are well known alkaloids with potent analgesic activity used for pain relief [45]. Some alkaloids such as vincristine and vinblastine have anticancer property; cocaine is used as an anesthetic while ephedrine relieves asthma and common cold [50]. Notably, alkaloids are also known for their neuro-protective activity against diseases such as epilepsy, dementia, depression, Parkinson's and Alzheimer's disease [51]. Alkaloids exert their neuroprotective action *via* inhibition of acetyl cholinesterase and increasing the level of gamma-aminobutyric acid among others [52, 53].

## 5.2. Flavonoids

Flavonoids have been reported to have potent antioxidant, anti-cancer, antidiabetic, anti-inflammatory, and antimicrobial activities [54]. For instance, kaempferol, quercetin and lutein isolated from different plants exhibit potent antioxidant activity through lipid peroxidation [55]. Other mechanisms of antioxidant action employed by flavonoids include scavenging of reactive oxygen species or suppression of its formation, and upregulation or protection of antioxidant defenses [56].

Flavonoids are known to be synthesized by plants in response to microbial attacks. It is therefore not surprising that they possess antimicrobial activity against a wide array of microorganisms including bacteria, viruses, and fungi. For instance, flavonoids extracted from different parts of *Sida acuta* showed antifungal activity against *Candida albicans* [57]. Their mode of antimicrobial action may be related to their ability to inactivate microbial adhesins, enzymes and cell envelope transport proteins. Most of the antiviral activity of flavonoids revolve around their ability to inhibit various enzymes associated with the life cycle of viruses.

Inflammation is a normal biological process that results from tissue injury, pathogenic infection, and chemical irritation. It is initiated by migration of immune cells from blood vessels and release of mediators at the site of damage. Certain members of flavonoids including hesperidin, apigenin, luteolin, and quercetin exhibit significant anti-inflammatory activity. Much of the anti-inflammatory activity of flavonoids is achieved through the biosynthesis of cytokines that mediate adhesion of circulating leukocytes to sites of injury. Some flavonoids also act by inhibiting the production of prostaglandins, which are powerful proinflammatory signaling molecules. Anthocyanins represent an important subset of flavonoids and they have been reported to slow down the aging process through their potent antioxidant/anti-inflammatory activities [58 - 60]. Catechins also possess strong anti-aging activity, hence consuming green tea rich in catechins, may delay the onset of aging [61]. Several other flavonoids such as apigenin, quercetin, naringenin, catechin, rutin, and venorutin have hepatoprotective activity through their ability to improve cell viability and inhibit cellular leakage of liver aspartate aminotransferase (AST) and alanine amino-transferase (ALT) caused by xenobiotics.

Several studies have implicated flavonoids like catechin, anthocyanin, epicatechin, epigallocatechin, epicatechin gallate, and isoflavones as potent antidiabetic agents [62, 63]. The mechanisms by which the antidiabetic activity is achieved include inhibition of glucose absorption in the gut, inhibition of glucose uptake by peripheral tissues [64], and inhibition of intestinal glycosidases and glucose transporter [65]. Flavonoids also demonstrate significant α-amylase inhibitory activity further indicative of their anti-diabetic potential [47 - 49, 66]. Quercetin, protocatechuic acid and anthocyanins showed strong antidiabetic activity by inhibiting lipid peroxidation [67] and attenuating diabetic nephropathy [68].

Flavonoids have been reported to improve blood circulation and lower blood pressure. For instance, quercetin prevents incidence of coronary heart disease by inhibiting the expression of metalloproteinase 1 and disruption of atherosclerotic plaques [69]. Catechins obtained from tea also prevent invasion and proliferation of smooth muscle cells in the arterial wall thereby slowing down the formation of atheromatous lesion [70].

Many flavonoids such as catechins, isoflavones, and flavanones showed protective effects in cancer cell lines by reducing the number and growth of tumor cells [71] although their mechanisms of action differ [72]. Theaflavins and thearubigins are prominent flavonoids in black tea with potent anticancer activity particularly against prostate carcinoma cells [73]. Quercetin is a potent flavonol that reduces the incidence of cancers of the prostate, lung, stomach, and breast. Quercetin has also been reported to possess anticancer property against benzo(a)pyrene induced lung carcinogenesis, an effect attributed to its free radical scavenging activity [74]. The major anticancer mechanisms of flavonoids include downregulation of mutant p53 protein, cell cycle arrest, inhibition of tyrosine kinase, inhibition of heat shock proteins, excretion of tumor cells by increasing the expression of phase II conjugating enzymes, and inhibition of expression of Ras proteins.

## 5.3. Terpenes

Terpenes are diverse naturally occurring organic compounds found widely in plants where they form the major constituent of essential oils. Their oxygen-containing derivatives are called terpenoids and they are formed when terpenes are modified chemically by such processes as oxidation or re-arrangement of carbon skeleton. Common sources of terpenes include tea, thyme, cannabis, lemon, and orange. They can be classified as mono, di, tri, tetra, and sesquiterpenes according to the number of isoprene units found in their structures. Terpenes have been reported to have a wide range of medicinal and health benefits among which are antiplasmodial, antiviral, anticancer, antidiabetic and antidepressant activities [75].

The potent antiplasmodial activity of terpenes can be exploited in the development of antimalarial drugs. The mechanism of action involves binding of terpenes to the hemin portion of infected erythrocytes which eventually kill the parasites without any serious side effects [76, 77]. Specifically, beta-myrcene, limonene and caryophyllene are powerful terpenoid compounds with proven antiplasmodial activity [78 - 81]. Thus, terpenes can be used as a safer and cost-effective alternative for the treatment of malaria.

Monoterpenes form a major constituent of essential oils in plants that have shown good results against viral diseases. These monoterpenoid oils namely carvone, carveol limonene, alpha- and beta-pinene, caryophylene, camphor, beta-ocimene, proved to be virucidal against three major human viruses namely herpes simplex virus-1 (HSV1), dengue virus type 2, and Junin virus [82]. The emergence of novel viral diseases has further necessitated the search for more effective antiviral agents from terpenes. This has led to the discovery of alpha- and beta-pinene, beta-ocimene, and 1,8-cineole used in the treatment of severe acute respiratory syndrome corona virus (SARS CoV) [83]. Different mechanisms of action have been proposed for the antiviral activity of these terpenes including direct inactivation of free viral particles and induced cell cycle arrest at G0 or G1 phase. This points to the fact that a combination of different terpenes may act as better antiviral agents rather than a single one [84].

The medicinal benefits of terpenes extend beyond antiplasmodial and antiviral activities as they are also known for their anticancer property. A combination of terpenes comprising monoterpenes, diterpenes and sesquiterpenes have been used for the treatment of colon, brain, and prostate cancers. For example, limonene has been reported to exhibit potent anticancer activity *via* different mechanisms of action. One of these is induction of transforming growth factor B-1 and mannose-6-phosphate/insulin-like growth factor II receptors [85]. Further studies also reported that limonene works by eliminating cancer cells through induction of apoptosis [86]. The lipophilic nature of limonene is also an indication that it can serve as a potent anticancer agent since it has the tendency to be stored in fatty tissues of the body [87]. Other terpenes with anticancer activity include thymoquinone, thermoquinone, alloocimene, camphor, beta-myrcene, pinene, alpha- and gamma-thujaplicin, terpinene, thymohydroquinone, carvone, camphene, and cymene [88 - 90].

The widespread use of terpenes in cancer treatment is hinged on the fact that it is unlikely to pose any serious side effect since it is a natural compound.

According to reports, terpenes also form the bulk of natural compounds used in the treatment of diabetes [91, 92]. Notable among the terpene compounds used as antidiabetics is a diterpenoid lactone called andrographolide which is obtained from *A. paniculata* leaves [93]. The compound enhances glucose utilization in the muscle by activating alpha-adrenoreceptors which causes the release of beta-endomorphin, thereby reducing plasma glucose concentration [93]. Another commonly used terpene in the treatment of diabetes and its complications is curcumin, popularly known as turmeric [94]. Curcumin acts as an antidiabetic by activating the enzymes that are essential for glycolysis in the liver [95].

Terpenes have also found relevance in the management of depression which is a major health challenge in both developed and developing countries [96, 97]. Some of the terpenes implicated as antidepressants include linalool and beta-pinene, beta-caryophyllene, hyperforin [98, 99]. These terpenes act by interacting with the 5HT1A receptors of the serotonergic pathway, adrenergic receptors, and dopaminergic receptors [99, 100].

## 5.4. Saponins

Saponins are naturally occurring plant glycosides with structures consisting of a sugar moiety linked to a hydrophobic aglycone called sapogenin. There are more than 100 plant families containing saponins belonging to different classes [101]. Saponins are known for their foaming properties in aqueous solutions and they generally impart bitter and astringent taste. Intravenous administration of saponins has been reported to be toxic due to their hemolytic activity on human erythrocytes [102]. Despite this untoward effect, saponins still offer several pharmacological properties, including anticancer, antidiabetic, antimicrobial, anti-obesity and hypoglycemic activities [103, 104].

Saponins from ginseng and soy have been reported to be effective against different cancer cell lines, including hepatocellular carcinoma cell line, fibrosarcoma cell line, HeLa, and promyelocytic leukemia cells [105, 106]. With respect to antidiabetic activity, saponin compounds such as saxifragifolin B and saxifragifolin D [107], α-hederin [108], glochierioside A [109] and filiasparoside C [110] demonstrate potent hypoglycemic effect. The mechanisms of action include restoration of insulin response, an increase in plasma insulin concentration, induction of insulin release from the pancreas as well as inhibition of α-amylase and α-glucosidase activities [111]. Saponins also act by delaying the transfer of glucose from stomach to small intestine [112] or by repairing pancreatic beta cells, thereby stimulating the release of insulin [113, 114].

Saponins also demonstrate a wide spectrum of antimicrobial activity against many harmful organisms. For instance, they showed potent antibacterial activity against *Staphylococcus aureus*, *Bacillus subtilis*, *Bacillus cereus* and *Klebsiella pneumoniae* [115]. In other studies, saponins also demonstrate biological activity against *Escherichia coli*, *Pseudomonas aeruginosa*, *Streptococcus faecalis*, *Candida albicans*, *Candida parapsilosis*, *Candida pseudotropicalis* and *Candida stellatoidea* [116, 117].

Investigation of anti-obesity activity of saponins indicates that they are potent modulators of body weight. A possible mechanism of action by which this is achieved is *via* inhibition of pancreatic lipase and modulation of adipogenesis [118]. Saponins also promote normal blood cholesterol levels by binding to bile causing cholesterol to be excreted rather than being reabsorbed back into the bloodstream [119]. The operation of many cholesterol drugs follows this pattern.

## CONCLUSION

Although PSM are primarily produced by plants to enhance their survival by providing protection against predators and microbial pathogens. These seemingly "toxic" compounds are being used in health management. It is a common practice in many parts of the world, particularly in developing countries, to use plants for the treatment of different ailments affecting humans. The therapeutic activity produced by these medicinal plants have been attributed to secondary metabolites, including alkaloids, flavonoids, terpenes, saponins, cardiac glycosides, fatty acids, steroids, and tannins. Of the different PSM, polyphenols particularly flavonoids seem to produce the widest range of pharmacological potential, including antioxidant, anti-cancer, antidiabetic, anti-inflammatory, and antimicrobial activities. In spite of the impressive use of PSM in health management, particularly at the traditional healthcare level, a multitude of plant species are yet to be screened for already known and novel secondary metabolites. Additionally, out of those that have been identified, many have not reached the stage of clinical trials for the development of new lead therapeutics for common ailments. This indicates that a lot still needs to be done in exploiting the full advantage of PSM in the management of health. Therefore, the continuous search for PSM is imperative with a view to isolating them for drug manufacture.

## CONSENT FOR PUBLICATION

Not applicable.

## CONFLICT OF INTEREST

The authors declare no conflict of interest, financial or otherwise.

## ACKNOWLEDGEMENTS

Declared none.

## REFERENCES

[1]     Jain C, Khatana S, Vijayvergia R. Bioactivity of secondary metabolites of various plants: a review. Int J Pharm Sci Res 2019; 10(2): 494-04.
[http://dx.doi.org/10.13040/IJPSR.0975-8232.10(2).494-04]

[2]     Ballhorn DJ, Kautz S, Heil M, Hegeman AD. Cyanogenesis of wild lima bean (*Phaseolus lunatus* L.) is an efficient direct defence in nature. Plant Signal Behav 2009; 4(8): 735-45.
[PMID: 19820319]

[3]     Rosenthal GA. The biochemical basis for the deleterious effects of L-canavanine. Phytochemistry 1991; 30: 1055-8.
[http://dx.doi.org/10.1016/S0031-9422(00)95170-7]

[4]     Pedral N, González L, Reigosa MJ. Allelopathy: A physiological process with ecological implication. Allelopathy and abiotic stress.Springer 2006; pp. 171-209.
[http://dx.doi.org/10.1007/1-4020-4280-9_9]

[5]     Waśkiewicz A, Muzalf-panek M, Galiński P. Phenolic content changes in plants under salt stress.Ahmad P, Azooz MM, Prasad MNV. Ecophysiology and Responses of Plants Under Salt Stress. Springer 2013; pp. 283-314.
[http://dx.doi.org/10.1007/978-1-4614-4747-4_11]

[6]     Weisshaar B, Jenkins GI. Phenylpropanoid biosynthesis and its regulation. Curr Opin Plant Biol 1998; 1(3): 251-7.
[http://dx.doi.org/10.1016/S1369-5266(98)80113-1] [PMID: 10066590]

[7]     Tsao R. Chemistry and biochemistry of dietary polyphenols. Nutrients 2010; 2(12): 1231-46.
[http://dx.doi.org/10.3390/nu2121231] [PMID: 22254006]

[8]     Ignat I, Volf I, Popa VI. A critical review of methods for characterisation of polyphenolic compounds in fruits and vegetables. Food Chem 2011; 126(4): 1821-35.
[http://dx.doi.org/10.1016/j.foodchem.2010.12.026] [PMID: 25213963]

[9]     Popa VI. Wood bark as valuable raw material for compounds with biological activity. Celulular:Si Hârtie 2015; 64: 5-17.

[10]    Naczk M, Shahidi F. Phenolics in cereals, fruits and vegetables: occurrence, extraction and analysis. J Pharm Biomed Anal 2006; 41(5): 1523-42.
[http://dx.doi.org/10.1016/j.jpba.2006.04.002] [PMID: 16753277]

[11]    Dopico-García MS, Fique A, Guerra L, *et al.* Principal components of phenolics to characterize red Vinho Verde grapes: anthocyanins or non-coloured compounds? Talanta 2008; 75(5): 1190-202.
[http://dx.doi.org/10.1016/j.talanta.2008.01.012] [PMID: 18585201]

[12]    Oprica L, Socaciu C. Metaboli‚ti Secundari din Plante: Origine, Structura, Func‚tii; Editura Universita‚tii" Alexandru Ioan Cuza: Iasi. Romania 2016; 16: 122-33.

[13]    Hardman WE. Diet components can suppress inflammation and reduce cancer risk. Nutr Res Pract 2014; 8(3): 233-40.
[http://dx.doi.org/10.4162/nrp.2014.8.3.233] [PMID: 24944766]

[14]    Pandey KB, Rizvi SI. Plant polyphenols as dietary antioxidants in human health and disease. Oxidative Medicine and Cellular Longevity, 2(5): 270-278. Oxid Med Cell Longev 2009; 2(5): 270-8.
[http://dx.doi.org/10.4161/oxim.2.5.9498] [PMID: 20716914]

[15]    Pereira D, Valentão P, Pereira J, Andrade P. Phenolics: From Chemistry to Biology. Molecules 2009; 14: 2202-11.

[http://dx.doi.org/10.3390/molecules14062202]

[16]   Bocalandro C, Sanhueza V, Gómez-Caravaca A M, *et al.* Comparison of the composition of Pinus adiate bark extracts obtained at bench-and pilot-scales. Industrial Crops Production 2012; 38: 21-6.

[17]   García-Pérez ME, Royer M, Herbette G, *et al.* Picea mariana bark: a new source of trans-resveratrol and other bioactive polyphenols. Food Chem 2012; 135(3): 1173-82.
[http://dx.doi.org/10.1016/j.foodchem.2012.05.050] [PMID: 22953840]

[18]   Maldini M, Sosa S, Montoro P, *et al.* Screening of the topical anti-inflammatory activity of the bark of *Acacia cornigera* Willdenow, *Byrsonima crassifolia Kunth, Sweetia panamensis Yakovlev* and the leaves of *Sphagneticola trilobata Hitchcock.* J Ethnopharmacol 2009; 122(3): 430-3.
[http://dx.doi.org/10.1016/j.jep.2009.02.002] [PMID: 19429307]

[19]   Adom KK, Liu RH. Antioxidant activity of grains. J Agric Food Chem 2002; 50(21): 6182-7.
[http://dx.doi.org/10.1021/jf0205099] [PMID: 12358499]

[20]   Chandrasekara A, Shahidi F. Content of insoluble bound phenolic in millets and their contribution to antioxidant capacity. J Sci Food Agric 2010; 58: 6706-14.

[21]   Ghasemzadeh A, Ghasemzadeh N. Flavonoids and phenolic acids: Role and biochemical activity in plants and human. J Med Plant Res 2011; 5: 31.

[22]   Gross M. Flavonoids and cardiovascular disease. Pharm Biol 2004; 4: 21-35.
[http://dx.doi.org/10.3109/13880200490893483]

[23]   Harborne JB, Williams CA. Advances in flavonoid research since 1992. Phytochemistry 2000; 55(6): 481-504.
[http://dx.doi.org/10.1016/S0031-9422(00)00235-1] [PMID: 11130659]

[24]   Chew K, Khoo M, Ng S, Thoo Y, Aida WW, Ho C. Effect of ethanol concentration, extraction time and extraction temperature on the recovery of phenolic compounds and antioxidant capacity of Orthosiphon stamineus extracts. Int Food Res J 2011; 1427.

[25]   Brusotti G, Andreola F, Sferrazza G, *et al. In vitro* evaluation of the wound healing activity of *Drypetes klainei* stem bark extracts. J Ethnopharmacol 2015; 175: 412-21.
[http://dx.doi.org/10.1016/j.jep.2015.09.015] [PMID: 26403594]

[26]   Keshari AK, Kumar G, Kushwaha PS, *et al.* Isolated flavonoids from *Ficus racemosa* stem bark possess antidiabetic, hypolipidemic and protective effects in albino Wistar rats. J Ethnopharmacol 2016; 181: 252-62.
[http://dx.doi.org/10.1016/j.jep.2016.02.004] [PMID: 26869543]

[27]   Tamashiro Filho P, Sikiru Olaitan B, Tavares de Almeida DA, *et al.* Evaluation of antiulcer activity and mechanism of action of methanol stem bark extract of Lafoensia pacari A. St.-Hil. (Lytraceae) in experimental animals. J Ethnopharmacol 2012; 144(3): 497-505.
[http://dx.doi.org/10.1016/j.jep.2012.09.019] [PMID: 23069941]

[28]   Prior RL, Lazarus SA, Cao G, Muccitelli H, Hammerstone JF. Identification of procyanidins and anthocyanins in blueberries and cranberries (Vaccinium spp.) using high-performance liquid chromatography/mass spectrometry. J Agric Food Chem 2001; 49(3): 1270-6.
[http://dx.doi.org/10.1021/jf001211q] [PMID: 11312849]

[29]   Manach C, Scalbert A, Morand C, Rémésy C, Jiménez L. Polyphenols: food sources and bioavailability. Am J Clin Nutr 2004; 79(5): 727-47.
[http://dx.doi.org/10.1093/ajcn/79.5.727] [PMID: 15113710]

[30]   Adlercreutz H, Mazur W. Phyto-oestrogens and Western diseases. Ann Med 1997; 29(2): 95-120.
[http://dx.doi.org/10.3109/07853899709113696] [PMID: 9187225]

[31]   Vitrac X, Moni JP, Vercauteren J, Deffieux G, Mérillon JM. Direct liquid chromatography analysis of resveratrol derivatives and flavanonols in wines with absorbance and fluorescence detection. Anal Chim Acta 2002; 458: 103-10.

[http://dx.doi.org/10.1016/S0003-2670(01)01498-2]

[32]   Aquilano K, Baldelli S, Rotilio G, Ciriolo MR. Role of nitric oxide synthases in Parkinson's disease: a review on the antioxidant and anti-inflammatory activity of polyphenols. Neurochem Res 2008; 33(12): 2416-26.
[http://dx.doi.org/10.1007/s11064-008-9697-6] [PMID: 18415676]

[33]   Singh M, Arseneault M, Sanderson T, Murthy V, Ramassamy C. Challenges for research on polyphenols from foods in Alzheimer's disease: bioavailability, metabolism, and cellular and molecular mechanisms. J Agric Food Chem 2008; 56(13): 4855-73.
[http://dx.doi.org/10.1021/jf0735073] [PMID: 18557624]

[34]   Markus MA, Morris BJ. Resveratrol in prevention and treatment of common clinical conditions of aging. Clin Interv Aging 2008; 3(2): 331-9.
[PMID: 18686754]

[35]   Athar M, Back JH, Tang X, *et al.* Resveratrol: a review of preclinical studies for human cancer prevention. Toxicol Appl Pharmacol 2007; 224(3): 274-83.
[http://dx.doi.org/10.1016/j.taap.2006.12.025] [PMID: 17306316]

[36]   Harikumar KB, Aggarwal BB. Resveratrol: a multitargeted agent for age-associated chronic diseases. Cell Cycle 2008; 7(8): 1020-35.
[http://dx.doi.org/10.4161/cc.7.8.5740] [PMID: 18414053]

[37]   Milne JC, Lambert PD, Schenk S, *et al.* Small molecule activators of SIRT1 as therapeutics for the treatment of type 2 diabetes. Nature 2007; 450(7170): 712-6.
[http://dx.doi.org/10.1038/nature06261] [PMID: 18046409]

[38]   Chen WP, Chi TC, Chuang LM, Su MJ. Resveratrol enhances insulin secretion by blocking K(ATP) and K(V) channels of beta cells. Eur J Pharmacol 2007; 568(1-3): 269-77.
[http://dx.doi.org/10.1016/j.ejphar.2007.04.062] [PMID: 17573071]

[39]   Gibbons S. An overview of plant extracts as potential therapeutics. Expert Opin Ther Pat 2003; 13(4): 489-97.
[http://dx.doi.org/10.1517/13543776.13.4.489]

[40]   Coley PD, Heller MV, Aizprua R, *et al.* Using ecological criteria to design plant collection strategies for drug discovery. Front Ecol Environ 2003; 1: 421-8.
[http://dx.doi.org/10.1890/1540-9295(2003)001[0421:UECTDP]2.0.CO;2]

[41]   Figueiredo MSL, Grelle CEV. Predicting global abundance of a threatened species from its occurrence: Implications for conservation planning. Divers Distrib 2009; 15: 117-21.
[http://dx.doi.org/10.1111/j.1472-4642.2008.00525.x]

[42]   Santosh MK, Sharanabasappa GK, Shaila D, Seetharam YN, Sanjeevarao I. Phytochemical studies on *Bauhinia racemosa* Lam., *Bauhinia purpurea* Linn. and *Hardwickia binate* Roxb. E-J Chem 2007; 4: 21-31.
[http://dx.doi.org/10.1155/2007/874721]

[43]   Harborne JB. Phytochemical Methods: A Guide to Modern Techniques of Plant Analysis. Chapman and Hall Ltd 1973.

[44]   Stary F. The Natural Guide to Medicinal Herbs and Plants. Barnes & Noble Inc 1996.

[45]   Wink M, Schmeller T, Latz-Briining B. Modes of action of allelochemical alkaloids: Interaction with neuroreceptors, DNA and other molecular targets. J Chem Ecol 1998; 24: 1888-937.

[46]   Okunade AL, Elvin-Lewis MP, Lewis WH. Natural antimycobacterial metabolites: current status. Phytochemistry 2004; 65(8): 1017-32.
[http://dx.doi.org/10.1016/j.phytochem.2004.02.013] [PMID: 15110681]

[47]   Jain C, Kumar P, Singh A. Hypoglycemic activity of flavonoids and alkaloids extracted from *Aloe vera* in two districts of Rajasthan: A comparative study. Elixir Int J 2013; 62: 17877-9.

[48]    Chitra J, Padma K, Archana S, Alka J. *In-vitro* comparisons of anti-diabetic activity of flavonoids and crude extracts of *Azadirachta indica* A Juss. International Journal of Drug Development and Research 2013; 5(1): 47-54.

[49]    Jain C, Singh A, Kumar P, Gautam K. Anti-diabetic potential of flavonoids and other crude extracts of stem bark of *Mangifera indica* Linn: a comparative study. J Sci Innov Res 2014; 3(1): 21-7.
[http://dx.doi.org/10.31254/jsir.2014.3105]

[50]    Rao RVK, Ali N, Reddy MN. Occurrence of both sapogenins and alkaloid lycorine in *Curculigo orchioides*. Indian J Pharm Sci 1978; 40: 104-5.

[51]    Amirkia V, Heinrich M. Alkaloids as drug leads – A predictive structural and biodiversity-based analysis. Phytochem Lett 2014; 10: 48-54.
[http://dx.doi.org/10.1016/j.phytol.2014.06.015]

[52]    Cushnie TPT, Cushnie B, Lamb AJ. Alkaloids: An overview of their antibacterial, antibiotic-enhancing and antivirulence activities. Vol. 44, International Journal of Antimicrobial Agents. Elsevier B 2014; 2014: 377-86.

[53]    Abhijit Dey AM. Plant-derived Alkaloids: A promising window for neuroprotective drug discovery.Discovery and development of neuroprotective agents from natural products. 2017; pp. 237-320.

[54]    Mills S, Bone K. Principles and Practice of Phytotherapy–Modern Herbal Medicine. New York: Churchill Livingstone 2000; pp. 31-4.

[55]    Vijayvargia P, Vijayvergia R. A Review on *Limonia acidissima* L.: Multipotential medicinal plant. Int J Pharm Sci Rev Res 2014; 28(1): 191-5.

[56]    Vijayvargia P, Vijayvergia R. Assesment of phytochemicals and antioxidant activity of *Murraya koenigii* Linn. Int J Pharm Sci Res 2016; 7(5): 2163-7.

[57]    Alka J, Padma K, Chitra J. Antifungal activity of flavonoids of *Sida acuta* Burm f. against *Candida albicans*. International Journal of Drug Development and Research 2016; 4(3): 92-6.

[58]    Cao G, Booth SL, Sadowski JA, Prior RL. Increases in human plasma antioxidant capacity after consumption of controlled diets high in fruit and vegetables. Am J Clin Nutr 1998; 68(5): 1081-7.
[http://dx.doi.org/10.1093/ajcn/68.5.1081] [PMID: 9808226]

[59]    Joseph JA, Shukitt-Hale B, Casadesus G. Reversing the deleterious effects of aging on neuronal communication and behavior: beneficial properties of fruit polyphenolic compounds. Am J Clin Nutr 2005; 81(1) (Suppl.): 313S-6S.
[http://dx.doi.org/10.1093/ajcn/81.1.313S] [PMID: 15640496]

[60]    Seeram NP, Cichewicz RH, Chandra A, Nair MG. Cyclooxygenase inhibitory and antioxidant compounds from crabapple fruits. J Agric Food Chem 2003; 51(7): 1948-51.
[http://dx.doi.org/10.1021/jf025993u] [PMID: 12643656]

[61]    Maurya PK, Rizvi SI. Protective role of tea catechins on erythrocytes subjected to oxidative stress during human aging. Nat Prod Res 2008; 1-8.
[PMID: 18846469]

[62]    Rizvi SI, Zaid MA. Insulin-like effect of (-)epicatechin on erythrocyte membrane acetylcholinesterase activity in type 2 diabetes mellitus. Clin Exp Pharmacol Physiol 2001; 28(9): 776-8.
[http://dx.doi.org/10.1046/j.1440-1681.2001.03513.x] [PMID: 11553037]

[63]    Rizvi SI, Zaid MA, Anis R, Mishra N. Protective role of tea catechins against oxidation-induced damage of type 2 diabetic erythrocytes. Clin Exp Pharmacol Physiol 2005; 32(1-2): 70-5.
[http://dx.doi.org/10.1111/j.1440-1681.2005.04160.x] [PMID: 15730438]

[64]    Matsui T, Ebuchi S, Kobayashi M, *et al.* Anti-hyperglycemic effect of diacylated anthocyanin derived from *Ipomoea batatas* cultivar Ayamurasaki can be achieved through the alpha-glucosidase inhibitory action. J Agric Food Chem 2002; 50(25): 7244-8.

[http://dx.doi.org/10.1021/jf025913m] [PMID: 12452639]

[65]    Matsui T, Ueda T, Oki T, Sugita K, Terahara N, Matsumoto K. alpha-Glucosidase inhibitory action of natural acylated anthocyanins. 2. alpha-Glucosidase inhibition by isolated acylated anthocyanins. J Agric Food Chem 2001; 49(4): 1952-6.
[http://dx.doi.org/10.1021/jf0012502] [PMID: 11308352]

[66]    Gautam K, Kumar P, Jain C. Comparative study of alpha-amylase inhibitory activity of flavonoids of *Vitex negundo* Linn. and *Andrographis paniculata* Nees. International Journal of Green Pharmacy 2013; 7(1): 25-8.
[http://dx.doi.org/10.4103/0973-8258.111602]

[67]    Rizvi SI, Mishra M. Anti-oxidant effect of quercetin on type 2 diabetic erythrocytes. J Food Biochem 2009; 33: 404-15.
[http://dx.doi.org/10.1111/j.1745-4514.2009.00228.x]

[68]    Lee WC, Wang CJ, Chen YH, *et al.* Polyphenol extracts from Hibiscus sabdariffa Linnaeus attenuate nephropathy in experimental type 1 diabetes. J Agric Food Chem 2009; 57(6): 2206-10.
[http://dx.doi.org/10.1021/jf802993s] [PMID: 19219995]

[69]    García-Lafuente A, Guillamón E, Villares A, Rostagno MA, Martínez JA. Flavonoids as anti-inflammatory agents: implications in cancer and cardiovascular disease. Inflamm Res 2009; 58(9): 537-52.
[http://dx.doi.org/10.1007/s00011-009-0037-3] [PMID: 19381780]

[70]    Maeda K, Kuzuya M, Cheng XW, *et al.* Green tea catechins inhibit the cultured smooth muscle cell invasion through the basement barrier. Atherosclerosis 2003; 166(1): 23-30.
[http://dx.doi.org/10.1016/S0021-9150(02)00302-7] [PMID: 12482547]

[71]    Yang CS, Landau JM, Huang MT, Newmark HL. Inhibition of carcinogenesis by dietary polyphenolic compounds. Annu Rev Nutr 2001; 21: 381-406.
[http://dx.doi.org/10.1146/annurev.nutr.21.1.381] [PMID: 11375442]

[72]    Johnson IT, Williamson G, Musk SRR. Anticarcinogenic factors in plant foods: a new class of nutrients? Nutr Res Rev 1994; 7(1): 175-204.
[http://dx.doi.org/10.1079/NRR19940011] [PMID: 19094297]

[73]    Sharma V, Rao LJ. A thought on the biological activities of black tea. Crit Rev Food Sci Nutr 2009; 49(5): 379-404.
[http://dx.doi.org/10.1080/10408390802068066] [PMID: 19399668]

[74]    Kamaraj S, Vinodhkumar R, Anandakumar P, Jagan S, Ramakrishnan G, Devaki T. The effects of quercetin on antioxidant status and tumor markers in the lung and serum of mice treated with benzo(a)pyrene. Biol Pharm Bull 2007; 30(12): 2268-73.
[http://dx.doi.org/10.1248/bpb.30.2268] [PMID: 18057710]

[75]    Cox-Georgian D, Ramadoss N, Dona C, Basu C. Therapeutic and Medicinal Uses of Terpenes. Medicinal Plants 2019; 333-59.

[76]    Nogueira CR, Lopes LMX. Antiplasmodial Natural Products. Molecules 2011; 16(12): 2146-90.
[http://dx.doi.org/10.3390/molecules16032146]

[77]    Kayembe JS, *et al. In vitro* antimalarial activity of 11 terpenes isolated from Ocimum gratissimum and Cassia alata leaves. Screening of their binding affinity with haemin. J Plant Stud 2012; 1(2)

[78]    Rodrigues Goulart H, Kimura EA, Peres VJ, Couto AS, Aquino Duarte FA, Katzin AM. Terpenes arrest parasite development and inhibit biosynthesis of isoprenoids in *Plasmodium falciparum*. Antimicrob Agents Chemother 2004; 48(7): 2502-9.
[http://dx.doi.org/10.1128/AAC.48.7.2502-2509.2004] [PMID: 15215101]

[79]    Kpadonou Kpoviessi BG, Kpoviessi SD, Yayi Ladekan E, *et al. In vitro* antitrypanosomal and antiplasmodial activities of crude extracts and essential oils of Ocimum gratissimum Linn from Benin and influence of vegetative stage. J Ethnopharmacol 2014; 155(3): 1417-23.

[http://dx.doi.org/10.1016/j.jep.2014.07.014] [PMID: 25058875]

[80]   Small E. Cannabis: a complete guide. Boca Raton: CRC Press 2017.

[81]   Kamaraj C, *et al.* Ag nanoparticles synthesized using β-caryophyllene isolated from *Murraya koenigii*: antimalarial (Plasmodium falciparum 3D7) and anticancer activity (A549 and HeLa cell lines). J Cluster Sci 2017; 28(3): 1667-84.
       [http://dx.doi.org/10.1007/s10876-017-1180-6]

[82]   Duschatzky CB, Possetto ML, Talarico LB, *et al.* Evaluation of chemical and antiviral properties of essential oils from South American plants. Antivir Chem Chemother 2005; 16(4): 247-51.
       [http://dx.doi.org/10.1177/095632020501600404] [PMID: 16130522]

[83]   Loizzo MR, Saab AM, Tundis R, *et al.* Phytochemical analysis and *in vitro* antiviral activities of the essential oils of seven Lebanon species. Chem Biodivers 2008; 5(3): 461-70.
       [http://dx.doi.org/10.1002/cbdv.200890045] [PMID: 18357554]

[84]   Pliego Zamora A, Edmonds JH, Reynolds MJ, Khromykh AA, Ralph SJ. The *in vitro* and *in vivo* antiviral properties of combined monoterpene alcohols against West Nile virus infection. Virology 2016; 495: 18-32.
       [http://dx.doi.org/10.1016/j.virol.2016.04.021] [PMID: 27152479]

[85]   Jirtle RL, Haag JD, Ariazi EA, Gould MN. Increased mannose 6-phosphate/insulin-like growth factor II receptor and transforming growth factor beta 1 levels during monoterpene-induced regression of mammary tumors. Cancer Res 1993; 53(17): 3849-52.
       [PMID: 8358708]

[86]   Rabi T, Bishayee A. D -Limonene sensitizes docetaxel-induced cytotoxicity in human prostate cancer cells: Generation of reactive oxygen species and induction of apoptosis. J Carcinog 2009; 8(1): 9.
       [http://dx.doi.org/10.4103/1477-3163.51368] [PMID: 19465777]

[87]   Miller JA, *et al.* -Limonene: a bioactive food component from citrus and evidence for a potential role in breast cancer prevention and treatment. Oncol Rev 2010; 5(1): 31-42.
       [http://dx.doi.org/10.1007/s12156-010-0066-8]

[88]   Taborsky J, *et al.* Identification of potential sources of thymoquinone and related compounds in Asteraceae, Cupressaceae, Lamiaceae, and Ranunculaceae families. Open Chem 2012; 10(6)
       [http://dx.doi.org/10.2478/s11532-012-0114-2]

[89]   Sobral MV, Xavier AL, Lima TC, de Sousa DP. Antitumor activity of monoterpenes found in essential oils. Sci World J 2014; 2014953451
       [http://dx.doi.org/10.1155/2014/953451] [PMID: 25401162]

[90]   Majdalawieh AF, Fayyad MW, Nasrallah GK. Anti-cancer properties and mechanisms of action of thymoquinone, the major active ingredient of *Nigella sativa*. Crit Rev Food Sci Nutr 2017; 57(18): 3911-28.
       [http://dx.doi.org/10.1080/10408398.2016.1277971] [PMID: 28140613]

[91]   Jung M, Park M, Lee HC, Kang YH, Kang ES, Kim SK. Antidiabetic agents from medicinal plants. Curr Med Chem 2006; 13(10): 1203-18.
       [http://dx.doi.org/10.2174/092986706776360860] [PMID: 16719780]

[92]   Bnouham M, Merhfour FZ, Ziyyat A, Aziz M, Legssyer A, Mekhfi H. Antidiabetic effect of some medicinal plants of Oriental Morocco in neonatal non-insulin-dependent diabetes mellitus rats. Hum Exp Toxicol 2010; 29(10): 865-71.
       [http://dx.doi.org/10.1177/0960327110362704] [PMID: 20154101]

[93]   Brahmachari G. Discovery and development of antidiabetic agents from natural products natural product drug discovery. Amsterdam: Elsevier 2017.

[94]   Nabavi SF, Thiagarajan R, Rastrelli L, *et al.* Curcumin: a natural product for diabetes and its complications. Curr Top Med Chem 2015; 15(23): 2445-55.
       [http://dx.doi.org/10.2174/1568026615666150619142519] [PMID: 26088351]

[95]  Zhang Y, Jiang P, Ye M, Kim SH, Jiang C, Lü J. Tanshinones: sources, pharmacokinetics and anti-cancer activities. Int J Mol Sci 2012; 13(10): 13621-66.
[http://dx.doi.org/10.3390/ijms131013621] [PMID: 23202971]

[96]  Holden C. Mental health. Global survey examines impact of depression. Science 2000; 288(5463): 39-40.
[http://dx.doi.org/10.1126/science.288.5463.39] [PMID: 10766633]

[97]  Bahramsoltani R, Farzaei MH, Farahani MS, Rahimi R. Phytochemical constituents as future antidepressants: a comprehensive review. Rev Neurosci 2015; 26(6): 699-719.
[http://dx.doi.org/10.1515/revneuro-2015-0009] [PMID: 26146123]

[98]  Guzmán-Gutiérrez SL, Gómez-Cansino R, García-Zebadúa JC, Jiménez-Pérez NC, Reyes-Chilpa R. Antidepressant activity of *Litsea glaucescens* essential oil: identification of β-pinene and linalool as active principles. J Ethnopharmacol 2012; 143(2): 673-9.
[http://dx.doi.org/10.1016/j.jep.2012.07.026] [PMID: 22867633]

[99]  Guzmán-Gutiérrez SL, Bonilla-Jaime H, Gómez-Cansino R, Reyes-Chilpa R. Linalool and β-pinene exert their antidepressant-like activity through the monoaminergic pathway. Life Sci 2015; 128: 24-9.
[http://dx.doi.org/10.1016/j.lfs.2015.02.021] [PMID: 25771248]

[100]  Chaouloff F. Serotonin, stress and corticoids. J Psychopharmacol 2000; 14(2): 139-51.
[http://dx.doi.org/10.1177/026988110001400203] [PMID: 10890308]

[101]  Man S, Gao W, Zhang Y, Huang L, Liu C. Chemical study and medical application of saponins as anti-cancer agents. Fitoterapia 2010; 81(7): 703-14.
[http://dx.doi.org/10.1016/j.fitote.2010.06.004] [PMID: 20550961]

[102]  Milgate J, Roberts D. The nutritional & biological significance of saponins. Nutr Res 1995; 15: 1223-49.
[http://dx.doi.org/10.1016/0271-5317(95)00081-S]

[103]  Francis G, Kerem Z, Makkar HP, Becker K. The biological action of saponins in animal systems: a review. Br J Nutr 2002; 88(6): 587-605. [CrossRef]. [PubMed].
[http://dx.doi.org/10.1079/BJN2002725] [PMID: 12493081]

[104]  Netala VR, Ghosh SB, Bobbu P, Anitha D, Tartte V. Triterpenoid saponins: A review on biosynthesis, applications and mechanism of their action. Int J Pharm Pharm Sci 2014; 7: 24-8.

[105]  Podolak I, Galanty A, Sobolewska D. Saponins as cytotoxic agents: a review. Phytochem Rev 2010; 9(3): 425-74. [CrossRef]. [PubMed].
[http://dx.doi.org/10.1007/s11101-010-9183-z] [PMID: 20835386]

[106]  Fuchs H, Bachran D, Panjideh H, *et al.* Saponins as tool for improved targeted tumor therapies. Curr Drug Targets 2009; 10(2): 140-51. [CrossRef]. [PubMed].
[http://dx.doi.org/10.2174/138945009787354584] [PMID: 19199910]

[107]  Park JH, Kwak JH, Khoo JH, *et al.* Cytotoxic effects of triterpenoid saponins from Androsace umbellata against multidrug resistance (MDR) and non-MDR cells. Arch Pharm Res 2010; 33(8): 1175-80. [CrossRef]. [PubMed].
[http://dx.doi.org/10.1007/s12272-010-0807-z] [PMID: 20803120]

[108]  Rooney S, Ryan MF. Effects of alpha-hederin and thymoquinone, constituents of *Nigella sativa*, on human cancer cell lines. Anticancer Res 2005; 25(3B): 2199-204. [PubMed].
[PMID: 16158964]

[109]  Kiem PV, Thu VK, Yen PH, *et al.* New triterpenoid saponins from Glochidion eriocarpum and their cytotoxic activity. Chem Pharm Bull (Tokyo) 2009; 57(1): 102-5. [CrossRef]. [PubMed].
[http://dx.doi.org/10.1248/cpb.57.102] [PMID: 19122328]

[110]  Zhou L-B, Chen T-H, Bastow KF, Shibano M, Lee K-H, Chen D-F. Filiasparosides A-D, cytotoxic steroidal saponins from the roots of *Asparagus filicinus*. J Nat Prod 2007; 70(8): 1263-7. [CrossRef].

[PubMed].
[http://dx.doi.org/10.1021/np070138w] [PMID: 17629328]

[111] Elekofehinti OO. Saponins: Anti-diabetic principles from medicinal plants - A review. Pathophysiology 2015; 22(2): 95-103. [CrossRef]. [PubMed].
[http://dx.doi.org/10.1016/j.pathophys.2015.02.001] [PMID: 25753168]

[112] Dembinska-Kiec A, Mykkänen O, Kiec-Wilk B, Mykkänen H. Antioxidant phytochemicals against type 2 diabetes. Br J Nutr 20 2008; 99: 109-17.
[http://dx.doi.org/10.1017/S000711450896579X]

[113] Abdel-Hassan IA, Abdel-Barry JA, Tariq Mohammeda S. The hypoglycaemic and antihyperglycaemic effect of *citrullus colocynthis* fruit aqueous extract in normal and alloxan diabetic rabbits. J Ethnopharmacol 2000; 71(1-2): 325-30.
[http://dx.doi.org/10.1016/S0378-8741(99)00215-9] [PMID: 10904181]

[114] Afolayan AJ, Sunmonu TO. Artemisia afra Jacq. ameliorates oxidative stress in the pancreas of streptozotocin-induced diabetic Wistar rats. Biosci Biotechnol Biochem 2011; 75(11): 2083-6.
[http://dx.doi.org/10.1271/bbb.100792] [PMID: 22056428]

[115] Khan H, Khan MA, Abdullah A. Antibacterial, antioxidant and cytotoxic studies of total saponin, alkaloid and sterols contents of decoction of Joshanda: identification of components through thin layer chromatography. Toxicol Ind Health 2015; 31(3): 202-8.
[http://dx.doi.org/10.1177/0748233712468023] [PMID: 23235996]

[116] Abbasolu U, Turkoz S. Antimicrobial activities of saponin extract from some indigenous plants of Turkey. Int J Pharmacogn 1995; 33(4): 293-6.
[http://dx.doi.org/10.3109/13880209509065381]

[117] Coleman JJ, Okoli I, Tegos GP, *et al.* Characterization of plant-derived saponin natural products against Candida albicans. ACS Chem Biol 2010; 5(3): 321-32.
[http://dx.doi.org/10.1021/cb900243b] [PMID: 20099897]

[118] Marrelli M, Conforti F, Araniti F, Statti GA. Effects of Saponins on Lipid Metabolism: A Review of Potential Health Benefits in the Treatment of Obesity. Molecules 2016; 21(10): 1404.
[http://dx.doi.org/10.3390/molecules21101404] [PMID: 27775618]

[119] Malinow MR, McLaughlin P, Papworth L, *et al.* Effect of alfalfa saponins on intestinal cholesterol absorption in rats. Am J Clin Nutr 1977; 30(12): 2061-7.
[http://dx.doi.org/10.1093/ajcn/30.12.2061] [PMID. 563169]

**CHAPTER 2**

# Medicinal Plants and Drug Discovery

## Emmanuel O. Ajani[1,*]

[1] *Department of Medical Biochemistry and Pharmacology, Kwara State University, Malete, P. M. B. 1530, Ilorin, Nigeria*

**Abstract:** Emerging communicable diseases, such as Ebola and Coronavirus Infection Disease (COVID-19), and non-communicable diseases related to diet and lifestyle, *e.g.*, diabetes, have been increasing over the last two decades, having a great negative impact on the health services, which are already over-stretched. This again has been compounded by some largely unresolved diseases, such as malaria and HIV/AIDS, which are common parasitic and infectious diseases in many developing countries. Over several years, natural medicine has been a dependable alternative in the prevention and treatment of diseases and has been widely recognized as important for drug discovery and development. Over the world, traditional medicine has largely depended on natural products. The structural diversity and biological activity of natural products have made them a valuable source of drugs and drug leads. Several active compounds have been isolated from natural products. Among them, some follow their traditional uses while some others do not. For many years, plant's bioactive compounds, otherwise referred to as secondary metabolites, have been the source of countless compounds and leads for drug discovery. The process of drug discovery includes the identification of a lead compound, which is then proposed for drug development. Drug discovery, therefore, encompasses moving from a screening hit to a compound becoming a therapeutic agent. It is a process that requires expertise and experience. In modern drug discovery research, techniques commonly employed include combinatorial chemistry, high-throughput screening, bioinformatics, proteomics and genomics.

**Keywords:** Drug development, Drug discovery, Drug leads, Natural products, Plant.

## 1. INTRODUCTION

As the world faces global health challenges, the importance of research into drug development through natural products has become increasingly important. Plants, animals and minerals are among the natural products that have been the basis for the treatment of many diseases for centuries [1].

---

[*] **Corresponding author Emmanuel O. Ajani:** Department of Medical Biochemistry and Pharmacology, Kwara State University, Malete, P. M. B. 1530, Ilorin, Nigeria; E-mail: emmanuel.ajani@kwasu.edu.ng

**Saheed Sabiu (Ed)**

Recently, much attention has been paid to pharmacognostic, phytochemical and pharmacological studies of traditional medicinal plants.

Medicinal plants are of vital value to the pharmacological systems since they possess multiple compounds, especially the lead molecules and thus have a number of advantages compared to synthetic molecules [2, 3]. Among natural products, plant metabolites have been revered for their usefulness as either drugs or drug precursors, being described as biosynthetic laboratories where chemical compounds could be extracted to serve multiple physiological functions [4]. Ethnopharmacological knowledge has offered a boost to the discovery and development of active and medicinally important compounds from plants. The approach is based on a body of work across several disciplines, including botany, chemistry, and pharmacology. Ethnopharmacology encompasses field observations, descriptions of the utilization and bioactivities of folk remedies, botanical identification of the plant material as well as phytochemical and pharmacological research. The study provides opportunity to explore the vast opportunities, chemical uniqueness and diversities that are present in the natural products, either as purified compounds or as crude extracts of the plant [2, 5]. The understanding of green pharmaceuticals is becoming increasingly popular and highly important as the world searches for new drugs [2]. The medicinal value of plants has come to recognition since ancient times, and available records have shown the use of many plants derived medicines for managing pathological conditions since time immemorial [6 - 8]. Literature search has shown that while some of these medicines have been used as concoctions, others have been used as crude plant extracts without the isolation of target active compounds that elicit the therapeutic function [8].

The isolation and application of bioactive plants' constituents in modern drug discovery started in the 19th century, and as of today, several active compounds with definite chemical structures have been identified in plants and are used globally as drugs [9, 10]. Compounds isolated from plants have shown some remarkable efficacy against some of the world's most challenging diseases and clinical conditions, including multi-drug resistance [11], cancer [12, 13], depressive disorders [14], diabetes [15], pest invasion [16], inflammation [17], and viral and other parasitic infections [18, 19]. The engagement of enthnobotanical and ethnopharmacological knowledge in the hunt for new medicines has offered a new route to further explore the different compounds in plants which could be important as a new class of drugs.

Despite the fact that ethnobotanical discoveries are essential factors for the development of modern medicine, globalization and urbanization have led to the disappearance of traditional medicinal plant knowledge [3, 20]. The adoption of plants in the making of edible vaccines poses a very interesting breakthrough with respect to the constraints of traditional vaccines [21]. Edible vaccine has the potential for global immunization against diseases that have been known to be pathogenic and their concrete exploration could bring a new evolution and approach to public health and medicine [21]. The decisive role played in pharmaceutics by plants since the prehistoric times could be further enhanced through the knowledge of phytomedicine and nanophytomedicine, and drugs could be developed from plant chemicals for specific targets in the system [22].

## 2. HISTORICAL USE OF PLANTS FOR PHARMACOLOGICAL PURPOSES

Life basically depends on plants as they occupy the central position in the ecosystem. The mankind has discovered the numerous benefits of the plant kingdom and has gainfully explored them not only as a source of food needed to survive but also as medicine [23]. How did man discover the therapeutic benefits of plants? Trial and errors may have acquainted man with the preparation of medicine and food from plants, and through this, he has mastered the act, built on the accumulation of experiences, and thus, is in a better position to harness the resources in his environment to meet his life needs [7, 23]. The experiences and information gathered have outlived every generation through information transmission. The evolution of the technologically driven generation, which gives prompt access to modern facilities, has brought an abundance of knowledge to human about natural resources and the use of the plant for multiple purposes [7]. Report from literature indicates that the use of plants for the treatment and prevention of diseases has its origin in the ancient Chinese, Egyptians, Indians, Greeks, Romans and the old Slavs, from where it spread across other nations of the world [23].

Traditional medicine generally describes knowledge about health, skills and practices that are peculiar to different cultures around the world, and this informs why early practices showed that there was diversity in drug development concepts [24]. Reports indicate that before the advent of the 20th century, man depended essentially on the use of crude and unpurified plants, animals and microbes' extracts for treating diseases. In the early 20th century, researchers were able to show that for medicinal activity, specific interactions occur between drug molecules and the living system [23]. This interaction is mediated by receptors which are cellular macromolecules, *i.e.*, proteins and nucleic acids. Thus, scientists have concluded that plant extracts contain chemical constituents generally referred to as bioactive compounds that elicit biological effects through interactions at target sites. In 1805, morphine, the first bioactive pharmacological compound, was isolated from opium by a German apothecary assistant Friedrich

Sertürner [25]. Following the discovery of opium, scientists began to evaluate other medicinal plants, and decades later, isolation of some other bioactive natural products, such as emetine (1817), quinine (1820), caffeine (1820), atropine (1819) and digitoxin (1841), was reported [26 - 28]. With this discovery, more studies targeted at the chemical synthesis of natural products were carried out. This facilitated their production at higher quality and at reduced costs.

The first natural compound to be produced by chemical synthesis was salicylic acid [28]. Since 1853 when salicylic acid was discovered, drug discovery from natural product has continued to play an immense role in revolutionizing the medicine. At a later time, the discovery of some other drugs, including artemisinin from *Artemisian afra* and cyclosporine from *Tolypocladium inflatum*, were reported [10, 29, 30]. The list of some plant-derived drugs, their biochemical action and plant source, is shown in (Table **1**). With these discoveries, attention has been shifted to the use of chemical compounds rather than extracts as a protocol for treating the diseases. This was what led scientists to intensify research to identify and elucidate the structures of these plant bioactive compounds identified to be responsible for medicinal activity of crude extracts.

**Table 1. Drugs derived from plants with their ethnomedical correlations and sources [16, 17].**

| **Drug Plant source Action or clinical use** |
|---|
| Acetyldigoxin *Digitalis lanata Ehrh.* Cardiotonic Digitalis |
| Adoniside *Adonis vernalis* L. Cardiotonic |
| Aescin *Aesculus hippocastanum* L. Anti-inflammatory |
| Aesculetin *Fraxinus rhynchophylla* Hance Antidysentery |
| Agrimophol *Agrimonia eupatoria* L Anthelmintic. |
| Ajmalicine *Rauvolfia serpentina* (L.) Benth ex. Kurz Circulatory disorders |
| Allyl isothiocyanate *Brassica nigra* (L.) Koch Rubefacient |
| Andrographolide *Andrographis paniculata* Nees Bacillary dysentery |
| Anisodamine *Anisodus tanguticus* (Maxim.) Pascher Anticholinergic |
| Anisodine *Anisodus tanguticus* (Maxim.) Pascher Anticholinergic |
| Arecoline *Areca catechu* L. Anthelmintic |
| Asiaticoside *Centella asiatica* (L.) Urban Vulnerary |
| Atropine *Atropa belladonna* L. Anticholinergic |
| Berberine *Berberis vulgaris* L. Bacillary dysentery |
| Bergenin *Ardisia japonica* Bl. Antitussive |
| Bromelain *Ananas comosus* (L.) Merrill Anti-inflammatory; proteolytic agent |
| Caffeine *Camellia sinensis* (L.) Kuntze CNS stimulant |

| Drug Plant source Action or clinical use |
| --- |
| (+)-Catechin *Potentilla fragaroides* L. Haemostatic |
| Chymopapain *Carica papaya* L. Proteolytic; mucolytic |
| Cocaine *Erythroxylum coca* Lamk. Local anaesthetic |
| Codeine *Papaver somniferum* L. Analgesic: Antitussive |
| Colchicine *Colchicum autumnale L.* Antitumor agent; antigout; anti-inflammatory |
| Convallotoxin *Convallaria majalis* L. Cardiotonic |
| Curcumin *Curcuma longa* L. Choleretic |
| Cynarin *Cynara scolymus* L. Choleretic |
| Danthron *Cassia spp.* Laxative |
| Deserpidine *Rauvolfia canescens* L. Antihypertensive; tranquilizer |

Studies have identified 310,000 plant species and, at the same time, stated that only about 6% of these plants have been investigated pharmacologically and 15% phytochemically [31, 32]. Corroborating these studies, a survey by Lautie *et al.* [10] reported that bioactive compounds from plants are derived from 165 different plant species, which include trees and ornamental plants. One interesting conclusion from this study is the fact that even to date, scientists are yet to fully explore a large proportion of plant species. Over the years, plants have been shown to be an important source of pharmacologically active compounds and directly or indirectly, plants are the source from which many novel therapeutic drugs are derived. In the dawn of the 21$^{st}$ century, the World Health Organization (WHO) recognized and classified two hundred and fifty-two drugs as basic and essential; 11% of these drugs were exclusively isolated from plant origin. Recent reports indicate that in the past few years, the use of medicinal plants in treating disease conditions has overshadowed modern medicine. This is not only reported in the developing countries, but it is also seen in the developed nations of the world [10, 33 - 35]. Integration of medicinal plants into modern medical practices to the extent of prescribing them as drugs has been well reported in countries, such as the UK, Germany, China and France [36, 37]. As of 2012, the world plant-derived drug market was estimated at US$ 22.1 billion, and this was also projected to grow to US$ 26.6 billion by 2017 at a compound yearly growth rate of 3.8% [38, 39]. Economically, the drastic herbal medicine development coupled with the increasing global demand for plant-based drugs has boosted the market outlook for pharma and pharma products with a market projection of $1.2 trillion by 2022 to meet global demand, and this is even further boosted by the endorsement of herbal medicine by the World Health Organization [40].

## 3. THE PROCESS AND TECHNIQUES OF DRUG DEVELOPMENT FROM PLANTS

The use of natural products, such as plants, for designing new leads in the process of drug synthesis is a task that is very challenging. This process includes the plant's phytochemical analysis, investigating the nature and structures of the bioactive compounds, characterizations, and pharmacological evaluation [38]. To start with, preliminary investigations must first be conducted on any novel therapeutic agent or plant-based drug compounds through diverse approaches that could include traditional, random ethnopharmacology, and zoopharmacognosy [39, 40].

It must be noted that not all plant products have the potential to be fully synthesized. The reasons, according to Issa *et al.* [41], include the fact that:

i. The complex nature of the structures of some natural products, such as penicillin, morphine, and paclitaxel, often makes it too difficult and expensive to synthesize them on an industrial scale. When it is difficult to synthesize a natural product, the alternative has always been to harvest it from its natural source. The process involved in doing this is often tedious, time-consuming, and expensive. It is also potentially unsustainable.

ii. Only a very limited number of structural analogues may be obtained from harvesting.

iii. Synthesized compounds may sometimes work in a different way from the original natural products.

iv. Drug development is an economically risky endeavor, and the final result from several trials may lead to the compound being discarded.

Averagely, reports indicate that the cost of developing a new therapeutic agent may be as much as $1.5 billion USD, and this may span several years depending on the disease complexity and the nature of the compound [42, 43]. It has also been reported that the failure rate in drug discovery process is about 90%, and that this failure could occur at any phase of the process [44, 45].

Koparde *et al.* [38] noted that the process of drug development from plants encompasses: (i) plant's collection and identification; (ii) literature survey and analysis; (iii) non-polar and polar extraction of the plant; (iv) extract preparation for phytochemical screening and investigation of biological activities; (v) chromatographic analysis of the extract; (vi) structural elucidation of the bioactive isolates; (vii) *in vitro* and *in vivo* testing of the bioactive compounds; (viii) molecular studies of the active compounds, and (ix) clinical trials (Fig. **1**).

The process begins with the identification of the lead compound and its optimization. For the identification of the lead compounds, the first step is to study the physical and biological properties of the target. This enables a prediction of the sorts of chemicals that might fit into an active site. After the establishment of a lead compound series that has sufficient target potency, is highly selective and that has favorable drug-like properties, one or two compounds may thereafter be proposed for use in drug development. The compound with the best property is generally referred to as the lead compound, and the other compound is then designated as the "backup". However, once a quality lead compound is obtained, it goes a long way in determining the success of the latter clinical trial phases [46]. Drug leads sometimes fail in the drug development process due to the poor understanding of the compound's properties and inadequate knowledge about the pathophysiology of the disease, failure to develop therapeutics that target overlapping dysregulated pathways, and the choice of irrelevant drug targets [45]. Koparde *et al.* [38] classified the process of drug discovery from plants into four phases.

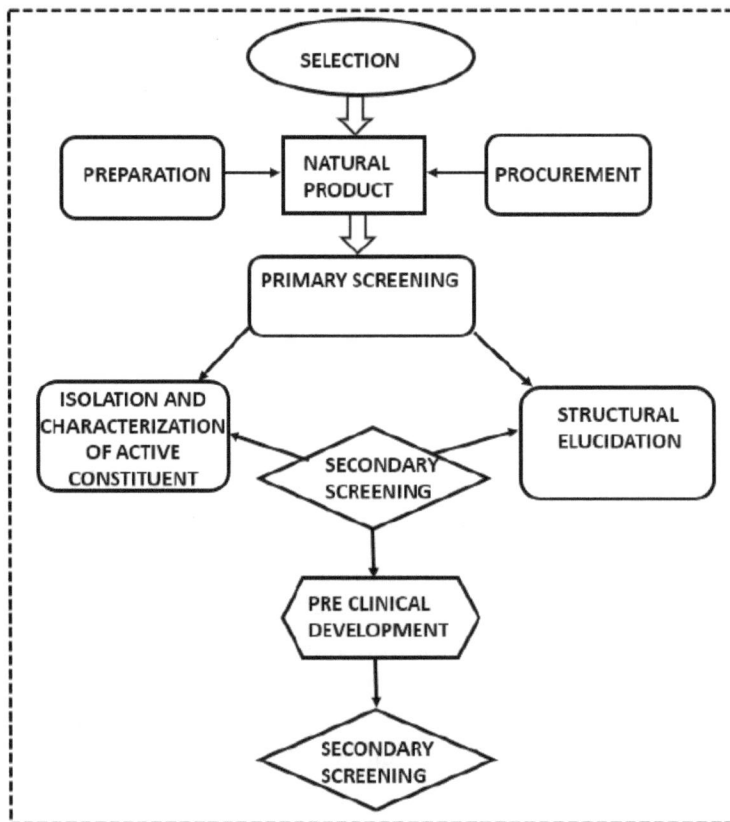

A

*(Fig. 1) contd.....*

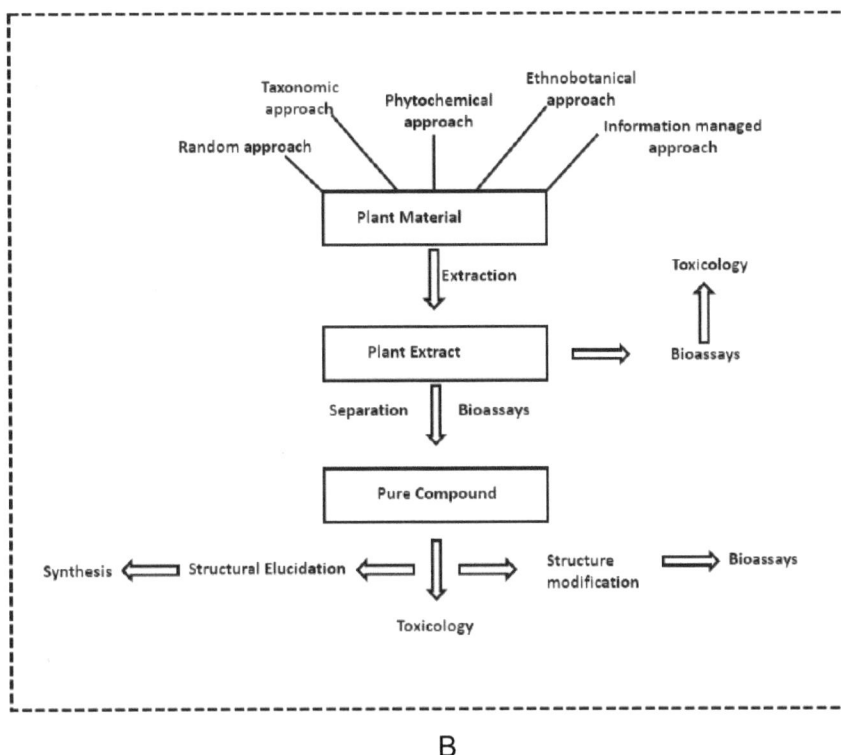

**Fig. (1). (A):** Summary of drug discovery strategies; **(B)**: General procedure for obtaining active principles from plant. **Source:** Koparde *et al.* [38].

## Phase 1: Collection and Identification

The process usually starts with plant collection, identification, authentication and sample deposition in the herbarium. Specific pharmacognosy procedures are used to identify, select and process plant products that show efficacy as medicinal plants. A report from Koparde *et al.* [38] suggested that a suitable plant selection method that suits the best interest of the drug intended to be developed should be adopted. The approach could be a random selection approach, taxonomic approach, ethnomedical approach, phytochemical (chemotaxonomic) approach, or information-managed approach. The selected plant possesses chemical constituents with biological activity, also referred to as bioactive compounds. Such a structure may act as a lead compound.

## Phase II: Isolation and Purification

High Throughput Screening (HTS) is a process involved in finding a new bioactive principle that can be used against a chosen target for a particular disease.

In this procedure, large libraries of chemicals are evaluated for their efficacy in modifying the target. Where a lead compound (or active principle) is seen to be present in a mixture that includes other compounds from a plant, the identified compound must first be isolated and purified. The structure, stability, and quantity of the lead compound determine the ease with which the active principle can be isolated and purified. The isolation process starts with solvent extraction, which is the preparation of the extracts to be used for phytochemical analysis and biological testing. Katiyar *et al.* [47] proposed two simplified extraction processes, including

a. **The parallel approach:** this method is built on prior experience of the biological activity of the plant through traditional use. To successfully isolate the compound of interest, three types of extract would be obtained if this approach is used, and they are 50% methanolic extract, 100% methanolic extract and 100% aqueous extract from the crude plant. Based on the result obtained from the primary screening, the extract that has the highest bioactivity will then be selected for further purification and evaluation.

b. **Sequential approach**: this method is used when there is no prior knowledge of the actual biological activity of the plant. What guides the extraction in this technique is the polarity of the solvents. The fractions are obtained in a sequential process by using solvents, such as hexane, chloroform, ethyl acetate and butanol.

For the purification process, techniques, such as chromatography-guided fractionation, including high-performance thin layer chromatography (HPTLC) and column chromatography (CC) [38, 47], are often used. Other notable techniques, including thin-layer chromatography (TLC) and high-performance liquid chromatography (HPLC), or non-chromatographic techniques, such as immunoassays, may also be used. This is then followed by monitoring each fraction obtained from the chromatography procedure, isolation of the compound, and calculation of Rf values. Katiyar *et al.* [47] opined that a further extraction that forms the purification stage is done where the individual compounds are structurally characterized. The determination of the structure of the biomolecules could be done using data from several spectroscopic techniques, such as UV-visible (UV-Vis), infrared (IR), nuclear magnetic resonance (NMR), and mass spectroscopic techniques [48]. Depending on the results obtained from these techniques, the structure of the various molecules can be identified [48].

### Phase III: Synthesis of the Bioactive Compound

The next stage is the synthesis of the active compound or large-scale re-isolation of the active compound of interest thorough pharmacological studies, which is initiated *in vitro* but concluded *in vivo*. It encompasses studies on molecular modeling and preparation of derivatives of the active compound of interest.

**Phase IV: Clinical Trials**

The purification and characterization of the drug molecule are then followed by testing of each purified and characterized compound in both *in vitro* and *in vivo* phyto-pharmacological investigation procedures. The purpose of the clinical trials is to evaluate the efficacy, safety and selectivity of the herbal extract or isolated compounds for drug discovery, and this is carried out in 3 phases. At the first phase, the highest dose that can be taken without serious side effects is determined in 20 to 80 people. At the second phase, the drug is administered to hundreds of people with the disease condition and monitored for months or years. The final clinical trial phase, which can last for many years, involves up to 3000 people with the disease condition. At this phase, the mode of action of the drug is monitored and compared with that of existing medication for the same condition.

## 4. PLANTS BIOACTIVE COMPOUNDS AND THEIR APPLICATIONS IN SOME DISEASES

The increasing popularity of phyto-compounds for use in drug discovery could be linked to their great bioavailability and high chemical diversity, making them new leads for the development of novel drugs [49]. The wide range of biological activities that can be exhibited by phyto-compounds include antioxidant, immunomodulatory, antimicrobial, cardiovascular, and anticancer. Quite a substantial number of drugs have been isolated from plants, and many of these drugs have found their use traditionally in ethnomedicine or ethnobotany. Some other drugs currently in use were initially discovered through random investigation of extracts from plants and animals, and subsequently, their biological activity has been investigated either *in vitro* or *in vivo* [50 - 54].

### 4.1. Plants Bioactive Compounds as Anticancer Agents

Considering the continuous rise in the incidence of cancer, the American Association for Cancer Research (AACR) projected that by 2030, 13 million people may die of this fatal disease. This report necessitated the need for research on natural products with anti-cancer properties. A study by Nirmala *et al.* [55] reported about thirty plant-derived anti-cancer compounds as efficacious in treating tumors of various types. Some of these plants are currently being used in clinical trials. Such compounds include podophyllotoxin from *Podophyllum pelltatum* [56] and 'vinca alkaloids', vinblastine and vincristine, from the Madagascan periwinkle, *Catharanthus roseus*. As the search for more anti-cancer drugs continues, the Pacific yew tree, *Taxus brevifolia*, has also been investigated.

From this plant, an active anticancer principle, paclitaxel (Taxol®), was discovered [57]. Paclitaxel, which has been shown to have a unique cytotoxic mechanism, is the first known anticancer drug that promotes the polymerization of microtubules by first stabilizing them. Paclitaxel is now known as a blockbuster drug used in the treatment of lung, ovarian, and breast cancer.

## 4.2. Plants Bioactive Compounds as Antimalarial Agents

For a long time, quinine, a constituent of *Cinchona officinalis* bark, was the first and only antimalarial drug [58]. Efforts to find a new antimalaria drug led to the emergence of chloroquine, now recognized as a highly efficacious antimalarial drug. However, with the emergence of chloroquine resistant *Plasmodium falciparum* strains, there was a consequent increase in malaria mortality rate [58]. The discovery of artemisinin in 1972 from the leaves of the traditional Chinese plant, *Artemisia annua*to, led to the most remarkable advances in the chemotherapy of malaria. It is significant to note that for over 2000 years before then, *Artemisia annua*to has been in use by the Chinese to treat malaria. Artemisinin, a sesquiterpene lactone, is highly effective, even in the cases that are incurable by chloroquine. However, its high lipophilicity is a major challenge in its administration [58, 59]. Attempts to prepare semi-synthetic derivatives of artemisinin by scientists have led to the existence of some active compounds, like artemether and sodium artesunate [58].

## 4.3. Plants Bioactive Compounds as Antiviral Agents

In 1987, an antiviral compound, coumarin calanolide A, was isolated from leaves and twigs extract of *Calophyllum lanigerum* (Clusiaceae) [60]. It was, however, in 1997 that the clinical development of calanolide A began. Presently, calanolide A is obtained by synthesis, and it is currently in Phase II trials. The National Cancer Institute (NCI), in one of the largest screening programs conducted between 1987-1996, in a *vitro* cell-based anti-HIV assay, investigated about 30,000 plants [60]. The study reported a considerable number of compounds that exhibited *in vitro* anti-HIV activity. Although no anti-HIV drug of plant origin is currently being marketed, the interesting outcome of the screening is that it has been proved that there are many plant compounds that may be valuable as lead compounds in HIV therapy. Studies have advanced to the preclinical and clinical phases on some of these compounds or their derivatives [61].

In a recent study, the presence of a wide array of plant-based bioactive oligosaccharides and polysaccharides that are potential candidates for the treatment of diseases, such as cancer, diabetes, influenza, tumor, inflammation, thrombosis, infections, and some other clinical conditions, was reported [62]. Allopathic medicine has leveraged the prescription of some of the plant-based phytochemical compounds for the treatment of severe and chronic health conditions like cancer. These compounds are not limited to aspirin, morphine, taxol, vinca alkaloids, artemisinin, yoga and acupuncture, all of which have been developed from plants [63, 64].

## 5. PLANT-BASED DRUG AND THE CHALLENGE OF EMERGING INFECTIOUS DISEASES: COVID-19 EXPERIENCE

COVID-19, a global pandemic that was first discovered in the Wuhan province of China [65], is a disease known to be caused by the Severe Acute Respiratory Syndrome Coronavirus 2 (SARS-CoV 2) [66]. The World Health Organization had declared public health emergency for global awareness of the COVID-19, which until now has no approved drug [67], but this has not stopped researchers from trying different natural and synthetic compounds as possible therapeutic agents for the disease that has claimed hundred thousands of lives over the world, including 14,750 in Africa; 367,934 in Americas; 41,601 in the East Mediterranean; 214,731 in Europe; 48,569 in South-East Asia; and 8,549 in Western Pacific [68]. Plant-based compounds have been used for antiviral purposes [61, 69, 70], and this could also form part of the reasons why the WHO is in the race for the development of therapeutic agents against the disease, openly showing its support for traditional medicines that are scientifically proven [71]. Prasad *et al.* reported, in a review, the synergistic antiviral effects against SARS-COV 2 of plant-based molecules and formulations, showing their efficacy in increasing immunity, and thereby, providing tolerance to infections from viruses. The drastic reduction in the number of recorded cases of SARS-COV-2 has been linked to the use of Traditional and Complementary Medicine (TCM) therapy [72]. *Sang Ju Yin* plus *Ping Feng San*, Chinese medicine extracts, have been reported to modulate the T-Cells in a manner that enhances the host defense capacity [73, 74]. This recorded progress, coupled with some others reported in the review by Yang *et al.* [75], is opined to be the motivation behind the rapid clinical trial of TCM for use against SARS-COV 2.

The high recovery rate at the inception of COVID-19 outbreak in Madagascar was multiple times linked to the well-publicized Madagascar tonic herbal mixture by the Nation's government, and it even prompted an early reopening of schools [76], but there was no sufficient evidence of scientific backings of clinical results to validate the claim by the Madagascar government of the efficacy of the herbal mixture. This led to its disapproval by the WHO for widespread use [77], but no death was initially recorded when it was used for COVID-19 management in Madagascar [78]. The mixture was, however, distributed to some African countries after a reported clinical trial by the concerned Madagascar Research Institute [79]. It soon became obvious that the herbal mixture may not have been responsible for the decline in the COVID-19 as was first observed in the African Nation, when as of July 2020, the WHO reported over 7049 confirmed cases with recorded 59 deaths [71].

The herbal mixture designated COVID-Organics and developed by the Malagasy Institute of Applied Research is believed to be developed from *Artemisia Annua* (sweet wormwood), from which the popular antimalarial drug artemisinin has been developed [80]. The unproven administration of herbal medicine could fuel multidrug resistance and possible toxicity effects [80], a cause of morbidity and mortality related to COVID-19 [81]. This development is not unexpected, as scientists have already reported that fear, quackery, false representations, anxiety and even paranoia could proliferate during a pandemic [82]. As COVID-19 has clearly shown many clinical, epidemiological and biological properties parallel to malaria, it may have informed the choice of the herbal development by the Madagascar Research Institute [83].

Africa has been a victim of several outbreaks of emerging and re-emerging infectious diseases, but COVID-19 pandemic has further prompted some observations, remarks and conclusions from scientists. Tangwa and Munung [84] made it clear that compared to previous pandemic and epidemic responses, many countries in Africa in the face of COVID-19 have displayed a sense of solidarity that demonstrates the departure from ethics dumping, which has further strengthened its research agenda and responses against COVID-19. Data from 20 African countries reported by Iwuoha *et al.* [85] explored as how COVID-19 responses affect the management of the pandemic in Africa, revealing that the dependence on herbal medicine in conjunction with other salient global initiatives for the management of COVID-19 proved effectiveness on the African continent. The study also admitted that the adopted global approach yielded positive outcomes as it increased the number of known COVID-19 patients that eventually recovered. Furthermore, it also, at the same time, scaled down the number of fatalities recorded in Africa when compared with those from other regions. This feat thoroughly caught the attention of the world because it was initially assumed that the pandemic would severely affect the Sub-Saharan Africa due to poverty and poor healthcare systems, but the obtainable has led to the whole situation being described as an African Miracle [86].

## 6. APPLICATION OF EMERGING TECHNOLOGIES IN PROMOTING DRUG DISCOVERY FROM PLANTS

The promotion of drug discovery from plants requires concerted efforts right from the gathering of information about plants to the documentation of such information on platforms where researchers and industries could access them for further development. The World Health Organization (WHO) is playing a lead role in this and has already published a list of more than 21,000 plant species that are in use all over the world as medicine [87]. The organization has equally given stringent conditions that would allow for the maximization of plant benefits through drug discovery without toxicological concerns. These include the WHO requirement, which stipulates that for a plant to be regarded as having health-promoting potentials, its assessment must be based on a valid scientific hypothesis and confirmed studies that support the hypothesis [88]. However, the needed rapid approvals by national organizations that could discourage vendor distribution of unapproved drugs have not been met [89].

Over the last decade, technologies, such as combinatorial chemistry, high-throughput screening, bioinformatics, proteomics and genomics, have been discovered and these are already being employed in drug discovery research. The potential of these new technologies lies in their ability to make use of the chemical diversity of natural products. In the last few years, some other new techniques have emerged, such as molecular diversity, compound library design, protein 3D-structures, NMR- based screening, and 3D QSAR in modern drug design. When using natural products to support high-throughput screening (HTS) in drug discovery programs, Lahlou [53] recommends that one must ensure that the process includes incorporating technologies that can effectively support the acquisition and inventory of the natural product sources.

In an attempt to contain the drug discovery studies costs, it becomes imperative to consider information on known natural products' chemistry. This generally requires recollection and dereplication. It may be easy to obtain the latitude-longitude location of a source organism by using satellite navigation technologies and then placing it on a map. In a similar manner, the position of past collections can also be mapped. The probability that the accuracy of the data obtained will vary is one major problem in this procedure. However, using a geographic information system (GIS), where computer-based mapped data are linked to traditional text/field database records, it is possible to map these positions. Researchers can easily visualize the spatial relationships between collection points to support decisions by using a comprehensive dataset of natural products' chemical discoveries within a GIS.

In addition to this, expeditions for new acquisition efforts could effectively be planned to target specific regions based on existing information, and to avoid duplicating past collections.

### (a). Proteomics, Genomics and Bioinformatics

Bioinformatics is a theoretical, computer-based science that is targeted at the extrapolation of biological knowledge obtained from biological information. One of the important tasks in biomedical research is to discover drugs that are scientifically proven, economically efficient, and socially acceptable [90]. Some recent studies on informatics, analytical and computational techniques have afforded great opportunities in processing complex natural products and using their structures in discovering new and novel drugs that may be efficacious against many clinical conditions [8].

Proteomics includes technologies that are used for the separation, purification and determining the quantity of proteins that are present in individual samples (protein mapping). It also includes techniques that are used for the identification of specific proteins and for characterization of both their three-dimensional structure and functions. The two-dimensional polyacrylamide gel electrophoresis (2D-PAGE) is the main protein mapping technology commonly used in drug discoveries. Through genomics, a large number of sequences are produced. These genetic sequences are further investigated, after which regions of similarity and/or identity are then identified to know the possible pharmaceutical interest. The traditional approach to discovering plant-based drugs is time and capital intensive, and it requires more struggle coupled with less results of success, but the inception of bioinformatics, coupled with a high generation of data in the past genomic era, has simplified the cumbersome process of drug designing and discovery [91]. Combined informatics approaches, including bioinformatics, chem-informatics, systems and other computational processes as well as engineering have been well-reviewed for their suitability for the rapid development of drugs from plants and these state-of-the-art techniques have helped researchers to validate medicinal plants based on knowledge other than mere myths or experience that could pose a threat to human health [3, 90, 92].

## (b). Combinatorial Chemistry

The drug discovery process is a long, time- and money-intensive process. Combinatorial chemistry is a key technology that allows large screening libraries to be generated efficiently for the needs of high-throughput screening. It is a technique that is used for creating huge numbers of biologically potent motif and their hybrids, then rapidly screening them for desirable properties. Combinatorial chemistry is a strategy that is currently being used by many pharmaceutical and agrochemical industries because of the potential for immensely reducing the time and cost. Presently, there are several drug candidates in clinical trials, which are the products of this methodology. Combinatorial chemistry allows larger libraries to be generated as different from the natural products' pool that gives a much higher hit-rate in high throughput screening along with high chemical diversity. From its early focus as a random strategy for generating molecular diversity, combinatorial chemistry has developed into a powerful design technology necessary to develop and optimize drug candidates. Molecular diversity of both natural and synthetic materials provides a valuable source of compounds for identifying and optimizing new drug leads. The rapidly evolving technology of combinatorial chemistry affords the possibility of producing libraries of small molecules to screen for novel bioactivities. This powerful new technology has begun to help pharmaceutical companies in finding new drug candidates quickly, saving significant dollars in preclinical development costs, and ultimately changing their fundamental approach to drug discovery. Lahlou [53] identified four main differences between compounds in combinatorial chemistry libraries and natural products:

i. The number of chiral centers is higher in natural compounds;
ii. Structure rigidity is lower in combinatorial chemistry libraries;
iii. The number of aromatic moieties is lower in natural compounds;
iv. Heteroatoms O and N and non-aromatic unsaturation are abundant in natural products, whereas S and halogen atoms are more often present in combinatorial chemistry libraries.

### (c). High-Throughput Screening (HTS)

This has been recognized as a standard procedure for hit discovery for scientific experimentation used especially in drug discovery, and has found relevance in the fields of biology and chemistry [93]. The technique allows an investigator to quickly carry out millions of biochemical, genetic or pharmacological tests through the use of robotics, data processing and control software, liquid handling devices, and sensitive detectors. High-throughput screening allows researchers to rapidly identify active compounds, antibodies or genes that modulate a particular biochemical pathway, thus providing starting points for drug design. This is needed to understand the nature of the interaction of a biochemical process. An HTS robot can usually prepare and analyze many plates simultaneously, thereby further speeding the data-collection process.

Computational molecular designs coupled with the use of computational software have been documented to contribute to both drug discovery, drug designs and the identification of drug targets using various computational approaches not limited to docking, pharmacophore and homology modeling [8, 94]. The predictive features, molecular modeling and relevant parameters, such as pharmacokinetics and pharmacodynamics, needed in drug development could easily be done using various computer software, databases and quantum computing, and this is the present and the future upon which green drug discovery could be built [8].

The drug development process is multifaceted, with each phase requiring some unique equipment and/or methods [37, 48]. Many novel techniques that can increase the efficiency of the drug discovery process are now available and are now an important part of the drug discovery process [95]. These techniques are crucial in both hit identification and optimization process. Other techniques, such as ligand- or structure-based virtual screening, are also very important in drug discovery efforts [95]. The study of protein is a unique molecular phase and very essential component of drug discovery process, since the target of lead compounds needs to be identified and studied [45]. Advances in technology have led to the development of equipment with rapid functions, easy usability and efficient performances. Solution-based nuclear magnetic resonance (NMR) spectroscopy has been developed as an essential tool necessary to investigate protein structure and its dynamics under physiological conditions. This has been recognized as very important in the target-based drug discovery process by revealing the ligand-binding information in the solution [96].

The advent of recent technologies has also brought automation to drug discovery. The use of artificial intelligence, 'organ-on-chip' and microfluidic technologies has also been identified as the game changer that could prompt rapid drug discovery from plant sources and also hasten the evaluation of their safety, pharmacokinetics, pharmacodynamics, and efficacy [8]. Artificial intelligence (AI) and machine learning (ML) tools have been identified as new technological innovations that could accelerate the drug discovery process, and when this is merged with automation and characterization, it has been hypothesized that the combination may disrupt the prolonged early-stage of drug discovery [46].

## 7. CHALLENGES TO DRUG DISCOVERY FROM PLANTS

Modern medicine requires that active compounds be isolated, purified and characterized from sources, and this involves very technical process and may be cost-intensive [8]. Extensive knowledge is required in the development of natural sources, but limited studies are available on the isolation and characterization of bioactive compounds from natural sources, especially plants [97, 98]. This may have contributed to why drugs that are developed from natural products form just 35% of the global medicine market, which is about 1.1 trillion US dollars [99]. The identification and isolation of lead compounds from plants, exploring the link between disease and cellular biology, understanding the pathway that is involved, associating the genes that are involved in these pathways, deciphering the roles of each of the genes in the pathway, pinpointing the critical gene involved, and eventually identifying suitable drug, constitute a very prolonged exercise that requires interdisciplinary approach majorly between a biologist and medicinal chemist, and it further makes drug development not very easy. Five key areas of challenges to the development of drugs from plant sources have been identified [45, 99].

i. **Regulatory status of herbal medicine:** Quality control ensures the quality of the products. Developing countries often have a great number of traditionally used herbal medicines and much folk knowledge about them, but have hardly any legislative criteria to establish these traditionally used herbal medicines as part of the drug legislation. Parven *et al.* reported that of the 11 member countries in the South-East Asia region, there are only four with national systems for monitoring the safety of traditional medicinal products. This is further worsened by insufficient sharing of regulatory information between regulatory authorities in different countries [99]. The challenge is that less documentation of efficacy and toxicity is available prior to marketing, which predisposes their consumers to inferior products. Although reports suggest that many countries already have established guidelines for herbal drug regulations [100 - 104], most regions have the regulations only at the developmental stage [105]. For the classification of herbal or traditional medicinal products, factors applied in regulatory systems include description in a pharmacopoeia monograph, prescription status, claim of a therapeutic effect, scheduled or regulated ingredients or substances, or periods of use [106].

ii. **Assessment of safety and efficacy**: The complexity of the efficacy and safety assessment protocols coupled with the nature of occurrence of active compounds in plants, which could widely vary, make it difficult to extract single active ingredients that elicit the therapeutic function [99]. Specifically, the US FDA [107] and Archdeacon *et al.* [108] reported that the United States' FDA has only approved two botanical drugs so far, and this has been linked to some commonly encountered complications, including insufficient evidence of efficacy, unrealistic goals and expectations, and insufficient funding that might have affected the development. While some studies claim that, like synthetic drugs, herbal drugs have no significant beneficial effect on clinical outcome but rather these increase the risk of bleeding [109], other studies, such as that of Lee *et al.* [110], suggest that herbal medicine may be safe and effective. These fluctuations call for the stringent evaluation of the safety and efficacy of herbal drugs.

iii. **Quality control of herbal medicines**: This is a major concern since the quality of medicinal plants for drug development depends not only on intrinsic factors but also on extrinsic factors, such as environmental conditions, acceptable agricultural practices, and good harvesting practices [99]. Since most of the world's herbal medicines are developed in the developing countries, Dhiman *et al.* [111] believed that the development of guiding principles through efforts of regulatory authorities, research organizations and botanical manufacturers is a way forward to ensure the standardization and quality control of botanical drugs. An increase in the use of herbal drugs has also led to a rise in the various forms of abuse and adulteration of the products, progressing to gross disappointment on the part of consumers and manufacturers coupled with increased fatality [112].

iv. **Safety monitoring of herbal medicine**: The adverse effects arising from the consumption of herbal medicine are multifactorial, and the racking could be very complex. Species selection, contamination, misuse or overdosage are some of the complex problems that could be difficult to tackle and solve [99].

v. One of the identified challenges to the development of druggable compounds from plants is poor communication among researchers regarding the use of herbal products in the local regions.

For drugs to be confirmed effective, their functionality against certain targets must be confirmed. However, the screening and testing of extracts against various pharmacological targets so as to harness their benefits constitute a challenge for many laboratories globally [113]. Lautie *et al.* [10] further expressed a concern on the rate of success of translation of the multiple researches on the numerous plants' bioactive compounds into new drug development. The reason for this low success rate has been explained by Dutra *et al.* [114], who confirmed that most of the publications related to the development of therapeutic agents from plants active compounds are preliminary and that they are only focused on reporting the *in vivo* and *in vitro* effects of non-purified extract, and that only very few studies are focused at investigating the mechanism of action of isolated plant compounds. To further buttress this, it was claimed that there is a paucity of studies dedicated to investigating the toxicity, pharmacokinetics and clinical trials, and all these are essential for the development of new therapeutic agents [114].

## 8. DRUG DISCOVERY FROM PLANTS: THE CHALLENGE FOR AFRICA

Africa is a continent with a very high disease burden. In Africa, the leading causes of morbidity and mortality are the neglected tropical diseases, including tuberculosis, malaria, diabetes, cancer, cardiovascular diseases, HIV and AIDS [115]. The continent, however, is equally endowed with a huge biodiversity that is capable of providing novel drugs for the treatment of these diseases, but which at the same time remain largely unexplored [115]. African traditional medicine is one of the many listed folklore medicinal practices that have existed since time immemorial [3, 116]. Many diseases, which may be endemic to the African region but with a low rate of treatment using synthetic medicine, may be approached using herbal formulations [3].

Africa is a home to numerous species of medicinal plants, some of which are being screened for use against parasitic infections [117]; notable is the *Trypanosoma brucei*, which is the causative agent of the Human African Trypanosomiasis (HAT) [118]. African botanicals have shown potential against some of the worlds' most threatening diseases, including cancer [119] and antibiotic resistance [118]. An important development in the drug discovery process from African botanicals was the creation of natural product database for over 4500 compounds, isolated mainly from plants between 1962 and 2016 [99]. The South African adoption of plant medicine for cure of local diseases was another major step forward [119]. Financial and infrastructural challenges have been identified as the major challenge to the robust development of plant-based medicine in Africa, and have led to the call for the development of the African scientific research capabilities of the African institutions through a global network [115]. Many evolving infections in the past decade, such as acquired immune deficiency syndrome, Ebola, and a few others, have no known cure, and all the chemotherapies have only shown suppressive effects other than curative effects, which calls for the consideration of plant-based drugs [119].

## 9. FUTURE PROSPECT OF PLANT-BASED DRUGS

The increasing demand and rapidly expanding market opportunities for plant-based drugs and other herbal healthcare products in both the developed and developing countries have led to a rapid development of herbal drugs [12]. In support of this view, Dutral *et al.* [114] earlier estimated the current world market of phytomedicine to be around US$27.5 billion, with the highest consumer being Europe. Due to increasing application, this is expected to rapidly increase. The availability of new methods and technologics offers great opportunities for the rapid development of herbal-based drugs in the nearest future. With the advent of recent methods for easy understanding of drug targets coupled with the extraction and characterization of bioactive compounds, there will be safer and faster development of lead molecules from plants [8]. Emerging fields, such as molecular phylogenetic [99], cyanotherapetics [120], nanomedicine [99], combinatorial chemistry and computer modeling [121], DNA sequencing, and computational drug design technologies [3] can facilitate the rates at which new molecular entities will be introduced into the market.

## CONCLUDING REMARKS AND FUTURE PERSPECTIVE

Drawing from available records, it has been well proven that plants have essential druggable compounds that could be explored to treat diverse emerging and persistent diseases. However, it is also well noted that the global medicinal plant diversities have not been well explored, and some of those that have been explored do not have adequate scientific backings to justify their efficacy or toxicity that will further prompt approval by concerned agencies. These conditions require holistic efforts so as to maximize the benefits that medicinal plants offer. Similarly, the challenges surrounding the development of druggable compounds are still numerous. These should be reviewed by concerned national and international agencies, and necessary regulations must be institutionalized to ensure the best practices involving the use of medicinal plants for drug development. Information about the already characterized medicinal plants is still hoarded in some regions; such information about medicinal plant extracts or lead molecules should be made available on open digital space for easy access by researchers and industries who would require them for further development. This will help reduce the cost of the drug development process, since the process will not be repeated from scratch, and it will further reduce the duration of the development. Modern equipment and methods that have proved to be efficient in recent times should be maximized as it will ensure efficiency in the drug development process.

## CONSENT FOR PUBLICATION

Not applicable.

## CONFLICT OF INTEREST

The authors declare no conflict of interest, financial or otherwise.

## ACKNOWLEDGEMENTS

Declared none.

## REFERENCES

[1]     Katiyar C, Gupta A, Kanjilal S, Katiyar S. Drug discovery from plant sources: An integrated approach. Ayu 2012; 33(1): 10-9.
        [http://dx.doi.org/10.4103/0974-8520.100295] [PMID: 23049178]

[2]     Süntar I. Importance of ethnopharmacological studies in drug discovery: role of medicinal plants. Phytochem Rev 2020; 19(5): 1199-209.
        [http://dx.doi.org/10.1007/s11101-019-09629-9]

[3]     Singh S, Sharma B, Kanwar SS, Kumar A. Lead phytochemicals for anticancer drug development. Front Plant Sci 2016; 7: 1667.
        [http://dx.doi.org/10.3389/fpls.2016.01667] [PMID: 27877185]

[4]     Sasidharan S, Saudagar P. Plant Metabolites as New Leads to Drug Discovery. Natural Bio-active Compounds. Singapore: Springer 2019; pp. 275-95.
        [http://dx.doi.org/10.1007/978-981-13-7205-6_12]

[5]     Jadid N, Kurniawan E, Himayani CES, *et al.* An ethnobotanical study of medicinal plants used by the Tengger tribe in Ngadisari village, Indonesia. PLoS One 2020; 15(7): e0235886.
        [http://dx.doi.org/10.1371/journal.pone.0235886] [PMID: 32658902]

[6]     Draye M, Chatel G, Duwald R. Ultrasound for Drug Synthesis: A Green Approach. Pharmaceuticals (Basel) 2020; 13(2): 23.
[http://dx.doi.org/10.3390/ph13020023] [PMID: 32024033]

[7]     Jamshidi-Kia F, Lorigooini Z, Amini-Khoei H. Medicinal plants: Past history and future perspective. J HerbMed Pharmacol 2018; 7: 1.

[8]     Thomford NE, Senthebane DA, Rowe A, *et al.* Natural products for drug discovery in the 21st century: innovations for novel drug discovery. Int J Mol Sci 2018; 19(6): 1578.
[http://dx.doi.org/10.3390/ijms19061578] [PMID: 29799486]

[9]     Fabricant DS, Farnsworth NR. The value of plants used in traditional medicine for drug discovery. Environ Health Perspect 2001; 109 (Suppl. 1): 69-75.
[PMID: 11250806]

[10]    Lautié E, Russo O, Ducrot P, Boutin JA. Unraveling plant natural chemical diversity for drug discovery purposes. Front Pharmacol 2020; 11: 397.
[http://dx.doi.org/10.3389/fphar.2020.00397] [PMID: 32317969]

[11]    Anand U, Jacobo-Herrera N, Altemimi A, Lakhssassi N. A comprehensive review on medicinal plants as antimicrobial therapeutics: potential avenues of biocompatible drug discovery. Metabolites 2019; 9(11): 258.
[http://dx.doi.org/10.3390/metabo9110258] [PMID: 31683833]

[12]    Datir SS. Plant Metabolites as New Leads to Anticancer Drug Discovery: Approaches and Challenges.Anticancer Plants: Natural Products and Biotechnological Implements. Singapore: Springer 2018; pp. 141-61.
[http://dx.doi.org/10.1007/978-981-10-8064-7_7]

[13]    Majolo F, Delwing LKD, Marmitt DJ, Bustamante-Filho IC, Goettert MI. Medicinal plants and bioactive natural compounds for cancer treatment: Important advances for drug discovery. Phytochem Lett 2019; 31: 196-207.
[http://dx.doi.org/10.1016/j.phytol.2019.04.003]

[14]    Dereli FTG, Ilhan M, Akkol EK. New drug discovery from medicinal plants and phytoconstituents for depressive disorders. CNS & Neurological Disorders-Drug Targets (Formerly Current Drug Targets-CNS & Neurological Disorders) 2019; 18(2): 92-102.
[http://dx.doi.org/10.2174/1871527317666181114141129]

[15]    Vivekanandarajah S. Plants used to treat diabetes in Sri Lankan Siddha Medicine 2018.

[16]    Lybrand DB, Xu H, Last RL, Pichersky E. How Plants Synthesize Pyrethrins: Safe and Biodegradable Insecticides. Trends Plant Sci 2020; 25(12): 1240-51.

[17]    Virshette SJ, Patil MK, Somkuwar AP. A review on medicinal plants used as anti-inflammatory agents. J Pharmacogn Phytochem 2019; 8(3): 1641-6.

[18]    Dhama K, Karthik K, Khandia R, *et al.* Medicinal and therapeutic potential of herbs and plant metabolites/extracts countering viral pathogens-current knowledge and future prospects. Curr Drug Metab 2018; 19(3): 236-63.
[http://dx.doi.org/10.2174/1389200219666180129145252] [PMID: 29380697]

[19]    Chaibou M, Hamadou HH, Moussa AN, *et al. In vitro* study of the anthelmintic effects of ethanolic extracts of *Bauhinia rufrescens* Lam.(Fabaceae) and *Chrozophora brocchiana* (Vis.) Schweinf (Euphorbiaceae) two plants used as antiparasitic in Azawagh area in Niger. J Pharmacogn Phytochem 2020; 9(1): 944-8.

[20]    Phumthum M, Srithi K, Inta A, *et al.* Ethnomedicinal plant diversity in Thailand. J Ethnopharmacol 2018; 214: 90-8.
[http://dx.doi.org/10.1016/j.jep.2017.12.003] [PMID: 29241674]

[21]    Concha C, Cañas R, Macuer J, *et al.* Disease prevention: an opportunity to expand edible plant-based

vaccines? Vaccines (Basel) 2017; 5(2): 14.
[http://dx.doi.org/10.3390/vaccines5020014] [PMID: 28556800]

[22]  Shukla R, Thok K, Alam I, Singh R. Nanophytomedicine Market: Global Opportunity Analysis and Industry Forecast.Nanophytomed. Singapore: Springer 2020; pp. 19-31.
[http://dx.doi.org/10.1007/978-981-15-4909-0_2]

[23]  Šantić Ž, Pravdić N, Bevanda M, Galić K. The historical use of medicinal plants in traditional and scientific medicine. Psychiatr Danub 2017; 29(Suppl 4) (Suppl. 4): 787-92.
[PMID: 29278625]

[24]  Sood M, Singh SK, Chadda RK. Relevance of traditional Indian medical concepts in psychosomatic medicine. Ann Natl Acad Med Sci 2017; 53(03): 148-55.
[http://dx.doi.org/10.1055/s-0040-1712757]

[25]  Yuan H, Ma Q, Ye L, Piao G. The traditional medicine and modern medicine from natural products. Molecules 2016; 21(5): 559.
[http://dx.doi.org/10.3390/molecules21050559] [PMID: 27136524]

[26]  Singh YD, Panda MK, Satapathy KB. Ethnomedicine for Drug Discovery.Advances in Pharmaceut Biotech. Singapore: Springer 2020; pp. 15-28.
[http://dx.doi.org/10.1007/978-981-15-2195-9_2]

[27]  Zenk MH, Juenger M. Evolution and current status of the phytochemistry of nitrogenous compounds. Phytochemistry 2007; 68(22-24): 2757-72.
[http://dx.doi.org/10.1016/j.phytochem.2007.07.009] [PMID: 17719615]

[28]  Newman DJ, Cragg GM. Natural products as sources of new drugs over the last 25 years. J Nat Prod 2007; 70(3): 461-77.
[http://dx.doi.org/10.1021/np068054v] [PMID: 17309302]

[29]  Newman DJ, Cragg GM. Natural products as sources of new drugs over the 30 years from 1981 to 2010 J Nat Prod 2012; 75(3): 311-35.
[http://dx.doi.org/10.1021/np200906s] [PMID: 22316239]

[30]  Cullen DR, Mocerino M. A brief review of drug discovery research for human African trypanosomiasis. Curr Med Chem 2017; 24(7): 701-17.
[http://dx.doi.org/10.2174/0929867324666170120160034] [PMID: 28117003]

[31]  Campbell IB, Macdonald SJF, Procopiou PA. Medicinal chemistry in drug discovery in big pharma: past, present and future. Drug Discov Today 2018; 23(2): 219-34.
[http://dx.doi.org/10.1016/j.drudis.2017.10.007] [PMID: 29031621]

[32]  Atanasov AG, Waltenberger B, Pferschy-Wenzig EM, *et al.* Discovery and resupply of pharmacologically active plant-derived natural products: A review. Biotechnol Adv 2015; 33(8): 1582-614.
[http://dx.doi.org/10.1016/j.biotechadv.2015.08.001] [PMID: 26281720]

[33]  Tansaz M, Tajadini H. Comparison of Leiomyoma of Modern Medicine and Traditional Persian Medicine. J Evid Based Complementary Altern Med 2016; 21(2): 160-3.
[http://dx.doi.org/10.1177/2156587215595299] [PMID: 26177818]

[34]  Ntie-Kang F, Telukunta KK, Döring K, *et al.* NANPDB: a resource for natural products from northern Afr sources. J Nat Prod 2017; 80(7): 2067-76.
[http://dx.doi.org/10.1021/acs.jnatprod.7b00283] [PMID: 28641017]

[35]  Nembo EN, Hescheler J, Nguemo F. Stem cells in natural product and medicinal plant drug discovery-An overview of new screening approaches. Biomed Pharmacother 2020; 131: 110730.
[http://dx.doi.org/10.1016/j.biopha.2020.110730] [PMID: 32920519]

[36]  Yahoo MT, Saxena A, Arumugan G, Mahmoud A, Kuldip P. Promising antidiabetic drugs, medicinal plant and herbs: an update. Int J Pharmacol 2017; 13(7): 732-45.
[http://dx.doi.org/10.3923/ijp.2017.732.745]

[37]   Ruhsam M, Hollingsworth PM. Authentication of Eleutherococcus and Rhodiola herbal supplement products in the United Kingdom. J Pharm Biomed Anal 2018; 149(149): 403-9.
[http://dx.doi.org/10.1016/j.jpba.2017.11.025] [PMID: 29154110]

[38]   Koparde AA, Doijad RC, Magdum CS. Natural products in drug discovery.Pharmacognosy-Medicinal Plants. 2019.

[39]   Naidoo D, Slavětínská LP, Aremu AO, *et al.* Metabolite profiling and isolation of biologically active compounds from Scadoxus puniceus, a highly traded South African medicinal plant. Phytother Res 2018; 32(4): 625-30.
[http://dx.doi.org/10.1002/ptr.6000] [PMID: 29226479]

[40]   Parvathaneni V, Kulkarni NS, Muth A, Gupta V. Drug repurposing: a promising tool to accelerate the drug discovery process. Drug Discov Today 2019; 24(10): 2076-85.
[http://dx.doi.org/10.1016/j.drudis.2019.06.014] [PMID: 31238113]

[41]   Issa NT, Wathieu H, Ojo A, Byers SW, Dakshanamurthy S. Drug metabolism in preclinical drug development: a survey of the discovery process, toxicology, and computational tools. Curr Drug Metab 2017; 18(6): 556-65.
[http://dx.doi.org/10.2174/1389200218666170316093301] [PMID: 28302026]

[42]   Dickson M, Gagnon JP. Key factors in the rising cost of new drug discovery and development. Nat Rev Drug Discov 2004; 3(5): 417-29.
[http://dx.doi.org/10.1038/nrd1382] [PMID: 15136789]

[43]   DiMasi JA, Grabowski HG, Hansen RW. Innovation in the pharmaceutical industry: New estimates of R&D costs. J Health Econ 2016; 47: 20-33.
[http://dx.doi.org/10.1016/j.jhealeco.2016.01.012] [PMID: 26928437]

[44]   Calcoen D, Laura E, Yu Xiaomeng. What does it take to produce a breakthrough drug? 2015; 161.
[http://dx.doi.org/10.1038/nrd4570]

[45]   Vaidya A, Roy A, Chaguturu R. How to rekindle drug discovery process through integrative therapeutic targeting? Expert Opin Drug Discov 2018; 13(10): 893-8.
[http://dx.doi.org/10.1080/17460441.2018.1514010] [PMID: 30146919]

[46]   Saikin SK, Kreisbeck C, Sheberla D, Becker JS, A AG. Closed-loop discovery platform integration is needed for artificial intelligence to make an impact in drug discovery. Expert Opin Drug Discov 2019; 14(1): 1-4.
[http://dx.doi.org/10.1080/17460441.2019.1546690] [PMID: 30488727]

[47]   Katiyar C, Gupta A, Kanjilal S, Katiyar S. Drug discovery from plant sources: An integrated approach. 2012; 33(1): 10.

[48]   Altemimi A, Lakhssassi N, Baharlouei A, Watson DG, Lightfoot DA. Phytochemicals: Extraction, isolation, and identification of bioactive compounds from plant extracts. Plants 2017; 6(4): 42.
[http://dx.doi.org/10.3390/plants6040042] [PMID: 28937585]

[49]   Rallabandi HR, Mekapogu M, Natesan K, *et al.* Computational Methods Used in Phytocompound-Based Drug Discovery.Plant-derived Bioactives. Singapore: Springer 2020; pp. 549-73.
[http://dx.doi.org/10.1007/978-981-15-2361-8_25]

[50]   Krause J, Tobin G. Discovery, development and regulation of natural products.Using old solutions to new problems- natural drug discovery in the 21st Century. 2013; pp. 3-35.

[51]   McChesney JD, Venkataraman SK, Henri JT. Plant natural products: back to the future or into extinction? Phytochemistry 2007; 68(14): 2015-22.
[http://dx.doi.org/10.1016/j.phytochem.2007.04.032] [PMID: 17574638]

[52]   Rout SP, Choudhary KA, Kar DM, Das L, Jain A. Plants in traditional medicinal system future source of new drugs. Internl J Pharmacy & Pharmaceurical Sci 2009; 1(1): 1-23.

[53]   Lahlou M. The Success of Natural Products in Drug Discovery. Pharmacol Pharm 2013; 4(3): 17-31.

[http://dx.doi.org/10.4236/pp.2013.43A003]

[54]  Aslam MS, Ahmad MS. Worldwide importance of medicinal plants: current and historical perspectives. Recent Adv Biol Med 2016; 2: 909.
[http://dx.doi.org/10.18639/RABM.2016.02.338811]

[55]  Nirmala C, Madho SB, Haorongbam S. Nutritional Properties of Bamboo Shoots: Potential and Prospects for Utilization as a Health Food. Compr Rev Food Sci Food Saf 2011; 10(3): 153-68.
[http://dx.doi.org/10.1111/j.1541-4337.2011.00147.x]

[56]  Hartwell JL, Shear JL. Classes of compounds under investigation and active components of podophyllin. Cancer Res 1947; 7: 716.

[57]  Wani MC, Taylor HL, Wall ME, Coggon P, McPhail AT. Plant antitumor agents. VI. The isolation and structure of taxol, a novel antileukemic and antitumor agent from Taxus brevifolia. J Am Chem Soc 1971; 93(9): 2325-7.
[http://dx.doi.org/10.1021/ja00738a045] [PMID: 5553076]

[58]  Potterat O, Hamburger M. Drug discovery and development with plant-derived compounds. Prog Drug Res 2008; 65: 45-118, 47-118.
[http://dx.doi.org/10.1007/978-3-7643-8117-2_2] [PMID: 18084913]

[59]  Ajani EO, Salau BA, Fagbohun TR, Ogun AO. Combined effect of chloroquine and insulin administration on some biochemical parameters in rats placed on high fat and calcium diet. Afr J Med Med Sci 2004; 33(4): 365-9.
[PMID: 15977446]

[60]  Cragg GM, Newman DJ. Plants as a source of anti-cancer and anti-HIV agents. Ann Appl Biol 2003; 143(2): 127-33.
[http://dx.doi.org/10.1111/j.1744-7348.2003.tb00278.x]

[61]  Salehi B, Kumar NVA, Şener B, *et al.* Medicinal Plants Used in the Treatment of Human Immunodeficiency Virus. Int J Mol Sci 2018; 19(5): 1459.
[http://dx.doi.org/10.3390/ijms19051459] [PMID: 29757986]

[62]  Kumar V, Nagar S, Sharma P. Opportunity of plant oligosaccharides and polysaccharides in drug development.Carbohydrates in Drug Discovery and Development. Elsevier 2020; pp. 587-639.
[http://dx.doi.org/10.1016/B978-0-12-816675-8.00015-4]

[63]  Trimble EL, Rajaraman P. Integrating traditional and allopathic medicine: An opportunity to improve global health in cancer. JNCI Monographs 2017; 2017(52)

[64]  Parasuraman S. Herbal drug discovery: Challenges and perspectives. Curr Pharmacogenomics Person Med 2018; 16(1): 63-8. [Formerly Current Pharmacogenomics].
[http://dx.doi.org/10.2174/1875692116666180419153313]

[65]  Halaji M, Farahani A, Ranjbar R, Heiat M, Dehkordi FS. Emerging coronaviruses: first SARS, second MERS and third SARS-CoV-2: epidemiological updates of COVID-19. Infez Med 2020; 28 (Suppl. 1): 6-17.
[PMID: 32532933]

[66]  Mirzaie A, Halaji M, Dehkordi FS, Ranjbar R, Noorbazargan H. A narrative literature review on traditional medicine options for treatment of corona virus disease 2019 (COVID-19). Complement Ther Clin Pract 2020; 40: 101214.
[http://dx.doi.org/10.1016/j.ctcp.2020.101214] [PMID: 32891290]

[67]  Fen Z, Chen L, Li J, Cheng X, Yang J, Tian C. Cheng features of COVID-19-related liver damage. Am J Respir Crit Care Med 2020; 201(10): 1299-300.
[PMID: 32228035]

[68]  WHO. Coronavirus disease (COVID-19): situation report. 2020; 182. Available from: https://www.afro.who.int/news/who-supports-scientifically-proven-traditional-

[69]   Czapar AE, Steinmetz NF. Plant viruses and bacteriophages for drug delivery in medicine and biotechnology. Curr Opin Chem Biol 2017; 38: 108-16.
[http://dx.doi.org/10.1016/j.cbpa.2017.03.013] [PMID: 28426952]

[70]   Shode FO, Idowu ASK, Uhomoibhi OJ, Sabiu S. Repurposing drugs and identification of inhibitors of integral proteins (Spike protein and Main protease) of SARS-CoV-2. 2021; 1-16.

[71]   World Health Organization. World Health Organization. Coronavirus disease (COVID-19) Situation Report Available from: https://www.google.com/url?sa=t&source=web&rct=j&url=https://www.who.int/docs/defaul-source/coronaviruse/situation-reports/20200805-covid-19-sitrep-2020

[72]   Chen Z, Nakamura T. Statistical evidence for the usefulness of Chinese medicine in the treatment of SARS. Phytother Res 2004; 18(7): 592-4.
[http://dx.doi.org/10.1002/ptr.1485] [PMID: 15305324]

[73]   Lau TF, Leung PC, Wong ELY, *et al.* Using herbal medicine as a means of prevention experience during the SARS crisis. Am J Chin Med 2005; 33(3): 345-56.
[http://dx.doi.org/10.1142/S0192415X05002965] [PMID: 16047553]

[74]   Poon PMK, Wong CK, Fung KP, *et al.* Immunomodulatory effects of a traditional Chinese medicine with potential antiviral activity: a self-control study. Am J Chin Med 2006; 34(1): 13-21.
[http://dx.doi.org/10.1142/S0192415X0600359X] [PMID: 16437735]

[75]   Yang Y, Islam MS, Wang J, Li Y, Chen X. Traditional Chinese medicine in the treatment of patients infected with 2019-new coronavirus (SARS-CoV-2): a review and perspective. Int J Biol Sci 2020; 16(10): 1708-17.
[http://dx.doi.org/10.7150/ijbs.45538] [PMID: 32226288]

[76]   Zafitsara J, Velo NMA. Madagascar's Responses to the COVID-19 Outbreak: Educational Perspectives from March to June 2020. Electronic Research Journal of Social Sciences and Humanities 2020; 2.

[77]   Vaughan A. No evidence 'Madagascar cure' for covid-19 works, says WHO. New scientistcom 2020; 15.

[78]   Jombo GTA, Onoja AM, Adigun KR, Udu C, Ojo BA. As Drugs Assemble to Treat SARS-COV-2, Which Drug will Prove Efficacious: A Search for Suitable Drug or Vaccine to Manage COVID-19 Pandemic. Western Journal of Medical and Biomedical Sciences 2020; 1(1): 1-18.
[http://dx.doi.org/10.46912/wjmbs.2]

[79]   Oxford Analytica. Madagascar's COVID-19'remedy'will prompt alarm. Emerald Expert Briefings 2020.
[http://dx.doi.org/10.1108/OXAN-ES252377]

[80]   Nordling L. Unproven herbal remedy against COVID-19 could fuel drug-resistant malaria, scientists warn 2020. Available from: www.sciencemag.org
[http://dx.doi.org/10.1126/science.abc6665]

[81]   Reihani H, Ghassemi M, Mazer-Amirshahi M, Aljohani B, Pourmand A. Non-evidenced based treatment: An unintended cause of morbidity and mortality related to COVID-19. Ame J of Emerg Med 2021; 39: 221-2.

[82]   Freckelton QI. COVID-19: Fear, quackery, false representations and the law. International J of Law and Psyc 2020; 101611.

[83]   Nghochuzie NN, Olwal CO, Udoakang AJ, Amenga-Etego LNK, Amambua-Ngwa A. Pausing the Fight Against Malaria to Combat the COVID-19 Pandemic in Africa: Is the Future of Malaria Bleak? Front Microbiol 2020; 11: 1476.
[http://dx.doi.org/10.3389/fmicb.2020.01476] [PMID: 32625198]

[84]   Tangwa GB, Munung NS. COVID-19: Africa's relation with epidemics and some imperative ethics considerations of the moment. Res Ethics Rev 2020; 16(3-4): 1-11.

[http://dx.doi.org/10.1177/1747016120937391]

[85]    Iwuoha VC, Ezeibe EN, Ezeibe CC. Glocalization of COVID-19 responses and management of the pandemic in Africa. Local Environ 2020; 25(8): 641-7.
[http://dx.doi.org/10.1080/13549839.2020.1802410]

[86]    Cambaza EM. The African miracle: why COVID-19 seems to spread slowly in Sub-Saharan Africa. Revista Científica da UEM: Série Ciências Biomédicas e Saúde Pública 2020; 1-8.

[87]    Kumar A, Mishra A, Sinha BN. Pharm Rev 2006; 6(1): 73-7.

[88]    Pérez-Sánchez H, den-Haan H, Peña-García J, *et al.* DIA-DB: A Database and Web Server for the Prediction of Diabetes Drugs. J Chem Inf Model 2020; 60(9): 4124-30.
[http://dx.doi.org/10.1021/acs.jcim.0c00107] [PMID: 32692571]

[89]    Ahn K. The worldwide trend of using botanical drugs and strategies for developing global drugs. BMB Rep 2017; 50(3): 111-6.
[http://dx.doi.org/10.5483/BMBRep.2017.50.3.221] [PMID: 27998396]

[90]    Romano JD, Tatonetti NP. Informatics and computational methods in natural product drug discovery: A review and perspectives. Front Genet 2019; 10: 368.
[http://dx.doi.org/10.3389/fgene.2019.00368] [PMID: 31114606]

[91]    Harishchander A. A review on application of bioinformatics in medicinal plant research. Bioinforma Proteomics Open Access J 2017; 1(1): 000104.

[92]    Mohd A, Jyoti DA. Current trends in drug discovery: target identification to clinical development of the drug. Int Res J Pharm 2012; 3(4): 23-37.

[93]    Littleton J. The future of plant drug discovery. Expert Opin Drug Discov 2007; 2(5): 673-83.
[http://dx.doi.org/10.1517/17460441.2.5.673] [PMID: 23488957]

[94]    Dali Y, Abbasi SM, Khan SAF, *et al.* Computational drug design and exploration of potent phytochemicals against cancer through in silico approaches. Biom Lett 2019; 5(1): 21-6.

[95]    Prada-Gracia D, Huerta-Yépez S, Moreno-Vargas LM. Application of computational methods for anticancer drug discovery, design, and optimization. Bol Méd Hosp Infant México 2016; 73(6): 411-23.
[http://dx.doi.org/10.1016/j.bmhimx.2016.10.006] [PMID: 29421286]

[96]    Li Y, Kang C. Solution NMR spectroscopy in target-based drug discovery. Molecules 2017; 22(9): 1399.
[http://dx.doi.org/10.3390/molecules22091399] [PMID: 28832542]

[97]    Sarsaiya S, Shi J, Chen J. A comprehensive review on fungal endophytes and its dynamics on Orchidaceae plants: current research, challenges, and future possibilities. Bioengineered 2019; 10(1): 316-34.
[http://dx.doi.org/10.1080/21655979.2019.1644854] [PMID: 31347943]

[98]    Ajani EO, Saheed S, Odufuwa KT, Ibrahim TB, Salau BA. Evaluation of Lens Aldose Reductase Inhibitory and Free Radical Scavenging Potential of Fractions of Lonchocarpus cyanescens Potential for Cataract Remediation. Pharmacogn J 2017; 9(1): 62-9.
[http://dx.doi.org/10.5530/pj.2017.1.12]

[99]    Bhardwaj S, Verma R, Gupta J. Challenges and future prospects of herbal medicine. International Research in Medical and Health Science 2018; 1(1): 12-5.
[http://dx.doi.org/10.36437/irmhs.2018.1.1.D]

[100]   Parveen A, Parveen B, Parveen R, Ahmad S. Challenges and guidelines for clinical trial of herbal drugs. J Pharm Bioallied Sci 2015; 7(4): 329-33.
[http://dx.doi.org/10.4103/0975-7406.168035] [PMID: 26681895]

[101]   Patwardhan B. Ayurvedic drugs in case: Claims, evidence, regulations and ethics. J Ayurveda Integr Med 2016; 7(3): 135-7.

[http://dx.doi.org/10.1016/j.jaim.2016.08.005] [PMID: 27640330]

[102]   Hooda R, Pandita D, Kumari P, Lather V. Regulatory and Quality Aspects of Herbal Drugs. Appl Clin Res Clin Trials Regul Aff 2017; 4(2): 107-13.
[http://dx.doi.org/10.2174/2213476X04666170619092022]

[103]   Giri RP, Gangawane AK, Giri SG. Regulation on herbal product used as medicine around the world: a review. Regulation 2018; 5: 10.

[104]   Bhat BB, Udupa N, Sreedhar D. Herbal Products Regulations in a few countries-A brief Overview. Curr Drug Discov Technol 2019; 16(4): 368-71.
[http://dx.doi.org/10.2174/1570163815666181105091254] [PMID: 30394210]

[105]   Onyambu MO, Gikonyo NK, Nyambaka HN, Thoithi GN. A review of trends in herbal drugs standardization, regulation and integration to the national healthcare systems in Kenya and the globe. International Journal of Pharmacognosy and Chinese Medicine 2019; 3(3): 13.

[106]   Kanwal H, Sherazi BA. Herbal medicine: Trend of practice, perspective, and limitations in Pakistan. Asian Pac J Health Sci 2017; 4(4): 6-8.
[http://dx.doi.org/10.21276/apjhs.2017.4.4.2]

[107]   US Food and Drug Administratione (Accessed, 02102020). 1997. Available from: http://www. fda. gov/cder/guidance/clin3

[108]   Archdeacon P, Grandinetti C, Vega JM, Balderson D, Kramer JM. Optimizing expedited safety reporting for drugs and biologics subject to an investigational new drug application. Ther Innov Regul Sci 2014; 48(2): 200-7.
[http://dx.doi.org/10.1177/2168479013509382] [PMID: 30227498]

[109]   Zeng L, Tang G, Wang J, *et al.* Safety and efficacy of herbal medicine for acute intracerebral hemorrhage (CRRICH): a multicentre randomised controlled trial. BMJ Open 2019; 9(5): e024932.
[http://dx.doi.org/10.1136/bmjopen-2018-024932] [PMID: 31076468]

[110]   Lee BC, Choi EJ, Lee BC, Choi EJ. The safety and efficacy of herbal medicine for 107 psoriasis patients: a retrospective chart review. Journal of Korean Medicine 2016; 37(1): 34-40.
[http://dx.doi.org/10.13048/jkm.16004]

[111]   Dhiman A, Sharma K, Sharma A, Sindhu P. A review on the status of quality control and standardization of herbal drugs in India. Drug Development & Therapeutics 2016; 7: 2.
[http://dx.doi.org/10.4103/2394-6555.191165]

[112]   Shulammithi R, Sharanya M, Tejaswini R, Kiranmai M. Standardization and quality evaluation of herbal drugs. J Pharm Biomed Sci 2016; 11(5): 89-100.

[113]   Chakraborty P. Herbal genomics as tools for dissecting new metabolic pathways of unexplored medicinal plants and drug discovery. Biochim Open 2018; 6(6): 9-16.
[http://dx.doi.org/10.1016/j.biopen.2017.12.003] [PMID: 29892557]

[114]   Dutraa RC, Campos MM, Adair RS. Santos d, João B. Calixto. Medicinal plants in Brazil: Pharmacological studies, drug discovery, challenges and perspectives. Pharmacol Res 2016; 112: 4-29.
[http://dx.doi.org/10.1016/j.phrs.2016.01.021]

[115]   Kyeremeh K, Flint A, Jaspars M, *et al.* Making North–South Collaborations Work: Facilitating Natural Product Drug Discovery in Africa.Africa and the Sustainable Development Goals. Cham: Springer 2020; pp. 257-66.
[http://dx.doi.org/10.1007/978-3-030-14857-7_24]

[116]   Blicharska N, Seidel V. Chemical diversity and biological activity of African propolis.Progress in the Chemistry of Organic Natural Products. 2019; pp. (109): 415-50.
[http://dx.doi.org/10.1007/978-3-030-12858-6_3]

[117]   Simoben CV, Ntie-Kang F, Akone SH, Sippl W. Compounds from African medicinal plants with activities against selected parasitic diseases: schistosomiasis, trypanosomiasis and leishmaniasis. Nat

Prod Bioprospect 2018; 8(3): 151-69.
[http://dx.doi.org/10.1007/s13659-018-0165-y] [PMID: 29744736]

[118] Boniface PK, Elizabeth FI. Flavonoid-derived Privileged Scaffolds in anti-Trypanosoma brucei Drug Discovery. Curr Drug Targets 2019; 20(12): 1295-314.
[http://dx.doi.org/10.2174/1389450120666190618114857] [PMID: 31215385]

[119] Kushwaha PP, Kumar A, Maurya S, Singh AK, Sharma AK, Kumar S. Bulbine frutescens phytochemicals as a promising anti-cancer drug discovery source: A computational study.Phytochemistry: An in-silico and in-vitro Update. Singapore: Springer 2019; pp. 491-510.
[http://dx.doi.org/10.1007/978-981-13-6920-9_26]

[120] Tiwari AK, Tiwari BS. Cyanotherapeutics: an emerging field for future drug discovery. Applied Phycol 2020; 1(1): 1-14.
[http://dx.doi.org/10.1080/26388081.2020.1744480]

[121] Prabu SL. Drug Discovery: Current State and Future Prospects. Computer Applications in Drug Discovery and Development. IGI Global 2019; pp. 1-46.

# CHAPTER 3

# Therapeutic Properties of Bioactive Secondary Metabolites in Essential Oil Crops

**Fikisiwe C. Gebashe[1], Adeyemi O. Aremu[2,3] and Stephen O. Amoo[1,2,4,\*]**

[1] *Agricultural Research Council – Vegetables, Industrial and Medicinal Plants, Pretoria, Private Bag X293, Pretoria 0001, South Africa*

[2] *Indigenous Knowledge Systems (IKS) Centre, Faculty of Natural and Agricultural Sciences, North-West University, Private Bag X2046, Mmabatho 2790, South Africa*

[3] *School of Life Sciences, University of KwaZulu-Natal Pietermaritzburg, Private Bag X01, Scottsville 3209, South Africa*

[4] *Department of Botany and Plant Biotechnology, Faculty of Science, University of Johannesburg, P.O. Box 524, Auckland Park 2006, South Africa*

**Abstract:** Medicinal herbs and their essential oils (EOs) are of commercial and industrial importance with diverse uses as forage and fiber crops, in food, cosmetics, perfumery and chemical industries, and in traditional medicine due to their phytochemical constituents and bioactivities. This chapter was aimed at documenting the therapeutic properties of major secondary metabolites in EOs extracted from six selected economically important medicinal herbs (*Achillea millefolium* L., *Melissa officinalis* L., *Origanum majorana* L., *Pelargonium graveolens* L'Hér. *Rosmarinus officinalis* L. and *Thymus vulgaris* L.). Forty-five compounds (mainly monoterpenes) were recorded as major compounds of the six medicinal herbs. The compounds possess varying biological activities, which include antimicrobial, anti-inflammatory, antioxidant and cytotoxicity properties. Other activities reported were antinociceptive, neuroprotective effects, acetylcholinesterase inhibition, anti-ulcerogenic, DNA protection, glutathione S-transferase activity, chemoprotective, anti-depressant and sedative effects. The compounds showed potential to be used as alternative agents as drugs, cosmetic ingredients and food additives. Though some scientific evidence has confirmed the use of these herbs in various industries, much work still needs to be done to comprehend the therapeutic application of their EOs and phytoconstituents to benefit from their full potential.

**Keywords:** Antimicrobial, Antioxidant, Cytotoxicity, Medicinal herbs, Phytochemicals.

---

\* **Corresponding author Stephen O. Amoo:** Agricultural Research Council – Vegetables, Industrial and Medicinal Plants, Pretoria, Private Bag X293, Pretoria 0001, South Africa, Indigenous Knowledge Systems (IKS) Centre, Faculty of Natural and Agricultural Sciences, North-West University, Private Bag X2046, Mmabatho 2790, South Africa and Department of Botany and Plant Biotechnology, Faculty of Science, University of Johannesburg, P.O. Box 524, Auckland Park 2006, South Africa; E-mail: AmooS@arc.agric.za

Saheed Sabiu (Ed)

# 1. INTRODUCTION

Plants are sources of secondary metabolites with curative properties. These secondary metabolites are distributed within limited taxonomic groups and are produced by plants in their interaction with the environment for adaptation and defense [1]. They are generally responsible for specific odours, tastes, and colours in plants [2], and are sources of food additives, flavors and industrially important pharmaceuticals [3]. Most of these compounds have imperative adaptive protection against herbivores, pests and microbial infections, while some serve as attractants for pollinators and seed-dispersing animals, and as allelopathic agents [4, 5]. On the other hand, primary metabolites (such as acyl lipids, nucleotides, amino acids, and organic acids) are produced by all plants and are essential for basic life functions such as cell division and growth, respiration, and reproduction [1, 6]. Secondary metabolites are classified according to their biosynthesis pathway into phenolics and phenylpropanoids, terpenes and steroids, and alkaloids [7]. The most common pathways for the production of secondary metabolites include pentose (glycosides); shikimic acid (phenols, tannins, aromatic alkaloids); acetate – malonate (phenols, alkaloids) and mevalonic acid (terpenes, steroids, alkaloids) [8].

For centuries, secondary metabolites have been used in traditional medicine for their therapeutic properties to relieve human ailments, including chronic diseases [6]. The production of secondary metabolites in plants is greatly influenced by environmental factors such as temperature, humidity, light intensity, moisture, and mineral nutrient availability [9] as well as biotic factors. Naturally, their production is very low and dependent on the physiological and development stage of the plant [10]. Currently, there are numerous biotechnology strategies (*e.g.* plant cell, tissue and organ cultures) that have been developed to increase the production of secondary metabolites *in vitro* to meet their commercial demand [6, 10]. Secondary metabolites demonstrate numerous biological activities that stimulate their use in pharmaceutical, cosmetics, aromatherapy and nutraceutical industries. The secondary metabolites in plant extracts and essential oils (EOs) are responsible for diverse biological properties [11], such as antidepressant [12], antimicrobial [13 - 18], anti-inflammatory [19], antimutagenic [20], chemoprotectant [21, 22], antioxidant [16, 23], DNA damage protection [23] and antiviral activities [24, 25].

This chapter was aimed at providing an appraisal of the therapeutic properties of major secondary metabolites in EOs extracted from six selected economically important medicinal herbs (*Achillea millefolium* L., *Melissa officinalis* L., *Origanum majorana* L., *Pelargonium graveolens* L'Hér., *Rosmarinus officinalis*

L. and *Thymus vulgaris* L.) as a case study. The majority of the selected herbs belong to the Lamiaceae family and are of great economic and industrial importance. They are widely used in the food industry for food flavoring or as seasoning agents and are popular as perfume ingredients in cosmetics and household cleaning products [26]. In addition, they are used in traditional medicine to treat many ailments, including asthma, indigestion, headache, rheumatism [22], as tonic, antispasmodic, carminative, diaphoretic, surgical dressing for wounds, sedative-hypnotic strengthening the memory, relief of stress-induced headache [27], against colds, and in functional disorders of the circulation [28].

## 2. SECONDARY METABOLITES AND THEIR ROLE IN PLANTS

Secondary metabolites in plants are the active components responsible for their therapeutic properties [29]. These compounds are produced for diverse purposes, such as protection against biotic and abiotic factors [30], to counteract or in response to environmental stimuli, and to tolerate certain stress conditions [31]. Abiotic stress triggers the generation of reactive oxygen species (ROS), which alter plant metabolic processes. Consequently, excessive ROS in plants can damage plant cells through the oxidation of biological components such as nucleic acids, proteins, and lipids [32]. Although plants possess antioxidant defense capacity and repair mechanisms, oxidative damage results from the imbalance between this capacity and the rate of ROS accumulation [33].

Plants develop antioxidant defense system and produce compounds such as brassinosteroids to scavenge the excessive accumulation of harmful ROS [32]. The intrinsic antioxidant defense system consists of many enzymatic, non-enzymatic, lipophilic and hydrophilic molecules, which allow for the adaptation of plants to different environments, maintain homeostasis and detoxify ROS. The secondary metabolites sustain plants through their stress regulatory and growth-promoting activity by directly quenching or removing ROS, or by indirectly influencing hormone-mediated signaling to up-regulate defense genes. Even though there will always be a standard level of secondary metabolites in a plant produced during biosynthesis, some plant parts may contain higher concentrations of secondary metabolites at different stages of plant growth.

Secondary metabolites serve as defense compounds against bacteria, fungi, viruses, herbivores and other competing plants [34]. Additionally, some plants can use secondary metabolites for communicating with other plants by sending signals, and between plants and symbiotic microorganisms [35]. They also serve as an attractant to pollinators and seed dispersal animals; and for these reasons, they have been explored for biopharmaceutical purposes [36]. Many secondary metabolites have been applied commercially in different industries and are known for various biological activities.

## 3. MAJOR BIOACTIVE SECONDARY METABOLITES FROM ESSENTIAL OILS OF SELECTED MEDICINAL HERBS

Forty-five compounds, including their isomers (mainly monoterpenes) were recorded as major compounds of the six selected medicinal herbs (Table 1; Fig. 1). The mass percentages of these major compounds in EOs extracted mainly from the leaves or aerial parts ranged from 1.52 - 49.10%. The concentrations of these compounds may however, be influenced by plant age, agronomic practice, environmental factors, genotype differences, postharvest management practice and oil extraction process. Linalool, for example, is a common compound present in three (*Origanum majorana*, *Pelargonium graveolens* and *Rosmarinus officinalis*) of the selected medicinal herbs. Linalool is a terpene alcohol, which is used as an ingredient in the perfumery industry and in household products. Besides their application in the food industry as flavourings, cosmetics additives (perfume industry) and cleaning detergents [37], EOs and their constituent compounds have low toxicity, are biologically active and cost effective [38, 39] with proven pharmacological properties.

**Table 1. Major secondary metabolites of essential oils (EOs) from six selected herbal plants.**

| Main Component of EOs | Mass Percentage (%) | Plant Source | Plant Part | References |
|---|---|---|---|---|
| Borneol | 16.35 | *Achillea millefolium* L. | Aerial parts | [40] |
| Bornyl acetate | 1.52–2.94 | *Origanum majorana* L. | Aerial parts | [41] |
| Caryophyllene | 4.99, 3.2 | *Origanum majorana* L., *Thymus vulgaris* L. | Leaves | [42, 43] |
| Caryophyllene oxide | 12.6–24.4, 1.7–7.3 | *Melissa officinalis* L., *Thymus vulgaris* L. | Leaves, Aerial parts | [28, 44] |
| Carvacrol | 10.14, 5.7–7.3, 45.5 | *Achillea millefolium* L., *Thymus vulgaris* L. | Aerial parts, Leaves | [40, 43, 44] |
| Camphene | 5.8, 11.52, 6.00 | *Rosmarinus officinalis* | Aerial parts, Leaves | [45-47] |
| Camphor | 13.2-39.7, 14.26, 17.1 | *Rosmarinus officinalis* | Aerial parts, Leaves | [46-48] |
| Citral | 33 | *Melissa officinalis* L. | Leaves | [27] |
| Citronellal | 39, 6.30 | *Melissa officinalis* L. | Leaves | [27, 49] |
| Citronellol | 30.2 | *Pelargonium graveolens* L'Hér. | Aerial parts | [50] |

*(Table 1) cont.....*

| Citronellyl formate | 9.3, 7.39 | *Pelargonium graveolens* L'Hér. | Aerial parts | [50, 51] |
|---|---|---|---|---|
| cis-Chrysanthenol | 27.3 | *Achillea millefolium* L. | Aerial parts | [52] |
| cis-Sabinene hydrate | 19.9–29.27, 17.5, | *Origanum majorana* L. | Aerial parts | [41, 53] |
| Endo-Borneol | 14.3 | *Thymus vulgaris* L. | Leaves | [43] |
| Eucalyptol (1,8-cineole) | 13.3-26.4, 27.23, 38.5 | *Rosmarinus officinalis* | Aerial parts, Leaves | [46-48] |
| Geranial | 2, 44.20 | *Melissa officinalis* L. | Leaves | [27, 49] |
| Geraniol | 7.6 | *Pelargonium graveolens* L'Hér. | Aerial parts | [50, 51] |
| Geranyl formate | 6.47 | *Pelargonium graveolens* L'Hér. | Leaves | [51] |
| Guai-6,9-diene | 5.4 | *Pelargonium graveolens* L'Hér. | Aerial parts | [50] |
| Limonene | 14.53, 6.23 | *Achillea millefolium* L., *Rosmarinus officinalis* | Aerial parts, Leaves | [40, 47] |
| Linalool | 12, 1.05–1.39, 5.70 | *Origanum majorana* L., *Pelargonium graveolens* L'Hér., *Rosmarinus officinalis* | Aerial parts, Leaves | [41, 45, 47, 51] |
| Neral | 30.20 | *Melissa officinalis* L. | Leaves | [49] |
| Sabinene | 6.9–17.4 | *Melissa officinalis* L. | Leaves | [28] |
| Sabinene hydrate | 37 | *Origanum majorana* L. | Leaves | [42] |
| Selin-11-en-4α-ol | 24.0 | *Achillea millefolium,* | Aerial parts | [52] |
| Spathulenol | 5.80 | *Origanum majorana* L. | Leaves | [42] |
| Terpinen-4-ol | 29.13–32.57, 30, 23.2, 12.81 | *Origanum majorana* L. | Aerial parts, Leaves | [41, 42, 45, 53] |
| Terpinene acetate | 16.20 | *Origanum majorana* L. | Leaves | [42] |
| Thymol | 26.47, 49.10, 46.2–67.5 | *Achillea millefolium* L., *Thymus vulgaris* L. | Aerial parts | [40, 44, 54] |
| Trans-sabinene hydrate | 3.5–11.61, 4.0, 7.41 | *Origanum majorana* L. | Aerial parts | [41, 42, 53] |
| Viridiflorol | 13.7 | *Achillea millefolium* L. | Aerial parts | [52] |
| 10-epi-γ-eudesmol | 10.0-15.6 | *Achillea millefolium* L. | Aerial parts | [52] |
| (E)-caryophyllene | 7.2–15.3 | *Melissa officinalis* L. | Leaves | [28] |
| α-pinene | 10.12, 5.9, 17.1-22.3, 19.43, 12.3 | *Achillea millefolium* L., *Rosmarinus officinalis* | Aerial parts | [40, 45-48] |
| α-Terpinene | 4.4, 3.2, 4.7 | *Origanum majorana* L. | Leaves | [45, 53] |

*(Table 1) cont.....*

| α-Terpineol | 5.6, 8.10, 22.9 | *Origanum majorana* L., *Thymus vulgaris* L. | Leaves | [42, 43, 53] |
|---|---|---|---|---|
| α-Terpinolene | 1.8 | *Origanum majorana* L. | Leaves | [45] |
| β-Citronellol | 16.24 | *Pelargonium graveolens* L'Hér. | Leaves | [51] |
| β-Caryophyllene | 1.8 | *Origanum majorana* L. | Aerial parts | [45] |
| β-Pinene | 6.4–18.2, 2.2, 6.71 | *Melissa officinalis* L., *Rosmarinus officinalis* | Leaves | [28, 45, 46] |
| l-Menthone | 4.13 | *Pelargonium graveolens* L'Hér. | Leaves | [51] |
| *p*-Cymene | 9, 20.01 | *Thymus vulgaris* L. | Aerial parts | [53, 54] |
| *p*-Cymol | 9.8 | *Origanum majorana* L. | Leaves | [45] |
| δ-Selinene | 8.69 | *Pelargonium graveolens* L'Hér. | Leaves | [51] |
| γ-Terpinene | 2.11–8.20, 10.5, 14 | *Origanum majorana* L. | Aerial parts | [41, 53] |

# 4. PHARMACOLOGICAL PROPERTIES OF ESSENTIAL OILS MAJOR COMPOUNDS

## 4.1. Antimicrobial Activity

Bacterial and fungal strains cause several human disease conditions, including meningitis, pneumonia, sexually transmitted diseases, urinary tract infections, food poisoning, upper respiratory tract infections, tuberculosis, and yeast infections [55, 56]. Conventional medicines are used to treat microbial infections; however, their toxicity coupled with increasing antimicrobial drug resistance has led to the search for effective alternative medicines [57]. Increasing drug resistance heightens the disease burden on the health care systems [58]. Drug resistance can be directed to a particular antibiotic or family of antibiotics and the resistant traits can be transferred between bacteria by exchanging genetic materials such as transposons, bacteriophages and plasmids [58]. Some antimicrobial resistance to human infections has been linked to foodborne pathogens of animal origin [59]. Common foodborne pathogens include some species from the genera *Campylobacter*, *Salmonella*, *Listeria*, *Escherichia*, *Yersinia*, and *Vibrio*. Some natural compounds have been proven to be effective antimicrobial agents with less toxicity, able to counteract some drug-resistant microbes [60, 61].

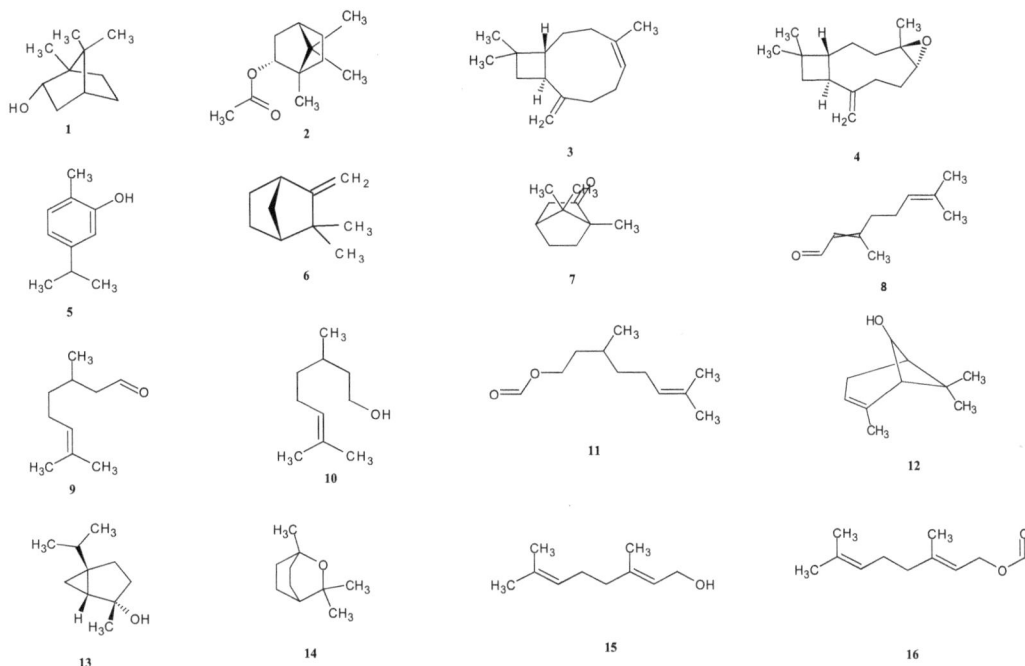

**Fig. (1).** Structural representation of some major compounds from essential oils (EOs) of selected medicinal herbs. 1 Borneol, 2 Bornyl acetate, 3 Caryophyllene, 4 Caryophyllene oxide, 5 Carvacrol, 6 Camphene, 7 Camphor, 8 Citral, 9 Citronellal, 10 Citronellol, 11 Citronellyl formate, 12 cis-Chrysanthenol, 13 cis-Sabinene hydrate, 14 Eucalyptol (1,8-cineole), 15 Geraniol, 16 Geranyl formate.

Compounds from EOs have been screened for antimicrobial activity using several methods (Tables **2** and **3**). Antimicrobial activity is one of the most common properties evaluated due to the availability of cost effective method, which allows for several compounds to be tested in a short time [62, 63]. For compounds to be regarded as active, their activities (minimum inhibitory concentration, MIC) should be ≤16 µg/mL, which is far less than the required activity of EOs (MIC ≤ 1000 µg/mL) and plant extracts (MIC ≤ 160 µg/mL) [64]. About 70% of the major compounds from the six selected medicinal herbs showed moderate antibacterial activity (MIC ≤ 1000 µg/mL) and did not meet the required criteria proposed for pure compounds to be regarded as active. Borneol, eucalyptol and thymol were amongst the compounds, which showed moderate activity against bacterial strains. These compounds were more effective against Gram-positive bacteria compared to Gram-negative bacteria. The frequently used methods to evaluate antimicrobial activities were broth micro-dilution and disc diffusion assay. Other methods such as well and agar diffusion, cytofluorometric and bioluminescent methods have also been utilised by researchers [65]. Broth micro-dilution is the most recommended method due to its simplicity, low cost, accuracy and efficiency [65, 66]. Evaluating compounds for their antimicrobial activities can result in the discovery of new effective antimicrobial agents to treat new microbial infections and resistant microbial strains.

**Table 2. Antibacterial activity of some major essential oil secondary metabolites.**

| Major Compound | Method | Test Microorganism | Antibacterial Effect* | Positive Control Response | Positive Control | Key Findings | Reference |
|---|---|---|---|---|---|---|---|
| Borneol | Microdilution | *Escherichia coli* | 250 µg/mL | 62.5 µg/mL | Chloramphenicol | Activity ranged from 125-250 µL/mL | [67] |
| | | *Staphylococcus aureus,* | 125 µg/mL | 7.81 µg/mL | | | |
| | | *Pseudomonas aeruginosa* | 125 µg/mL | 250 µg/mL | | | |
| | | *Enterobacter aerogenes,* | 125 µg/mL | 125 µg/mL | | | |
| | | *Proteus vulgaris* | 125 µg/mL | 31.25 µg/mL | | | |
| | | *Salmonella typhimurium* | 125 µg/mL | 62.5 µg/mL | | | |
| | Disc diffusion | *Staphylococcus aureus* | 26.1 mm | 28.4 mm | Chloramphenicol | Varying degree of activity against all of the tested microorganisms | [68] |
| | | *Bacillus subtilis* | 24.3 mm | 25.5 mm | | | |
| | | *Pseudomonas aeruginosa* | 22.1 mm | 21.5 mm | | | |
| | | *Escherichia coli* | 26.3 mm | 28.7 mm | | | |
| | Broth dilution | *Staphylococcus aureus* | 0.97 mg/mL | 10.08 µg/mL | | | |
| | | *Bacillus subtilis* | 1.53 mg/mL | 15.06 µg/mL | | | |
| | | *Pseudomonas aeruginosa* | 1.75 mg/mL | 100 µg/mL | | | |
| | | *Escherichia coli* | 1.05 mg/mL | 10.3 µg/mL | | | |
| | Disc diffusion | *Staphylococcus aureus* | 6 mm | - | Chloramphenicol | Weak activity | [69] |
| | | *Escherichia coli* | 7 mm | 22 mm | | | |
| | - | *Gardnerella vaginalis* | 0.125% (v/v) | 0.06% (v/v) | Clotrimazole | Active against *Gardnerella vaginalis* | [70] |
| Bornyl acetate | Broth micro-dilution | *Campylobacter jejuni* | 0.10% | 0.00006% | Gentamycin | Weak activity against most of the tested bacterial strains | [71] |
| | | *Escherichia coli* | >0.67% | 0.00012% | | | |
| | | *Salmonella enterica* | >0.67% | 0.00006% | | | |
| | | MR 2388 *Listeria monocytogenes* | >0.67% | 0.016% | Chloramphenicol | | |
| | | MR 2199 *Listeria monocytogenes* | >0.67% | 0.020% | | | |
| Camphor | Micro-broth dilution | *Bacillus cereus* | 312 µg/mL | 1.22 µg/mL | Gentamicin sulfate | Significantly inhibit growth rate *against B. cereus* | [72] |
| | | *Staphylococcus aureus* | 1250 µg/mL | 0.61 µg/mL | | | |
| | | *Escherichia coli* | 625 µg/mL | 1.22 µg/mL | | | |
| | | *Pseudomonas aeruginosa* | 625 µg/mL | 2.44 µg/mL | | | |

(Table 2) cont.....

| Compound | Method | Organism | Value | CPN | LDM | TCH | Standard value | Standard drug | Outcome | Ref |
|---|---|---|---|---|---|---|---|---|---|---|
| Carvacrol | Disc diffusion | *Escherichia coli* | 31.5 mm | | | | 28.4 mm | Chloramphenicol | -Carvacrol standard and a fraction with highest carvacrol was most effective | [68] |
| | | *Bacillus subtilis* | 30.5 mm | | | | 25.5 mm | | | |
| | | *Pseudomonas aeruginosa* | 24.4 mm | | | | 21.5 mm | | | |
| | | *Staphylococcus aureus* | 31.4 mm | | | | 28.7 mm | | | |
| | Broth dilution | *Escherichia coli* | 0.52 mg/mL | | | | 10.08 µg/mL | | | |
| | | *Bacillus subtilis* | 0.75 mg/mL | | | | 15.06 µg/mL | | | |
| | | *Pseudomonas aeruginosa* | 1.53 mg/mL | | | | 100 µg/mL | | | |
| | | *Staphylococcus aureus* | 0.75 mg/mL | | | | 10.3 µg/mL | | | |
| | Broth micro-dilution | *Campylobacter jejuni* | 0.011% | | | | 0.00006% | Gentamycin | Active against all tested bacterial strains | [71] |
| | | *Escherichia coli* | 0.057% | | | | 0.00012% | | | |
| | | *Salmonella enterica* | 0.054% | | | | 0.00006% | | | |
| | | MR 2388 *Listeria monocytogenes* | 0.086% | | | | 0.016% | Chloramphenicol | | |
| | | MR 2199 *Listeria monocytogenes* | 0.083% | | | | 0.020% | | | |
| Citronellol | Disc diffusion | *Staphylococcus aureus* | 25 mm | 35 mm | 27 mm | 15 mm | | | | |
| | | *Enterococcus faecalis* | 18 mm | 33 mm | 27 mm | 22 mm | | | | |
| | | *Escherichia coli* | na | 22 mm | 11 mm | 11 mm | | | | |
| | | *Proteus vulgaris* | 8 mm | 25 mm | 23 mm | 13 mm | | | | |
| | | *Pseudomonas aeruginosa* | na | 32 mm | na | 15 mm | | | | |
| | | *Salmonella* sp. | 7 mm | 10 mm | 8 mm | 10 mm | | | | |
| | | *Klebsiella pneumoniae* | na | 25 mm | na | 20 mm | | | | |
| Eucalyptol (1,8-cineole) | Broth micro-dilution | *Staphylococcus aureus* | 600 ppm | 600 ppm | 600 ppm | 600 ppm | | Ciproxin (CPN), Lidaprim (LDM), Tetracycline hydrochloride (TCH) | Effective against all tested microorganisms | [37] |
| | | *Enterococcus faecalis.* | 60 ppm | 600 ppm | 600 ppm | 600 ppm | | | | |
| | | *Escherichia coli* | na | 600 ppm | 60 ppm | 600 ppm | | | | |
| | | *Proteus vulgaris* | 600 ppm | 600 ppm | 600 ppm | 600 ppm | | | | |
| | | *Pseudomonas aeruginosa* | na | 600 ppm | na | 600 ppm | | | | |
| | | *Salmonella* sp. | 600 ppm | 600 ppm | 60 ppm | 600 ppm | | | | |
| | | *Klebsiella pneumoniae* | na | 600 ppm | na | 600 ppm | | | | |
| | - | *Gardnerella vaginalis* | 0.125% (v/v) | | | | 0.06% (v/v) | Clotrimazole | Inhibited microbial growths | [70] |
| | Broth micro-dilution | *Bacillus cereus* | 312 µg/mL | | | | 1.22 µg/mL | Gentamicin sulfate | Exhibited good activity against *B. cereus* | [72] |
| | | *Staphylococcus aureus* | 1250 µg/mL | | | | 0.61 µg/mL | | | |
| | | *Escherichia coli* | 625 µg/mL | | | | 1.22 µg/mL | | | |
| | | *Pseudomonas aeruginosa* | 625 µg/mL | | | | 2.44 µg/mL | | | |

*(Table 2) cont.....*

| | | | | | | | |
|---|---|---|---|---|---|---|---|
| Geranial (Citral) | Disc diffusion | *Bacillus subtilis* | 31 mm | 14 mm | Ampicillin | Showed good to moderate activity | [73] |
| | | *Staphylococcus epidermidis* | 24 mm | 19 mm | | | |
| | | *Staphylococcus aureus* | 30 mm | 13 mm | | | |
| | | *Enterococcus faecalis* | 19 mm | 11 mm | | | |
| | | *Klebsiella pneumoniae* | 14 mm | na | | | |
| | | *Escherichia coli* | 22 mm | 12 mm | | | |
| | Broth micro-dilution | *Bacillus subtilis* | 1.8 mg/mL | nt | Ampicillin | Showed weak activity | |
| | | *Staphylococcus epidermidis* | 3.6 mg/mL | nt | | | |
| | | *Staphylococcus aureus* | 1.8 mg/mL | nt | | | |
| | | *Enterococcus faecalis* | 7.2 mg/mL | nt | | | |
| | | *Klebsiella pneumoniae* | 14.2 mg/mL | nt | | | |
| | | *Escherichia coli* | 7.2 mg/mL | nt | | | |
| | Broth micro-dilution | *Campylobacter jejuni* | 0.21% | 0.00006% | Gentamycin | Active against all tested bacterial strains | [71] |
| | | *Escherichia coli* | 0.22% | 0.00012% | | | |
| | | *Salmonella enterica* | 0.023% | 0.00006% | | | |
| | | MR 2388 *Listeria monocytogenes* | 0.20% | 0.016% | Chloramphenicol | | |
| | | MR 2199 *Listeria monocytogenes* | 0.099% | 0.020% | | | |

*(Table 2) cont.....*

| | | | | | | | |
|---|---|---|---|---|---|---|---|
| Geraniol | Disc diffusion | *Bacillus subtilis* | 16 mm | 14 mm | | Ampicillin | Showed good activity against most of the bacterial strains, comparable with the ampicillin | [73] |
| | | *Staphylococcus epidermidis* | 22 mm | 19 mm | | | | |
| | | *Staphylococcus aureus* | 14 mm | 13 mm | | | | |
| | | *Enterococcus faecalis* | 11 mm | 11 mm | | | | |
| | | *Klebsiella pneumoniae* | na | na | | | | |
| | | *Escherichia coli* | 14 mm | 12 mm | | | | |
| | Broth micro-dilution | *Bacillus subtilis* | 7.2 mg/mL | nt | | Ampicillin | Showed weak activity | |
| | | *Staphylococcus epidermidis* | 3.6 mg/mL | nt | | | | |
| | | *Staphylococcus aureus* | 14.4 mg/mL | nt | | | | |
| | | *Enterococcus faecalis* | 14.4 mg/mL | nt | | | | |
| | | *Klebsiella pneumoniae* | nt | nt | | | | |
| | | *Escherichia coli* | 14.4 mg/mL | nt | | | | |

| | | | | **Imipenem** | **Chlorhexidine** | | | |
|---|---|---|---|---|---|---|---|---|
| | Agar-diffusion | *Staphylococcus aureus* | 19 mm | 59 mm | 25 mm | Imipenem and Chlorhexidine | Compound showed moderate activity to most tested microorganisms. | [74] |
| | | *Staphylococcus epidermidis* | 19 mm | 52 mm | 18 mm | | | |
| | | *Enterococcus faecalis* | 11 mm | 35 mm | 14 mm | | | |
| | | *Streptococcus pyogenes* | 10 mm | 38 mm | 17 mm | | | |
| | | *Escherichia coli* | 10 mm | 32 mm | 17 mm | | | |
| | | *Pseudomonas aeruginosa* | 15 mm | 19 mm | 18 mm | | | |
| | Broth micro-dilution | *Staphylococcus aureus* | 0.25 | nt | | - | Showed moderate activity against *S. aureus* | |
| | | *Escherichia coli* | >8 | nt | | | | |
| | Broth micro-dilution | *Campylobacter jejuni* | 0.10% | 0.00006% | | Gentamycin | Active against all tested bacterial strains | [71] |
| | | *Escherichia coli* | 0.15% | 0.00012% | | | | |
| | | *Salmonella enterica* | 0.15% | 0.00006% | | | | |
| | | MR 2388 *Listeria monocytogenes* | 0.51% | 0.016% | | Chloramphenicol | | |
| | | MR 2199 *Listeria monocytogenes* | 0.28% | 0.020% | | | | |
| | Disc diffusion | *Escherichia coli* | 11.78 mm | nt | | - | Potent antimicrobial activity | [75] |
| | | *Listeria innocua* | 13.83 mm | nt | | | | |
| | | *Pseudomonas lundensis* | 12.50 mm | nt | | | | |

*(Table 2) cont.....*

| | | | | CPN | LDM | TCH | | | |
|---|---|---|---|---|---|---|---|---|---|
| Geranyl formate | Disc diffusion | *Staphylococcus aureus* | 10 mm | 35 mm | 27 mm | 15 mm | | | |
| | | *Enterococcus faecalis.* | 9 mm | 33 mm | 27 mm | 22 mm | | | |
| | | *Escherichia coli* | 7 mm | 22 mm | 11 mm | 11 mm | | | |
| | | *Proteus vulgaris* | 8 mm | 25 mm | 23 mm | 13 mm | | | |
| | | *Pseudomonas aeruginosa* | 8 mm | 32 mm | nt | 15 mm | | | |
| | | *Salmonella* sp. | 7 mm | 10 mm | 8mm | 10 mm | | | |
| | | *Klebsiella pneumoniae* | 7 mm | 25 mm | nt | 20 mm | | | |
| | Broth micro-dilution | *Staphylococcus aureus* | 600 ppm | 600 ppm | 600 ppm | 600 ppm | Ciproxin (CPN), Lidaprim (LDM), Tetracycline hydrochloride (TCH) | Effective against all tested microorganisms | [37] |
| | | *Enterococcus faecalis.* | 600 ppm | 600 ppm | 600 ppm | 600 ppm | | | |
| | | *Escherichia coli,* | 600 ppm | 600 ppm | 60 ppm | 600 ppm | | | |
| | | *Proteus vulgaris* | 600 ppm | 600 ppm | 600 ppm | 600 ppm | | | |
| | | *Pseudomonas aeruginosa* | 600 ppm | 600 ppm | nt | 600 ppm | | | |
| | | *Salmonella* sp. | 600 ppm | 600 ppm | 60 ppm | 600 ppm | | | |
| | | *Klebsiella pneumoniae* | 600 ppm | 600 ppm | nt | 600 ppm | | | |

*(Table 2) cont.....*

| | | | | | | | | | |
|---|---|---|---|---|---|---|---|---|---|
| Linalool | Disc diffusion | *Escherichia coli* | 26.5 mm | | | | 28.4 mm | Chloramphenicol | Activity against all of the tested microorganisms | [68] |
| | | *Bacillus subtilis* | 26.4 mm | | | | 25.5 mm | | | |
| | | *Pseudomonas aeruginosa* | 21.9 mm | | | | 21.5 mm | | | |
| | | *Staphylococcus aureus* | 25.5 mm | | | | 28.7 mm | | | |
| | Broth dilution | *Escherichia coli* | 1.10 mg/mL | | | | 10.08 µg/mL | | | |
| | | *Bacillus subtilis* | 1.25 mg/mL | | | | 15.06 µg/mL | | | |
| | | *Pseudomonas aeruginosa* | 1.75 mg/mL | | | | 100 µg/mL | | | |
| | | *Staphylococcus aureus* | 1.04 mg/mL | | | | 10.3 µg/mL | | | |
| | Disc diffusion | *Escherichia coli* | 18.32 mm | | | | nt | - | Potent antimicrobial activity | [75] |
| | | *Listeria innocua* | 16.50 mm | | | | nt | | | |
| | | *Pseudomonas lundensis* | 14.55 mm | | | | nt | | | |
| | Broth micro-dilution | *Campylobacter jejuni* | 0.35% | | | | 0.00006% | Gentamycin | | [71] |
| | | *Escherichia coli* | 0.40% | | | | 0.00012% | | | |
| | | *Salmonella enterica* | 0.37% | | | | 0.00006% | | | |
| | | MR 2388 *Listeria monocytogenes* | >0.67% | | | | 0.016% | Chloramphenicol | | |
| | | MR 2199 *Listeria monocytogenes* | >0.67% | | | | 0.020% | | | |
| | | *Escherichia coli* | 100 µL/mL | | | | nt | - | Inhibitory and bactericidal effect on tested microorganisms except *P. citrinum* | [76] |
| | | *Staphylococcus aureus* | 50 µL/mL | | | | nt | | | |
| | Broth micro-dilution | *Porphylomonas gingivalis* ATCC 33277 | 0.8 mg/mL | | | | - | Ampicillin | Compound showed good activity against periodontopathic and cariogenic bacteria | [77] |
| | | *P. gingivalis* ATCC 49417 | 0.1 mg/mL | | | | - | | | |
| | | *P. gingivalis* ATCC 53978 | 0.1 mg/mL | | | | - | | | |
| | | *Prevotella intermedia* ATCC 25611 | 0.2 mg/mL | | | | - | | | |
| | | *P. intermedia* ATCC 49046 | 1.6 mg/mL | | | | - | | | |
| | | *Prevotella nigrescens* ATCC 33563 | 0.8 mg/mL | | | | - | | | |
| | | *P. nigrescens* ATCC 25261 | 0.8 mg/mL | | | | - | | | |
| | | *Fusobacterium nucleatum* ATCC 25586 | 0.2 mg/mL | | | | - | | | |
| | | *F. nucleatum* ATCC 10953 | 0.2 mg/mL | | | | - | | | |
| | | *F. nucleatum* ATCC 49046 | 0.1 mg/mL | | | | - | | | |
| | | *F. nucleatum* ATCC 51190 | 0.2 mg/mL | | | | - | | | |
| | | *F. nucleatum* ATCC 51191 | 0.2 mg/mL | | | | - | | | |
| | | *Aggregatibacter actinomycetemcomitans* ATCC 33384 | 0.1 mg/mL | | | | - | | | |
| | | *A. actinomycetemcomitans* ATCC 43717 | 0.1 mg/mL | | | | - | | | |
| | | *A. actinomycetemcomitans* ATCC 43718 | 0.1 mg/mL | | | | - | | | |
| | Disc diffusion | | | **T** | **O** | **E** | | | | |
| | | *Staphylococcus aureus* | 13 mm | 24mm | 35mm | 39mm | | Tetracycline (T) Ofloxacin (O) Erythromycin (E) | Was significantly active against *E. coli* and *C. albicans* | [78] |
| | | *Pseudomonas aeruginosa* | 8 mm | 36mm | 24mm | 35mm | | | | |
| | | *Escherichia coli* | 21 mm | 29mm | 39mm | 16mm | | | | |

(Table 2) cont.....

| | | | | | | | |
|---|---|---|---|---|---|---|---|
| Limonene | Broth micro-dilution | *Campylobacter jejuni* | >0.67% | 0.00006% | Gentamycin | Compound had moderate activity against | [71] |
| | | *Escherichia coli* | >0.67% | 0.00012% | | | |
| | | *Salmonella enterica* | 0.35% | 0.00006% | | | |
| | | MR 2388 *Listeria monocytogenes* | >0.67% | 0.016% | Chloramphenicol | | |
| | | MR 2199 *Listeria monocytogenes* | 0.25% | 0.020% | | | |
| Thymol | Broth micro-dilution | *Bacillus cereus,* | 312 µg/mL | 1.22 µg/mL | Gentamicin sulfate | Exhibited good activity against *B. cereus* and *C. albicans* | [72] |
| | | *Staphylococcus aureus* | 1250 µg/mL | 0.61 µg/mL | | | |
| | | *Escherichia coli* | 625 µg/mL | 1.22 µg/mL | | | |
| | | *Pseudomonas aeruginosa* | 625 µg/mL | 2.44 µg/mL | | | |
| | Broth micro-dilution | *Campylobacter jejuni* | 0.024% | 0.00006% | Gentamycin | Active against all tested bacterial strains | [71] |
| | | *Escherichia coli* | 0.060% | 0.00012% | | | |
| | | *Salmonella enterica* | 0.034% | 0.00006% | | | |
| | | MR 2388 *Listeria monocytogenes* | 0.077% | 0.016% | Chloramphenicol | | |
| | | MR 2199 *Listeria monocytogenes* | 0.077% | 0.020% | | | |
| Trans-sabinene hydrate | Disc diffusion | *Escherichia coli* | 25.3 mg/mL | 28.4 µg/mL | Chloramphenicol | showed the weak antimicrobial activity | [68] |
| | | *Bacillus subtilis* | 22.7 mg/mL | 25.5 µg/mL | | | |
| | | *Pseudomonas aeruginosa* | 21.4 mg/mL | 21.5 µg/mL | | | |
| | | *Staphylococcus aureus* | 24.7 mg/mL | 28.7 µg/mL | | | |
| | Broth dilution | *Escherichia coli* | 1.25 mg/mL | 10.08 µg/mL | Chloramphenicol | | |
| | | *Bacillus subtilis* | 1.74 mg/mL | 15.06 µg/mL | | | |
| | | *Pseudomonas aeruginosa* | 1.75 mg/mL | 100 µg/mL | | | |
| | | *Staphylococcus aureus* | 1.25 mg/mL | 10.3 µg/mL | | | |

*(Table 2) cont.....*

| | | | | | | | |
|---|---|---|---|---|---|---|---|
| | | *Gardnerella vaginalis* | 0.06% (v/v) | 0.06% (v/v | Clotrimazole. | Antimicrobial activity was comparable to that of clotrimazole. | [70] |
| | Broth micro-dilution | *Campylobacter jejuni* | 0.10% | 0.00006% | Gentamycin | Active against all tested bacterial strains | [71] |
| | | *Escherichia coli* | 0.39% | 0.00012% | | | |
| | | *Salmonella enterica* | 0.18% | 0.00006% | | | |
| | | MR 2388 *Listeria monocytogenes* | >0.67% | 0.016% | Chloramphenicol | | |
| | | MR 2199 *Listeria monocytogenes* | 0.56% | 0.020% | | | |
| α–Terpineol (terpineol) | Broth micro-dilution | *Porphylomonas gingivalis* ATCC 33277 | 0.4 mg/mL | - | Ampicillin | Compound showed good activity against periodontopathic and cariogenic bacteria | [77] |
| | | *P. gingivalis* ATCC 49417 | 0.1 mg/mL | - | | | |
| | | *P. gingivalis* ATCC 53978 | 0.4 mg/mL | - | | | |
| | | Prevotella intermedia ATCC 25611 | 0.4 mg/mL | - | | | |
| | | *P. intermedia* ATCC 49046 | 0.8 mg/mL | - | | | |
| | | *Prevotella nigrescens* ATCC 33563 | 0.4 mg/mL | - | | | |
| | | *P. nigrescens* ATCC 25261 | 0.4 mg/mL | - | | | |
| | | *Fusobacterium nucleatum* ATCC 25586 | 0.4 mg/mL | - | | | |
| | | *F. nucleatum* ATCC 10953 | 0.4 mg/mL | - | | | |
| | | *F. nucleatum* ATCC 49046 | 0.1 mg/mL | - | | | |
| | | *F. nucleatum* ATCC 51190 | 0.2 mg/mL | - | | | |
| | | *F. nucleatum* ATCC 51191 | 0.4 mg/mL | - | | | |
| | | *Aggregatibacter actinomycetemcomitans* ATCC 33384 | 0.2 mg/mL | - | | | |
| | | *A. actinomycetemcomitans* ATCC 43717 | 0.2 mg/mL | - | | | |
| | | *A. actinomycetemcomitans* ATCC 43718 | 0.2 mg/mL | - | | | |

(-)= not reported, na= not active, nt= not tested, *Antibacterial effect reported as minimal inhibitory concentration (microdilution/broth dilution assay), percentage inhibition (microdilution/broth dilution assay), or zone of inhibition in disc diffusion assay.

For antifungal activity, citronella and geraniol showed good activity with MICs ≤16 μg/mL, while 60% of the compounds demonstrated moderate activity with MICs ≤ 1000 μg/mL (Table **3**). These compounds are potential antifungal agents, which can be used as alternative compounds in different industries.

**Table 3. Antifungal activity of some major essential oil secondary metabolites.**

| Major Compound | Method | Test Microorganism | Antifungal Effect* | Positive Control Response | Positive Control | Key Findings | Reference |
|---|---|---|---|---|---|---|---|
| Borneol | Microdilution | *Candida albicans* | 250 µg/mL | 125 µg/mL | Ketoconazole | Activity ranged from 125-250 µl/mL | [67] |
| | Disc diffusion | *Candida albicans* | 27.1 mm | 24.4 mm | Amphotericin B | Showed activity against all the microorganisms tested | [68] |
| | | *Aspergillus niger* | 23.5 mm | 21.9 mm | | | |
| | Broth dilution | *Candida albicans* | 0.75 mg/mL | 100 µg/ml | | | |
| | | *Aspergillus niger* | 2.25 mg/mL | 100 µg/ml | | | |
| | Disc diffusion | *Candida albicans* | 19 mm | - | - | (-)borneol showed high activity | [69] |
| | - | *Candida albicans* | > 1% (v/v) | 0.03% (v/v) | Clotrimazole | Active against *Gardnerella vaginalis* | [70] |
| Camphor | Micro-broth dilution | *Candida albicans* | 625 µg/mL | 0.61µg/mL | Amphotericin B | Significantly inhibit growth rate against *B. cereus* | [72] |
| | | *Aspergillus niger* | 625 µg/mL | 1.22µg/mL | | | |
| Camphene | Broth micro-dilution | *Trichophyton mentagrophytes* | >735 µmol/L | 5 µmol/L | Fluconazole | Camphene alone exhibited weak activity | [79] |
| | | | Minimum inhibitory concentration: 55 µmol/L; Minimum fungicidal concentration: 110 µmol/L. | | | Its derivative showed the strongest effect against *T. mentagrophytes* | |
| | Broth micro-dilution | *Candida albicans* strains | 8-32 mM | >128 µg/mL | Fluconazole | -Inhibited planktonic growth and were fungistatic -Inhibited morphogenesis significantly and exhibited considerable activity against biofilm formation. | [80] |
| Carvacrol | Disc diffusion | *Candida albicans* | 30.5 mm | 24.4 mm | Amphotericin B | -Carvacrol standard and a fraction with highest carvacrol was most effective | [68] |
| | | *Aspergillus niger* | 24.4 mm | 21.9 mm | | | |
| | Broth dilution | *Candida albicans* | 0.53 mg/mL | 100 µg/mL | | | |
| | | *Aspergillus niger* | 2.03 mg/mL | 100 µg/mL | | | |

*(Table 3) cont.....*

| | | | | | | | |
|---|---|---|---|---|---|---|---|
| Citronellol | Broth micro-dilution | *Trichophyton rubrum* strains | 8-1024 µg/mL | 16 µg/mL | Ketoconazole | -Inhibited the mycelial growth, conidia germination, and fungal growth on nail fragments -Act on cell wall and cell membrane of *T. rubrum* | [81] |
| | Disc diffusion | *Candida albicans* | na | - | Ciproxin (CPN), Lidaprim (LDM), Tetracycline hydrochloride (TCH) | Not effective against *C. albicans* | [37] |
| | Broth micro-dilution | *Candida albicans* | na | - | | | |
| Eucalyptol (1,8-cineole) | - | *Candida albicans* | 1% (v/v) | 0.03% (v/v) | Clotrimazole | Inhibited microbial growths | [70] |
| | Diffusion Method | *Fusarium cerealis* | 0.0-4.54 cm | -ve control 5.2 cm | - | 0.1% of the compound inhibited fungal growth | [82] |
| | Broth micro-dilution | *Candida albicans* | 625 µg/mL | 0.61µg/mL | Amphotericin B | Exhibited moderate activity | [72] |
| | | *Aspergillus niger* | 625 µg/mL | 1.22µg/mL | | | |
| Geranial (Citral) | Disc diffusion | *Candida albicans* | 22 mm | 18 mm | Nystatin | Showed good to moderate activity | [73] |
| | | *Saccharomyces cerevisae* | 21 mm | 18 mm | | | |
| | | *Aspergillus niger* | 15 mm | 16 mm | | | |
| | Broth micro-dilution | *Candida albicans* | 2.5 mg/mL | nt | Nystatin | Showed weak activity | |
| | | *Saccharomyces cerevisae* | 2.5 mg/mL | nt | | | |
| | | *Aspergillus niger* | 5.0 mg/mL | nt | | | |

*(Table 3) cont.....*

| | | | | | | | | | |
|---|---|---|---|---|---|---|---|---|---|
| Geraniol | Disc diffusion | *Candida albicans* | 12 mm | 18mm | | | Nystatin | Showed good activity against most of the bacterial strains, comparable with the poisitive control | [73] |
| | | *Saccharomyces cerevisae* | 13 mm | 18mm | | | | | |
| | | *Aspergillus niger* | 11 mm | 16 mm | | | | | |
| | Broth micro-dilution | *Candida albicans* | 10.0 mg/mL | nt | | | Nystatin | Showed weak activity | |
| | | *Saccharomyces cerevisae* | 10.0 mg/mL | nt | | | | | |
| | | *Aspergillus niger* | 10.0 mg/mL | nt | | | | | |
| | Broth micro-dilution | *Candida albicans* | 16 µg/mL | 2 µg/mL | | | Amphotericin B | Showed good activity | [83] |
| | Broth micro-dilution | *Trichophyton rubrum* strains | 16-256 µg/mL | 16 µg/mL | | | Ketoconazole | -Inhibited the mycelial growth, conidia germination and fungal growth on nail fragments -Acted on cell wall and cell membrane of *T. rubrum* | [81] |
| Geranyl formate | Disc diffusion | *Candida albicans* | 15 mm | CPN | LDM | TCH | Ciproxin (CPN), Lidaprim (LDM), Tetracycline hydrochloride (TCH) | Effective against all tested fungal strains | [37] |
| | | | | nt | nt | nt | | | |
| | Broth micro-dilution | *Candida albicans* | 600 ppm | nt | nt | nt | | | |

(Table 3) cont.....

| Compound | Method | Microorganism | Value | Control | | | | | Control drug | Comments | Ref |
|---|---|---|---|---|---|---|---|---|---|---|---|
| Linalool | Disc diffusion | *Candida albicans* | 27.2 mm | 24.4 mm | | | | | Amphotericin B | Showed activity against all the microorganisms tested | [68] |
| | | *Aspergillus niger* | 20.3 mm | 21.9 mm | | | | | | | |
| | Broth dilution | *Candida albicans* | 0.75 mg/mL | 100 µg/mL | | | | | | | |
| | | *Aspergillus niger* | 2.54 mg/mL | 100 µg/mL | | | | | | | |
| | | *Saccharomyces cerivisiae* | 50 µL/mL | nt | | | | | - | Showed inhibitory and bactericidal effect on test microorganisms except *P. citrinum* | [76] |
| | | *Penicillium citrinum* | >400 µL/mL | nt | | | | | | | |
| | | *Aspergillus niger* | 50 µL/mL | nt | | | | | | | |
| | Disc diffusion | *Candida albicans* | 21 mm | T | O | E | M | F | Tetracycline (T) Ofloxacin (O) Erythromycin (E) Miconazole (M) Fluconazole (F) | Was significantly active against *E. coli* and *C. albicans* | [78] |
| | | | | nt | nt | nt | 20mm | 16mm | | | |
| | | *Aspergillus brasiliensis* | na | nt | nt | nt | 20mm | na | | | |
| Limonene | Broth micro-dilution | *Trichophyton mentagrophytes* | >735 µmol/L | 5 µmol/L | | | | | Fluconazole | Limonene alone had weak activity, it derivative, showed moderate activity, with MIC and MFC values of 110 µmol/L and 220 µmol/L | [79] |
| Terpinen-4-ol | Diffusion Method | *Fusarium cerealis* | 0.0-2.18 cm | -ve control 5.2 cm | | | | | - | 0.1% of the compound inhibited fungal growth | [82] |
| | Broth micro-dilution | *Candida albicans* | 312 µg/mL | 0.61µg/mL | | | | | Amphotericin B | Exhibited good activity against *B. cereus* and *C. albicans* | [72] |
| | | *Aspergillus niger.* | 625 µg/mL | 1.22µg/mL | | | | | | | |
| Thymol | Diffusion Method | *Fusarium cerealis* | 0.0-3.47 cm | -ve control 5.2 cm | | | | | - | 0.1% of the compound inhibited fungal growth | [82] |
| Trans-sabinene hydrate | Disc diffusion | *Candida albicans* | 26.9 mg/mL | 24.4 µg/mL | | | | | Amphotericin B | Sabinene hydrate showed weak antimicrobial activity | [68] |
| | | *Aspergillus niger* | 18.8 mg/mL | 21.9 µg/mL | | | | | | | |
| | Broth dilution | *Candida albicans* | 0.75 mg/mL | 100 µg/mL | | | | | | | |
| | | *Aspergillus niger* | 2.75 mg/mL | 100 µg/mL | | | | | | | |

(Table 3) cont.....

| | | | | | | | |
|---|---|---|---|---|---|---|---|
| α–terpineol (terpineol) | | Candida albicans | 0.125% (v/v) | 0.03% (v/v | Clotrimazole. | Antimicrobial activity was comparable to that of clotrimazole. | [70] |

(-)= not reported, na= not active, nt= not tested, *Antifungal effect reported as minimal inhibitory concentration (microdilution or broth dilution assay), percentage inhibition (microdilution or broth dilution assay), or zone of inhibition in disc diffusion assay

## 4.2. Anti-inflammatory

Inflammation reaction frequently occurs in living tissues, in response to injury, chemical irritant and infections. It is characterized by heat, itchiness, pain, swelling, redness and loss of function [84]. Inflammation is associated with the pathogenesis of acute/chronic diseases such as cancer, atherosclerosis, diabetes mellitus, obesity, multiple sclerosis, asthma and arthritis [85]. Inflammation reactions are commonly treated with steroids or non-steroidal anti-inflammatory drugs, depending on the severity. Like most synthetic drugs, anti-inflammatory drugs have undesirable side effects, necessitating the search for alternatives with less side effects [86]. The side effects of some non-steroidal anti-inflammatory drugs include increased blood pressure, risk of congestive heart failure, thrombosis and gastrointestinal erosion [87]. Steroidal drugs are associated with immunosuppressing effects and disease resistance.

*In vitro* and *in vivo* methods have been used to evaluate anti-inflammatory activity of essential oil compounds (Table **4**). *In vitro* methods include inhibition of targeted inflammatory mediators and testing for immune-modulation, while *in vivo* methods include using an antigen or adjuvant to stimulate the immune system in animal models for delayed-type hypersensitivity, paw edema, ear edema and colitis. Essential oil secondary metabolites such as eucalyptol and bornyl acetate have demonstrated potent anti-inflammatory activity in *in vitro* and *in vivo* assays. Eucalyptol is one of the main constituents of *Rosmarinus officinalis* [85], which was evaluated for its potential as an anti-inflammatory agent in a clinical trial [88]. Findings from the clinical trials indicated that *R. officinalis* effectively reduced inflammation in patients with osteoarthritis and rheumatoid arthritis. Suppression of inflammatory cytokines expression was a major mechanism of action of many evaluated compounds. Overall, the reviewed compounds have noteworthy anti-inflammatory activity with potential as alternative compounds to current anti-inflammatory drugs.

**Table 4. Anti-inflammatory properties of some major essential oil secondary metabolites.**

| Major Compound | Method/Model | Inducer/Dose | Mode | System | Positive Control | Key Findings | Reference |
|---|---|---|---|---|---|---|---|
| Borneol | Peritonitis | Carrageenan-induced peritonitis (500 μg/cavity, 500 μL, i.p.) | *In vivo* | Leukocytes | Morphine (10 mg/kg), Indomethacin (20 mg/kg) | Reduced leukocyte migration induced by inflammatory agent | [89] |
| | Colitis | TNBS (70 mg/kg) | *In vivo* | Male mice (ICR strain) | Thymoquinone (0.05%) | Borneol significantly suppressed pro-inflammatory cytokine mRNA expression in colonic inflammation | [90] |
| Bornyl acetate | Haemocytometer | Lipopolysaccharide (1mg/L) | *In vivo* | Male BALB/c mice/ | Penicillin and streptomycin, (100 U/mL) | Significant lowering of the number of total cells, neutrophils, and macrophages. Preventive agent for lung inflammatory diseases. | [91] |
| | ELISA kit | Lipopolysaccharide (1mg/L) | *In vitro* | RAW 264.7 cells | | Significantly decreased concentrations of TNF-α, IL-1β, and IL-6 compared with the LPS group in a dose-dependent manner | |
| Bornyl acetate | Femoral heads | IL-1b (5 ng/mL) | *In vitro* | Human primary chondrocytes. | Antimycotic solution (1%) Penicillin–streptomycin (1%) | Exerts anti-inflammatory effects on IL-1b-stimulated chondrocyte | [92] |
| Bornyl acetate | Endothelium | ox-LDL (100 mg/L) | *In vitro* | Human umbilical vein endothelial cells, THP-1 cells | Antimycotic solution (1%) | Attenuated production of the pro-inflammatory cytokines TNF-α and IL-1β, both of which are essential regulators in the pathogenesis of atherosclerosis (comprehensive anti-inflammatory effect) | [93] |
| Eucalyptol (1,8-cineole) | Vaginal cavities | G. vaginalis | *In vivo* | Male and Female ICR mice | Clotrimazole (10% w/w) | Inhibited the expressions of pro-inflammatory cytokines (IL-1β, IL-6, TNF-α), COX-2, iNOS, and the activation of NF-κB and increased expression of the anti-inflammatory cytokine IL10. | [70] |
| | | C. albicans | | | | | |

*(Table 4) cont.....*

| | | | | | | | |
|---|---|---|---|---|---|---|---|
| Eucalyptol (1,8-cineole) | Ear edema | Croton oil | *In vivo* | Swiss (*Mus musculus*) male mice | Dexamethasone (4 mg/mL/v.t) | 34.97% inhibition (69.44% +ve control), Significantly reduced inflammation | [94] |
| | Paw edema | Carrageenan, Dextran Histamine Arachidonic acid | | | Indomethacin (10 mg/kg/s.c.) Promethazine (6 mg/kg/v.o.) | Reduced edema 79.8%-80.50% (78.07 and 89.94% +ve control) Statistically reduced paw edema induced by carrageenan, dextran, histamine and arachidonic acid | |
| | Granuloma | Cotton pellets | | | Dexamethasone (5 mg/kg/v.o.) | Reduced granulomatous 20% (66.66%+ve control) Significantly reduced granulomatous tissue | |
| | Gastric mucosa | Indomethacin (30 mg/kg) | *In vivo* | Male and female Wistar rats | Pantoprazole (40 mg/kg) | 58.3 % reduction of lesions and ulcers (91.2% +ve control)  Inhibited indomethacin-induced gastric lesions and reduced ulcers | [95] |
| Geraniol | Colitis | Dextran sulfate sodium (DSS) | *In vivo* | Male C57BL/6 mice | Hydrocortisone (2.5 mg kg$^{-1}$) | Significantly reduced cyclooxygenase-2 (COX-2) expression in colonocytes and in the gut wall | [96] |
| Linalool | Liver tissues | Lipopolysaccharide (LPS, 50 μg/kg) and GalN)/d-galactosamine (GalN, 800 mg/kg). | *In vivo* | Male BALB/c mice | NR | Suppressed iNOS and COX-2 expression, by NF-κB inhibition | [97] |
| | BALF(Bronchoalveolar lavage fluid) and lung tissues | Cigarette smoke (CS) | *In vivo* | Male C57BL/6 mice | NR | Inhibited inflammatory cytokines | [98] |
| | Paw edema | Carrageenin | *In vivo* | Male albino Wistar rats | Aspirin (AsA, 150 mg/kg) | 25-60% inhibition against edema (52-64% +ve control)  Protect against lung inflammation through inhibiting CS-induced NF-κB activation | [99] |

NR= Not recorded

## 4.3. Antioxidants

Antioxidants are defense molecules produced to reduce cell damage caused by free radicals, which are implicated in the pathogenesis of several diseases [100]. Natural antioxidants can be acquired through diets, and if obtained in sufficient amounts, they can help in the prevention of vascular diseases. They play an important role in the treatment of neurodegenerative diseases [101]. Due to safety concerns regarding synthetic antioxidants, the search for natural antioxidants is gaining momentum. Natural antioxidants have low toxicity and similar or higher antioxidant activity when compared to synthetic antioxidants [102].

The most commonly used method for *in vitro* antioxidant activity is 2, 2-dipheny--1-picrylhydrazyl (DPPH) free radical scavenging assay. The method is preferred due to its simplicity, cost effectiveness and rapidness when compared to other free radical scavenging methods [100]. Among the reported compounds, eucalyptol demonstrated a relatively potent *in vivo* antioxidant activity (Table **5**). Generally, most of the compounds demonstrated weak antioxidant activity *in vitro*, although the EOs from which they were isolated possessed good antioxidant activity. This could be due to the combined activity or synergism of the phytochemicals in the EOs [103].

In order to better explore the antioxidant activity of a substance, the use of more than one test systems/models has been recommended [100]. Test models comprise of hydrogen transfer reactions (such as oxygen radical absorbance capacity (ORAC), β-carotene/linoleic acid model system and inhibition of phospholipid peroxidation assays) and single electron transfer reactions (Folin-Ciocalteu (Folin-C), DPPH free radical scavenging, Trolox equivalent antioxidant capacity (TEAC) and ferric reducing ability of plasma (FRAP) assays) [100]. As depicted in Table **5**, citronellol and α-pinene showed good antioxidant activity based on DPPH test, while exhibiting weak activity in ABTS assay. Although both DPPH and ABTS assays are classified in the single electron transfer reactions, the compounds demonstrated different activities [104]. This emphasizes the importance of evaluating antioxidants using more than one test method considering the complexities involved in antioxidant processes.

**Table 5. Antioxidant activity of some major essential oil secondary metabolites.**

| Major Compound | Method | Mode | Result/IC$_{50}$ | Positive Control | Key Finding | Reference |
|---|---|---|---|---|---|---|
| Citronellol | DPPH | *In vitro* | 40 µg/mL | Trolox 1.9 µg/mL | Had strong antioxidant activity | [105] |
|  | ABTS | *In vitro* | >1000 µg/mL | Trolox 10.2 µg/mL | Exhibited weak antioxidant activity | |

(Table 5) cont.....

| | | | | | | |
|---|---|---|---|---|---|---|
| Eucalyptol (1,8-cineole) | na | *In vivo* | Negative control: 147.2 ±7.5 μg/g Induced ulcer: 64.2 μg/g of tissue 1,8-cineole: 104.4 ±7.3 μg/g Positive control: 147.9 μg/g of tissue | N-acetylcysteine (NAC, 750 mg/kg) | Restored the antioxidant system through levels of sulfhydryl groups | [95] |
| Linalool | DPPH assay | *In vitro* | 108.90 mg/mL | NR | Showed less antioxidant activity compared to the oil | [76] |
| | Reducing power assay | *In vitro* | Abs. 0.55 (137.5 mg/mL conc.) | | | |
| Limonene | DPPH | *In vitro* | >1000 μg/mL | Trolox 1.9 μg/mL | Exhibited weak antioxidant activity | [105] |
| | ABTS | *In vitro* | >1000 μg/mL | Trolox 10.2 μg/mL | | |
| α-pinene | DPPH | *In vitro* | 310 μg/mL | Trolox 1.9 μg/mL | Had good antioxidant activity | [105] |
| | ABTS | *In vitro* | >1000 μg/mL | Trolox 10.2 μg/mL | Exhibited weak antioxidant activity | |

na= not applicable, NR= not recorded, DPPH= 2,2-diphenyl-1-picrylhydrazyl, ABTS = 2,2-azinobis (3-ethy--benzothiazoline-6-sulfonic acid)

## 4.4. Cytotoxicity

Cytotoxicity determination employs biological test that uses tissue cells to evaluate compound toxicity. *In vitro* cytotoxicity test is simple, fast and has high sensitivity as an indicator for toxicity evaluation of pharmaceutical compounds [106]. Cytotoxicity is a primary method that establishes safety of a test compound [107] and its importance cannot be over emphasised, especially in determining the safety of compounds that are to be used as pharmaceuticals. To be considered safe, compounds must be critically tested and adhere to standards of the International Organization for Standardization (ISO) and their recommendations must be applied for clinical use [108]. Therefore, cytotoxicity status determines the fate of the compounds to be used as health products.

MTT (3-[4,5- dimethylthiazol-2-yl]-2,5 diphenyl tetrazolium bromide) assay was used to detect cell cytotoxicity against compounds from essential oils (Table 6). Although some of these compounds maybe toxic at high dosages, they are used at lower concentrations, which are safer for human consumption. Therefore, a critical evaluation of the safety/therapeutic window, also called therapeutic index, of the compounds is imperative for their application in different industries.

**Table 6. Cytotoxic activity of some major essential oil secondary metabolites.**

| Major Compound | Tested Concentration | Method | Cell Line | Result | Positive Control | Key Finding | Reference |
|---|---|---|---|---|---|---|---|
| Bornyl acetate | 0–500 µg/mL | MTT | RAW 264.7 cells | Control (OD): 2.3 LPS: 2.3 Bornyl acetate: ≥ 2.2 | NR | No toxicity observed | [91] |
| Camphor | 0.05-15 mM | MTT | MRC-5 | $IC_{50}$ 11.0 mM | NR | HCT116 and HT-29 cells were most sensitive | [109] |
| | | | HT-29 | 5.5 mM | | | |
| | | | HCT116 | 4.5 mM | | | |
| Citronellol | 1.56–200 µg/mL | MTT | T98G cells | 18.2 µg/mL | Cisplatin: 2.3 µg/mL | Exhibited strong inhibitory effect against all the cell lines | [105] |
| | | | MDA-MB 231 cells | 10.7 µg/mL | 2.1 µg/mL | | |
| | | | A375 cells | 8.4 µg/mL | 0.2 µg/mL | | |
| | | | HCT116 cells | 13.5 µg/mL | 2.6 µg/mL | | |
| Eucalyptol (1,8-cineole) | 0.05-15 mM | MTT | MRC-5 | $IC_{50}$ 11.0 mM | NR | most significant inhibitory effect against HCT116 cell | [109] |
| | | | HT-29 | 7.5 mM | | | |
| | | | HCT116 | 4.0 mM | | | |
| Geraniol | 1.56–200 µg/mL | MTT | T98G cells | 10.8 µg/mL | Cisplatin: 2.3 µg/mL | Exhibited strong inhibitory effect against all the cell lines | [105] |
| | | | MDA-MB 231 cells | 21.6 µg/mL | 2.1 µg/mL | | |
| | | | A375 cells | 3.6 µg/mL | 0.2 µg/mL | | |
| | | | HCT116 cells | 6.2 µg/mL | 2.6 µg/mL | | |
| Linalool | 4, 6, 8, 16, 24, and 32 mg/mL | MTT | Hela cells | 3.24 µg/mL | NR | Showed significant cytotoxicity aginst the cell lines | [76] |

(Table 6) cont.....

| | 1.56–200 µg/mL | MTT | T98G cells | 45.4 µg/mL | Cisplatin: 2.3 µg/mL | Had significant inhibitory effect against A375 cells | [105] |
|---|---|---|---|---|---|---|---|
| Limonene | | | MDA-MB 231 cells | 124.0 µg/mL | 2.1 µg/mL | | |
| | | | A375 cells | 18.4 µg/mL | 0.2 µg/mL | | |
| | | | HCT116 cells | 83.4 µg/mL | 2.6 µg/mL | | |
| | 1.56–200 µg/mL | MTT | T98G cells | 44.6 µg/mL | Cisplatin: 2.3 µg/mL | Compound showed weak inhibitory activity against all cell lines | [105] |
| α-pinene | | | MDA-MB 231 cells | 27.3 µg/mL | 2.1 µg/mL | | |
| | | | A375 cells | 44.8 µg/mL | 0.2 µg/mL | | |
| | | | HCT116 cells | 63.1 µg/mL | 2.6 µg/mL | | |

NR= not recorded, MTT = 3-[4,5-dimethylthiazol-2-yl]-2,5 diphenyl tetrazolium bromide)

## CONCLUDING REMARKS

The benefit of compounds from EOs is their diverse biological activities including antimicrobial, anti-inflammatory, antioxidants and cytotoxicity properties. These compounds have potential to be used as alternative agents in drugs, cosmetic ingredients and as food additives. Extensive research work may be required with some compounds to ascertain their therapeutic index for their diverse non-toxic applications. While studies have investigated the chemical composition of the EOs and demonstrated their biological activities, there is a dearth of information on the therapeutic effects of the active compounds when combined for different applications. Therapeutic data on these compounds will contribute to drug discovery and application as alternative compounds in different industries.

## CONSENT FOR PUBLICATION

Not applicable.

## CONFLICT OF INTEREST

The authors declare no conflict of interest, financial or otherwise.

## ACKNOWLEDGEMENTS

We gratefully acknowledge funding from the EU-GBS programme through the Department of Science and Innovation, South Africa (DST/CON 0092/2019),

National Research Foundation (NRF: Grant no. 128 102:2020) for postdoctoral fellowship award to the first author, the institutional support of the Agricultural Research Council (ARC), and the North-West University, South Africa.

# REFERENCES

[1]    Croteau R, Kutchan TM, Lewis NG. Natural products (secondary metabolites).Biochemistry and Molecular Biology of Plants. 2nd ed. New York: American Society of Plant Physiologists 2000; pp. 1250-319.

[2]    Bennett RN, Wallsgrove RM. Secondary metabolites in plant defence mechanisms. New Phytol 1994; 127(4): 617-33.
[http://dx.doi.org/10.1111/j.1469-8137.1994.tb02968.x] [PMID: 33874382]

[3]    Ravishankar G, Rao S. Biotechnological Production of Phyto-Pharmaceuticals. J Biochem Mol Biol Biophys 2000; 4: 73-102.

[4]    Crozier A, Jaganath IB, Clifford MN. Phenols, Polyphenols and Tannins: An Overview.Plant Secondary Metabolites: Occurrence, Structure and Role in the Human Diet. Oxford: Blackwell Publishing 2006; pp. 1-22.
[http://dx.doi.org/10.1002/9780470988558.ch1]

[5]    Avoseh O, Oyedeji O, Rungqu P, Nkeh-Chungag B, Oyedeji A. *Cymbopogon* species; ethnopharmacology, phytochemistry and the pharmacological importance. Molecules 2015; 20(5): 7438-53.
[http://dx.doi.org/10.3390/molecules20057438] [PMID: 25915460]

[6]    Bourgaud F, Gravot A, Milesi S. Gontier. Production of plant secondary metabolites: a historical perspective. Plant Sci 2001; 161: 839-51.
[http://dx.doi.org/10.1016/S0168-9452(01)00490-3]

[7]    Harborne J. Classes and functions of secondary products from plants.Chemicals from Plants, Perspectives on Secondary Plant Products. London: Imperial College Press 1999; pp. 1-25.
[http://dx.doi.org/10.1142/9789812817273_0001]

[8]    Pengelly A, Bone K. The Constituents of Medicinal Plants: An Introduction to the Chemistry and Therapeutics of Herbal Medicine. 1st ed., New York: Routledge 2020.
[http://dx.doi.org/10.4324/9781003117964]

[9]    Ramakrishna A, Ravishankar GA. Influence of abiotic stress signals on secondary metabolites in plants. Plant Signal Behav 2011; 6(11): 1720-31.
[http://dx.doi.org/10.4161/psb.6.11.17613] [PMID: 22041989]

[10]   Rao SR, Ravishankar GA. Plant cell cultures: Chemical factories of secondary metabolites. Biotechnol Adv 2002; 20(2): 101-53.
[http://dx.doi.org/10.1016/S0734-9750(02)00007-1] [PMID: 14538059]

[11]   Pesavento G, Calonico C, Bilia A, *et al.* Antibacterial activity of *Oregano, Rosmarinus* and *Thymus* essential oils against *Staphylococcus aureus* and *Listeria monocytogenes* in beef meatballs. Food Control 2015; 54: 188-99.
[http://dx.doi.org/10.1016/j.foodcont.2015.01.045]

[12]   Lin S-H, Chou M-L, Chen W-C, *et al.* A medicinal herb, *Melissa officinalis* L. ameliorates depressive-like behavior of rats in the forced swimming test *via* regulating the serotonergic neurotransmitter. J Ethnopharmacol 2015; 175: 266-72.
[http://dx.doi.org/10.1016/j.jep.2015.09.018] [PMID: 26408043]

[13]   Park E-S, Moon W-S, Song M-J, *et al.* Antimicrobial activity of phenol and benzoic acid derivatives. Int Biodeterior Biodegradation 2001; 47: 209-14.
[http://dx.doi.org/10.1016/S0964-8305(01)00058-0]

[14]    Choi WH, Jiang M. Evaluation of antibacterial activity of hexanedioic acid isolated from *Hermetia illucens* larvae. J Appl Biomed 2014; 12: 179-89.
[http://dx.doi.org/10.1016/j.jab.2014.01.003]

[15]    Cueva C, Moreno-Arribas MV, Martín-Alvarez PJ, *et al.* Antimicrobial activity of phenolic acids against commensal, probiotic and pathogenic bacteria. Res Microbiol 2010; 161(5): 372-82.
[http://dx.doi.org/10.1016/j.resmic.2010.04.006] [PMID: 20451604]

[16]    Gutiérrez-Larraínzar M, Rúa J, Caro I, *et al.* Evaluation of antimicrobial and antioxidant activities of natural phenolic compounds against foodborne pathogens and spoilage bacteria. Food Control 2012; 26: 555-63.
[http://dx.doi.org/10.1016/j.foodcont.2012.02.025]

[17]    Lou Z, Wang H, Rao S, *et al. p*-Coumaric acid kills bacteria through dual damage mechanisms. Food Control 2012; 25: 550-4.
[http://dx.doi.org/10.1016/j.foodcont.2011.11.022]

[18]    Puupponen-Pimiä R, Nohynek L, Meier C, *et al.* Antimicrobial properties of phenolic compounds from berries. J Appl Microbiol 2001; 90(4): 494-507.
[http://dx.doi.org/10.1046/j.1365-2672.2001.01271.x] [PMID: 11309059]

[19]    Mohammed MS, Osman WJ, Garelnabi EA, *et al.* Secondary metabolites as anti-inflammatory agents. J Phytopharmacol 2014; 3: 275-85.
[http://dx.doi.org/10.31254/phyto.2014.3409]

[20]    Gulluce M, Karadayi M, Guvenalp Z, *et al.* Isolation of some active compounds from *Origanum vulgare* L. ssp. *vulgare* and determination of their genotoxic potentials. Food Chem 2012; 130: 248-53.
[http://dx.doi.org/10.1016/j.foodchem.2011.07.024]

[21]    Torres Y Torres JL, Rosazza JP. Microbial transformations of *p*-coumaric acid by *Bacillus megaterium* and *Curvularia lunata.* J Nat Prod 2001; 64(11): 1408-14.
[http://dx.doi.org/10.1021/np010238g] [PMID: 11720522]

[22]    Jun WJ, Han BK, Yu KW, *et al.* Antioxidant effects of *Origanum majorana* L. on superoxide anion radicals. Food Chem 2001; 75: 439-44.
[http://dx.doi.org/10.1016/S0308-8146(01)00233-3]

[23]    Sevgi K, Tepe B, Sarikurkcu C. Antioxidant and DNA damage protection potentials of selected phenolic acids. Food Chem Toxicol 2015; 77: 12-21.
[http://dx.doi.org/10.1016/j.fct.2014.12.006] [PMID: 25542528]

[24]    Wang Y, Chen M, Zhang J, *et al.* Flavone C-glycosides from the leaves of *Lophatherum gracile* and their in vitro antiviral activity. Planta Med 2012; 78(1): 46-51.
[http://dx.doi.org/10.1055/s-0031-1280128] [PMID: 21870321]

[25]    Zhang X-L, Guo Y-S, Wang C-H, *et al.* Phenolic compounds from *Origanum vulgare* and their antioxidant and antiviral activities. Food Chem 2014; 152: 300-6.
[http://dx.doi.org/10.1016/j.foodchem.2013.11.153] [PMID: 24444941]

[26]    Sarrou E, Chatzopoulou P, Dimassi-Theriou K, *et al.* Effect of melatonin, salicylic acid and gibberellic acid on leaf essential oil and other secondary metabolites of bitter orange young seedlings. J Essent Oil Res 2015; 27: 487-96.
[http://dx.doi.org/10.1080/10412905.2015.1064485]

[27]    Moradkhani H, Sargsyan E, Bibak H, *et al. Melissa officinalis L.*, a valuable medicine plant: A review. J Med Plants Res 2010; 4: 2753-9.

[28]    Basta A, Tzakou O, Couladis M. Composition of the leaves essential oil of *Melissa officinalis* sl from Greece. Flavour Fragrance J 2005; 20: 642-4.
[http://dx.doi.org/10.1002/ffj.1518]

[29]    Rungsung W, Ratha KK, Dutta S, *et al.* Secondary metabolites of plants in drugs discovery. World J Pharm Res 2015; 4: 604-13.

[30]    Mazid M, Khan T, Mohammad F. Role of secondary metabolites in defense mechanisms of plants. Biol Med (Aligarh) 2011; 3: 232-49.

[31]    Yang L, Wen K-S, Ruan X, Zhao YX, Wei F, Wang Q. Response of plant secondary metabolites to environmental factors. Molecules 2018; 23(4): 762.
[http://dx.doi.org/10.3390/molecules23040762] [PMID: 29584636]

[32]    Bartwal A, Mall R, Lohani P, *et al.* Role of secondary metabolites and brassinosteroids in plant defense against environmental stresses. J Plant Growth Regul 2013; 32: 216-32.
[http://dx.doi.org/10.1007/s00344-012-9272-x]

[33]    Metcalfe NB, Alonso-Alvarez C. Oxidative stress as a life-history constraint: the role of reactive oxygen species in shaping phenotypes from conception to death. Funct Ecol 2010; 24: 984-96.
[http://dx.doi.org/10.1111/j.1365-2435.2010.01750.x]

[34]    Wink M. Plant secondary metabolism: diversity, function and its evolution. Nat Prod Commun 2008; 3
[http://dx.doi.org/10.1177/1934578X0800300801]

[35]    Pagare S, Bhatia M, Tripathi N, *et al.* Secondary metabolites of plants and their role: Overview. Curr Trends Biotechnol Pharm 2015; 9: 293-304.

[36]    Wink M. Evolution of secondary plant metabolism. eLS 2016; 1-11.

[37]    Jirovetz L, Eller G, Buchbauer G, *et al.* Chemical composition, antimicrobial activities and odor descriptions of some essential oils with characteristic floral-rosy scent and of their principal aroma compounds. Recent Res Dev Agron Hortic 2006; 2: 1-12.

[38]    Polonio T, Efferth T. Leishmaniasis: drug resistance and natural products (review). Int J Mol Med 2008; 22(3): 277-86.
[PMID: 18698485]

[39]    Kanduluru A, Manasa S, Reddy MT, Anusha V. Essential oils as therapeutics. Int J Oral Care Res 2013; 1: 409-11.

[40]    Kazemi M. Chemical composition and antimicrobial, antioxidant activities and anti-inflammatory potential of *Achillea millefolium* L., *Anethum graveolens* L., and *Carum copticum* L. essential oils. J Herb Med 2015; 5: 217 22.
[http://dx.doi.org/10.1016/j.hermed.2015.09.001]

[41]    Sellami IH, Maamouri E, Chahed T, *et al.* Effect of growth stage on the content and composition of the essential oil and phenolic fraction of sweet marjoram (*Origanum majorana* L.). Ind Crops Prod 2009; 30: 395-402.
[http://dx.doi.org/10.1016/j.indcrop.2009.07.010]

[42]    Arranz E, Jaime L, de las Hazas ML, *et al.* Supercritical fluid extraction as an alternative process to obtain essential oils with anti-inflammatory properties from marjoram and sweet basil. Ind Crops Prod 2015; 67: 121-9.
[http://dx.doi.org/10.1016/j.indcrop.2015.01.012]

[43]    Fachini-Queiroz FC, Kummer R, Estevao-Silva CF, *et al.* Effects of thymol and carvacrol, constituents of Thymus vulgaris L essential oil, on the inflammatory response. Evid-Based Complementary Altern Med 2012.

[44]    Mancini E, Senatore F, Del Monte D, *et al.* Studies on chemical composition, antimicrobial and antioxidant activities of five *Thymus vulgaris* L. essential oils. Molecules 2015; 20(7): 12016-28.
[http://dx.doi.org/10.3390/molecules200712016] [PMID: 26140436]

[45]    Vági E, Simándi B, Suhajda A, Hethelyi E. Essential oil composition and antimicrobial activity of *Origanum majorana* L. extracts obtained with ethyl alcohol and supercritical carbon dioxide. Int Food Res J 2005; 38: 51-7.

[http://dx.doi.org/10.1016/j.foodres.2004.07.006]

[46] Wang W, Wu N, Zu YG, Fu YJ. Antioxidative activity of *Rosmarinus officinalis* L. essential oil compared to its main components. Food Chem 2008; 108(3): 1019-22.
[http://dx.doi.org/10.1016/j.foodchem.2007.11.046] [PMID: 26065766]

[47] Hussain AI, Anwar F, Chatha SAS, Jabbar A, Mahboob S, Nigam PS. *Rosmarinus officinalis* essential oil: antiproliferative, antioxidant and antibacterial activities. Braz J Microbiol 2010; 41(4): 1070-8.
[http://dx.doi.org/10.1590/S1517-83822010000400027] [PMID: 24031588]

[48] Jordán MJ, Lax V, Rota MC, *et al.* Effect of bioclimatic area on the essential oil composition and antibacterial activity of *Rosmarinus officinalis* L. Food Control 2013; 30: 463-8.
[http://dx.doi.org/10.1016/j.foodcont.2012.07.029]

[49] Abdellatif F, Boudjella H, Zitouni A, Hassani A. Chemical composition and antimicrobial activity of the essential oil from leaves of Algerian *Melissa officinalis* L. EXCLI J 2014; 13: 772-81.
[PMID: 26417300]

[50] Boukhatem MN, Kameli A, Saidi F. Essential oil of Algerian rose-scented geranium (*Pelargonium graveolens*): Chemical composition and antimicrobial activity against food spoilage pathogens. Food Control 2013; 34: 208-13.
[http://dx.doi.org/10.1016/j.foodcont.2013.03.045]

[51] Boukhris M, Bouaziz M, Feki I, Jemai H, El Feki A, Sayadi S. Hypoglycemic and antioxidant effects of leaf essential oil of *Pelargonium graveolens* L'Hér. in alloxan induced diabetic rats. Lipids Health Dis 2012; 11: 81.
[http://dx.doi.org/10.1186/1476-511X-11-81] [PMID: 22734822]

[52] Judzentiene A. Atypical chemical profiles of wild yarrow (*Achillea millefolium* L.) essential oils. Rec Nat Prod 2016; 10: 262.

[53] Hajlaoui H, Mighri H, Aouni M, Gharsallah N, Kadri A. Chemical composition and *in vitro* evaluation of antioxidant, antimicrobial, cytotoxicity and anti-acetylcholinesterase properties of Tunisian *Origanum majorana* L. essential oil. Microb Pathog 2016; 95: 86-94.
[http://dx.doi.org/10.1016/j.micpath.2016.03.003] [PMID: 26997648]

[54] Nicolás C, Hermosa R, Rubio B, Mukherjee PK, Monte E. *Trichoderma* genes in plants for stress tolerance- status and prospects. Plant Sci 2014; 228: 71-8.
[http://dx.doi.org/10.1016/j.plantsci.2014.03.005] [PMID: 25438787]

[55] Morens DM, Fauci AS. Emerging infectious diseases: threats to human health and global stability. PLoS Pathog 2013; 9(7): e1003467.
[http://dx.doi.org/10.1371/journal.ppat.1003467] [PMID: 23853589]

[56] Baumgardner DJ. Soil-related bacterial and fungal infections. J Am Board Fam Med 2012; 25(5): 734-44.
[http://dx.doi.org/10.3122/jabfm.2012.05.110226] [PMID: 22956709]

[57] Ahmadian E, Samiei M, Hasanzadeh A, *et al.* Monitoring of drug resistance towards reducing the toxicity of pharmaceutical compounds: Past, present and future. J Pharm Biomed Anal 2020; 186: 113265.
[http://dx.doi.org/10.1016/j.jpba.2020.113265] [PMID: 32283481]

[58] Ballal M. Trends in Antimicrobial Resistance Among Enteric Pathogens: A Global Concern.Antibiotic Resistance: Mechanisms and New Antimicrobial Approaches. New York, USA: Elsevier Science 2016; pp. 63-92.
[http://dx.doi.org/10.1016/B978-0-12-803642-6.00004-6]

[59] Swartz MN. Human diseases caused by foodborne pathogens of animal origin. Clin Infect Dis 2002; 34 (Suppl. 3): S111-22.
[http://dx.doi.org/10.1086/340248] [PMID: 11988881]

[60] Kouidhi B, Al Qurashi YMA, Chaieb K. Drug resistance of bacterial dental biofilm and the potential

use of natural compounds as alternative for prevention and treatment. Microb Pathog 2015; 80: 39-49.
[http://dx.doi.org/10.1016/j.micpath.2015.02.007] [PMID: 25708507]

[61]   Ferreira J, Ramos AA, Almeida T, Azqueta A, Rocha E. Drug resistance in glioblastoma and cytotoxicity of seaweed compounds, alone and in combination with anticancer drugs: A mini review. Phytomedicine 2018; 48: 84-93.
[http://dx.doi.org/10.1016/j.phymed.2018.04.062] [PMID: 30195884]

[62]   Klančnik A, Piskernik S, Jeršek B, Možina SS. Evaluation of diffusion and dilution methods to determine the antibacterial activity of plant extracts. J Microbiol Methods 2010; 81(2): 121-6.
[http://dx.doi.org/10.1016/j.mimet.2010.02.004] [PMID: 20171250]

[63]   Hostettmann K, Wolfender J-L, Rodriguez S. Rapid detection and subsequent isolation of bioactive constituents of crude plant extracts. Planta Med 1997; 63(1): 2-10.
[http://dx.doi.org/10.1055/s-2006-957592] [PMID: 17252325]

[64]   Van Vuuren S, Holl D. Antimicrobial natural product research: A review from a South African perspective for the years 2009-2016. J Ethnopharmacol 2017; 208: 236-52.
[http://dx.doi.org/10.1016/j.jep.2017.07.011] [PMID: 28694104]

[65]   Balouiri M, Sadiki M, Ibnsouda SK. Methods for *in vitro* evaluating antimicrobial activity: A review. J Pharm Anal 2016; 6(2): 71-9.
[http://dx.doi.org/10.1016/j.jpha.2015.11.005] [PMID: 29403965]

[66]   Eloff JN. Avoiding pitfalls in determining antimicrobial activity of plant extracts and publishing the results. BMC Complement Altern Med 2019; 19(1): 106.
[http://dx.doi.org/10.1186/s12906-019-2519-3] [PMID: 31113428]

[67]   Tabanca N, Kirimer N, Demirci B, Demirci F, Başer KH. Composition and antimicrobial activity of the essential oils of *Micromeria cristata* subsp. *phrygia* and the enantiomeric distribution of borneol. J Agric Food Chem 2001; 49(9): 4300-3.
[http://dx.doi.org/10.1021/jf0105034] [PMID: 11559128]

[68]   Santoyo S, Cavero S, Jaime L, Ibañez E, Señoráns FJ, Reglero G. Supercritical carbon dioxide extraction of compounds with antimicrobial activity from *Origanum vulgare* L.: determination of optimal extraction parameters. J Food Prot 2006; 69(2): 369-75.
[http://dx.doi.org/10.4315/0362-028X-69.2.369] [PMID: 16496578]

[69]   Al-Farhan K, Warad I, Al-Resayes S, *et al.* Synthesis, structural chemistry and antimicrobial activity of–(−) borneol derivative. Open Chem 2010; 8: 1127-33.
[http://dx.doi.org/10.2478/s11532-010-1093-0]

[70]   Trinh H-T, Lee I-A, Hyun Y-J, Kim D-H. *Artemisia princeps* Pamp. Essential oil and its constituents eucalyptol and α-terpineol ameliorate bacterial vaginosis and vulvovaginal candidiasis in mice by inhibiting bacterial growth and NF-κB activation. Planta Med 2011; 77(18): 1996-2002.
[http://dx.doi.org/10.1055/s-0031-1280094] [PMID: 21830186]

[71]   Friedman M, Henika PR, Mandrell RE. Bactericidal activities of plant essential oils and some of their isolated constituents against *Campylobacter jejuni, Escherichia coli, Listeria monocytogenes*, and *Salmonella enterica.* J Food Prot 2002; 65(10): 1545-60.
[http://dx.doi.org/10.4315/0362-028X-65.10.1545] [PMID: 12380738]

[72]   Setzer WN, Vogler B, Schmidt JM, Leahy JG, Rives R. Antimicrobial activity of *Artemisia douglasiana* leaf essential oil. Fitoterapia 2004; 75(2): 192-200.
[http://dx.doi.org/10.1016/j.fitote.2003.12.019] [PMID: 15030924]

[73]   Sonboli A, Mojarrad M, Gholipour A, *et al.* Biological activity and composition of the essential oil of *Dracocephalum moldavica* L. grown in Iran. Nat Prod Commun 2008; 3.

[74]   Pontes EKU, Melo HM, Nogueira JWA, *et al.* Antibiofilm activity of the essential oil of citronella (*Cymbopogon nardus*) and its major component, geraniol, on the bacterial biofilms of *Staphylococcus aureus.* Food Sci Biotechnol 2018; 28(3): 633-9.

[http://dx.doi.org/10.1007/s10068-018-0502-2] [PMID: 31093420]

[75]    Balta I, Brinzan L, Stratakos AC, *et al.* Geraniol and linalool loaded nanoemulsions and their antimicrobial activity. Bull Univ Agric Sci Vet Med Cluj Napoca 2017; 74: 157-61.
[http://dx.doi.org/10.15835/buasvmcn-asb:0025]

[76]    Liu K, Chen Q, Liu Y, Zhou X, Wang X. Isolation and biological activities of decanal, linalool, valencene, and octanal from sweet orange oil. J Food Sci 2012; 77(11): C1156-61.
[http://dx.doi.org/10.1111/j.1750-3841.2012.02924.x] [PMID: 23106968]

[77]    Park S-N, Lim YK, Freire MO, Cho E, Jin D, Kook JK. Antimicrobial effect of linalool and α-terpineol against periodontopathic and cariogenic bacteria. Anaerobe 2012; 18(3): 369-72.
[http://dx.doi.org/10.1016/j.anaerobe.2012.04.001] [PMID: 22537719]

[78]    Herman A, Tambor K, Herman A. Linalool affects the antimicrobial efficacy of essential oils. Curr Microbiol 2016; 72(2): 165-72.
[http://dx.doi.org/10.1007/s00284-015-0933-4] [PMID: 26553262]

[79]    Yamaguchi MU, Barbosa da Silva AP, Ueda-Nakamura T, Dias Filho BP, Conceição da Silva C, Nakamura CV. Effects of a thiosemicarbazide camphene derivative on *Trichophyton mentagrophytes.* Molecules 2009; 14(5): 1796-807.
[http://dx.doi.org/10.3390/molecules14051796] [PMID: 19471200]

[80]    Thakre AD, Mulange SV, Kodgire SS, *et al.* Effects of cinnamaldehyde, ocimene, camphene, curcumin and farnesene on *Candida albicans.* Adv Microbiol 2016; 6: 627-43.
[http://dx.doi.org/10.4236/aim.2016.69062]

[81]    Pereira FdeO, Mendes JM, Lima IO, Mota KS, Oliveira WA, Lima EdeO. Antifungal activity of geraniol and citronellol, two monoterpenes alcohols, against *Trichophyton rubrum* involves inhibition of ergosterol biosynthesis. Pharm Biol 2015; 53(2): 228-34.
[http://dx.doi.org/10.3109/13880209.2014.913299] [PMID: 25414073]

[82]    Morcia C, Malnati M, Terzi V. *In vitro* antifungal activity of terpinen-4-ol, eugenol, carvone, 1,8-cineole (eucalyptol) and thymol against mycotoxigenic plant pathogens. Food Addit Contam Part A Chem Anal Control Expo Risk Assess 2012; 29(3): 415-22.
[PMID: 22257275]

[83]    Leite MCA, de Brito Bezerra AP, de Sousa JP, de Oliveira Lima E. Investigating the antifungal activity and mechanism(s) of geraniol against *Candida albicans* strains. Med Mycol 2015; 53(3): 275-84.
[http://dx.doi.org/10.1093/mmy/myu078] [PMID: 25480017]

[84]    Yuan G, Wahlqvist ML, He G, Yang M, Li D. Natural products and anti-inflammatory activity. Asia Pac J Clin Nutr 2006; 15(2): 143-52.
[PMID: 16672197]

[85]    Ghasemian M, Owlia S, Owlia MBJAips. Review of anti-inflammatory herbal medicines. Adv Pharmacol Sci 2016; 2016: 9130979.

[86]    Saudagar RB, Saokar S. Anti-inflammatory natural compounds from herbal and marine origin. J Drug Deliv Ther 2019; 9: 669-72.

[87]    Brune K, Patrignani P. New insights into the use of currently available non-steroidal anti-inflammatory drugs. J Pain Res 2015; 8: 105-18.
[http://dx.doi.org/10.2147/JPR.S75160] [PMID: 25759598]

[88]    Lukaczer D, Darland G, Tripp M, *et al.* A pilot trial evaluating Meta050, a proprietary combination of reduced iso-alpha acids, rosemary extract and oleanolic acid in patients with arthritis and fibromyalgia. Phytother Res 2005; 19(10): 864-9.
[http://dx.doi.org/10.1002/ptr.1709] [PMID: 16261517]

[89]    Almeida JRGdS, Souza GR, Silva JC, *et al.* Borneol, a bicyclic monoterpene alcohol, reduces nociceptive behavior and inflammatory response in mice. Sci World J 2013; 2013.

[90]    Juhás S, Cikos S, Czikková S, *et al.* Effects of borneol and thymoquinone on TNBS-induced colitis in mice. Folia Biol (Praha) 2008; 54(1): 1-7.
[PMID: 18226358]

[91]    Chen N, Sun G, Yuan X, *et al.* Inhibition of lung inflammatory responses by bornyl acetate is correlated with regulation of myeloperoxidase activity. J Surg Res 2014; 186(1): 436-45.
[http://dx.doi.org/10.1016/j.jss.2013.09.003] [PMID: 24120240]

[92]    Yang H, Zhao R, Chen H, Jia P, Bao L, Tang H. Bornyl acetate has an anti-inflammatory effect in human chondrocytes *via* induction of IL-11. IUBMB Life 2014; 66(12): 854-9.
[http://dx.doi.org/10.1002/iub.1338] [PMID: 25545915]

[93]    Yang L, Liu J, Li Y, Qi G. Bornyl acetate suppresses ox-LDL-induced attachment of THP-1 monocytes to endothelial cells. Biomed Pharmacother 2018; 103: 234-9.
[http://dx.doi.org/10.1016/j.biopha.2018.03.152] [PMID: 29655164]

[94]    Martins AOBPB, Rodrigues LB, Cesário FRAS, *et al.* Anti-edematogenic and anti-inflammatory activity of the essential oil from *Croton rhamnifolioides* leaves and its major constituent 1,8-cineole (eucalyptol). Biomed Pharmacother 2017; 96: 384-95.
[http://dx.doi.org/10.1016/j.biopha.2017.10.005] [PMID: 29031196]

[95]    Rocha Caldas GF, Oliveira AR, Araújo AV, *et al.* Gastroprotective mechanisms of the monoterpene 1, 8-cineole (eucalyptol). PLoS One 2015; 10(8): e0134558.
[http://dx.doi.org/10.1371/journal.pone.0134558] [PMID: 26244547]

[96]    De Fazio L, Spisni E, Cavazza E, *et al.* Dietary geraniol by oral or enema administration strongly reduces dysbiosis and systemic inflammation in dextran sulfate sodium-treated mice. Front Pharmacol 2016; 7: 38.
[http://dx.doi.org/10.3389/fphar.2016.00038] [PMID: 26973525]

[97]    Li J, Zhang X, Huang H. Protective effect of linalool against lipopolysaccharide/D-galactosamin--induced liver injury in mice. Int Immunopharmacol 2014; 23(2): 523-9.
[http://dx.doi.org/10.1016/j.intimp.2014.10.001] [PMID: 25311666]

[98]    Ma J, Xu H, Wu J, Qu C, Sun F, Xu S. Linalool inhibits cigarette smoke-induced lung inflammation by inhibiting NF-κB activation. Int Immunopharmacol 2015; 29(2): 708-13.
[http://dx.doi.org/10.1016/j.intimp.2015.09.005] [PMID: 26432179]

[99]    Peana AT, D'Aquila PS, Panin F, Serra G, Pippia P, Moretti MD. Anti inflammatory activity of linalool and linalyl acetate constituents of essential oils. Phytomedicine 2002; 9(8): 721-6.
[http://dx.doi.org/10.1078/094471102321621322] [PMID: 12587692]

[100]   Alam MN, Bristi NJ, Rafiquzzaman M. Review on *in vivo* and *in vitro* methods evaluation of antioxidant activity. Saudi Pharm J 2013; 21(2): 143-52.
[http://dx.doi.org/10.1016/j.jsps.2012.05.002] [PMID: 24936134]

[101]   Kinsella J, Frankel E, German B, Kanner J. Possible mechanisms for the protective role of antioxidants in wine and plant foods: physiological mechanisms by which flavonoids, phenolics, and other phytochemicals in wine and plant foods prevent or ameliorate some common chronic diseases are discussed. Food Technol 1993; 47: 85-9.

[102]   Velioglu Y, Mazza G, Gao L, Oomah B. Antioxidant activity and total phenolics in selected fruits, vegetables, and grain products. J Agric Food Chem 1998; 46: 4113-7.
[http://dx.doi.org/10.1021/jf9801973]

[103]   Antolovich M, Prenzler PD, Patsalides E, McDonald S, Robards K. Methods for testing antioxidant activity. Analyst (Lond) 2002; 127(1): 183-98.
[http://dx.doi.org/10.1039/b009171p] [PMID: 11827390]

[104]   Prior RL, Wu X, Schaich K. Standardized methods for the determination of antioxidant capacity and phenolics in foods and dietary supplements. J Agric Food Chem 2005; 53(10): 4290-302.
[http://dx.doi.org/10.1021/jf0502698] [PMID: 15884874]

[105] Fogang HP, Tapondjou LA, Womeni HM, *et al.* Characterization and biological activity of essential oils from fruits of *Zanthoxylum xanthoxyloides* Lam. and *Z. leprieurii* Guill. & Perr., two culinary plants from Cameroon. Flavour Fragrance J 2012; 27: 171-9.
[http://dx.doi.org/10.1002/ffj.3083]

[106] Li W, Zhou J, Xu Y. Study of the *in vitro* cytotoxicity testing of medical devices. Biomed Rep 2015; 3(5): 617-20.
[http://dx.doi.org/10.3892/br.2015.481] [PMID: 26405534]

[107] Lorge E, Hayashi M, Albertini S, Kirkland D. Comparison of different methods for an accurate assessment of cytotoxicity in the *in vitro* micronucleus test. I. Theoretical aspects. Mutat Res 2008; 655(1-2): 1-3.
[http://dx.doi.org/10.1016/j.mrgentox.2008.06.003] [PMID: 18602494]

[108] Srivastava GK, Alonso-Alonso ML, Fernandez-Bueno I, *et al.* Comparison between direct contact and extract exposure methods for PFO cytotoxicity evaluation. Sci Rep 2018; 8(1): 1425.
[http://dx.doi.org/10.1038/s41598-018-19428-5] [PMID: 29362382]

[109] Nikolić B, Vasilijević B, Mitić-Ćulafić D, Vuković-Gačić B, Knežević-Vukćević J. Comparative study of genotoxic, antigenotoxic and cytotoxic activities of monoterpenes camphor, eucalyptol and thujone in bacteria and mammalian cells. Chem Biol Interact 2015; 242: 263-71.
[http://dx.doi.org/10.1016/j.cbi.2015.10.012] [PMID: 26482939]

# CHAPTER 4

# Bioactive Compounds as Therapeutic Intervention in Cancer Therapy

**Depika Dwarka**[1], **Himansu Baijnath**[2] and **John Jason Mellem**[1,*]

[1] *Durban University of Technology, Department of Biotechnology and Food Science, Durban, KwaZulu-Natal, South Africa*

[2] *University of KwaZulu-Natal, School of Biological Sciences, Durban, South Africa*

**Abstract:** Neither transmittable nor communicable, painstakingly the second most fatal disease worldwide, cancer has gained the interest of scientists who are attempting with tenacity to decrypt its unknown facets, discover new diagnosis techniques, as well as to create improved and more efficient treatment methods. A major impediment to effective cancer therapy is the inability to destroy the complete malignant tumour growth and evolution of tumour resistance. Chemotherapeutic drugs are known for their cell death mode of action, thereby incapacitating non-cancerous cells in the process. A successful anti-cancer drug should kill or debilitate cancer cells without causing unnecessary damage to normal cells. Administration of natural bioactive compounds exemplifies an alternative technique as they are associated with lower toxicities. These bioactive molecules are effective and demonstrate great specificity as they possibly operate as potent anti-oxidants and apoptosis inducers. Moderating apoptosis might be helpful in managing, treating, or deterring cancer. Significantly, bioactive compounds are providing such templates. Plants have a long history in cancer treatment. More than 3000 species have been known for their anti-cancer potential. Over 60% of currently used anti-cancer agents are derived in one way or another from higher plants. This chapter describes the roles and advancements of the use of bioactive compounds in the treatment of cancer.

## 1. INTRODUCTION

Cancer is ranked as the second most cause of death globally. A major challenge for effective treatment of cancer is the absence of obliteration of the entire tumour cell population and the subsequent development of chemoresistance. In the past 50 years, considerable progress has been made in recognizing the molecular basis of cancer. Some anti-cancer regimens do exist, although they are linked with excessive toxicity. During the 1960s, the National Cancer Institute (USA) started to screen plant extracts with antitumor activity [1].

* **Corresponding author John Jason Mellem:** Durban University of Technology, Department of Biotechnology and Food Science, Durban, KwaZulu-Natal, South Africa ; E-mail: johnm@dut.ac.za

**Saheed Sabiu (Ed)**

Bioactive compounds isolated from medicinal plants, as powerful foundations of new anti-cancer drugs, were found to be of growing interest from then on. Administration of these bioactive compounds in low concentrations can be fatal for microorganisms and small animals however, in larger organisms, including humans, they might explicitly alter the fastest-growing tissues like the tumours [2].

We stand at a turning point in cancer therapy. The last 60 years have been dominated by drugs, which are not limited to cancer cells. Being non-specific, these drugs also destroy normal cells and can cause serious and often deadly adverse outcomes during the process. However, the future does look promising for possible success in the struggle against cancer. As a science, the use of bioactive compounds from plants acts as an anti-oxidant and can contribute to inducing signalling pathways, including apoptosis. From many natural compounds investigated, several have been shown to be promising based on their anti-cancer effects related to apoptosis. This ultimately may lead to a greater impact on tumours specifically, thus leading to the development of successful treatment.

## 2. CANCER AND APOPTOSIS

### 2.1. Global Prevalence of Cancer

Cancer is a massive hurdle in improving the average lifespan in all countries of the globe in the 21st century. In the year 2018, an estimated 9.6 million deaths occurred due to cancer [3]. On a global scale, the collective probability of prevalence indicates that 1 in 8 men and 1 in 10 women are going to develop the illness during their lifespan. By 2050, the global burden is expected to grow to 27 million new cancer cases and 17.5 million cancer deaths [4].

Cancer morbidity and mortality rates are increasing precipitously. The common rationalizations are aging and expansion of the populace, as well as socio-economic development [5]. Environmental factors, such as tobacco use, urban development, and its associated pollution, as well as changing diet patterns, also contribute immensely to the cause of this disease. The most diagnosed cancers worldwide are lung, breast, and colorectal cancers (Fig. **1**). The most common causes of cancer-causing deaths are lung, stomach, and liver cancers.

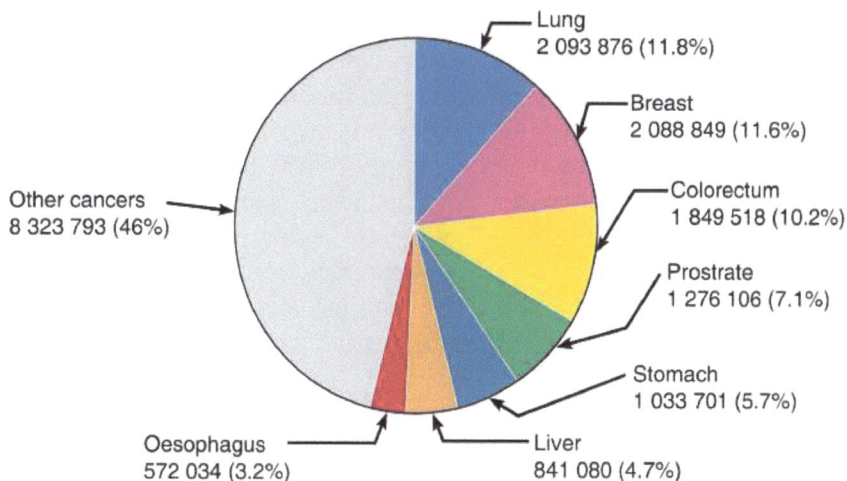

**Fig. (1).** The distribution of all-cancer types as well as incidence and mortality globally, for both sexes combined [3].

## 2.2. General Features of Cancer

Cancer is a disease in which abnormal cells divide without being regulated and can invade other tissues. This is not just one disease but many diseases. Cancer cells may spread to other components of the body through the bloodstream and lymph systems. There are more than 100 different types of cancer. Most cancers are named for the organ or type of cell in which they start.

Cancer occurs when a cell obtains adequate mutations to allow it to survive and multiply free from its normal regulation by soluble extracellular factors and by interaction with its neighbours. The genes that become deregulated are the key proteins that manage these processes. These proteins can be placed into three overlapping categories: (i) those that control signal transduction of extracellular signals regulating cell division; (ii) those that control processes associated with cell invasion; and (iii) those that affect processes associated with the cell cycle and apoptosis. In some cases, the proteins that control these processes become mutated, and they function inappropriately [2].

## 2.3. Pathophysiology of the Carcinogenic Process

The loss of self-controlled expansion is the enduring effect of the build-up of anomalies in various regulatory systems. This, therefore, results in alterations of cell mechanisms that differentiate cancerous cells from normal healthy cells [6]. The carcinogenic process that arises by the accumulation of mutations in these crucial genes follows a stepwise sequence [7]. Initially, tumor is triggered when mutations free the cell from growth restraints, and build-up of small cells occurs. As increased cell division accelerates the accumulation of further mutations, tumor promotion leads to cells that are more dysfunctional and have lost further growth controls, which will lead to uncontrolled growth. As the colonies of these cells grow, it must procure its own blood supply by the growth of blood vessels into the tumor; this process is called angiogenesis. The colonies grow to be aggressive when they developthe capability to break down local structures. During metastasis, cells from the tumor mass travel around the body to create cell colonies at other locations. The last two processes are elements of progression and are shown in Fig. (**2**). The extent of this determines the tumor type.

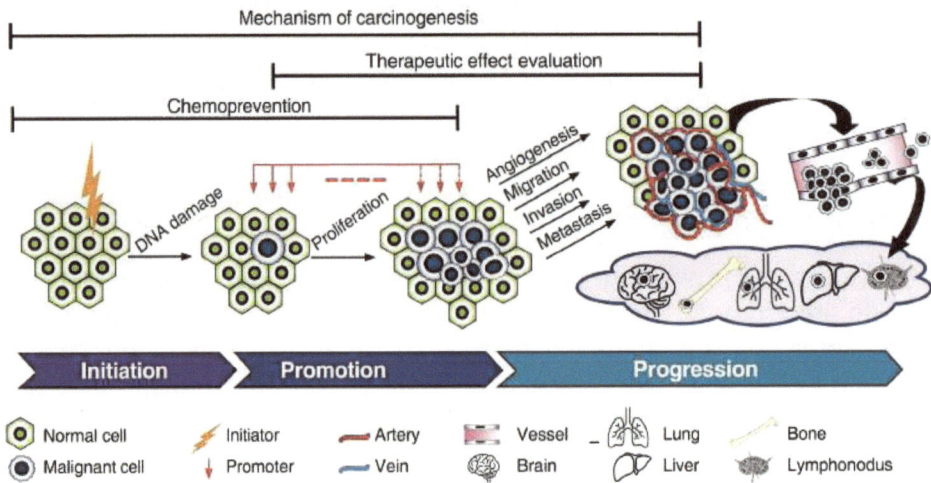

**Fig. (2).** Cancer initiation, promotion, and progression and the various research applications based on models of primary cancers [9].

In carcinogenesis, reactive oxygen species are responsible for initiating the multistage progression beginning with DNA damage and accumulation of genetic events in one or few cell lines, which leads to progressively dysplastic cellular appearance, deregulated cell growth, and finally carcinoma [8].

Currently, there are four general strategies for cancer treatment. Chemotherapy (use of chemicals), Radiotherapy (use x-rays/gamma rays), Surgery (physical extraction of tumour) and Immunotherapy (Harnesses the immune system, enabling it to fight against cancer). Unfortunately, these treatments damage cancer cells as well as healthy cells, which lead to numerous damage [10]. Therefore, scientists are concentrating on developing anti-cancer drugs from plant bioactive compounds, which in all hopes, do not implement adverse effects on the normal functioning of the body [11].

## 2.4. Apoptosis: Hallmark of Cancer Development and Progression

Apoptosis is a vital component of natural growth. The homeostatic equilibrium sandwiched between cell proliferation and cell death is crucial for the preservation of conventional physiological activities. Currently, the development of apoptosis targeting anti-cancer drugs has gained much interest since cell death prompted by apoptosis causes minimal inflammation. An ideal anti-cancer agent should be able to induce apoptosis in cancer cells while not affecting normal cells. Genetic changes resulting in loss of apoptosis or derangement of apoptosis-signaling pathways in the transformed cells are likely the determining factors of carcinogenesis [12].

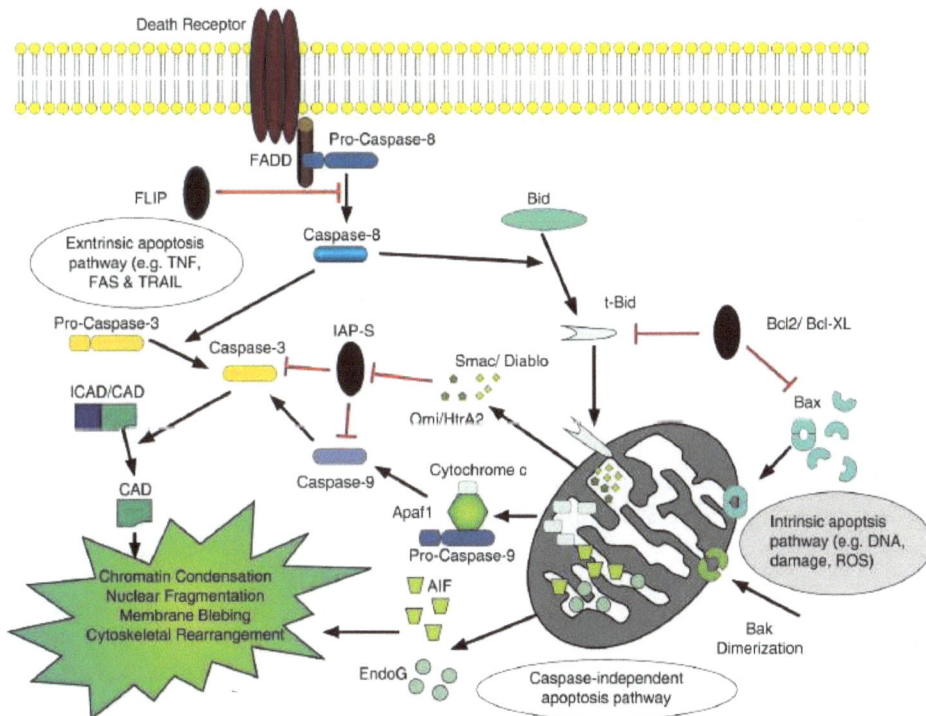

**Fig. (3).** The extrinsic and intrinsic pathways of apoptotic signalling. In both pathways, signalling results in the activation of a family of cys (cysteine) proteases, named caspases (caspase 8) that act in a proteolytic cascade to take apart and eliminate the dying cell. In the intrinsic pathway, cells in stress undergo compartmental changes involving the mitochondrion and endoplasmic reticulum permeability controlled by the Bcl-2 family, which cause the activation of initiator caspases, either caspase-9 in an apoptosome complex upon release of cytochrome C, or caspase-12 release *via* transmembrane channels across the mitochondrial outer membrane [14].

Apoptosis can be initiated through one of two pathways (Fig. **3**). In the intrinsic pathway, the cell kills itself or "commits suicide" because it senses cell stress. While in the extrinsic pathway, the cell kills itself because of signals from other cells (Fig. **3**). Both pathways induce cell death by activating caspases, which are proteases; enzymes that degrade proteins [13].

Various plants and their bioactive compounds have been proven to have anti-carcinogenic and anti-proliferative influences on the various types of cancers. Scientists have also described a positive association between the anti-oxidant activity of plants and their anti-proliferative effects, indicating the possible action of anti-oxidants in hindering cancer cell growth [15].

## 2.5. Free Radicals and Anti-oxidants in Relation to Cancer Inflammation

The recent profusion of evidence proposing the contribution of oxidative stress in the pathogenesis of cancer attracted a lot of interest in the role of anti-oxidants in the maintenance of human health and the prevention and treatment of cancer. Oxidative stress alludes to the overproduction of reactive oxygen species (ROS) in the cells as well as the tissues, whereby the anti-oxidant system does not have the ability to offset them, consequently leaving behind highly reactive free radicals in the cells. An imbalance in this defensive system may lead to the mutation of cellular molecules such as DNA, proteins, and lipids [16]. Reactive oxygen species are typically manufactured in the body in limited amounts and are essential compounds implicated in the regulation of various processes, including the maintenance of cell homeostasis and events like signal transduction, gene expression, and activation of receptors [17]. The destruction of these such mechanisms results in a permanent alteration of genetic material, representing the first stage in carcinogenesis [18]. Free radicals are deactivated by anti-oxidants. Even at small concentrations, anti-oxidants impede oxidation reactions and therefore have several critical physiological roles in the body.

Anti-oxidants can be divided into three categories of defence mechanisms, as seen in Fig. (**4**). The first category of anti-oxidants has been implicated in averting the formation of new free radicals, for example, reducing hydrogen peroxide and lipid hydroperoxides to water and lipid hydroxides, respectively, or by sequestering metal ions such as iron and copper. The second category captures existing free radicals to prevent oxidative chain reactions. Superoxide dismutase (SOD) converts superoxide to hydrogen peroxide, while carotenoids scavenge singlet oxygen either physically or chemically. The third category is solely responsible for repairing the harm caused by free radicals to biomolecules, such as lipases, proteases, DNA repair enzymes and transferases [19]. Additionally, the revision mechanism functions as the fourth line protection, where suitable anti-oxidants are created at exactly the right moment and moved to the correct position in the appropriate concentration.

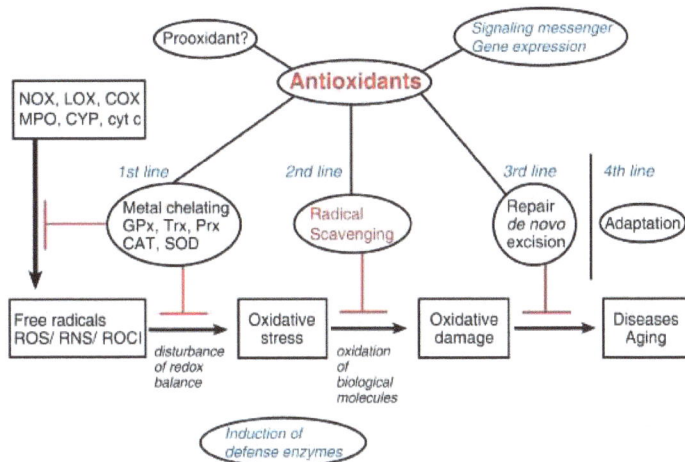

**Fig. (4).** Defence network *in vivo* against oxidative stress. Various anti-oxidants with different functions play their roles in the defence network, the free radical scavenging anti-oxidants being one of the players [20].

Anti-oxidant constituents of plant materials act as radical scavengers, and convert the radicals to less reactive species [21]. Over the last few years, scientific and research interest has been diverted towards sources of natural anti-oxidants that encourage apoptosis, as opposed to synthetic anti-oxidants. This is due to its cost efficiency as they are abundant in nature and purportedly have fewer side effects than synthetic anti-oxidants.

## 3. MEDICINAL PLANTS: THEIR USE IN ANTI-CANCER TREATMENT

The anti-cancer properties of plants have been acknowledged for centuries. In the 1950's the search for anti-cancer agents from plant sources began. As an outcome, in the 1960's the National Cancer Institute (NCI) introduced an all-encompassing plant compilation database [22]. The program resulted in the breakthrough of novel chemotypes that demonstrated a variety of cytotoxic potential, but their evolution into clinically active agents lasted over 30 years from the early 1960s to the 1990s. In 1982 the plant collection program was terminated. In 1986 the collection of plants and other organisms was revived due to technological advancement [23].

The Plant Kingdom produces naturally occurring secondary metabolites, which are being investigated for their anti-cancer activities leading to the development of new clinical drugs. Novel natural compounds from plants can be isolated by fractionation and isolation using modern analytical and chemical techniques [23]. Recent reports published by the World Health Organization (WHO) showed that although many advanced countries have considered the traditional herbal treatment as an official treatment for cancer, only 5–15% of these herbs have been examined to identify their bioactive compounds, *i.e.*, anti-cancer compounds [24].

## 3.1. Plant Based Chemotherapeutics

There are various classes of plant-derived anti-cancer agents in the market today. For example, the vinca alkaloids (vinblastine, vincristine and vindesine), the epipodophyllotoxins (etoposide and teniposide), the taxanes (paclitaxel and docetaxel) and the camptothecin derivatives (camptothecin and irinotecan) [25].

### *3.1.1. Camptothecin*

During a screening program led by the NCI in the late 50s, it was confirmed that a compound from *Camptotheca acuminata* (Fig. **5**) had anti-cancer properties [26]. Later, in 1966, a quinoline alkaloid camptothecin (CPT) (Fig. **5**), was extracted from bark (and wood), by Wall and other researchers of the Research Triangle Institute [27]. After that CPTs became the second most important source of anti-cancer drugs [28].

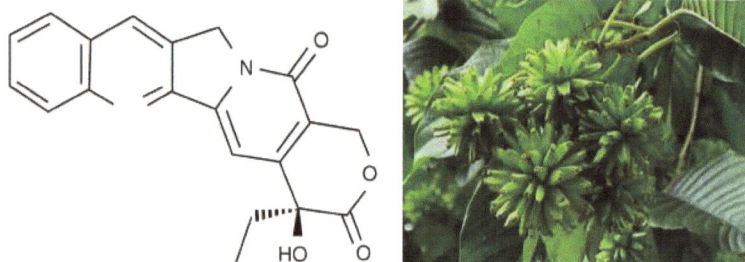

**Fig. (5).** Camptothecin (A), a monoterpene indole alkaloid, is isolated from the bark and stems of *Camptotheca acuminata* [29].

Camptothecin and its close chemical relatives aminocamptothecin, CPT-11 [irinotecan], DX-8951f, and topotecan are S phase specific anti-cancer agents that inhibit the activity of the enzyme DNA topoisomerase I (Fig. **6**) [30].

The significant limitations of the drug is the inadequate solubility and inactivity at physiological conditions, preventing full clinical application. Additionally, interpatient variability has been detected in numerous cases using the CPTs. The incapability to precisely ascertain an optimal dose for all patients has restricted the value of these drugs until improved methods for patient-specific therapies have been developed [32].

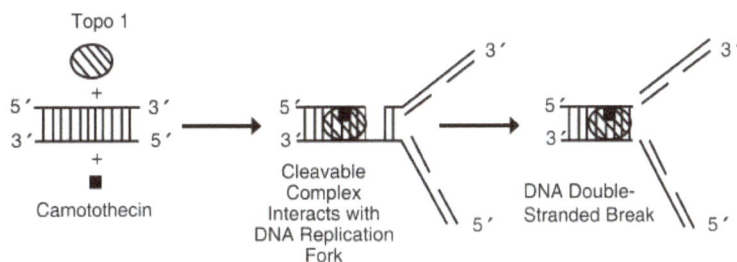

**Fig. (6).** Mechanism of action of camptothecin. Topo I is an enzyme that causes transient DNA single strand breaks that are re-joined a complex with the broken DNA strand during replication and transcription in normal cells. CPT binds to the topo I–DNA complex, thereby inhibiting re-joining of the broken strand [31].

## 3.1.2. Paclitaxel and Docetaxel

Paclitaxel (Taxol) illustrated in Fig. (**7B**) and docetaxel (Taxotere) are diterpenoids originally isolated from the bark of the *Taxus brevifolius* (Fig. **7A**) by Mansukh Wani and Monroe Wall [27]. Although taxol is presently isolated from the dried bark, it is implemented that it could not be required to supply enough of the drug. It necessitates the bark from about three matured 100-year-old trees to supply one gram of taxol. Usually, a course of treatment might require 2 grams of taxol. Present demand for taxol is in the region of 100–200 kg per annum [33].

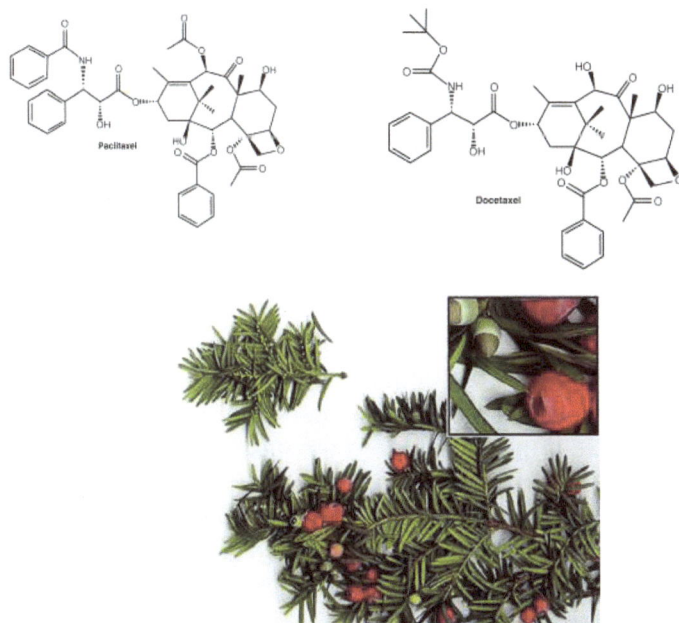

**Fig. (7).** Paclitaxel and docetaxel (**A**) were first isolated in 1971 from *Taxus brevifolius* (**B**) [34].

Paclitaxel binds to the microtubules and inhibits their depolymerization (Fig. **8**) into tubulin [35]. This obstructs the cells' capability to break down the mitotic spindle through mitosis and therefore prevents cells from dividing into two daughter cells triggering G2-M arrest [36, 35]. Paclitaxel is an intravenous drug the most efficient against ovarian carcinomas and advanced breast carcinomas.

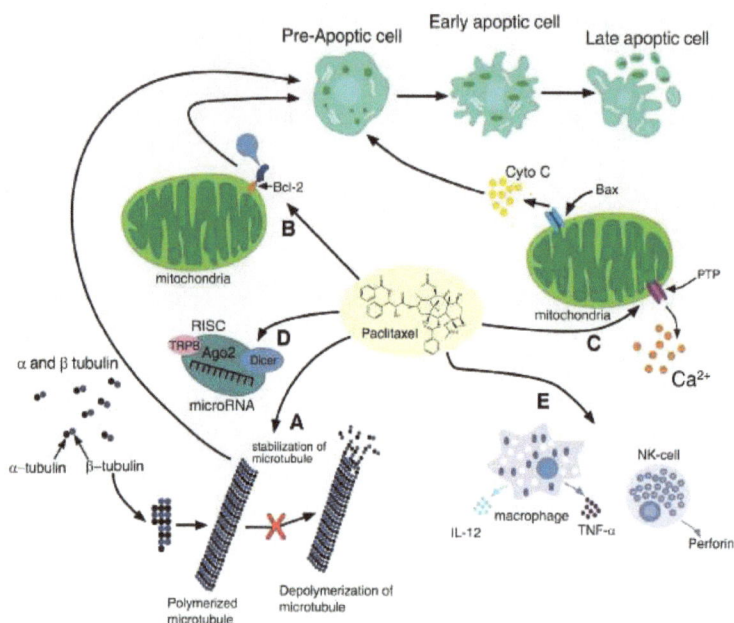

**Fig. (8).** Mode of action of Taxol. Anti-tumor mechanism of action of taxol leads to the steadiness of microtubules, cell arrest, and ensuing apoptosis **(A)**. Taxol also triggers an immune response supporting tumour annihilation **(B)**. Taxol inactivates Bcl-2 *via* phosphorylation of the anti-apoptotic protein, which leads to apoptosis **(C)**. It also contributes to the regulation of certain miRNAs linked with the adjustment of tumour progression **(D)**. Taxol also releases cyto C from the mitochondria [37].

### 3.1.3. Colchicine

Colchicine (Fig. **9A**), a water-soluble alkaloid, was isolated from the *Colchicum autumnale* (Fig. **9B**) in 1820 by Pellétier and Caventou. The margin between therapy and toxicity was only found towards the end of the nineteenth century. Colchicine is inadequately immersed from the gastrointestinal tract. The drug and its metabolites experience massive transformation in enterohepatic circulation, and it is believed that this recirculation might contribute substantially to the severe injury to the gut that happens after an overdose [38].

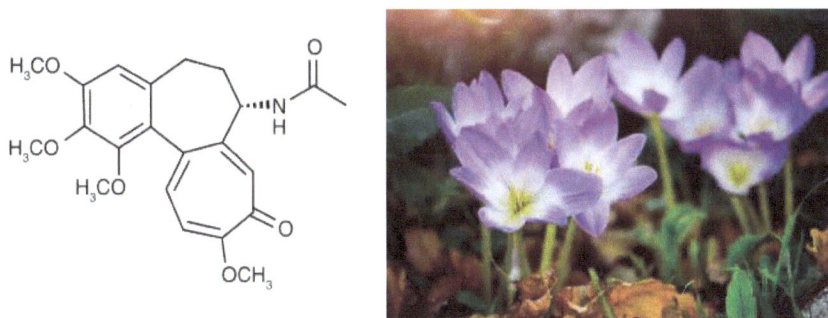

**Fig. (9).** The chemical structure of colchicine was isolated from *Colchicum autumnale* [39].

Colchicine suppresses cell division by blocking mitosis by binding with the tubulin molecule, thus preventing its assemblage into microtubules and as a result inhibiting the further development of spindles as the nuclei are dividing (Fig. **10**). It is used in veterinary medicine to treat animal cancers and used to treat gastric cancers in humans [40]. Colchicine can also enhance cellular free tubulin to limit mitochondrial metabolism in cancer cells through the inhibition of the voltage-dependent anion channels of the mitochondrial membrane [41]. The clinical use of colchicine has remained limited due to its severe toxicity, even though oral colchicine is a safe medication when properly used and contraindications were excluded [42].

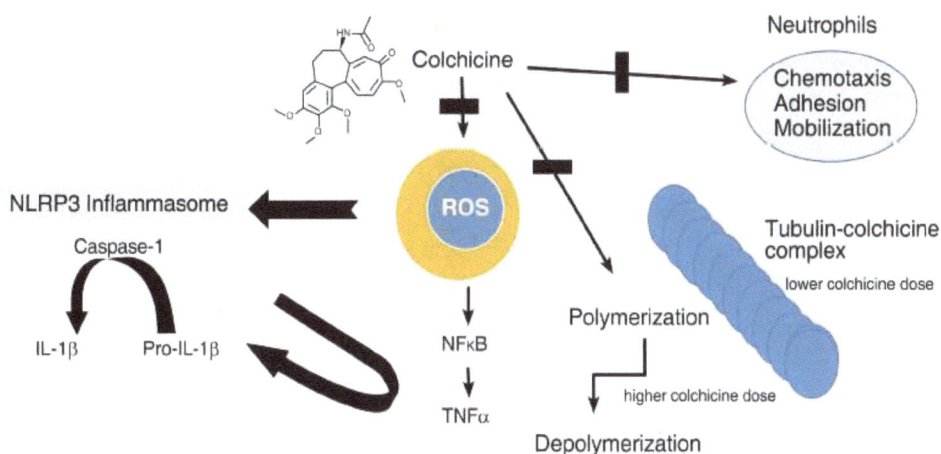

**Fig. (10).** Colchicine anti-inflammatory and tubulin depolymerization effects [43].

### 3.1.4. Vinca Alkaloids

During 1955–1960, Canadian researchers discovered the extracts of the leaves of *Catharanthus roseus* (Fig. **11**) produced leukopenic actions in rats.

Approximately 150 alkaloids were isolated from *C. roseus*, however, only six showed effectiveness in this cancer treatment [33], which contains those having antineoplastic activity, including leurocristine (vincristine) and vincaleukoblastine (vinblastine).

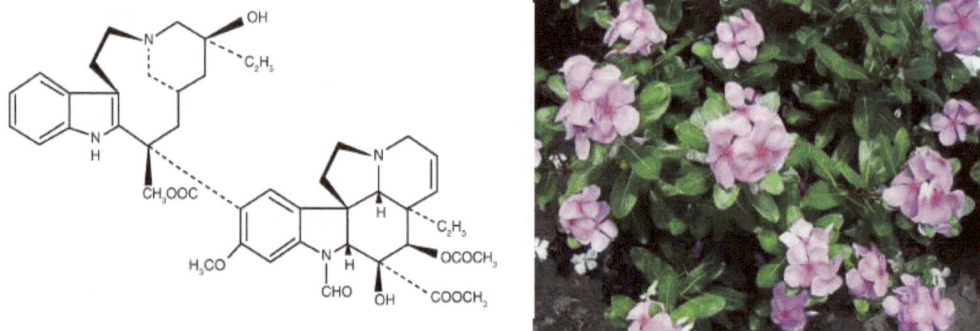

**Fig. (11).** Molecular structure of vincristine **(A)** isolated from the leaves of *Catharanthus roseus* **(B)**.

Vinca alkaloids inhibit cell proliferation through binding microtubules, which results in mitotic blockages and apoptosis. Vincristine and related compounds induce the destabilization of microtubules. Exposure of cells to vinca alkaloids influences the induction of tumour protein p53 and cyclin-dependent kinase inhibitor 1A as well as rapidly alters protein kinase events. However, the vinca alkaloids as well as the other antimicrotubule vehicles also have an impact on both non-malignant and malignant cells in the non-mitotic cell cycle since microtubules are engaged in many non-mitotic events [44]. Vinca alkaloids have been utilized as an essential component of medicinal treatment regimens for testicular carcinoma and both Hodgkin and non-Hodgkin lymphomas. It has also been used in breast cancer and germ cell tumours [45].

### 3.1.5. Homoharringtonine

Homoharringtonine (Fig. **12A**) is an alkaloid isolated from the bark of *Cephalotaxus harringtonii* (Fig. **12B**). Homoharringtonine is indicated for use as a treatment for patients with chronic myeloid leukaemia [46].

Homoharringtonine is a first-in-class protein translation inhibitor, which implies that it suppresses the elongation step of protein synthesis. Furthermore, homoharringtonine binds to the A-site of the larger ribosomal subunit, an operation that stops the entry of the charged tRNA and subsequently the peptide bond development [48]. Given that this chemical is not aimed at a specific protein, its success has primarily been due to the fact that this may interfere with proteins with speedy turnover for *e.g.*, the leukemic cells upregulated short-lived oncoproteins BCR-ABL1 and antiapoptotic proteins (Mcl-1, Myc) leading to cell apoptosis [49].

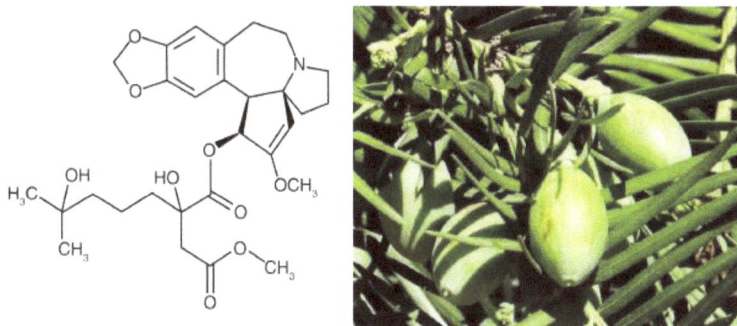

**Fig. (12).** Homoharringtonine (**A**) isolated a cytotoxic alkaloid initially isolated from the evergreen tree, *Cephalotaxus hainanensis* (**B**) [47].

### 3.1.6. Podophyllotoxin

In the 1880's, podophyllotoxin was first isolated by Podwyssotzki from the North American plant *Podophyllum peltatum* L., commonly referred to as the American mandrake or May apple. This compound is the most common lignan in podophyllin (Fig. **13**), a resin generated by species of the genus *Podophyllum* [50]. Clinical trials on the use of podophyllotoxin showed that the use of this natural product could be helpful in the treatment of some cancers, especially lung cancer [51].

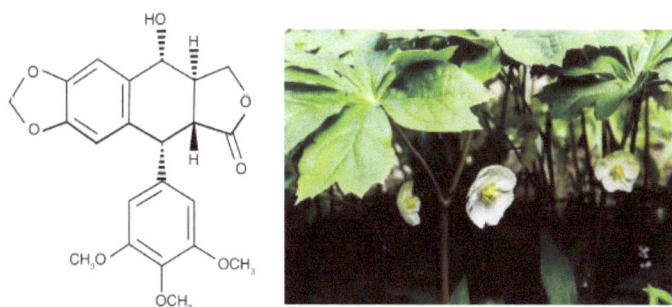

**Fig. (13).** The structure of podophyllotoxin (**A**) isolated from *Podophyllum peltatum* (**B**).

Abad [52] showed that the podophyllotoxin mechanism could be anti-neoplastic, whereby it blocks the construction of tubulin into microtubules and thereby encourages apoptosis. This was in line with studies by Passarella [53]. They showed that podophyllotoxin works by preventing the polymerization of tubulin, thus inducing cell cycle arrest at mitosis and impeding the formation of the mitotic-spindles microtubules. Chen [54], confirmed that preclinical studies demonstrated that podophyllotoxin blocked the polymerization of microtubules which has resulted in mitotic detention as shown by the accumulation of mitosis-related proteins, BIRC5 and aurora B. Severe multiple organ toxicity has been noted with the use of this natural compound; therefore the user is limited.

## 3.2. Other Plant-based Compounds of Importance in Cancer Treatment

There are many new plant compound-based drug candidates in active preclinical trials. Inputs from traditional medicinal knowledge and using modern techniques to speed up the bioactive plant compound- based drug discovery; have now made us consider beyond the mere 10–15% of plant diversity that has been explored for their pharmaceutical purpose so far. Over 100 compounds are currently under way, as anti-cancer drugs alone, from plant sources. Even though some natural compounds possess unique anti-cancer influences, their application in clinical practice may not be possible owing to their physio-chemical characteristics (*e.g.,* limited bioavailability) and/or their toxicity. The following are grouped according to their class of bioactivity.

### 3.2.1. Phenolic Compounds

Phenolic compounds are a category of plant secondary metabolites that contain a polyhydroxylated phytochemical. Polyphenolic compounds that are thought to have anti-cancer activity consist of flavonoids, stilbenes, and phenolic acids [55]. Research has shown that the cytotoxic effect of phenols against various tumours is transmitted through apoptosis. Tannic acid and caffeic acid are phenols that prompted DNA disintegration only in HL-60 cells [56]. Gallic acid-induced apoptosis in HL-60 RG cells through reactive oxygen species generation, Ca2+ influx and activation of calmodulin. Curcumin, a phenolic compound that was identified as a key pigment in turmeric, stimulates apoptosis in altered rodent and human cells in culture. Curcumin facilitated the chemopreventive action by preventing the formation of cyclooxygenase (COX) metabolites, which might provide a mechanism for the initiation of apoptosis [57].

#### 3.2.1.1. Flavonoids

Flavonoids are the biggest and most diverse sub-group of polyphenolic compounds that are manufactured as plant secondary metabolites. In past etiological studies, the consumption of particular kinds of polyhydroxy phenols such as flavonoids or lignans in the diet has been associated with low incidence of colon cancer. The position of hydroxyl groups and other features in the chemical structure of flavonoids are essential to their anti-oxidant and anti-cancer activities. A flow cytometric analysis suggested that genistein (a hydroxyisoflavone) induced apoptosis in human pro-myelocytic HL-60 leukaemic cells.

Genistein is also reported to inhibit tyrosine kinase, angiogenesis, and cell-cycle progression [58]. Other flavonoids in clinical trials are listed in Table 1.

**Table 1. Bioactive flavonoids in cancer treatment.**

| Bioactive Flavanoid | Structure | Source | Mode of Action | Reference |
|---|---|---|---|---|
| Quercetin (Flavonol) | | Different vegetables and fruits, seeds, nuts, tea as well as red wine. | Quercetin downregulates Bcl-2 through the inhibition of NF-κB and inhibits phosphorylation of EGFR suppressing downstream signalling in colon carcinoma cells. | [59, 60] |
| Flavopiridol (Flavone) | | First reported from *Amoora rohituka* and later from *Dysoxylum binectariferum*) and *Schumanniophyton problematicum* | Flavopiridol inhibits phosphokinases. Its activity is strongest on cyclin dependent kinases (cdk-1, -2, -4, -6, -7) and less on receptor tyrosine kinases (EGFR), receptor associates tyrosine kinases (pp60 Src) and signal transducing kinases (PKC and Erk-1). | [61] |
| Apigenin (Flavone) | | Apigenin is present in fruits and vegetables but found abundantly in the flowers of chamomile | Inhibits proliferation by activating apoptosis, stimulating autophagy and modulating the cell cycle. Apigenin also reduces cancer cell motility and inhibits cancer cell migration and invasion. | [62, 63] |

(Table 1) cont.....

| Bioactive Flavanoid | Structure | Source | Mode of Action | Reference |
|---|---|---|---|---|
| **Catechin (Flavanol)** | | Catechin is isolated from green tea (Camellia sinensis). | Catechins protect against oxidative stress and cause cellular DNA breakage, therefore inducing apoptosis. | [64, 65]. |
| **Hesperetin (Flavanone)** | | Hesperetin is found in large amounts in the rinds of some citrus species | Reported as an anti-oxidant and anti-inflammatory agent. Studies suggest that hesperetin inhibits tumor cell metastasis, angiogenesis, and chemoresistance. | [66, 67] |
| **Cyanidin (Anthocyanin)** | | Found in grapes, berries, pomegranate, red cabbage, corn, and apples | The potential antitumour effects are reported to be based on a wide variety of biological activities, including anti-oxidant, inhibiting proliferation by modulating signal transduction pathways, inducing cell cycle arrest and stimulating apoptosis or autophagy of cancer cells as well as anti-invasion and anti-metastasis | [68, 69] |

## 3.2.1.2. Stilbenes

Natural stilbenes are an important group of nonflavonoid phytochemicals of polyphenolic structure categorized by the presence of a 1,2-diphenylethylene nucleus. There are over 400 naturally occurring stilbenes [70]. The natural stilbene, resveratrol, is found in multiple foods, for example, mulberries, peanuts, grapes, and red wine. Its potential anti-cancer activity was originally reported by Jang [71]. It has been tested against various types of cancers. According to Singh

[72], resveratrol acts through multiple mechanisms, including pro-apoptotic, anti-proliferative, anti-inflammatory, and anti-angiogenesis mechanisms.

### 3.2.1.3. Phenolic Acids

Phenolic acids are secondary metabolites that are available in almost all plant-derived foods. These compounds may be divided into two major groups, hydroxybenzoic and hydroxycinnamic acids, which have been derived from the non-phenolic benzoic and cinnamic acids [55]. Phenolics acid's effectiveness as anti-cancer compounds is mostly ascribed to them being durable radical scavengers, modifiers of superoxide dismutase (SOD), catalase (CAT), glutathione peroxidases (GPx), enhancers of glutathione (GSH) redox status, and regulators of diverse proteins and transcriptional factors such as nuclear factor erythroid related factor (NRF2) [73]. Furthermore, their anti-carcinogenic potential is related to their ability to inhibit cell proliferation (extracellular signal-regulated kinase (Erk)1/2, D-type cyclins, and cyclin-dependent kinases (CDKs)), angiogenic factors (vascular endothelial growth factor (VEGF) and MIC-1), oncogenic signalling cascades (phosphoinositide 3-kinase (PI3K) and protein kinase B (Akt)), inducing apoptosis, and preventing cellular migration and metastasis [74]. Phenolic acids such as hydroxybenzoic and hydroxycinnamic acids and their derivatives play a crucial role in not only the treatment of cancer but contribute immensely to the prevention.

### 3.2.2. Alkaloids

Alkaloids are the principal group of low molecular weight organic nitrogenous compounds isolated from terrestrial and marine sources. The structural diversity of this compound occurs; due to the broad number of amino acids used as building blocks [75]. Some of the well-known alkaloids that induce apoptosis, as discussed in the previous sections, are vinblastine, topotecan, taxol, and vincristine which are used clinically in cancer therapy globally. Other studies showed that solamargine, an alkaloid obtained from the Chinese herb *Solanum incanum*, has been observed to promote apoptosis in human hepatocyte (Hep-3B) and normal skin fibroblast cells in culture. Additionally, Chang [76], has shown that the gene expression of TNF receptor I was up-regulated within 30 min of solamargine treatment. Whilst TNF receptor I have been engaged in apoptosis, its over-expression may be linked to the mechanism of cytotoxicity of solamargine.

### 3.2.3. Polysaccharides

The anti-cancer potential of polysaccharides has been identified for the first time by Nauts [77]. These researchers found that certain polysaccharides may possibly prompt full remission in with cancer suffers. Nevertheless, due to their structural complexity and certain redundant structures that stimulate a function, the therapeutic capacity of polysaccharides has not been well exploited [78].

Xu [78], proposed that polysaccharides elicit their effects on cancer cells by induction of tumor cell apoptosis, cell cycle arrest, anti-angiogenesis, preventing the synthesis of protein and nucleic acid, inhibiting tumor invasion, adhesion, and metastasis. Very recently, the underlying anti-tumour mechanism has been revealed that certain polysaccharides trigger immune response to induce tumour cell apoptosis through caspase 3-dependent signalling pathway and inhibit tumour cell proliferation through targeting p53 *via* enhancement of p21, as well as anti-angiogenesis. He [79], investigated the *in vitro* and *in vivo* anti-cancer effects of *Cyclocarya paliurus* polysaccharide on thyroid carcinoma. They showed that the polysaccharide exerts an anti-cancer effect on thyroid cancer cells through p-Akt, Akt, Bcl-2, and Bax pathways.

### 3.2.4. Terpenoids

As the most abundant class of natural raw materials, terpenoids comprise roughly 25,000 chemical compositions with possible practical use in the pharmaceutical and chemical industries specifically [80]. Terpenoids are structure-wise encompassing monoterpenoids, sesquiterpenoids, diterpenoids, triterpenoids and tetraterpenoids, where triterpenoids are among the most widely studied in anti-cancer research [81]. The table below (Table **2**) summarizes the potential anti-cancer activities and mechanisms of some of the classes of terpenoids.

**Table 2. Terpenoids that possess anti-cancer activity.**

| Class | Name of Compound | Structure | Mechanism of Action | Reference |
|---|---|---|---|---|
| **Monoterpenoid** | D-limonene (isolated from *Citrus limon* L.) | | In an orthotopic a mouse model for human gastric cancer, D-limonene inhibits tumor growth and metastasis, probably *via* its antiangiogenic, pro-apoptotic, and anti-oxidant effects. | [82] |

*(Table 2) cont.....*

| Class | Name of Compound | Structure | Mechanism of Action | Reference |
|---|---|---|---|---|
| **Sesquiterpenoid** | Artemisinin (isolated from *Artemisia annua* L) | | The anti-cancer mechanisms of artemisinin are associated to the cleavage of iron- or heme-mediated peroxide bridge | [83] |
| **Diterpenoids** | Triptolide (isolated from *Tripterygium wilfordii* Hook.f.) | | Triptolide disrupts several transcription factors, including NF-kB, p53, NF-AT, and HSF-1 | [84] |
| | Pseudolaric acid B (isolated from *Pseudolarix kaempferi)* | | Contributes to microtubule blocking and hence apoptosis | [85] |

*(Table 2) cont.....*

| Class | Name of Compound | Structure | Mechanism of Action | Reference |
|---|---|---|---|---|
| **Triterpenoids** | Celastrol | | Celastrol inactivates the Cdc37 and p23 proteins and inhibits AKT/mTOR/P70S6K signalling to mediate the tumor growth suppression and angiogenesis | [86] |
| | Alisol | | Alisol B 23-acetate mediates G2/M cell cycle arrest and evokes apoptosis in cancer cells as well as the inhibition of PI3K/Akt signaling pathway, upregulation of Bax/Bcl-2 ratio, and activation of caspases which contribute to its anti-cancer effect | [87] |

### 3.2.5. Quinones

Quinones are plant-derived secondary metabolites that are a class of compounds with the quinone structure and are primarily divided into four categories, conferring to the number of benzene rings in the structure, explicitly, benzoquinone, naphthoquinone, phenanthrenequinone, and anthraquinon. Aloe-emodin is a bioactive hydroxyanthraquinone that is isolated from *Rheum palmatum* L. This quinone unusually inhibits chorioallantoic membrane angiogenesis at low concentrations and inhibits tubule recognition of endothelial cells on Matrigel. Aloe-emodin inhibits cancer cell migration, invasion, and metastasis. Shikonin, a quinone ingredient of *Lithospermum erythrorhizon* Siebole & Zucc. prompted apoptosis in HL-60 leukaemia cell line. The surge of apoptotic cells by shikonin treatment was headed by the activation of caspase-3, which plays a pivotal role in the apoptotic process [89]. Thymoquinone is an effective benzoquinone isolated from *Nigella sativa* L. The anti-cancer properties of thymoquinone are facilitated across the various mechanisms of action, involving antiproliferation, apoptosis induction, cell cycle arrest, anti-metastasis, and anti-angiogenesis [90].

## CONCLUSION

Conventional drugs employed in cancer treatment have been proven to provoke resistance in tumour eradication, resulting in the number of cells multiplying explicitly, perhaps through the modulation of tumour cell mechanisms such as proliferative or anti-apoptotic proteins. Different statistics are presented on the anti-cancer potential of bioactive compounds in cancer treatment. Higher plants linger to hold their historical worth as imperative foundations of new composites used directly as anti-cancer drugs or as sources of building blocks for generations of synthetic drugs. The plant bioactive compounds depicted in the above review and numerous other examples help illuminate the ongoing significance of plant derived secondary metabolites as practical compounds of modern anti-cancer drug development. The research that is summarized strongly indicates that natural metabolites from plants perform a substantial role as being the greatest leading foundation of anti-cancer treatments.

## CONSENT FOR PUBLICATION

Not applicable.

## CONFLICT OF INTEREST

The authors declare no conflict of interest, financial or otherwise.

## ACKNOWLEDGEMENTS

Declared none.

## REFERENCES

[1]     Monks NR, Bordignon SA, Ferraz A, *et al.* Anti-tumour screening of Brazilian plants. Pharm Biol 2002; 40(8): 603-16.
[http://dx.doi.org/10.1076/phbi.40.8.603.14658]

[2]     Boik J. Natural compounds in cancer therapy. Princeton, MN: Oregon Medical Press 2001.

[3]     World Health Organization. Cancer Geneva 2019. Available from: https://www. who. int/news-room/fact-sheets/detail/cancer

[4]     Bray F, Ferlay J, Soerjomataram I, Siegel RL, Torre LA, Jemal A. Global cancer statistics 2018: GLOBOCAN estimates of incidence and mortality worldwide for 36 cancers in 185 countries. CA Cancer J Clin 2018; 68(6): 394-424.
[http://dx.doi.org/10.3322/caac.21492] [PMID: 30207593]

[5]     Omran AR. The epidemiologic transition. A theory of the Epidemiology of population change. 1971. Bull World Health Organ 2001; 79(2): 161-70.
[PMID: 11246833]

[6]     Cancer. 1996. Available from: https://www.mdpi.com/journal/cancers/sections/Cancer_ Pathophysiology (accessed 17 November 2020).

[7]     Perera F, Hemminki K, Jedrychowski W, *et al.* In utero DNA damage from environmental pollution is

associated with somatic gene mutation in newborns. Cancer Epidemiol Biomarkers Prev 2002; 11(10 Pt 1): 1134-7.
[PMID: 12376523]

[8]    Van Cruchten S, Van Den Broeck W. Morphological and biochemical aspects of apoptosis, oncosis and necrosis. Anat Histol Embryol 2002; 31(4): 214-23.
[http://dx.doi.org/10.1046/j.1439-0264.2002.00398.x] [PMID: 12196263]

[9]    Liu Y, Yin T, Feng Y, *et al.* Mammalian models of chemically induced primary malignancies exploitable for imaging-based preclinical theragnostic research. Quant Imaging Med Surg 2015; 5(5): 708-29.
[PMID: 26682141]

[10]   Pearce A, Haas M, Viney R, *et al.* Incidence and severity of self-reported chemotherapy side effects in routine care: A prospective cohort study. PLoS One 2017; 12(10): e0184360.
[http://dx.doi.org/10.1371/journal.pone.0184360] [PMID: 29016607]

[11]   Dwarka D, Thaver V, Naidu M, Koorbanally NA, Baijnath AH. *In vitro* chemo-preventative activity of Strelitzia nicolai aril extract containing bilirubin. Afr J Tradit Complement Altern Med 2017; 14(3): 147-56.
[http://dx.doi.org/10.21010/ajtcam.v14i3.16] [PMID: 28480426]

[12]   Kaufmann SH, Vaux DL. Alterations in the apoptotic machinery and their potential role in anticancer drug resistance. Oncogene 2003; 22(47): 7414-30.
[http://dx.doi.org/10.1038/sj.onc.1206945] [PMID: 14576849]

[13]   Slattery J, Frye RE. Application of N-Acetylcysteine in Psychiatric Disorders.The Therapeutic Use of N-Acetylcysteine (NAC) in Medicine. Singapore: Adis 2019; pp. 203-18.
[http://dx.doi.org/10.1007/978-981-10-5311-5_12]

[14]   Ghavami S, Hashemi M, Ande SR, *et al.* Apoptosis and cancer: mutations within caspase genes. J Med Genet 2009; 46(8): 497-510.
[http://dx.doi.org/10.1136/jmg.2009.066944] [PMID: 19505876]

[15]   Bostan M, Mihaila M, Hotnog C, *et al.* Modulation of Apoptosis in Colon Cancer Cells by Bioactive Compounds. Colorectal Cancer From Pathogenesis to Treatment 2016; 1174-446.
[http://dx.doi.org/10.5772/63382]

[16]   Ďuračková Z. Some current insights into oxidative stress. Physiol Res 2010; 59(4): 459-69.
[http://dx.doi.org/10.33549/physiolres.931844] [PMID: 19929132]

[17]   Hussain T, Tan B, Yin Y, Blachier F, Tossou MC, Rahu N. Oxidative stress and inflammation: what polyphenols can do for us?. Oxidative medicine and cellular longevity 2016; 2016

[18]   Woo RA, McLure KG, Lees-Miller SP, Rancourt DE, Lee PW. DNA-dependent protein kinase acts upstream of p53 in response to DNA damage. Nature 1998; 394(6694): 700-4.
[http://dx.doi.org/10.1038/29343] [PMID: 9716137]

[19]   Sun H, Mu B, Song Z, Ma Z, Mu T. The *in vitro* anti-oxidant activity and inhibition of intracellular reactive oxygen species of sweet potato leaf polyphenols. Oxid Med Cell Longev 2018; •••: 2018.

[20]   Niki E. Assessment of antioxidant capacity *in vitro* and *in vivo*. Free Radic Biol Med 2010; 49(4): 503-15.
[http://dx.doi.org/10.1016/j.freeradbiomed.2010.04.016] [PMID: 20416370]

[21]   Mandal S, Yadav S, Yadav S, Nema RK. Anti-oxidants: a review. J Chem Pharm Res 2009; 1(1): 102-4.

[22]   Cai Y, Luo Q, Sun M, Corke H. Antioxidant activity and phenolic compounds of 112 traditional Chinese medicinal plants associated with anticancer. Life Sci 2004; 74(17): 2157-84.
[http://dx.doi.org/10.1016/j.lfs.2003.09.047] [PMID: 14969719]

[23]   Svejda B, Aguiriano-Moser V, Sturm S, *et al.* Anticancer activity of novel plant extracts from

Trailliaedoxa gracilis (W. W. Smith & Forrest) in human carcinoid KRJ-I Cells. Anticancer Res 2010; 30(1): 55-64.
[PMID: 20150617]

[24] Hassan B. Plants and Cancer Treatment. Med Plants Use Prev Treat Dis 2019; 1-11.

[25] Desai AG, Qazi GN, Ganju RK, *et al.* Medicinal plants and cancer chemoprevention. Curr Drug Metab 2008; 9(7): 581-91.
[http://dx.doi.org/10.2174/138920008785821657] [PMID: 18781909]

[26] Pettit GR. Progress in the discovery of biosynthetic anticancer drugs. J Nat Prod 1996; 59(8): 812-21.
[http://dx.doi.org/10.1021/np9604386] [PMID: 8792630]

[27] Duke JA, Ayensu ES. Medicinal plants of China. Reference Publications 1985.

[28] Kintzios SE. Nature's pharmacy for cancer treatment.Plants that fight cancer. CRC Press 2019.

[29] Epharmacognosy 2020. Available from: http://www.epharmacognosy.com/ 2020/04/camptotheca-acuminata-decne.html

[30] Cragg GM. Paclitaxel (Taxol): a success story with valuable lessons for natural product drug discovery and development. Med Res Rev 1998; 18(5): 315-31.
[http://dx.doi.org/10.1002/(SICI)1098-1128(199809)18:5<315::AID-MED3>3.0.CO;2-W] [PMID: 9735872]

[31] Rajasekharan PE, Kareem VA, Kavitha P. Enhancement of Camptothecin Production in Nothapodytes nimmoniana, Graham., an Anticancerous Medicinal Plant: Current and Future Perspective. DNA 2011; 5(3): 5.

[32] Venditto VJ, Simanek EE. Cancer therapies utilizing the camptothecins: a review of the *in vivo* literature. Mol Pharm 2010; 7(2): 307-49.
[http://dx.doi.org/10.1021/mp900243b] [PMID: 20108971]

[33] Pezzuto JM. Plant-derived anticancer agents. Biochem Pharmacol 1997; 53(2): 121-33.
[http://dx.doi.org/10.1016/S0006-2952(96)00654-5] [PMID: 9037244]

[34] Nrem 2020. Available from: https://www.nrem.iastate.edu/class/for356/species/Taxus_brevifolia.html (Accessed 21 November 2020).

[35] Schiff PB, Horwitz SB. Taxol assembles tubulin in the absence of exogenous guanosine 5′-triphosphate or microtubule-associated proteins. Biochemistry 1981; 20(11): 3247-52.
[http://dx.doi.org/10.1021/bi00514a041] [PMID: 6113842]

[36] Schiff PB, Fant J, Horwitz SB. Promotion of microtubule assembly *in vitro* by taxol. Nature 1979; 277(5698): 665-7.
[http://dx.doi.org/10.1038/277665a0] [PMID: 423966]

[37] Abu Samaan TM, Samec M, Liskova A, Kubatka P, Büsselberg D. Paclitaxel's mechanistic and clinical effects on breast cancer. Biomolecules 2019; 9(12): 789.
[http://dx.doi.org/10.3390/biom9120789] [PMID: 31783552]

[38] Lee MR. Colchicum autumnale and the gout. Naked ladies and portly gentlemen. Proc R Coll Physicians Edinb 1999; 29(1): 65-70.
[http://dx.doi.org/10.1177/147827159902900113] [PMID: 11623671]

[39] Plant-identification 2020.(Accessed 18 November 2020). Available from: https://plant-identification.net/perennials/colchicum-autumnale/

[40] Vacca A, Ribatti D, Iurlaro M, *et al.* Docetaxel *versus* paclitaxel for antiangiogenesis. J Hematother Stem Cell Res 2002; 11(1): 103-18.
[http://dx.doi.org/10.1089/152581602753448577] [PMID: 11847007]

[41] Maldonado EN, Patnaik J, Mullins MR, Lemasters JJ. Free tubulin modulates mitochondrial membrane potential in cancer cells. Cancer Res 2010; 70(24): 10192-201.

[http://dx.doi.org/10.1158/0008-5472.CAN-10-2429] [PMID: 21159641]

[42]    Kallinich T, Haffner D, Niehues T, *et al.* Colchicine use in children and adolescents with familial Mediterranean fever: literature review and consensus statement. Pediatrics 2007; 119(2): e474-83.
[http://dx.doi.org/10.1542/peds.2006-1434] [PMID: 17242135]

[43]    Schlesinger N, Firestein BL, Brunetti L. Colchicine in COVID-19: an old drug, new use. Curr Pharmacol Rep 2020; 6(4): 137-45.
[http://dx.doi.org/10.1007/s40495-020-00225-6] [PMID: 32837853]

[44]    Gidding CE, Kellie SJ, Kamps WA, de Graaf SS. Vincristine revisited. Crit Rev Oncol Hematol 1999; 29(3): 267-87.
[http://dx.doi.org/10.1016/S1040-8428(98)00023-7] [PMID: 10226730]

[45]    Moudi M, Go R, Yien CY, Nazre M. Vinca alkaloids. Int J Prev Med 2013; 4(11): 1231-5.
[PMID: 24404355]

[46]    Chang Y, Meng FC, Wang R, Wang CM, Lu XY, Zhang QW. Chemistry, Bioactivity, and the Structure-Activity Relationship of Cephalotaxine-Type Alkaloids From Cephalotaxus sp. Studies in Natural Products Chemistry. Elsevier 2017; 53: pp. 339-73.

[47]    Royal Botanic Gradens 2018. Available from: http://www.plantsoftheworldonline. org/taxon/urn:lsid:ipni.org:names:261818-1

[48]    Seca AML, Pinto DCGA. Plant secondary metabolites as anti-cancer agents: successes in clinical trials and therapeutic application. Int J Mol Sci 2018; 19(1): 263.
[http://dx.doi.org/10.3390/ijms19010263] [PMID: 29337925]

[49]    Gandhi V, Plunkett W, Cortes JE. Omacetaxine: a protein translation inhibitor for treatment of chronic myelogenous leukemia. Clin Cancer Res 2014; 20(7): 1735-40.
[http://dx.doi.org/10.1158/1078-0432.CCR-13-1283] [PMID: 24501394]

[50]    Kusari S, Lamshöft M, Spiteller M. Aspergillus fumigatus Fresenius, an endophytic fungus from Juniperus communis L. Horstmann as a novel source of the anticancer pro-drug deoxypodophyllotoxin. J Appl Microbiol 2009; 107(3): 1019-30.
[http://dx.doi.org/10.1111/j.1365-2672.2009.04285.x] [PMID: 19486398]

[51]    Ardalani H, Avan A, Ghayour-Mobarhan M. Podophyllotoxin: a novel potential natural anticancer agent. Avicenna J Phytomed 2017; 7(4): 285-94.
[PMID: 28884079]

[52]    Abad A, López-Pérez JL, del Olmo E, *et al.* Synthesis and antimitotic and tubulin interaction profiles of novel pinacol derivatives of podophyllotoxins. J Med Chem 2012; 55(15): 6724-37.
[http://dx.doi.org/10.1021/jm2017573] [PMID: 22607205]

[53]    Passarella D, Peretto B, Blasco y Yepes R, *et al.* Synthesis and biological evaluation of novel thiocolchicine-podophyllotoxin conjugates. Eur J Med Chem 2010; 45(1): 219-26.
[http://dx.doi.org/10.1016/j.ejmech.2009.09.047] [PMID: 19880222]

[54]    Chen JY, Tang YA, Li WS, Chiou YC, Shieh JM, Wang YC. A synthetic podophyllotoxin derivative exerts anti-cancer effects by inducing mitotic arrest and pro-apoptotic ER stress in lung cancer preclinical models. PLoS One 2013; 8(4): e62082.
[http://dx.doi.org/10.1371/journal.pone.0062082] [PMID: 23646116]

[55]    Shin SA, Moon SY, Kim WY, Paek SM, Park HH, Lee CS. Structure-based classification and anti-cancer effects of plant metabolites. Int J Mol Sci 2018; 19(9): 2651.
[http://dx.doi.org/10.3390/ijms19092651] [PMID: 30200668]

[56]    Hutchings A. A survey and analysis of traditional medicinal plants as used by the Zulu; Xhosa and Sotho. Bothalia 1989; 19(1): 112-23.
[http://dx.doi.org/10.4102/abc.v19i1.947]

[57]    Kiuchi F, Shibuya M, Sankawa U. Inhibitors of prostaglandin biosynthesis from Alpinia officinarum.

Chem Pharm Bull (Tokyo) 1982; 30(6): 2279-82.
[http://dx.doi.org/10.1248/cpb.30.2279]

[58]    Adlercreutz H, Fotsis T, Heikkinen R, *et al.* Excretion of the lignans enterolactone and enterodiol and of equol in omnivorous and vegetarian postmenopausal women and in women with breast cancer. Lancet 1982; 2(8311): 1295-9.
[http://dx.doi.org/10.1016/S0140-6736(82)91507-0] [PMID: 6128595]

[59]    Kim YH, Lee DH, Jeong JH, Guo ZS, Lee YJ. Quercetin augments TRAIL-induced apoptotic death: involvement of the ERK signal transduction pathway. Biochem Pharmacol 2008; 75(10): 1946-58.
[http://dx.doi.org/10.1016/j.bcp.2008.02.016] [PMID: 18377872]

[60]    Ren W, Qiao Z, Wang H, Zhu L, Zhang L. Flavonoids: promising anticancer agents. Med Res Rev 2003; 23(4): 519-34.
[http://dx.doi.org/10.1002/med.10033] [PMID: 12710022]

[61]    Sedlacek HH. Mechanisms of action of flavopiridol. Crit Rev Oncol Hematol 2001; 38(2): 139-70.
[http://dx.doi.org/10.1016/S1040-8428(00)00124-4] [PMID: 11311660]

[62]    Yan X, Qi M, Li P, Zhan Y, Shao H. Apigenin in cancer therapy: anti-cancer effects and mechanisms of action. Cell Biosci 2017; 7(1): 50.
[http://dx.doi.org/10.1186/s13578-017-0179-x] [PMID: 29034071]

[63]    Ravishankar D, Rajora AK, Greco F, Osborn HM. Flavonoids as prospective compounds for anti-cancer therapy. Int J Biochem Cell Biol 2013; 45(12): 2821-31.
[http://dx.doi.org/10.1016/j.biocel.2013.10.004] [PMID: 24128857]

[64]    Farhan M, Khan HY, Oves M, *et al.* Cancer therapy by catechins involves redox cycling of copper ions and generation of reactive oxygen species. Toxins (Basel) 2016; 8(2): 37.
[http://dx.doi.org/10.3390/toxins8020037] [PMID: 26861392]

[65]    Lecumberri E, Dupertuis YM, Miralbell R, Pichard C. Green tea polyphenol epigallocatechin-3-gallate (EGCG) as adjuvant in cancer therapy. Clin Nutr 2013; 32(6): 894-903.
[http://dx.doi.org/10.1016/j.clnu.2013.03.008] [PMID: 23582951]

[66]    Aggarwal V, Tuli HS, Thakral F, *et al.* Molecular mechanisms of action of hesperidin in cancer: Recent trends and advancements. Exp Biol Med (Maywood) 2020; 245(5): 486-97.
[http://dx.doi.org/10.1177/1535370220903671] [PMID: 32050794]

[67]    Wolfram J, Scott B, Boom K, *et al.* Hesperetin liposomes for cancer therapy. Curr Drug Deliv 2016; 13(5): 711-9.
[http://dx.doi.org/10.2174/1567201812666151027142412] [PMID: 26502889]

[68]    Lin BW, Gong CC, Song HF, Cui YY. Effects of anthocyanins on the prevention and treatment of cancer. Br J Pharmacol 2017; 174(11): 1226-43.
[http://dx.doi.org/10.1111/bph.13627] [PMID: 27646173]

[69]    Bracone F, De Curtis A, Di Castelnuovo A, *et al.* Skin toxicity following radiotherapy in patients with breast carcinoma: is anthocyanin supplementation beneficial? Clin Nutr 2021; 40(4): 2068-77.
[http://dx.doi.org/10.1016/j.clnu.2020.09.030] [PMID: 33051045]

[70]    Sirerol JA, Rodríguez ML, Mena S, Asensi MA, Estrela JM, Ortega AL. Role of natural stilbenes in the prevention of cancer. Oxid Med Cell Longev 2016; 3128951.
[http://dx.doi.org/10.1155/2016/3128951]

[71]    Jang M, Cai L, Udeani GO, *et al.* Cancer chemopreventive activity of resveratrol, a natural product derived from grapes. Science 1997; 275(5297): 218-20.
[http://dx.doi.org/10.1126/science.275.5297.218] [PMID: 8985016]

[72]    Singh CK, Ndiaye MA, Ahmad N. Resveratrol and cancer: Challenges for clinical translation. Biochimica et Biophysica Acta (BBA)-. Biochim Biophys Acta Mol Basis Dis 2015; 1852(6): 1178-85.
[http://dx.doi.org/10.1016/j.bbadis.2014.11.004]

[73]    Abotaleb M, Liskova A, Kubatka P, Büsselberg D. Therapeutic potential of plant phenolic acids in the treatment of cancer. Biomolecules 2020; 10(2): 221.
[http://dx.doi.org/10.3390/biom10020221] [PMID: 32028623]

[74]    Rosa LD, Silva NJ, Soares NC, Monteiro MC, Teodoro AJ. Anti-cancer properties of phenolic acids in colon cancer–a review. J Nutr Food Sci 2016; 6(2): 1-7.

[75]    Habli Z, Toumieh G, Fatfat M, Rahal ON, Gali-Muhtasib H. Emerging cytotoxic alkaloids in the battle against cancer: overview of molecular mechanisms. Molecules 2017; 22(2): 250.
[http://dx.doi.org/10.3390/molecules22020250] [PMID: 28208712]

[76]    Chang LC, Tsai TR, Wang JJ, Lin CN, Kuo KW. The rhamnose moiety of solamargine plays a crucial role in triggering cell death by apoptosis. Biochem Biophys Res Commun 1998; 242(1): 21-5.
[http://dx.doi.org/10.1006/bbrc.1997.7903] [PMID: 9439603]

[77]    Nauts HC, Swift WE, Coley BL. The treatment of malignant tumors by bacterial toxins as developed by the late William B. Coley, M.D., reviewed in the light of modern research. Cancer Res 1946; 6(4): 205-16.
[PMID: 21018724]

[78]    Xu H, Xu X. Polysaccharide, a potential anti-cancer drug with high efficacy and safety. Adv Oncol Res Treat 2016; 1: 1-2.

[79]    He Z, Lv F, Gan Y, Gu J, Que T. Anticancer effects of Cyclocarya paliurus polysaccharide (CPP) on thyroid carcinoma *in vitro* and *in vivo*. Int J Polym Sci 2018; 2018.
[http://dx.doi.org/10.1155/2018/2768120]

[80]    Gershenzon J, Dudareva N. The function of terpene natural products in the natural world. Nat Chem Biol 2007; 3(7): 408-14.
[http://dx.doi.org/10.1038/nchembio.2007.5] [PMID: 17576428]

[81]    Huang M, Lu JJ, Huang MQ, Bao JL, Chen XP, Wang YT. Terpenoids: natural products for cancer therapy. Expert Opin Investig Drugs 2012; 21(12): 1801-18.
[http://dx.doi.org/10.1517/13543784.2012.727395] [PMID: 23092199]

[82]    Rabi T, Bishayee A. d -Limonene sensitizes docetaxel-induced cytotoxicity in human prostate cancer cells: Generation of reactive oxygen species and induction of apoptosis. J Carcinog 2009; 8(1): 9.
[http://dx.doi.org/10.4103/1477-3163.51368] [PMID: 19465777]

[83]    Lu JJ, Meng LH, Cai YJ, *et al.* Dihydroartemisinin induces apoptosis in HL-60 leukemia cells dependent of iron and p38 mitogen-activated protein kinase activation but independent of reactive oxygen species. Cancer Biol Ther 2008; 7(7): 1017-23.
[http://dx.doi.org/10.4161/cbt.7.7.6035] [PMID: 18414062]

[84]    Chang WT, Kang JJ, Lee KY, *et al.* Triptolide and chemotherapy cooperate in tumor cell apoptosis. A role for the p53 pathway. J Biol Chem 2001; 276(3): 2221-7.
[http://dx.doi.org/10.1074/jbc.M009713200] [PMID: 11053449]

[85]    Aparicio LM, Pulido EG, Gallego GA. Vinflunine: a new vision that may translate into antiangiogenic and antimetastatic activity. Anticancer Drugs 2012; 23(1): 1-11.
[http://dx.doi.org/10.1097/CAD.0b013e32834d237b] [PMID: 22027536]

[86]    Pang X, Yi Z, Zhang J, *et al.* Celastrol suppresses angiogenesis-mediated tumor growth through inhibition of AKT/mammalian target of rapamycin pathway. Cancer Res 2010; 70(5): 1951-9.
[http://dx.doi.org/10.1158/0008-5472.CAN-09-3201] [PMID: 20160026]

[87]    Chou CC, Pan SL, Teng CM, Guh JH. Pharmacological evaluation of several major ingredients of Chinese herbal medicines in human hepatoma Hep3B cells. Eur J Pharm Sci 2003; 19(5): 403-12.
[http://dx.doi.org/10.1016/S0928-0987(03)00144-1] [PMID: 12907291]

[88]    Elgass S, Cooper A, Chopra M. Lycopene inhibits angiogenesis in human umbilical vein endothelial cells and rat aortic rings. Br J Nutr 2012; 108(3): 431-9.

[http://dx.doi.org/10.1017/S0007114511005800] [PMID: 22142444]

[89]  Yoon Y, Kim YO, Lim NY, Jeon WK, Sung HJ. Shikonin, an ingredient of Lithospermum erythrorhizon induced apoptosis in HL60 human premyelocytic leukemia cell line. Planta Med 1999; 65(6): 532-5.
[http://dx.doi.org/10.1055/s-1999-14010] [PMID: 10483373]

[90]  Lu JJ, Bao JL, Wu GS, *et al.* Quinones derived from plant secondary metabolites as anti-cancer agents. Anti-Cancer Agents in Medicinal Chemistry (Formerly Current Medicinal Chemistry-Anti-Cancer Agents) 2013; 13(3): 456-63.

# CHAPTER 5

# Bioactive Compounds as Therapeutic Intervention in Mucocutaneous Cancers

**Henry A. Adeola**[1,2,*], **Rashmi Bhardwaj**[3], **Aderonke F. Ajayi-Smith**[4], **Afsareen Bano**[3], **Tayo A. Adekiya**[5], **Michael C. Ojo**[6], **Raphael T. Aruleba**[7], **Adeniyi C. Adeola**[8], **Babatunji E. Oyinloye**[6,9] and **Chinedu E. Udekwu**[10]

[1] *Department of Oral and Maxillofacial Pathology, Faculty of Dentistry, University of the Western Cape and Tygerberg Hospital, Cape Town, South Africa*

[2] *Division of Dermatology, Department of Medicine, Faculty of Health Sciences and Groote Schuur Hospital, University of Cape Town, Cape Town, South Africa*

[3] *Centre for Medical Biotechnology, Maharshi Dayanand University, Rohtak, Haryana, India*

[4] *International Centre for Genetic Engineering and Biotechnology (ICGEB), Cape Town, South Africa*

[5] *Wits Advanced Drug Delivery Platform Research Unit, Department of Pharmacy and Pharmacology, School of Therapeutic Science, Faculty of Health Sciences, University of the Witwatersrand, Johannesburg, York Road, Parktown, South Africa*

[6] *Department of Biochemistry and Microbiology, University of Zululand, KwaDlangezwa, South Africa*

[7] *Department of Molecular and Cell Biology, Faculty of Science, University of Cape Town, Cape Town, South Africa*

[8] *State Key Laboratory of Genetic Resources and Evolution, and Yunnan Laboratory of Molecular Biology of Domestic Animals, Kunming Institute of Zoology, Chinese Academy of Sciences, Kunming, China*

[9] *Phytomedicine, Biochemical Toxicology and Biotechnology Research Laboratories, Department of Biochemistry, Faculty of Sciences, Afe Babalola University, Ado Ekiti, Nigeria*

[10] *Department of Biochemistry, College of Natural Sciences, Michael Okpara University of Agriculture, Umudike, Abia State, Nigeria*

**Abstract:** There are several beneficial effects of plant bioactive compounds in the evidence-based prevention and treatment of mucocutaneous cancers. For instance, several bioactive compounds *via* various antioxidant and immunomodulatory mechanisms have been shown to positively improve different diseases, including cancer. Considering the complex, multifactorial processes that regulate genetic and cellular function in cancer development, the use of small phytochemical molecules capable of targeting multiple carcinogenetic genes and pathways is plausible.

* **Corresponding author Henry A. Adeola**: Division of Dermatology, Department of Medicine, Faculty of Health Sciences and Groote Schuur Hospital, University of Cape Town, Observatory 7925, Cape Town, South Africa; E-mail: henry.adeola@uct.ac.za

Furthermore, the identification of molecular targets and cognate dietary bioactive molecules in mucocutaneous cancer, using applied combinatorial chemistry approaches, potentially presents a key complementary ancillary tool for developing robust, physiologically bioavailable, diversity-oriented, and cost-effective therapies. These systems biology and omics-based theragnostic tools are crucial for the management of cancers that affect the oral mucous membranes and skin in a resource-limited setting. Natural products and nutraceuticals are poised to ameliorate the burden of mucocutaneous cancers and improve the drug discovery pipelines if state-of-the-art research techniques are used to elucidate their therapeutic values in the era of precision medicine. Hence, this review focuses on the currently available and potential therapeutic benefits of plant bioactive compounds in the prevention and management of mucocutaneous cancers.

**Keywords:** Bioactive compounds, Mucocutaneous cancers, Oral cancer, Phytocompounds, Skin cancer, Therapy.

# 1. INTRODUCTION TO MUCOSAL AND SKIN CANCERS

The human surface covering (skin) adapts to the physiological demand of its local environment to either form mucosa or skin [1]. Furthermore, there are different physiological, anatomical and histological modifications of skin (*e.g.*, acral, non-acral) depending on the requisite function of the skin [2]. Even within the oral mucosa, there are functional transitions and keratinization changes [1, 3] from mucosa to the gingiva, at the muco-gingival junction [4 - 6]. The junction where skin transitions to form mucosa is known as mucocutaneous junctions [7 - 9], and has been shown to be a source of mitotically active transient amplifying cells [7]. In addition, reticular and papillary micro-vascularization networks with extensive capillary looping with the deep reticular networks have been identified as characteristic of the mucocutaneous junctions of the eyelids and lips [9]. The anatomical contiguity of skin and mucosa structures, and the spatio-physiological adaptation of the skin and mucosa structures, demand a holistic approach to a systematic understanding of its pathologies and effective personalized and targeted therapies.

A report has shown that melanoma skin cancers affect about 132,000 people globally, and non-melanoma skin cancer has an estimated incidence of *ca.* 2-3 million people every year worldwide [10]. Skin cancers are typically divided into two major groups: melanoma and non-melanoma skin cancer (NMSC). The most common NMSCs are SCC and basal BCC [11]. Other NMSCs include cutaneous lymphoma, Merkel cell carcinoma, and Kaposi's sarcoma [11]. Using available literature evidence, we discuss in this chapter the role of bioactive compounds in three common mucocutaneous cancers, *viz*: malignant melanomas (MM), basal cell carcinomas (BCC) and squamous cell carcinomas (SCC).

## 1.1. Melanomas

Melanoma is a malignant melanocytic neoplasm that occurs as a result of accumulated genetic dysregulation [12]. Melanomas arise from dendritic melanocytes, which are neuroectodermal-derived cells situated in the basal layers of the skin, skin, eye, mucosal epithelial and meninges [13, 14]. Melanomas can develop from both cutaneous and mucosal surfaces [15]. Frequent melanoma sites include the head, neck, and lower extremities. Less frequent sites are oral and genital mucosa, nail beds, conjunctiva, oesophagus, nasal mucosa, vagina and leptomeninges [13].

*Mucosal melanomas* are tumours that arise from the melanocytes situated in the epithelia of the nasal cavity, oropharynx, gastrointestinal tract, and genitourinary tract [16]. Mucosal melanomas are uncommon and account for approximately 1.3% of all melanomas [17]. Approximately 50% of mucosal melanomas affect the head and neck region accounting for about 9% of all malignant head and neck tumours [14]. Mucosal melanomas are more aggressive than cutaneous melanomas, and approximately one-third of patients with mucosal melanoma present with advanced disease [16, 17]. Cutaneous melanoma is linked to exposure to ultraviolet light, but the anatomic location of mucosal melanoma excludes ultraviolet light exposure as a risk factor [17]. The overall 5-year survival rate is 25% despite the aggressive surgical intervention and adjuvant treatment therapies [16]. The aggressiveness of mucosal melanoma may be clarified by its late presentation and late diagnosis, vascularity of the mucous membranes, which promotes hematogenous metastases [16].

## 1.2. Basal Cell Carcinoma

Basal cell carcinoma (BCC) is a non-melanoma skin cancer. Approximately 80% of non-melanoma skin cancers are BCC [18], making it the most common skin cancer type globally [19]. BCCs arise from basal keratinocytes of the epidermis, hair follicles and eccrine sweat ducts [18]. BCCs are basophilic with large nuclei, and they require surrounding stroma for support during growth [18]. BCCs are usually slow-growing, and they rarely metastasise; however, delayed or inadequate treatment may lead to significant morbidity arising from destroyed skin, tissue, cartilage and bone [20]. There are five main histologic patterns of BCC: nodular, micronodular, superficial, infiltrative and morpheaform [18]. Risk factors for the development of BCC include ultraviolet radiation, immunosuppression, genetic disorders and age [19]. Most patients affected by BCC are middle-aged or the elderly [20]. Approaches for treating BCC can be surgical or non-surgical. Surgical techniques include curettage and cautery, cryosurgery, excision and Mohs micrographic surgery [20].

## 1.3. Squamous Cell Carcinoma

Squamous cell carcinoma (SCC) is the skin cancer most commonly associated with a significant risk of metastasis [21, 22]. The main precursor of squamous cell carcinoma (SCC) is actinic keratosis. Actinic keratosis occurs when there is a neoplastic transformation of epidermal keratinocytes, usually initiated by UV radiation [18]. The extension of actinic keratosis into the dermis is termed SCC [18]. Other risk factors for SCC include chronic ulcers, burns and post-traumatic scars [21]. Some genetic syndromes such as albinism and xeroderma pigmentosum are also associated with a high risk for SCC development [11]. Cutaneous SCC spreads by local infiltration and expansion through nerves and vessels. Distant metastasis by hematogenous dissemination occurs in approximately 5% of cases. Large tumours are three times more likely to metastasize than smaller tumours [18]. SCC usually appears as a firm, smooth or hyperkeratotic papule, mostly with central ulcerations. Patients report a non-healing lesion that bleeds with minimum trauma [18].

## 2. CONVENTIONAL MUCOCUTANEOUS CANCER THERAPY

Over the years, several conventional approaches have been employed in the treatment and management of mucocutaneous cancers. Notwithstanding, the choice of therapeutic interventions depends on the kind of cancers, the location of the tumour, stages of the tumour and the overall health condition of an individual involved. In this section, these therapeutic interventions will be highlighted.

Numerous treatment approaches are available for the treatment of skin cancer such as surgical removal, radiotherapy, immunotherapy and the use of chemotherapeutic agents [23, 24] such as doxorubicin, cisplatin, bleomycin, cyclophosphamide and 5-FU [24]. Both 5-FU and imiquimod are topical chemotherapies used in the treatment of BCC and SCC while only imiquimod is approved for the topical treatment of cutaneous malignant melanoma 14. The greatest risk factor for all types of skin cancers is overexposure to sunlight, which induces DNA damage by ultraviolet rays-A and B (UVA and UVB) on different genes [10]. The most prominent of which are *p53* gene, rapidly accelerated fibrosarcoma homolog B (*BRAF*) proto-oncogene (which turns oncogenic upon activation by mutation), and nucleotide excision repair genes as occurs in xeroderma pigmentosum [25].

Several treatment procedures are available for curing different types of skin cancer. These include photodynamic therapy (which involves the destruction of cancer cells with photoactivation of antioxidants molecules), targeted molecular therapy (which uses molecules designed to interact with specific proteins that play a key role in cancer development and growth), chemotherapy (which may involve the use of purine/pyrimidine analogues like 5-fluorouracil (5-FU) to block protein synthesis in cancer cells); and surgical procedures, some of which are (a) cryosurgery, which uses the production of extreme cold by liquid nitrogen to destroy abnormal tissues, (b) laser surgery, which uses a laser light beam to heat and destroy cancer cells, (c) curettage and electrodesiccation (C&D), in which curettage using a sharp curette is followed by dehydration of cells [26].

## 2.1. Surgical Excision of Mucocutaneous Cancers

This is the most frequently conventional therapeutic intervention employed in the treatment of both NMSC (BCC & SCC) and melanoma. Examples of surgical approaches used over the years include Mohs micrographic surgery (MMS), conventional excision (excisional surgery), curettage and electrodesiccation (electrosurgery), cryosurgery and laser surgery. Amongst these surgical therapeutic interventions, MMS remains the best standard approach in the treatment of diverse mucocutaneous cancers due to its ability to provide complete histological analysis of tumour margins [27]. In this surgical approach, the smallest margin of tumour is removed, thereby preserving the maximum amount of normal or healthy tissue; it also has the highest cure rate [27, 28]. In MMS technique, the serial horizontal sections of tumour tissues are mapped, processed and removed layer by layer until cancer-free tissue is attained through a frozen section in an enface fashion and evaluated using microscopes [27, 28]. The most common types of stain used during the MMS routine process are hematoxylin and eosin stain, on the other hand, some surgeons use toluidine blue when performing MMS. Although, other surgical approaches, for instance, electrodesiccation and curettage or excision, could be the treatment option in some cases due to their effectiveness and low cost involved in carrying out the procedures.

## 2.2. Non-surgical Treatment of Mucocutaneous Cancers

In the treatment of mucocutaneous cancers, several other conventional therapeutic interventions have been employed over the years, which are non-surgical methods. These types of interventions are suitable in certain patients in order to avoid some shortcomings associated with surgical procedures such as inherent risks and functional impairment and disfigurement.

*Anticancer chemotherapeutic agents* who happen to be the major target for apoptosis have been used in specific circumstances because most cancer cells take advantage of defective apoptosis mechanisms or develop ways to evade apoptosis, which in turn results in uncontrollable cell growth [29]. Examples of these chemotherapies include imiquimod [30] and 5-fluorouracil [31], which are employed in topical chemotherapies in both basal and squamous cell carcinoma.

Imiquimod, dacarbazine and temozolomide are approved therapy for melanoma [23, 32].

*Radiation therapy* is another conventional treatment for mucocutaneous cancers, which can either be used as a primary or adjuvant therapy after surgery. Radiation treatment is appropriate and helpful in debilitated patients. In this type of therapy, fractionated doses of radiation are delivered in the form of electron-beam therapy, orthovoltage or deep X-rays, or superficial X-rays to kill cancer cells. During mucocutaneous radiation therapy treatments, the fractionation of the dosage allows the recovery of the normal tissue, thereby decreasing the possibility of damaging the normal surrounding tissue without hampering the efficacy of the treatment [33, 34]. Radiation therapy would have been an efficient treatment option for non-surgical cases of mucocutaneous cancers, but the cost and side effects of this technique limit its usefulness. More so, some patients may suffer from initial dermatological adverse effects, some of which include alopecia, and (paradoxically) mucositis, pruritus, atrophy, depigmentation, telangiectasia and radionecrosis in the areas with thin skin, which can in turn result to other side effects as time goes by [27].

*Immunotherapy* has also been employed in the treatment of mucocutaneous cancers. In this type of therapy, an immunotherapy-based drug is used to stimulate the patient immune system to fight cancer cells. This approach has led to significant progress in treating patients with advanced mucocutaneous cancers. Examples of immunotherapy-based drugs include ipilimumab which inhibits cytotoxic-T-lymphocyte antigen-4 (CTLA-4), a protein on the T cell that regulates the activation of the immune system [35, 36]. The inhibition of CTLA-4 results in the destruction of tumour cells by T cells [37, 38]. Sometimes, it is used in combination with programmed death-1 (PD-1) inhibitors such as nivolumab and pembrolizumab [37, 38]. The blockade of PD-1, a protein receptor found on T cells that binds to the ligand PD-L1 on the T cells' surface, helps keep the immune response in check [39, 40].

*Oncolytic virotherapy and other immunomodulatory therapy for mucocutaneous cancers.* Other examples of immunotherapy drugs for mucocutaneous cancers are talimogene laherparepvec (T-VEC; Imlygic™), a genetically modified herpes simplex virus (HSV1) which is the first FDA approved oncolytic virotherapeutic agent for the management of advances melanoma [41, 42], interferon α-2b [43], interleukin-2 [44] and pegylated interferon α-2b [45], which are mostly used as early immunotherapy in the treatment of mucocutaneous cancers.

However, all these procedures are limited by their side effects, as detailed below. Additionally, these conventional therapeutic interventions have become less effective due to tumor resistance, tumor relapse and cancer metastasis [46 - 48]. In this section, insights into several treatment approaches for mucocutaneous cancers have been reported with surgical techniques as frequently and widely used. Nevertheless, several other alternatives and non-invasive treatments have been employed, some of which have come with success stories, in the treatment of mucocutaneous cancers by selectively inhibiting the tumours' growth. Also, reducing the morbidity of the disease as well as lessens several limitations associated with the surgical, chemotherapies and radiation methods, such as dermatological toxicity, which results in skin changes, mucosal changes, nail changes and hair changes. However, there is a need to develop relevant future or next-generation treatment strategies in which bioactive compounds could act as a basis for a better alternative therapeutic candidate for mucocutaneous cancers. Therefore, novel therapeutic modalities, preferably of natural origin, are of paramount necessity.

## 3. TARGETED MUCOCUTANEOUS CANCER THERAPIES

### 3.1. Purine/Pyrimidine Analogues

The characteristic that constitutes the ability of a chemotherapeutic agent to kill tumour cells is the fact that they can potentially sustain inhibition of DNA replication or function [49]. Different chemical agents have different mechanisms of action. 5-fluorouracil (5-FU) is a pyrimidine analogue. It functions as an antimetabolite where it interferes with DNA, and to a lesser extent, RNA synthesis by blocking the methylation of deoxyuridylic acid into thymidylic acid [50]. 5-FU may be used for the chemical destruction of many superficial lesions present on the face and head. Also, since the purine and pyrimidine analogues have a direct effect on DNA which can only be repaired in a case of damage, it can potentially lead to continuous apoptosis [50]. Other factors leading to chemotherapy resistance may include defective drug transport system and changes in enzymatic systems that mediate cellular metabolic machinery [51]. Therefore, these issues have demanded the need for more research on structurally modified nucleosides.

### 3.2. Photodynamic Therapy (using Antioxidants)

Photodynamic therapy application uses a photosensitive compound capable of accumulating within the tumour cell and thereafter activate by a source of light [52, 53]. Photodynamic therapy involves a two-part therapeutic process. Firstly, the application of an exogenous photosensitizing agent, which is selectively taken up by malignant or premalignant cells. The target cells convert the prodrug to protoporphyrin IX (PpIX) *via* the haem synthesis pathway. Secondly, the introduction of a light source causes activation of PpIX, leading to the formation of reactive oxygen species, which causes cytotoxicity of malignant cells [54]. Proinflammatory cytokines are induced secondary to PDT, and this causes neutrophil migration to the treated tumour cells [54]. Some PDT photosensitive compounds used in this technique includes photosensitizing porphyrin 5-aminolevulinic acid (ALA) and methyl aminolevulinate (MAL), which, when both are absorbed into the skin, they get converted to protoporphyrin IX; an endogenous photosensitizer that accumulates in the intracellular membranes of organelles. The depth of penetration of the photosensitive agent can limit the effectiveness of this technique against thicker tumours, interestingly, methyl aminolevulinate has been shown to be more lipophilic than 5-aminolevulinic acid, thus allowing more deep penetration into tissues [55]. The main limitation of conventional PDT is pain and burning, which can be intolerable for some patients.

## 3.3. Bioactive Compound and Photodynamic Therapy-carotenoids, Flavonoids and Terpenoids

A bioactive compound is a compound having biological activity. Bioactive compounds have direct physiological or cellular effects on a living organism. These effects may be positive or negative depending on the type of substance, dose, and bioavailability [24].

Carotenoids, flavonoids and terpenoids have been proven to be among the phytochemicals that potentially serve as anti-cancer agents due to their ability to scavenge reactive oxygen species on usage [56]. Selected flavonoids like quercetin, kaempferol, Epigallocatechin-3-gallate, apigenin and daidzein all act by either cell survival-promoting proteins or down-regulation of apoptosis inhibiting proteins, and through tumour suppressor proteins induction. Also, these phytochemicals have photo-protective activity on ultra-violate B (UVB) rays, thus preventing sunburn that ultimately leads to cell proliferation [57]. Vitamins such as C, D and E all play a crucial role in down-regulating Type 1 insulin-like growth factor receptor (IGF-1R) and COX-2 expression, resulting in anti-proliferative effects, as observed by [58]. Also, oral tretinoin (retinoids) can also act as a chemopreventive or chemotherapeutic agent for the treatment of all kinds of mucocutaneous cancers [59].

## 3.4. Emerging Targeted Molecular Therapies-Obstacles and Opportunities

Certain key proteins play a significant role in cancer development, and molecular research has shown that targeted molecular skin cancer therapies can be performed using molecules designed to interact with these proteins. Novel therapies that target the mammalian target of rapamycin (mTOR) and phosphatidyl-inositol 3-kinase (PI3K)/protein kinase B (Akt) are beginning to emerge in the management of melanoma and non-melanoma skin cancers [60]. For example, vismodegib is a targeted molecular therapy developed from the study of the genetic basis of nevoid basal cell carcinoma syndrome, a condition where numerous basal cell carcinomas develop [61]. Targeted therapy has also been used in treating skin cancer *via* inhibiting the Hedgehog pathway through inhibitors such as posaconazole and itraconazole [24]. Also, therapies such as vemurafenib are being used in the treatment of cutaneous malignant melanoma that often arises from the V600E mutation that activates an oncogene called BRAF1 [62]. Currently, targeted molecular therapies are used in advanced or metastatic cases of skin cancer, where surgical resection is inappropriate [63]. Targeted therapy has been used in specific circumstances for the treatments of several kinds of mucocutaneous cancers and the emergence of targeted therapy has marked the new beginning in the personalized drug for the treatment of mucocutaneous cancers in which tumours are targeted with minimal or without damage to the normal cells. These targeted therapeutic agents attack mucocutaneous cancers by inhibiting the action of defective molecules and genes, for instance, *MEK* and *BRAF,* which play an essential role in proliferating the growth and spread of mucocutaneous cancers, especially melanoma cells [64, 65]. Examples of approved targeted therapeutic drugs from mucocutaneous cancers include vemurafenib, dabrafenib and encorafenib, which help to interrupt and deactivate the tumour growth pathway stimulated by the genetic change in BRAF [66 - 68]. Common novel targeted therapies for skin cancer is listed in Table **1**. While targeted molecular therapies should target cancerous cells specifically in contrast to the cytotoxic brushstroke of chemotherapy, their many side effect profiles still limit use. The STEVIE trial investigating vismodegib for advanced BCC (where surgery was contraindicated or inoperable) found that 98% of patients experienced at least one adverse event from the drug, such as muscle spasms, alopecia, dysgeusia and weight loss [69]. Most of these treatment modalities have some limitations that reduce the potential of these treatment methods. This has resulted in searching for treatment strategies with little or no side effects.

## 4. BIOACTIVE COMPOUNDS AS POTENTIAL TARGETS FOR MUCOCUTANEOUS CANCERS

Medicinal plants are believed to be rich sources of bioactive compounds (phytochemicals) with vast and diverse chemical space that serves as an ideal springboard for the prevention and development of novel therapeutic drugs for the management and treatment of various human diseases [84]. It has been established that bioactive compounds possess the capacity to regulate various pathways that have been implicated in cancer [85]. The various anti-carcinogenic mechanisms of phytochemicals are a result of their anti-oxidative, anti-inflammatory, anti-proliferative, and anti-angiogenic potentials [86]. A few promising phytochemicals have been identified from medicinal plants (fruits, seeds, vegetables, roots, and herbs) [87, 88]. Of interest are epigallocatechin--gallate, resveratrol, curcumin, proanthocyanidins, silymarin, apigenin, capsaicin, genistein, indole-3-carbinol, and luteolin, just to mention a few [86].

**Table 1. Examples of targeted molecular therapies for different skin cancer types.**

| Skin Cancer Type | Target Molecule | Targeted Therapy | References |
|---|---|---|---|
| Melanoma | BRAF V600E<br>MEK<br>C-Kit | Vemurafenib<br>Encorafenib<br>Dabrafenib<br>Trametinib<br>Binimetinib<br>Cobimentinib<br>Imatinib<br>Nilotinib<br>Sorafenib | [70 - 72]<br>[70, 73, 74]<br>[75 - 77] |
| Basal cell carcinoma | Smoothened (SMO)<br>EGFR | Vismodegib<br>Sonidegib<br>Cetuximab<br>Panitumumab | [69, 78, 79]<br>[80, 81] |
| Squamous cell carcinoma | EGFR | Cetuximab | [80 - 83] |

Considering the adverse effects and limitations of targeted therapies, tackling mucocutaneous cancers with adjunctive phytochemicals has three distinct advantages, *inter alia*. Firstly, because various neoplastic dermatological lesions, with malignant transformation potential to mucocutaneous cancers, are easily accessible, hence, topical agents developed from phytochemicals can be selectively applied to the lesional area, and this is believed to be accompanied by negligible damage to normal skin [86, 89]. The second advantage is that the treatment efficacy of phytochemicals on dermatological growths can be monitored or evaluated effortlessly by physicians and patients. Lastly, if there are any adverse effects as a result of the application of the topical agents, it can be easily noticed by patients; this is a great advantage as it will reduce discomfort, possibly from long-term damage of further severe side effects in patients [86]. These phytochemicals act *via* multiple mechanisms, notably by inhibiting angiogenesis, metastasis, proliferation, apoptosis induction and cell cycle arrest [86, 90]. Currently, bioavailability, target specificity and dosing are some of the major challenges with the use of phytochemicals as cancer therapies [86, 91]. To improve the specificity of bioactive compounds, many novel state-of-the-art instrumentations, omics approaches, artificial intelligence and machine learning approaches have been employed to improve the targeting ability of bioactive compounds in cancer therapy [92 - 98].

## 5. BIOACTIVE COMPOUNDS AND OMICS APPROACH IN MUCOCUTANEOUS CANCERS

About 70% of anti-cancer agents have their origin from natural sources, which include animals, plants, marine life and plants [23]. Bioactive compounds include flavonoids, antracyanins, tannins, carotenoids, betalains and glucosinates [99]. Non-nutrient plant chemical compounds or bioactive components obtained from plants are known as phytochemicals [100]. Numerous promising phytochemicals have played vital roles in the prevention and treatment of skin cancer by regulating various molecular processes [24]. Phytochemicals such as curcumin, genistein, piperine and Epigallocatechin-3-Gallate (EGCG) have been shown to inhibit proliferation, induce apoptosis and cell cycle arrest in skin cancer [24]. Fucoxanthin is a marine-derived carotenoid with major sources, including brown algae, edible seaweeds and heterokonts. Fucoxanthin has been shown to suppress the metastatic potential of melanoma cells by downregulating proteins involved in cell migration and cell adhesion [23]. By targeting numerous signalling pathways necessary for carcinogenesis, these bioactive compounds may serve as important complementary therapeutic options in the treatment of melanoma and NMSCs.

It is generally known that natural products are a major source of new chemical entities with potential applications in drug discovery [101], however, one of the major challenges of modern medicine is the identification of biomarkers that allow for early diagnosis, enable relevant clinical intervention and also predict responses to treatment [102]. Discovering the molecular targets of bioactive compounds has been made easier because of recent innovations in genomics, proteomics, transcriptomics and metabolomics [103]. Pharmacogenomics focuses on defining genetic markers that predict individual responses to drugs. Pharmacoproteomics has many roles in drug development, including identification and validation of drug targets, assay development for the screening of leads and generation of *in vitro* and *in vivo* biomarkers as proxy endpoints for efficacy, toxicology and disease stratification [104]. Metabolomics is a key player in the development of new molecular entities into effective therapeutic medicines. Metabolomics bridges the gap between animal and human studies, as there is a large attrition rate when drugs move from animal models into human studies. Furthermore, drug safety may also be investigated using metabolomics techniques [104]. Mass spectrometry and nuclear magnetic resonance-based techniques associated with bioinformatics tools have been crucial in designing and developing natural products. These models are used to evaluate the molecular content of biological systems with exceptional precision and sensitivity [101]. Omics high throughput techniques provide a synopsis of the biochemical changes happening during pathogenic processes as well as response to the application of therapy [102]. The combination of information obtained from all Omics platforms will improve the knowledge of the molecular mechanisms of different bioactive compounds, which will promote the discovery of newer and more effective skin cancer treatments.

## 6. BIOACTIVE COMPOUNDS AND IMPORTANCE IN THE TREATMENT OF MUCOCUTANEOUS CANCERS

Over the years, the management of skin cancer has relied on chemotherapy, surgery, radiotherapy and cryotherapy. However, most of these techniques come with serious side effects and can damage normal cells instead of proliferating cancerous cells. Based on these reasons, researchers are now investigating natural products as alternative medicine or supplement for concurrent use. This stems from the fact that natural supplements can significantly reduce side effects like hepatotoxicity, oral mucositis, hematopoietic system injury, gastrointestinal toxicity, neurotoxicity and cardiotoxicity which are associated with pharmacological treatments. In line with this, several bioactive compounds are now being investigated in the management of skin cancer. Although different cancer types possess morphological and phenotypical peculiarities, diverse contributory factors with common underlying mechanisms have been implicated in their pathophysiology [105, 106]. Plant-derived phytochemicals or phytoconstituents is also known as secondary metabolites, are the bioactive substances in plant extracts that have been known over centuries to possess diverse biological activities, among which are anti-inflammatory, antioxidant, anti-diabetic, neuroprotective and anti-cancer properties [107 - 111]. It is worth noting that these bioactive compounds halt skin carcinogenesis by targeting one or more molecules that mediate cellular processes, including inflammation, immunity, cell cycle progression and apoptosis [105, 106, 112]. Our focus in this book chapter will be on plant-derived bioactive compounds with potential therapeutic benefit against mucocutaneous cancers.

### 6.1. Bioactive Compounds with Anti-skin Cancer Property

#### *6.1.1. Curcumin*

Curcumin, also known as diferuloylmethane, is a bioactive component derived predominantly from a plant endemic in East India called *Curcuma longa* [113, 114]. Its synthetic and phenolic analogues have also been reported to possess numerous bioactivities. Curcumin is known to have low bioavailability, but its systemic circulation longevity has been enhanced using nanoparticles such as piperine, liposomes *etc* [115, 116]. Studies have reported that curcumin exerts anti-cancer activities on different cancer types including skin melanoma by inhibiting angiogenesis, cell proliferation, cell growth and metastasis through several mechanisms, including decreased expression of NF-*k*B and metalloproteinase-9 (MMP9), inhibition of phosphatidylinositol-2,4,5-triphophate kinase (*PI3K*)/*Akt* pathway as well as enhanced apoptosis through upregulating *p53* and *Bax* [117 - 121].

### 6.1.2. Myricetin

Myricetin whose IUPAC name is 3,5,7,3',4',5'-hexahydroxy flavone cannabiscetin is a biflavonoid that was first isolated from the bark of *Myrica nagi Thunb* [114]. Myricetin is abundant in vegetables, tea, berries, medicinal plants, and red wines [114, 122]. Myricetin is pH and temperature sensitive, hydrophobic, but dissolves in organic solvents such as acetone, dimethylformamide, and tetrahydrofuran [123]. However, its solubility can be enhanced with microemulsion formulation [124]. Myricetin has been reported to possess therapeutic effect against skin cancer [125] and other cancer type [126 - 128], mainly by inducing cell cycle arrest, apoptosis and attenuating tumor progression as well as metastasis through the following mechanisms; downregulation of cyclin B1 and cyclin-dependent kinase *cdc 2*, metalloproteinases 2 and 9 (*MMP 2* and *MMP9*), and the *Bcl* protein family, as well as activation of the caspase 3 pathways and inhibition of the *p21* activated kinase-1 (*Pak1*) [129 - 132].

### 6.1.3. Tocotrienol

Tocotrienol is a fat-soluble antioxidant that is a component of vitamin E [133]. Food sources such as palm oil, rice bran oil and palm kernel oil are enriched with tocotrienol mainly in the tocotrienol-rich- fraction [134, 135]. Studies have reported that this bioactive compound display diverse biological activities, including neuroprotective, cardio protective, immunomodulation, antioxidant, and anti-thrombotic activities [136 - 140]. Furthermore, several cell-based and experimental models have revealed that tocotrienol and its isoforms' tumor efficacy against different cancer types, including skin cancer is by attenuation of tumor cell proliferation, angiogenesis, and *NF-kB* transcription faction as well as immunomodulation and apoptosis enhancement [140 - 142].

## 7. NOVEL APPLICATIONS OF BIOACTIVE FLAVONOID COMPOUNDS FOR MUCOCUTANEOUS CANCER MANAGEMENT

Although there are various challenges to overcome before their druggability can be established, these compounds have been documented to be involved in various signal transduction pathways [143]. In this context, flavonoids have been documented to possess broad-spectrum activity such as chemoprevention and inhibition, migration and invasion of skin cancer [144, 145]. These secondary metabolites play a significant role in signal transduction pathways associated with angiogenesis, cellular proliferation, apoptosis, inflammation and metastasis [146, 147]. For instance, diosmin, a glycosylated flavonoid, induced apoptosis in A431 (skin cancer cell line) by increasing the expression of caspases 3 and 9 [148]. After treatment with this compound, the A431 cell line showed decreased expression of MMP-2 and MMP-9; both associated with poor clinical outcomes [148]. Hence, diosmin could act as an anti-invasive agent. Other studies have shown the antimetastatic effect of this compound when combined with interferon α (IFN-α), a highly toxic cytokine that tends to be one of the most significant treatments for melanoma [149].

Luteolin, a common flavone, has been shown to present potential for anticancer as it induces apoptosis in human melanoma cells A2058 *via* a mechanism related to reactive oxygen species mediated endoplasmic reticulum stress [150]. Apigenin is another natural dietary flavonoid that has been shown to have a potential role in melanoma treatment and prevention due to its anti-proliferative activity [151]. Similar to diosmin, apigenin downregulated the expression and activity of STAT3 target genes MMP-2 and MMP-9 [151]. Epigallocatechin-3-gallate (EGCG) is the most abundant catechins in green tea [152] and its anti-cancer potentials have been broadly studied in *in-vitro, in vivo* and human studies. In skin cancer, it has been shown to significantly impair proliferation and metastasis by suppressing activation of *NF-κB* pathway *via* binding to TRAF6 and blocking its E3 ligase enzymatic activity [153]. Hence, targeting TRAF6 using ECGC holds great potential for the prevention or chemotherapy of skin cancer. This compound inhibits cell viability and induces cytotoxicity in human skin cancer cells A431 and SSC13 by impairing the activation of β-catenin signalling.

Resveratrol (RES), a polyphenolic phytoalexin found in grapes and other fruits have been demonstrated to delay ultraviolet B induced skin carcinogenesis in p53+/− hairless SKH-1 mice [154]. Also, RES suppressed the malignant transition of benign papillomas to squamous cell carcinoma [155, 156]. Nichols and Katiyar (2010) highlighted that the topical application of this polyphenolic compound impairs the initiation, promotion, and progression of UVB-induced skin cancer [157]. Similarly, the topical application of sulforaphane derived from broccoli sprouts protected against UVR-inflicted inflammation in mouse and human skin and decreased susceptibility to erythema developing from UVR in humans [158]. This compound is highly unstable and completely degrades when added to the conventional topical formulation [159]. In light of this shortcoming, Cristiano and co-workers (2020) loaded sulforaphane into an ultradeformable vesicle (ethosomes) in order to enhance its penetration and percutaneous diffusion [160]. Interestingly, ethosomes increased the anti-cancer activity of sulforaphane against human SK-MEL 28 malignant melanoma cells as most cells were not viable at 50μM drug concentration. Thus, the vesicle allowed cell permeation and direct drug release into the cytoplasm [160]. An overview of common bioactive compounds with potential for management of mucocutaneous cancers is presented in Table **2** below.

**Table 2. Common bioactive compounds for management of mucocutaneous cancers.**

| Bioactive Phytocompound | Mechanism of Action | Plant Source | Type of Mucocutaneous Tumour | Experimental Evidence | Reference |
|---|---|---|---|---|---|
| **Curcumin** | Inhibits proliferation, induces apoptosis and cell cycle arrest | *Curcuma longa* plant | Melanoma | *In-vivo* | [24] |
| **Luteolin** | Antoxidant and inflammatory activity, inihibits angiogenesis and pro-apoptosis | Celery, peppers, Olives, carrots | Melanoma | *In-vitro* | [24, 86, 150] |
| **Diosmin** | Anti-inflammatory, antimetastatic, antioxidant, downmodulates matrix metalloproteinases (MMPs), pro-apoptotic by increasing expression of caspases 3 and 9, | Olive leaves, citrus species | Non-melanoma skin cancer | *In-vitro* | [148, 149] |
| **Myricetin** | Induces cell cycle arrest, apoptosis & attenuates tumor progression and as metastasis, antoxidant effects | vegetables, tea, berries, medicinal plants, and red wines, bark of *Myrica nagi Thunb* | Melanoma and inflammation associated skin cancers | *In-vitro* | [114, 122, 125] |
| **Tocotrienol** | Fat-soluble antioxidant that is a component of vitamin E | palm oil, rice bran oil and palm kernel oil | Melanoma | *In-vitro and in-vivo* | [133 - 142] |
| **Resveratrol** | Anti-inflammatory, antioxidant and anti-proliferative | Mulberries, grapes, peanuts, red wine | Squamous cell carcinoma | *In-vivo* | [24, 86, 154, 157] |

(Table 2) cont.....

| Bioactive Phytocompound | Mechanism of Action | Plant Source | Type of Mucocutaneous Tumour | Experimental Evidence | Reference |
|---|---|---|---|---|---|
| Silymarin | Proapoptotic | Seeds of Milk thistle | Melanoma, squamous cell carcinoma | *In-vivo* | [24, 86] |
| Genistein | Antioxidant and anti-proliferative, induces apoptosis and cell cycle arrest | Soybean | Non-melanoma skin cancer and melanoma | *In-vitro, in-vivo* | [24] |
| Epigallocatechin-3-Gallate (EGCG) | Anti-inflammatory and antioxidant, inhibits proliferation, induce apoptosis, and cell cycle arrest | Green tea *Camellia sinensis* | Papilloma, actinic keratosis | *In-vivo* | [24] |
| Apigenin | Anti-proliferative and anti-inflammatory activity | Parsley, sweet pepper, celery, thyme, tea, onions | Non-melanoma skin cancers | *In-vivo* | [86, 151] |
| Fucoxanthin | suppresses the metastatic potential by downregulating proteins involved in cell migration and cell adhesion | Brown algae, edible seaweeds and heterokonts | Melanoma | *In vitro* | [23] |
| Capsaicin | Anti-proliferative, antimigratory effect, induction of apoptosis and cell cycle arrest | Jalapeno, red chilli pepper | Melanoma | *In-vivo* | [24, 86] |
| Grape seeds proanthocyanidins (GSPs) | Anti-inflammatory and antioxidant activity, inhibits epithelial-mesenchymal transition (EMT), improved DNA repair | Grape seed *Vitis Vinifera*, fruits, vegetables, flowers, seeds, flowers, bark, nuts | Non-melanoma skin cancer | *In vitro, In-vivo* | [86, 157] |
| Indole-3-carbinol | Pro-apoptotic, Anti-proliferative by regulation of PTEN degradation | Vegetables (family Cruciferae)-Cauliflower, broccoli, Brussels sprouts | Melanoma | *In-vitro and in-vivo* | [24, 86] |

## CONCLUSION AND FUTURE PERSPECTIVES

Overall, lots of interesting studies have investigated how various bioactive entities could work independently or as adjuvants on skin cancer. Despite cumulative and excellent results both *in vitro* and *in vivo*, non as translated well into clinical settings. Holistically, modes of action, safety profile and selectivity are basic considerations for translation; hence, the role of bioactive compounds in melanoma warrants further research to move from bench to bedside. On the other hand, several synthetic products (analogues) of natural products from plants (phytochemicals) have been synthesized, and procedures for improving their solubility and targeting specific tumours have also been developed [161]. Taken together, there is overwhelming evidence that plant phytochemicals and synthetic products possess a huge potential for personalized and non-toxic management of mucocutaneous cancers, particularly in resource-limited settings. In the era of precision medicine, the adjunctive use of omics technology to isolate bioactive compounds has a tremendous scope for the management of skin and mucosal cancers.

## CONSENT FOR PUBLICATION

Not applicable.

## CONFLICT OF INTEREST

The authors declare no conflict of interest, financial or otherwise.

## ACKNOWLEDGEMENTS

H. A. A. would like to thank the South African Medical Research Council (SAMRC) for a mid-career scientist and self-initiated research grants and the South African National Research Foundation (NRF) for a research development grant for rated researchers. AFA thank the International Centre for Genetic Engineering and Biotechnology (ICGEB) Arturo Falaschi Post-doctoral Fellowship Programme.

## AUTHORS' CONTRIBUTIONS

HAA conceptualized, designed, prepared, and critically revised the manuscript, table and figure. RB, AFA, CEU, TAA, MCO, RTA, ACA, BEO and AB were involved in the design and critical intellectual revision of the paper. All authors were involved in preparing the manuscript and had final approval of the submitted version.

# REFERENCES

[1] Liu J, Bian Z, Kuijpers-Jagtman AM, Von den Hoff JW. Skin and oral mucosa equivalents: construction and performance. Orthod Craniofac Res 2010; 13(1): 11-20.
[http://dx.doi.org/10.1111/j.1601-6343.2009.01475.x] [PMID: 20078790]

[2] Elstad M, Vanggaard L, Lossius AH, Walløe L, Bergersen TK. Responses in acral and non-acral skin vasomotion and temperature during lowering of ambient temperature. J Therm Biol 2014; 45: 168-74.
[http://dx.doi.org/10.1016/j.jtherbio.2014.09.003] [PMID: 25436967]

[3] Squier CA, Kremer MJ. Biology of oral mucosa and esophagus. J Natl Cancer Inst Monogr 2001; 2001(29): 7-15.
[http://dx.doi.org/10.1093/oxfordjournals.jncimonographs.a003443] [PMID: 11694559]

[4] Lozdan J. Studies on the mucogingival junction. Dent Pract Dent Rec 1970; 20(11): 379-84.
[PMID: 4990009]

[5] Schroeder HE, Amstad-Jossi M. Epithelial differentiation at the mucogingival junction: a stereological comparison of the epithelia of the vestibular gingiva and alveolar mucosa. Cell Tissue Res 1979; 202(1): 75-97.
[http://dx.doi.org/10.1007/BF00239222] [PMID: 509505]

[6] Lozdan J, Squier CA. The histology of the muco-gingival junction. J Periodontal Res 1969; 4(2): 83-93.
[http://dx.doi.org/10.1111/j.1600-0765.1969.tb01950.x] [PMID: 4242747]

[7] Wirtschafter JD, Ketcham JM, Weinstock RJ, Tabesh T, McLoon LK. Mucocutaneous junction as the major source of replacement palpebral conjunctival epithelial cells. Invest Ophthalmol Vis Sci 1999; 40(13): 3138-46.
[PMID: 10586935]

[8] Heilman E. Histology of the mucocutaneous junctions and the oral cavity. Clin Dermatol 1987; 5(2): 10-6.
[http://dx.doi.org/10.1016/0738-081X(87)90003-4] [PMID: 3607702]

[9] Wolfram-Gabel R, Sick H. Microvascularization of the mucocutaneous junctions of the head in fetuses and neonates. Cells Tissues Organs 2002; 171(4): 250-9.
[http://dx.doi.org/10.1159/000063126] [PMID: 12169822]

[10] Narayanan DL, Saladi RN, Fox JL. Ultraviolet radiation and skin cancer. Int J Dermatol 2010; 49(9): 978-86.
[http://dx.doi.org/10.1111/j.1365-4632.2010.04474.x] [PMID: 20883261]

[11] Kallini JR, Hamed N, Khachemoune A. Squamous cell carcinoma of the skin: epidemiology, classification, management, and novel trends. Int J Dermatol 2015; 54(2): 130-40.
[http://dx.doi.org/10.1111/ijd.12553] [PMID: 25428226]

[12] Natarajan E. Black and Brown Oro-facial Mucocutaneous Neoplasms. Head Neck Pathol 2019; 13(1): 56-70.
[http://dx.doi.org/10.1007/s12105-019-01008-2] [PMID: 30693458]

[13] Gilain L, Houette A, Montalban A, Mom T, Saroul N. Mucosal melanoma of the nasal cavity and paranasal sinuses. Eur Ann Otorhinolaryngol Head Neck Dis 2014; 131(6): 365-9.
[http://dx.doi.org/10.1016/j.anorl.2013.11.004] [PMID: 24906226]

[14] Papaspyrou G, Garbe C, Schadendorf D, Werner JA, Hauschild A, Egberts F. Mucosal melanomas of the head and neck: new aspects of the clinical outcome, molecular pathology, and treatment with c-kit inhibitors. Melanoma Res 2011; 21(6): 475-82.
[http://dx.doi.org/10.1097/CMR.0b013e32834b58cf] [PMID: 21897303]

[15] Yde SS, Sjoegren P, Heje M, Stolle LB. Mucosal Melanoma: a Literature Review. Curr Oncol Rep 2018; 20(3): 28.
[http://dx.doi.org/10.1007/s11912-018-0675-0] [PMID: 29569184]

[16]    O'Regan K, Breen M, Ramaiya N, *et al.* Metastatic mucosal melanoma: imaging patterns of metastasis and recurrence. Cancer Imaging 2013; 13(4): 626-32.
[http://dx.doi.org/10.1102/1470-7330.2013.0055] [PMID: 24434078]

[17]    Spencer KR, Mehnert JM. Mucosal Melanoma: Epidemiology, Biology and Treatment. Cancer Treat Res 2016; 167: 295-320.
[http://dx.doi.org/10.1007/978-3-319-22539-5_13] [PMID: 26601869]

[18]    Firnhaber JM. Diagnosis and treatment of Basal cell and squamous cell carcinoma. Am Fam Physician 2012; 86(2): 161-8.
[PMID: 22962928]

[19]    Migden MR, Chang ALS, Dirix L, Stratigos AJ, Lear JT. Emerging trends in the treatment of advanced basal cell carcinoma. Cancer Treat Rev 2018; 64: 1-10.
[http://dx.doi.org/10.1016/j.ctrv.2017.12.009] [PMID: 29407368]

[20]    Stanoszek LM, Wang GY, Harms PW. Histologic Mimics of Basal Cell Carcinoma. Arch Pathol Lab Med 2017; 141(11): 1490-502.
[http://dx.doi.org/10.5858/arpa.2017-0222-RA] [PMID: 29072946]

[21]    Kubo Y, Matsudate Y, Fukui N, *et al.* Molecular tumorigenesis of the skin. J Med Invest 2014; 61(1-2): 7-14.
[http://dx.doi.org/10.2152/jmi.61.7] [PMID: 24705742]

[22]    Kubo Y, Murao K, Matsumoto K, Arase S. Molecular carcinogenesis of squamous cell carcinomas of the skin. J Med Invest 2002; 49(3-4): 111-7.
[PMID: 12322999]

[23]    Chinembiri TN, du Plessis LH, Gerber M, Hamman JH, du Plessis J. Review of natural compounds for potential skin cancer treatment. Molecules 2014; 19(8): 11679-721.
[http://dx.doi.org/10.3390/molecules190811679] [PMID: 25102117]

[24]    Iqbal J, Abbasi BA, Ahmad R, *et al.* Potential phytochemicals in the fight against skin cancer: Current landscape and future perspectives. Biomed Pharmacother 2019; 109: 1381-93.
[http://dx.doi.org/10.1016/j.biopha.2018.10.107] [PMID: 30551389]

[25]    Heinzerling L, Kühnapfel S, Meckbach D, *et al.* Rare BRAF mutations in melanoma patients: implications for molecular testing in clinical practice. Br J Cancer 2013; 108(10): 2164-71.
[http://dx.doi.org/10.1038/bjc.2013.143] [PMID: 23579220]

[26]    Kauvar AN, Arpey CJ, Hruza G, Olbricht SM, Bennett R, Mahmoud BH. Consensus for Nonmelanoma Skin Cancer Treatment, Part II: Squamous Cell Carcinoma, Including a Cost Analysis of Treatment Methods. Dermatol Surg 2015; 41(11): 1214-40.
[http://dx.doi.org/10.1097/DSS.0000000000000478] [PMID: 26445288]

[27]    Neville JA, Welch E, Leffell DJ. Management of nonmelanoma skin cancer in 2007. Nat Clin Pract Oncol 2007; 4(8): 462-9.
[http://dx.doi.org/10.1038/ncponc0883] [PMID: 17657251]

[28]    Mosterd K, Krekels GA, Nieman FH, *et al.* Surgical excision *versus* Mohs' micrographic surgery for primary and recurrent basal-cell carcinoma of the face: a prospective randomised controlled trial with 5-years' follow-up. Lancet Oncol 2008; 9(12): 1149-56.
[http://dx.doi.org/10.1016/S1470-2045(08)70260-2] [PMID: 19010733]

[29]    Pfeffer CM, Singh ATK. Apoptosis: A Target for Anticancer Therapy. Int J Mol Sci 2018; 19(2): 19.
[http://dx.doi.org/10.3390/ijms19020448] [PMID: 29393886]

[30]    Bubna AK. Imiquimod - Its role in the treatment of cutaneous malignancies. Indian J Pharmacol 2015; 47(4): 354-9.
[http://dx.doi.org/10.4103/0253-7613.161249] [PMID: 26288465]

[31]    Zhang N, Yin Y, Xu SJ, Chen WS. 5-Fluorouracil: mechanisms of resistance and reversal strategies.

Molecules 2008; 13(8): 1551-69.
[http://dx.doi.org/10.3390/molecules13081551] [PMID: 18794772]

[32]   Robert C, Thomas L, Bondarenko I, *et al.* Ipilimumab plus dacarbazine for previously untreated metastatic melanoma. N Engl J Med 2011; 364(26): 2517-26.
[http://dx.doi.org/10.1056/NEJMoa1104621] [PMID: 21639810]

[33]   Fischbach AJ, Sause WT, Plenk HP. Radiation therapy for skin cancer. West J Med 1980; 133(5): 379-82.
[PMID: 7467294]

[34]   Locke J, Karimpour S, Young G, Lockett MA, Perez CA. Radiotherapy for epithelial skin cancer. Int J Radiat Oncol Biol Phys 2001; 51(3): 748-55.
[http://dx.doi.org/10.1016/S0360-3016(01)01656-X] [PMID: 11697321]

[35]   Wang XY, Zuo D, Sarkar D, Fisher PB. Blockade of cytotoxic T-lymphocyte antigen-4 as a new therapeutic approach for advanced melanoma. Expert Opin Pharmacother 2011; 12(17): 2695-706.
[http://dx.doi.org/10.1517/14656566.2011.629187] [PMID: 22077831]

[36]   Buchbinder E, Hodi FS. Cytotoxic T lymphocyte antigen-4 and immune checkpoint blockade. J Clin Invest 2015; 125(9): 3377-83.
[http://dx.doi.org/10.1172/JCI80012] [PMID: 26325034]

[37]   Robert C, Schachter J, Long GV, *et al.* Pembrolizumab *versus* Ipilimumab in Advanced Melanoma. N Engl J Med 2015; 372(26): 2521-32.
[http://dx.doi.org/10.1056/NEJMoa1503093] [PMID: 25891173]

[38]   Wolchok JD, Kluger H, Callahan MK, *et al.* Nivolumab plus ipilimumab in advanced melanoma. N Engl J Med 2013; 369(2): 122-33.
[http://dx.doi.org/10.1056/NEJMoa1302369] [PMID: 23724867]

[39]   Alsaab HO, Sau S, Alzhrani R, *et al.* PD-1 and PD-L1 Checkpoint Signaling Inhibition for Cancer Immunotherapy: Mechanism, Combinations, and Clinical Outcome. Front Pharmacol 2017; 8: 561.
[http://dx.doi.org/10.3389/fphar.2017.00561] [PMID: 28878676]

[40]   Zou W, Wolchok JD, Chen L. PD-L1 (B7-H1) and PD-1 pathway blockade for cancer therapy: Mechanisms, response biomarkers, and combinations. Sci Transl Med 2016; 8(328): 328rv4.
[http://dx.doi.org/10.1126/scitranslmed.aad7118] [PMID: 26936508]

[41]   Dommareddy PK, Patel A, Hossain S, Kaufman HL. Talimogene Laherparepvec (T-VEC) and Other Oncolytic Viruses for the Treatment of Melanoma. Am J Clin Dermatol 2017; 18(1): 1-15.
[http://dx.doi.org/10.1007/s40257-016-0238-9] [PMID: 27988837]

[42]   Johnson DB, Puzanov I, Kelley MC. Talimogene laherparepvec (T-VEC) for the treatment of advanced melanoma. Immunotherapy 2015; 7(6): 611-9.
[http://dx.doi.org/10.2217/imt.15.35] [PMID: 26098919]

[43]   Asmana Ningrum R. Human interferon alpha-2b: a therapeutic protein for cancer treatment. Scientifica (Cairo) 2014; 2014: 970315.
[http://dx.doi.org/10.1155/2014/970315] [PMID: 24741445]

[44]   Rosenberg SA, Lotze MT, Mulé JJ. NIH conference. New approaches to the immunotherapy of cancer using interleukin-2. Ann Intern Med 1988; 108(6): 853-64.
[http://dx.doi.org/10.7326/0003-4819-108-6-853] [PMID: 3285747]

[45]   Eggermont AM, Suciu S, Santinami M, *et al.* Adjuvant therapy with pegylated interferon alfa-2b *versus* observation alone in resected stage III melanoma: final results of EORTC 18991, a randomised phase III trial. Lancet 2008; 372(9633): 117-26.
[http://dx.doi.org/10.1016/S0140-6736(08)61033-8] [PMID: 18620949]

[46]   Shehzad A, Lee J, Lee YS. Curcumin in various cancers. Biofactors 2013; 39(1): 56-68.
[http://dx.doi.org/10.1002/biof.1068] [PMID: 23303705]

[47]    Devassy JG, Nwachukwu ID, Jones PJ. Curcumin and cancer: barriers to obtaining a health claim. Nutr Rev 2015; 73(3): 155-65.
[http://dx.doi.org/10.1093/nutrit/nuu064] [PMID: 26024538]

[48]    Tao F, Zhang Y, Zhang Z. The Role of Herbal Bioactive Components in Mitochondria Function and Cancer Therapy. Evid Based Complement Alternat Med 2019; 2019: 3868354.
[http://dx.doi.org/10.1155/2019/3868354] [PMID: 31308852]

[49]    Kitao H, Iimori M, Kataoka Y, *et al.* DNA replication stress and cancer chemotherapy. Cancer Sci 2018; 109(2): 264-71.
[http://dx.doi.org/10.1111/cas.13455] [PMID: 29168596]

[50]    Parker WB. Enzymology of purine and pyrimidine antimetabolites used in the treatment of cancer. Chem Rev 2009; 109(7): 2880-93.
[http://dx.doi.org/10.1021/cr900028p] [PMID: 19476376]

[51]    Kalal BS, Upadhya D, Pai VR. Chemotherapy Resistance Mechanisms in Advanced Skin Cancer. Oncol Rev 2017; 11(1): 326-6.
[http://dx.doi.org/10.4081/oncol.2017.326] [PMID: 28382191]

[52]    Agostinis P, Berg K, Cengel KA, *et al.* Photodynamic therapy of cancer: an update. CA Cancer J Clin 2011; 61(4): 250-81.
[http://dx.doi.org/10.3322/caac.20114] [PMID: 21617154]

[53]    Dougherty TJ, Gomer CJ, Henderson BW, *et al.* Photodynamic therapy. J Natl Cancer Inst 1998; 90(12): 889-905.
[http://dx.doi.org/10.1093/jnci/90.12.889] [PMID: 9637138]

[54]    Griffin LL, Lear JT. Photodynamic Therapy and Non-Melanoma Skin Cancer. Cancers (Basel) 2016; 8(10): 8.
[http://dx.doi.org/10.3390/cancers8100098] [PMID: 27782094]

[55]    Dolmans DEJGJ, Fukumura D, Jain RK. Photodynamic therapy for cancer. Nat Rev Cancer 2003; 3(5): 380-7.
[http://dx.doi.org/10.1038/nrc1071] [PMID: 12724736]

[56]    Batra P, Sharma A K. Anti-cancer potential of flavonoids: recent trends and future perspectives. 3 Biotech 2013; 3: 439-59.

[57]    Sevin A, Oztaş P, Senen D, *et al.* Effects of polyphenols on skin damage due to ultraviolet A rays: an experimental study on rats. J Eur Acad Dermatol Venereol 2007; 21(5): 650-6.
[http://dx.doi.org/10.1111/j.1468-3083.2006.02045.x] [PMID: 17447979]

[58]    Harborne JB, Williams CA. Advances in flavonoid research since 1992. Phytochemistry 2000; 55(6): 481-504.
[http://dx.doi.org/10.1016/S0031-9422(00)00235-1] [PMID: 11130659]

[59]    Weinstock MA, Bingham SF, Digiovanna JJ, *et al.* Tretinoin and the prevention of keratinocyte carcinoma (Basal and squamous cell carcinoma of the skin): a veterans affairs randomized chemoprevention trial. J Invest Dermatol 2012; 132(6): 1583-90.
[http://dx.doi.org/10.1038/jid.2011.483] [PMID: 22318383]

[60]    Chamcheu JC, Roy T, Uddin MB, *et al.* Role and Therapeutic Targeting of the PI3K/Akt/mTOR Signaling Pathway in Skin Cancer: A Review of Current Status and Future Trends on Natural and Synthetic Agents Therapy. Cells 2019; 8(8): 8.
[http://dx.doi.org/10.3390/cells8080803] [PMID: 31370278]

[61]    Tang JY, Mackay-Wiggan JM, Aszterbaum M, *et al.* Inhibiting the hedgehog pathway in patients with the basal-cell nevus syndrome. N Engl J Med 2012; 366(23): 2180-8.
[http://dx.doi.org/10.1056/NEJMoa1113538] [PMID: 22670904]

[62]    Kim A, Cohen MS. The discovery of vemurafenib for the treatment of BRAF-mutated metastatic

melanoma. Expert Opin Drug Discov 2016; 11(9): 907-16.
[http://dx.doi.org/10.1080/17460441.2016.1201057] [PMID: 27327499]

[63]    Leonardi GC, Falzone L, Salemi R, *et al.* Cutaneous melanoma: From pathogenesis to therapy (Review). Int J Oncol 2018; 52(4): 1071-80. [Review].
[http://dx.doi.org/10.3892/ijo.2018.4287] [PMID: 29532857]

[64]    Cheepala SB, Yin W, Syed Z, *et al.* Identification of the B-Raf/Mek/Erk MAP kinase pathway as a target for all-trans retinoic acid during skin cancer promotion. Mol Cancer 2009; 8: 27.
[http://dx.doi.org/10.1186/1476-4598-8-27] [PMID: 19432991]

[65]    Flaherty KT, Robert C, Hersey P, *et al.* Improved survival with MEK inhibition in BRAF-mutated melanoma. N Engl J Med 2012; 367(2): 107-14.
[http://dx.doi.org/10.1056/NEJMoa1203421] [PMID: 22663011]

[66]    Robert C, Karaszewska B, Schachter J, *et al.* Improved overall survival in melanoma with combined dabrafenib and trametinib. N Engl J Med 2015; 372(1): 30-9.
[http://dx.doi.org/10.1056/NEJMoa1412690] [PMID: 25399551]

[67]    Shelledy L, Roman D. Vemurafenib: First-in-Class BRAF-Mutated Inhibitor for the Treatment of Unresectable or Metastatic Melanoma. J Adv Pract Oncol 2015; 6(4): 361-5.
[PMID: 26705496]

[68]    Roskoski R Jr. Allosteric MEK1/2 inhibitors including cobimetanib and trametinib in the treatment of cutaneous melanomas. Pharmacol Res 2017; 117: 20-31.
[http://dx.doi.org/10.1016/j.phrs.2016.12.009] [PMID: 27956260]

[69]    Basset-Seguin N, Hauschild A, Grob JJ, *et al.* Vismodegib in patients with advanced basal cell carcinoma (STEVIE): a pre-planned interim analysis of an international, open-label trial. Lancet Oncol 2015; 16(6): 729-36.
[http://dx.doi.org/10.1016/S1470-2045(15)70198-1] [PMID: 25981813]

[70]    Hamid O, Cowey CL, Offner M, Faries M, Carvajal RD. Efficacy, Safety, and Tolerability of Approved Combination BRAF and MEK Inhibitor Regimens for *BRAF*-Mutant Melanoma. Cancers (Basel) 2019; 11(11): 11.
[http://dx.doi.org/10.3390/cancers11111642] [PMID: 31653096]

[71]    Koelblinger P, Thuerigen O, Dummer R. Development of encorafenib for BRAF-mutated advanced melanoma. Curr Opin Oncol 2018; 30(2): 125-33.
[http://dx.doi.org/10.1097/CCO.0000000000000426] [PMID: 29356698]

[72]    Warburton L, Meniawy TM, Calapre L, *et al.* Stopping targeted therapy for complete responders in advanced BRAF mutant melanoma. Sci Rep 2020; 10(1): 18878.
[http://dx.doi.org/10.1038/s41598-020-75837-5] [PMID: 33139839]

[73]    Johnson D. Is there a role for single-agent MEK inhibition in melanoma? Clinical advances in hematology & oncology : H&O 2016; 14: 976-8.

[74]    Greco A, Safi D, Swami U, Ginader T, Milhem M, Zakharia Y. Efficacy and Adverse Events in Metastatic Melanoma Patients Treated with Combination BRAF Plus MEK Inhibitors *versus* BRAF Inhibitors: A Systematic Review. Cancers (Basel) 2019; 11(12): 11.
[http://dx.doi.org/10.3390/cancers11121950] [PMID: 31817473]

[75]    Carvajal RD, Lawrence DP, Weber JS, *et al.* Phase II Study of Nilotinib in Melanoma Harboring KIT Alterations Following Progression to Prior KIT Inhibition. Clin Cancer Res 2015; 21(10): 2289-96.
[http://dx.doi.org/10.1158/1078-0432.CCR-14-1630] [PMID: 25695690]

[76]    Han Y, Gu Z, Wu J, *et al.* Repurposing Ponatinib as a Potent Agent against *KIT* Mutant Melanomas. Theranostics 2019; 9(7): 1952-64.
[http://dx.doi.org/10.7150/thno.30890] [PMID: 31037149]

[77]    Handolias D, Hamilton AL, Salemi R, *et al.* Clinical responses observed with imatinib or sorafenib in melanoma patients expressing mutations in KIT. Br J Cancer 2010; 102(8): 1219-23.

[http://dx.doi.org/10.1038/sj.bjc.6605635] [PMID: 20372153]

[78]   Dummer R, Ascierto PA, Basset-Seguin N, *et al.* Sonidegib and vismodegib in the treatment of patients with locally advanced basal cell carcinoma: a joint expert opinion. J Eur Acad Dermatol Venereol 2020; 34(9): 1944-56.
[http://dx.doi.org/10.1111/jdv.16230] [PMID: 31990414]

[79]   Odom D, Mladsi D, Purser M, *et al.* A Matching-Adjusted Indirect Comparison of Sonidegib and Vismodegib in Advanced Basal Cell Carcinoma. J Skin Cancer 2017; 2017: 6121760.
[http://dx.doi.org/10.1155/2017/6121760] [PMID: 28607774]

[80]   Holcmann M, Sibilia M. Mechanisms underlying skin disorders induced by EGFR inhibitors. Mol Cell Oncol 2015; 2(4): e1004969.
[http://dx.doi.org/10.1080/23723556.2015.1004969] [PMID: 27308503]

[81]   Diociaiuti A, Steinke H, Nyström A, *et al.* EGFR inhibition for metastasized cutaneous squamous cell carcinoma in dystrophic epidermolysis bullosa. Orphanet J Rare Dis 2019; 14(1): 278.
[http://dx.doi.org/10.1186/s13023-019-1262-7] [PMID: 31796084]

[82]   Capalbo C, Belardinilli F, Filetti M, *et al.* Effective treatment of a platinum-resistant cutaneous squamous cell carcinoma case by EGFR pathway inhibition. Mol Clin Oncol 2018; 9(1): 30-4.
[http://dx.doi.org/10.3892/mco.2018.1634] [PMID: 29977536]

[83]   Tischer B, Huber R, Kraemer M, Lacouture M E. Dermatologic events from EGFR inhibitors: the issue of the missing patient voice. Supportive care in cancer : official journal of the Multinational Association of Supportive Care in Cancer 2017; 25: 651-60.

[84]   Mohanraj K, Karthikeyan BS, Vivek-Ananth RP, *et al.* IMPPAT: A curated database of Indian Medicinal Plants, Phytochemistry And Therapeutics. Sci Rep 2018; 8(1): 4329.
[http://dx.doi.org/10.1038/s41598-018-22631-z] [PMID: 29531263]

[85]   Puccinelli MT, Stan SD. Dietary Bioactive Diallyl Trisulfide in Cancer Prevention and Treatment. Int J Mol Sci 2017; 18(8): 18.
[http://dx.doi.org/10.3390/ijms18081645] [PMID: 28788092]

[86]   Ng CY, Yen H, Hsiao HY, Su SC. Phytochemicals in Skin Cancer Prevention and Treatment: An Updated Review. Int J Mol Sci 2018; 19(4): 19.
[http://dx.doi.org/10.3390/ijms19040941] [PMID: 29565284]

[87]   Ahmad U, Ahmad RS. Anti diabetic property of aqueous extract of Stevia rebaudiana Bertoni leaves in Streptozotocin-induced diabetes in albino rats. BMC Complement Altern Med 2018; 18(1): 179.
[http://dx.doi.org/10.1186/s12906-018-2245-2] [PMID: 29890969]

[88]   Ranjan A, Ramachandran S, Gupta N, *et al.* Role of Phytochemicals in Cancer Prevention. Int J Mol Sci 2019; 20(20): 20.
[http://dx.doi.org/10.3390/ijms20204981] [PMID: 31600949]

[89]   Forni C, Facchiano F, Bartoli M, *et al.* Beneficial Role of Phytochemicals on Oxidative Stress and Age-Related Diseases. BioMed Res Int 2019; 2019: 8748253.
[http://dx.doi.org/10.1155/2019/8748253] [PMID: 31080832]

[90]   George BP, Chandran R, Abrahamse H. Role of Phytochemicals in Cancer Chemoprevention: Insights. Antioxidants 2021; 10(9): 1455.
[http://dx.doi.org/10.3390/antiox10091455] [PMID: 34573087]

[91]   Zubair H, Azim S, Ahmad A, *et al.* Cancer Chemoprevention by Phytochemicals: Nature's Healing Touch. Molecules 2017; 22(3): 22.
[http://dx.doi.org/10.3390/molecules22030395] [PMID: 28273819]

[92]   Dos Santos BS, da Silva LC, da Silva TD, *et al.* Application of Omics Technologies for Evaluation of Antibacterial Mechanisms of Action of Plant-Derived Products. Front Microbiol 2016; 7: 1466.
[http://dx.doi.org/10.3389/fmicb.2016.01466] [PMID: 27729901]

[93]    Ferguson LR, Barnett MP. Why Are Omics Technologies Important to Understanding the Role of Nutrition in Inflammatory Bowel Diseases? Int J Mol Sci 2016; 17(10): 17.
[http://dx.doi.org/10.3390/ijms17101763] [PMID: 27775675]

[94]    Paananen J, Fortino V. An omics perspective on drug target discovery platforms. Brief Bioinform 2020; 21(6): 1937-53.
[http://dx.doi.org/10.1093/bib/bbz122] [PMID: 31774113]

[95]    Patel-Murray NL, Adam M, Huynh N, Wassie BT, Milani P, Fraenkel E. A Multi-Omics Interpretable Machine Learning Model Reveals Modes of Action of Small Molecules. Sci Rep 2020; 10(1): 954.
[http://dx.doi.org/10.1038/s41598-020-57691-7] [PMID: 31969612]

[96]    Chen JT. Phytochemical Omics in Medicinal Plants. Biomolecules 2020; 10(6): 10.
[http://dx.doi.org/10.3390/biom10060936] [PMID: 32575904]

[97]    Meeran SM, Ahmed A, Tollefsbol TO. Epigenetic targets of bioactive dietary components for cancer prevention and therapy. Clin Epigenetics 2010; 1(3-4): 101-16.
[http://dx.doi.org/10.1007/s13148-010-0011-5] [PMID: 21258631]

[98]    Turanli B, Karagoz K, Bidkhori G, et al. Multi-Omic Data Interpretation to Repurpose Subtype Specific Drug Candidates for Breast Cancer. Front Genet 2019; 10: 420.
[http://dx.doi.org/10.3389/fgene.2019.00420] [PMID: 31134131]

[99]    Walia A. G. A., Sharma V, Role of Bioactive Compounds in Human Health. Acta Sci Med Sci 2019; 3: 25-33.

[100]   Mousavi L, Salleh RM, Murugaiyah V. Phytochemical and bioactive compounds identification of Ocimum tenuiflorum leaves of methanol extract and its fraction with an anti-diabetic potential. Int J Food Prop 2018; 21: 2390-9.
[http://dx.doi.org/10.1080/10942912.2018.1508161]

[101]   Wolfender J-L, Litaudon M, Touboul D, Queiroz EF. Innovative omics-based approaches for prioritisation and targeted isolation of natural products - new strategies for drug discovery. Nat Prod Rep 2019; 36(6): 855-68.
[http://dx.doi.org/10.1039/C9NP00004F] [PMID: 31073562]

[102]   Odriozola L, Corrales FJ. Discovery of nutritional biomarkers: future directions based on omics technologies. Int J Food Sci Nutr 2015; 66 (Suppl. 1): S31-40.
[http://dx.doi.org/10.3109/09637486.2015.1038224] [PMID: 26241009]

[103]   Ashraf MA. Phytochemicals as Potential Anticancer Drugs: Time to Ponder Nature's Bounty. BioMed Res Int 2020; 2020: 8602879.
[http://dx.doi.org/10.1155/2020/8602879] [PMID: 32076618]

[104]   Matthews H, Hanison J, Nirmalan N. "Omics"-Informed Drug and Biomarker Discovery: Opportunities, Challenges and Future Perspectives. Proteomes 2016; 4(3): 4.
[http://dx.doi.org/10.3390/proteomes4030028] [PMID: 28248238]

[105]   Whiteside TL. The tumor microenvironment and its role in promoting tumor growth. Oncogene 2008; 27(45): 5904-12.
[http://dx.doi.org/10.1038/onc.2008.271] [PMID: 18836471]

[106]   Todoric J, Antonucci L, Karin M. Targeting Inflammation in Cancer Prevention and Therapy. Cancer Prev Res (Phila) 2016; 9(12): 895-905.
[http://dx.doi.org/10.1158/1940-6207.CAPR-16-0209] [PMID: 27913448]

[107]   Dinkova-Kostova AT. Chemoprotection against cancer by isothiocyanates: a focus on the animal models and the protective mechanisms. Top Curr Chem 2013; 329: 179-201.
[http://dx.doi.org/10.1007/128_2012_337] [PMID: 22752581]

[108]   Liu RH. Health-promoting components of fruits and vegetables in the diet. Adv Nutr 2013; 4(3): 384S-92S.

[http://dx.doi.org/10.3945/an.112.003517] [PMID: 23674808]

[109]  Shahidi F, Yeo J. Bioactivities of Phenolics by Focusing on Suppression of Chronic Diseases: A Review. Int J Mol Sci 2018; 19(6): 19.
[http://dx.doi.org/10.3390/ijms19061573] [PMID: 29799460]

[110]  Peng J, Zheng TT, Li X, *et al.* Plant-Derived Alkaloids: The Promising Disease-Modifying Agents for Inflammatory Bowel Disease. Front Pharmacol 2019; 10: 351.
[http://dx.doi.org/10.3389/fphar.2019.00351] [PMID: 31031622]

[111]  Bungau S, Abdel-Daim MM, Tit DM, *et al.* Health Benefits of Polyphenols and Carotenoids in Age-Related Eye Diseases. Oxid Med Cell Longev 2019; 2019: 9783429.
[http://dx.doi.org/10.1155/2019/9783429] [PMID: 30891116]

[112]  Singh M, Suman S, Shukla Y. New Enlightenment of Skin Cancer Chemoprevention through Phytochemicals: *In Vitro* and *In Vivo* Studies and the Underlying Mechanisms. BioMed Res Int 2014; 2014: 243452.
[http://dx.doi.org/10.1155/2014/243452] [PMID: 24757666]

[113]  Chattopadhyay I, Biswas K, Bandyopadhyay U, Banerjee RK. Turmeric and curcumin: Biological actions and medicinal applications. Curr Sci 2004; 87: 44-53.

[114]  Subramaniam S, Selvaduray KR, Radhakrishnan AK. Bioactive Compounds: Natural Defense Against Cancer? Biomolecules 2019; 9(12): 9.
[http://dx.doi.org/10.3390/biom9120758] [PMID: 31766399]

[115]  Stohs SJ, Chen O, Ray SD, Ji J, Bucci LR, Preuss HG. Highly Bioavailable Forms of Curcumin and Promising Avenues for Curcumin-Based Research and Application: A Review. Molecules 2020; 25(6): 25.
[http://dx.doi.org/10.3390/molecules25061397] [PMID: 32204372]

[116]  Dei Cas M, Ghidoni R. Dietary Curcumin: Correlation between Bioavailability and Health Potential. Nutrients 2019; 11(9): 11.
[http://dx.doi.org/10.3390/nu11092147] [PMID: 31500361]

[117]  Guo LD, Chen XJ, Hu YH, Yu ZJ, Wang D, Liu JZ. Curcumin inhibits proliferation and induces apoptosis of human colorectal cancer cells by activating the mitochondria apoptotic pathway. Phytother Res 2013; 27(3): 422-30.
[http://dx.doi.org/10.1002/ptr.4731] [PMID: 22628241]

[118]  Li W, Wang Y, Song Y, Xu L, Zhao J, Fang B. A preliminary study of the effect of curcumin on the expression of p53 protein in a human multiple myeloma cell line. Oncol Lett 2015; 9(4): 1719-24.
[http://dx.doi.org/10.3892/ol.2015.2946] [PMID: 25789029]

[119]  Jee SH, Shen SC, Tseng CR, Chiu HC, Kuo ML. Curcumin induces a p53-dependent apoptosis in human basal cell carcinoma cells. J Invest Dermatol 1998; 111(4): 656-61.
[http://dx.doi.org/10.1046/j.1523-1747.1998.00352.x] [PMID: 9764849]

[120]  Abusnina A, Keravis T, Zhou Q, Justiniano H, Lobstein A, Lugnier C. Tumour growth inhibition and anti-angiogenic effects using curcumin correspond to combined PDE2 and PDE4 inhibition. Thromb Haemost 2015; 113(2): 319-28.
[http://dx.doi.org/10.1160/TH14-05-0454] [PMID: 25230992]

[121]  Kunnumakkara AB, Bordoloi D, Harsha C, Banik K, Gupta SC, Aggarwal BB. Curcumin mediates anticancer effects by modulating multiple cell signaling pathways. Clin Sci (Lond) 2017; 131(15): 1781-99.
[http://dx.doi.org/10.1042/CS20160935] [PMID: 28679846]

[122]  Perkin AG, Hummel JJ. LXXVI.—The colouring principle contained in the bark of Myrica nagi. Part I. J Chem Soc Trans 1896; 69: 1287-94.
[http://dx.doi.org/10.1039/CT8966901287]

[123]  Yao Y, Lin G, Xie Y, *et al.* Preformulation studies of myricetin: a natural antioxidant flavonoid.

Pharmazie 2014; 69(1): 19-26.
[PMID: 24601218]

[124]  Guo RX, Fu X, Chen J, Zhou L, Chen G. Preparation and Characterization of Microemulsions of Myricetin for Improving Its Antiproliferative and Antioxidative Activities and Oral Bioavailability. J Agric Food Chem 2016; 64(32): 6286-94.
[http://dx.doi.org/10.1021/acs.jafc.6b02184] [PMID: 27455843]

[125]  George VC, Vijesh VV, Amararathna DIM, *et al.* Mechanism of Action of Flavonoids in Prevention of Inflammation- Associated Skin Cancer. Curr Med Chem 2016; 23(32): 3697-716.
[http://dx.doi.org/10.2174/0929867323666160627110342] [PMID: 27356537]

[126]  Xu Y, Xie Q, Wu S, *et al.* Myricetin induces apoptosis *via* endoplasmic reticulum stress and DNA double-strand breaks in human ovarian cancer cells. Mol Med Rep 2016; 13(3): 2094-100.
[http://dx.doi.org/10.3892/mmr.2016.4763] [PMID: 26782830]

[127]  Sangwan V, Banerjee S, Jensen KM, *et al.* Primary and liver metastasis-derived cell lines from KrasG12D; Trp53R172H; Pdx-1 Cre animals undergo apoptosis in response to triptolide. Pancreas 2015; 44(4): 583-9.
[http://dx.doi.org/10.1097/MPA.0000000000000317] [PMID: 25875797]

[128]  Jayakumar JK, Nirmala P, Praveen Kumar BA, Kumar AP. Evaluation of protective effect of myricetin, a bioflavonoid in dimethyl benzanthracene-induced breast cancer in female Wistar rats. South Asian J Cancer 2014; 3(2): 107-11.
[http://dx.doi.org/10.4103/2278-330X.130443] [PMID: 24818105]

[129]  Sun F, Zheng XY, Ye J, Wu TT, Wang Jl, Chen W. Potential anticancer activity of myricetin in human T24 bladder cancer cells both *in vitro* and *in vivo*. Nutr Cancer 2012; 64(4): 599-606.
[http://dx.doi.org/10.1080/01635581.2012.665564] [PMID: 22482362]

[130]  Yi JL, Shi S, Shen YL, *et al.* Myricetin and methyl eugenol combination enhances the anticancer activity, cell cycle arrest and apoptosis induction of cis-platin against HeLa cervical cancer cell lines. Int J Clin Exp Pathol 2015; 8(2): 1116-27.
[PMID: 25972998]

[131]  Iyer SC, Gopal A, Halagowder D. Myricetin induces apoptosis by inhibiting P21 activated kinase 1 (PAK1) signaling cascade in hepatocellular carcinoma. Mol Cell Biochem 2015; 407(1-2): 223-37.
[http://dx.doi.org/10.1007/s11010-015-2471-6] [PMID: 26104578]

[132]  Ci Y, Zhang Y, Liu Y, *et al.* Myricetin suppresses breast cancer metastasis through down-regulating the activity of matrix metalloproteinase (MMP)-2/9. Phytother Res 2018; 32(7): 1373-81.
[http://dx.doi.org/10.1002/ptr.6071] [PMID: 29532526]

[133]  Traber MG, Packer L, Vitamin E. Vitamin E: beyond antioxidant function. Am J Clin Nutr 1995; 62(6) (Suppl.): 1501S-9S.
[http://dx.doi.org/10.1093/ajcn/62.6.1501S] [PMID: 7495251]

[134]  Ong ASH, Goh SH. Palm oil: a healthful and cost-effective dietary component. Food Nutr Bull 2002; 23(1): 11-22.
[http://dx.doi.org/10.1177/156482650202300102] [PMID: 11975364]

[135]  Aggarwal BB, Sundaram C, Prasad S, Kannappan R. Tocotrienols, the vitamin E of the 21st century: its potential against cancer and other chronic diseases. Biochem Pharmacol 2010; 80(11): 1613-31.
[http://dx.doi.org/10.1016/j.bcp.2010.07.043] [PMID: 20696139]

[136]  Mensink RP, van Houwelingen AC, Kromhout D, Hornstra G. A vitamin E concentrate rich in tocotrienols had no effect on serum lipids, lipoproteins, or platelet function in men with mildly elevated serum lipid concentrations. Am J Clin Nutr 1999; 69(2): 213-9.
[http://dx.doi.org/10.1093/ajcn/69.2.213] [PMID: 9989682]

[137]  Packer L, Weber SU, Rimbach G. Molecular aspects of alpha-tocotrienol antioxidant action and cell signalling. J Nutr 2001; 131(2): 369S-73S.

[http://dx.doi.org/10.1093/jn/131.2.369S] [PMID: 11160563]

[138]  Das S, Nesaretnam K, Das DK. Vitamins & Hormones. Academic Press 2007; pp. 419-33.

[139]  Frank J, Chin XWD, Schrader C, Eckert GP, Rimbach G. Do tocotrienols have potential as neuroprotective dietary factors? Ageing Res Rev 2012; 11(1): 163-80.
[http://dx.doi.org/10.1016/j.arr.2011.06.006] [PMID: 21763788]

[140]  Radhakrishnan AK, Mahalingam D, Selvaduray KR, Nesaretnam K. Supplementation with natural forms of vitamin E augments antigen-specific TH1-type immune response to tetanus toxoid. BioMed Res Int 2013; 2013: 782067.
[http://dx.doi.org/10.1155/2013/782067] [PMID: 23936847]

[141]  Wali VB, Sylvester PW. Synergistic antiproliferative effects of gamma-tocotrienol and statin treatment on mammary tumor cells. Lipids 2007; 42(12): 1113-23.
[http://dx.doi.org/10.1007/s11745-007-3102-0] [PMID: 17701065]

[142]  Weng-Yew W, Selvaduray KR, Ming CH, Nesaretnam K. Suppression of tumor growth by palm tocotrienols *via* the attenuation of angiogenesis. Nutr Cancer 2009; 61(3): 367-73.
[http://dx.doi.org/10.1080/01635580802582736] [PMID: 19373610]

[143]  Wang H, Khor TO, Shu L, *et al.* Plants vs. cancer: a review on natural phytochemicals in preventing and treating cancers and their druggability. Anticancer Agents Med Chem 2012; 12(10): 1281-305.
[http://dx.doi.org/10.2174/187152012803833026] [PMID: 22583408]

[144]  Ginwala R, Bhavsar R, Chigbu DI, Jain P, Khan ZK. Potential Role of Flavonoids in Treating Chronic Inflammatory Diseases with a Special Focus on the Anti-Inflammatory Activity of Apigenin. Antioxidants 2019; 8(2): 8.
[http://dx.doi.org/10.3390/antiox8020035] [PMID: 30764536]

[145]  Lin Y, Shi R, Wang X, Shen HM. Luteolin, a flavonoid with potential for cancer prevention and therapy. Curr Cancer Drug Targets 2008; 8(7): 634-46.
[http://dx.doi.org/10.2174/156800908786241050] [PMID: 18991571]

[146]  Mirossay L, Varinská L, Mojžiš J. Antiangiogenic Effect of Flavonoids and Chalcones: An Update. Int J Mol Sci 2017; 19(1): 19.
[http://dx.doi.org/10.3390/ijms19010027] [PMID: 29271940]

[147]  Gupta SC, Kim JH, Prasad S, Aggarwal BB. Regulation of survival, proliferation, invasion, angiogenesis, and metastasis of tumor cells through modulation of inflammatory pathways by nutraceuticals. Cancer Metastasis Rev 2010; 29(3): 405-34.
[http://dx.doi.org/10.1007/s10555-010-9235-2] [PMID: 20737283]

[148]  Buddhan R, Manoharan S. Diosmin reduces cell viability of A431 skin cancer cells through apoptotic induction. J Cancer Res Ther 2017; 13(3): 471-6.
[PMID: 28862211]

[149]  Alvarez N, Vicente V, Martínez C. Synergistic effect of diosmin and interferon-alpha on metastatic pulmonary melanoma. Cancer Biother Radiopharm 2009; 24(3): 347-52.
[http://dx.doi.org/10.1089/cbr.2008.0565] [PMID: 19538057]

[150]  Kim JK, Kang KA, Ryu YS, *et al.* Induction of Endoplasmic Reticulum Stress *via* Reactive Oxygen Species Mediated by Luteolin in Melanoma Cells. Anticancer Res 2016; 36(5): 2281-9.
[PMID: 27127134]

[151]  Cao HH, Chu JH, Kwan HY, *et al.* Inhibition of the STAT3 signaling pathway contributes to apigenin-mediated anti-metastatic effect in melanoma. Sci Rep 2016; 6: 21731.
[http://dx.doi.org/10.1038/srep21731] [PMID: 26911838]

[152]  Du GJ, Zhang Z, Wen XD, *et al.* Epigallocatechin Gallate (EGCG) is the most effective cancer chemopreventive polyphenol in green tea. Nutrients 2012; 4(11): 1679-91.
[http://dx.doi.org/10.3390/nu4111679] [PMID: 23201840]

[153]  Zhang J, Lei Z, Huang Z, *et al.* Epigallocatechin-3-gallate(EGCG) suppresses melanoma cell growth and metastasis by targeting TRAF6 activity. Oncotarget 2016; 7(48): 79557-71.
[http://dx.doi.org/10.18632/oncotarget.12836] [PMID: 27791197]

[154]  Kim KH, Back JH, Zhu Y, *et al.* Resveratrol targets transforming growth factor-β2 signaling to block UV-induced tumor progression. J Invest Dermatol 2011; 131(1): 195-202.
[http://dx.doi.org/10.1038/jid.2010.250] [PMID: 20720562]

[155]  Aziz SW, Aziz MH. Protective molecular mechanisms of resveratrol in UVR-induced Skin carcinogenesis. Photodermatol Photoimmunol Photomed 2018; 34(1): 35-41.
[http://dx.doi.org/10.1111/phpp.12336] [PMID: 28767162]

[156]  Ko JH, Sethi G, Um JY, *et al.* The Role of Resveratrol in Cancer Therapy. Int J Mol Sci 2017; 18(12): 18.
[http://dx.doi.org/10.3390/ijms18122589] [PMID: 29194365]

[157]  Nichols JA, Katiyar SK. Skin photoprotection by natural polyphenols: anti-inflammatory, antioxidant and DNA repair mechanisms. Arch Dermatol Res 2010; 302(2): 71-83.
[http://dx.doi.org/10.1007/s00403-009-1001-3] [PMID: 19898857]

[158]  Talalay P, Fahey JW, Healy ZR, *et al.* Sulforaphane mobilizes cellular defenses that protect skin against damage by UV radiation. Proc Natl Acad Sci USA 2007; 104(44): 17500-5.
[http://dx.doi.org/10.1073/pnas.0708710104] [PMID: 17956979]

[159]  Franklin SJ, Dickinson SE, Karlage KL, Bowden GT, Myrdal PB. Stability of sulforaphane for topical formulation. Drug Dev Ind Pharm 2014; 40(4): 494-502.
[http://dx.doi.org/10.3109/03639045.2013.768634] [PMID: 23611476]

[160]  Cristiano MC, Froiio F, Spaccapelo R, *et al.* Sulforaphane-Loaded Ultradeformable Vesicles as A Potential Natural Nanomedicine for the Treatment of Skin Cancer Diseases. Pharmaceutics 2019; 12(1): 12.
[http://dx.doi.org/10.3390/pharmaceutics12010006] [PMID: 31861672]

[161]  Cragg GM, Pezzuto JM. Natural Products as a Vital Source for the Discovery of Cancer Chemotherapeutic and Chemopreventive Agents. Med Princ Pract 2016; 25 (Suppl. 2): 41-59.
[http://dx.doi.org/10.1159/000443404] [PMID: 26679767]

# CHAPTER 6

# Bioactive Compounds as Therapeutic Intervention in Bacterial Infections

**Kazeem A. Alayande[1,2,\*], Abdulwakeel A. Ajao[3] and Mariam O. Oyedeji-Amusa[3]**

[1] *Antibiotic Resistance and Phage Biocontrol Research Group, Department of Microbiology, North-West University, Mmabatho 2745, South Africa*

[2] *Unit for Environmental Sciences and Managements, North-West University, Potchefstroom, South Africa*

[3] *Department of Botany and Plant Biotechnology, University of Johannesburg, PO Box 524, Auckland Park 2006, Johannesburg, South Africa*

**Abstract:** This study highlights the significance of drug resistance towards difficulties in the treatment of infectious diseases, the essence of bioactive compounds in therapeutic intervention, and the unique approach employed by bioactive compounds away from conventional synthetic drugs. Literature was gathered from different online databases to retrieve the required information. Bacterial resistance to antibiotics is a major concern that threatens clinical efforts in treating bacterial infections. This has grossly reduced clinical success on previously curable infections and/or sometimes results in a prolonged hospital stay. Antibiotics provide protection and remedy against infectious diseases. But the emergence of multi-drug resistance strains has inflicted untold loss of effectiveness on virtually every conventional antibiotic. Hence, scientific communities are propelled into seeking alternative therapies in a bid to mitigate the overwhelming consequence on public health. Bioactive molecules are important sources of newly derived therapeutic agents. They have minimal likelihood of inducing unintended immune reactions, reduced level of toxicity; are structurally diverse in nature, exhibit broad-spectrum therapeutic effects. Bioactive molecules are commonly present in small amounts in plant-based foods; and provide health benefits in addition to the basic nutritional values expected in foods. Several plant-based bioactive principles serve as inhibitors for drug resistance in order to enhance the effective delivery of the antibacterial compounds. Meat products are a good source of non-plant bioactive molecules, which are expressed in the form of peptides, vitamins, minerals and fatty acids. Other important sources include endophytic bacteria, endophytic fungi, probiotic bacteria, actinomycetes and marine organisms. Natural products are relatively

---

**\* Corresponding author Kazeem A. Alayande:** Antibiotic Resistance and Phage Biocontrol Research Group, Department of Microbiology, North-West University, Mmabatho 2745, South Africa; Tel: +2763 033 3574; E-mail: jkadekunle2@gmail.com

**Saheed Sabiu (Ed)**
**All rights reserved-© 2022 Bentham Science Publishers**

safe when compared to their synthetic counterparts. As newly manufactured potent antibiotics become increasingly unavailable and/or unaffordable, bioactive compounds present viable alternatives. They are readily available and are derived from inexpensive raw materials *via* cheap technology.

**Keywords:** Alkaloids, Antimicrobials, Bacteriocins, Natural products, Phenols, Super burgs.

# 1. INTRODUCTION

The resurgence of multi-drug resistant bacterial pathogens of infectious diseases has significantly reduced therapeutic options in the clinics, hence propelling the scientific communities into seeking alternative therapy in a bid to mitigate the overwhelming consequence on public health. The resurgence has led to reduced clinical success on previously curable infections and in some cases, results in a prolonged stay in hospitals [1, 2]. Antibiotics, as natural or synthetic organic molecules, are lethal to microorganisms; and provide protections and remedies against infections caused by bacteria pathogens. However, the emergence of multi-drug resistance strains has inflicted untold loss of effectiveness on virtually every conventional, including the frontline, antibiotics [3].

Bioactive compounds are secondary metabolites produced by some living cells and are capable of therapeutic potentials; exhibit prophylactic and immunomodulatory activities; mitigate toxin effects; reduce oxidative stress; and enhance effective metabolism [4, 5]. Bioactive molecules are commonly present, in small amounts, in plant-based foods and provide health benefits in addition to the basic nutritional values expected in foods; hence, they are said to be non-nutrient food components that exhibit medicinal effects in living systems when ingested [6]. The presence of these molecules has been speculated to be responsible for the evidenced-based potential health benefits attributed to the adequate consumption of fruits and vegetables [7].

Moreover, there has been increasing interest in the medicinal advantages of these bioactive molecules. Plant-based foods and traditional medicinal plants employed in folklore remedies have been the primary source of these active molecules [5, 8]. Though in recent times, more considerations have equally been given to the non-plant entities, such as microorganisms and meat products, as other rich sources of bioactive agents of therapeutic importance [9]. The increasing awareness of the valuable medicinal features of the bioactive compounds has warranted the need for a collective effort among stakeholders to provide an accessible database containing required basic information on these compounds. The available public database in this respect includes USDA flavonoid content of selected foods [10]; Phenol-Explorer: database for polyphenols in foods [11]; and EuroFIR eBASIS: Bioactive Substances in Food Information Systems [12].

Natural products have been the most important source of bioactive molecules while plants and microbes have been the centre of this for valuable drug discovery [13, 14]. Bioactive compounds are made up of extremely heterogeneous classes of compounds with structurally diverse chemical compositions and are widely distributed in nature. They have a different range of concentrations in both plants and animals; they also have specific sites of action for their biological activities and are equally effective against reactive oxygen species [15]. Meat products are a good source of non-plant bioactive molecules where they are expressed in the form of proteins/peptides, vitamins, minerals and fatty acids [16]. Other important sources include, endophytic bacterial [17], endophytic fungi [18], probiotic bacteria [2], actinomycetes [19] and marine organisms [20] (Fig. **1**). Several organisms in the oceanic ecosystems are indispensable sources of natural products endowed with ranges of structural diversities and significant bioactivities for human applications [21]. The marine environment is highly rich in biological and chemical diversity. Due to the extremity, aggressiveness and competitiveness associated with the marine environment, organisms therein produce several secondary metabolites with promising potential therapeutic agents, nutritional supplements and agrochemicals [20].

Polyphenols are among the most prevalent and diverse groups of secondary metabolites, produced by plants and other organisms and are noted for their potential against quorum sensing, detoxification and formation of biofilm by pathogens [22]. Alkaloids, on the other hand, provide the underlying structures for the development of a great variety of antibiotics with a wider range of actions [23]. The bacteriocidal effect of tannins against pathogens is not limited to plasma membrane destabilization; it also involves inhibition of extracellular enzymes, disruption of metabolic pathways and blockage of the trace-nutrients required for cell growth [24]. Terpenoids are another abundant group of valuable natural products that play important roles in plant defence against pathogens and pest attacks and are widely used in pharmaceuticals for drug discoveries [25]. Moreover, saponins, due to their amphipathic property, have also been a valuable natural product employed in the development of drugs, cosmetics, and surface disinfectants against bacterial contamination, while several studies have also reported their activities against bacterial pathogens [26, 27]. The ability of some of these metabolites, and several others in their category, to modify resistance features in a pathogen provides a hedge in the combat against the spread of bacterial resistance [23].

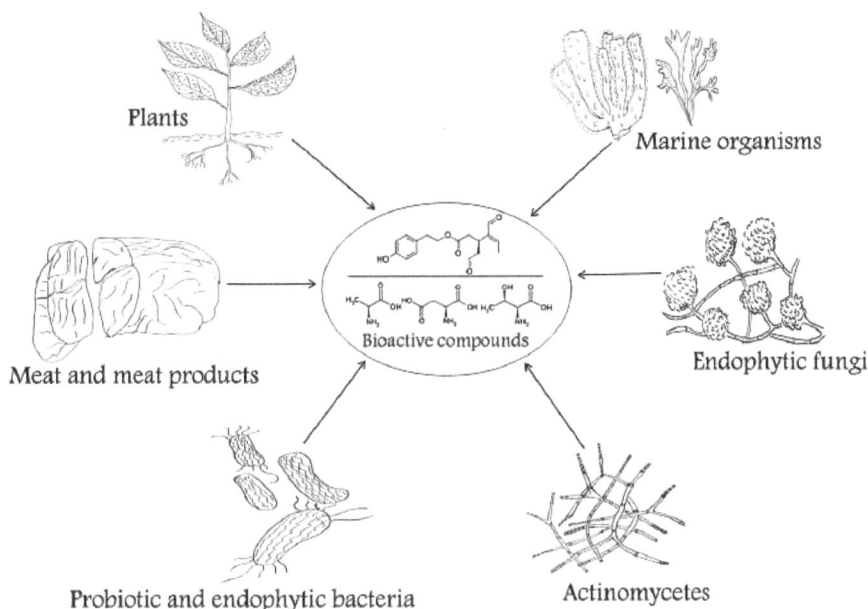

**Fig. (1).** Important sources of bioactive compounds.

Hence, in this study, we have put together the significance of the daily increase in the occurrence of multi-drug resistant bacterial pathogens and their contributions to the galvanised difficulties the world is experiencing in the treatment of bacterial infections. We equally highlight essence of the bioactive compounds in therapeutic intervention towards the rescue of this unpleasant condition which has impacted a huge setback on clinical success. We also mentioned a number of unique approaches employed by these compounds away from the conventional synthetic drugs and finally dwelled on specific antibacterial activities of some of these active secondary metabolites, which substantiate their efficacy as an alternative therapeutic option.

Relevant articles used in this study were gathered from different online databases (these are: Scopus, Web of Science, ScienceDirect, Google Scholar and PubMed) in order to retrieve information on specific scientific reports that investigate bioactive compounds and their therapeutic intervention in the combat against bacterial infections. The online searches were carried out between August 2020 and February 2021 with no exclusion of any period, and no language restrictions were as well applied. The abstracts for all retrieved articles were carefully read to determine their relevance and eligibility. Articles from 2015 and before were only considered if no recent study had closely related contents.

## 2. DIFFICULTIES IN THE TREATMENT OF BACTERIAL INFECTIONS

Bacterial resistance to antibiotics is a major concern that threatens clinical efforts in the treatment of common bacterial infections [28]. The increasing frequency and ease of acquiring drug resistance genes among bacteria of the same or different species have made the infections caused by bacteria extremely difficult to treat because the resistance is often not limited to a specific class of antibiotic. And many recognized highly potent antibiotics have become clinically insignificant within a short period of time [29]. A bacterial strain that has acquired resistance genes could eventually become resistant to every commonly prescribed, and even the last-resort, clinical antimicrobials. Thereby results in protracted ailment and may aggravate the risk of spreading the multi-resistant strain across communities. This could result in an outbreak that may consequently be expensive and difficult to eradicate, therefore, increasing the risk of death [30].

In early 2017, the World Health Organization [31] released a list of antimicrobial drug-resistant priority pathogens referred to as the "threat list," which comprises 12 groups of bacteria; prioritized in ranking as critical, high and medium sub-categories (Table **1**). The highest-ranked bacterial pathogen is carbapenem-resistant *Acinetobacter baumannii*. The bacterial species causes severe infection with almost no treatment in existence and mainly affects individuals with the compromised immune system. Its resistance to carbapenem antibiotics, which serve as the last line of clinical drug prescription, would further worsen the precarious condition [32].

In addition, multi-drug resistant strains of *Pseudomonas aeruginosa* have been reportedly spread within and outside several communities and hospital environments; often leading to severe outbreaks and therapeutic impasse [33]. Several scientific studies have indicated a plethora of resistance genes common with *P. aeruginosa*; this include β-lactamase resistance genes, *blaPAO* and *blaOXA50*; *rmtB*, a 16S rRNA methylase known to confer resistance against almost all aminoglycosides; aminoglycosides phosphotransferases (*aph(3')-IIbI*); efflux pump systems and resistance-nodulation-division family; tetracyclin class B and class C; fosfomycin *fosA*; vancomycin B-type (*vanW*); and phenicols *catB7* [34 - 40]. It has been equally established that insertion of *blaOXA50 in Pseudomonas aeruginosa* drastically reduces its sensitivity towards ticarcillin, ampicillin, meropenem and moxalactam [41].

**Table 1. The threat list ranking according to World Health Organization.**

| Sub-categories | Priority Pathogens | Important Resistance Profile |
|---|---|---|
| Priority 1: Critical | *Acinetobacter baumannii* | Carbapenem resistance |
| - | *Pseudomonas aeruginosa* | Carbapenem resistance |
| - | *Enterobacteriaceae* | Carbapenem resistance, Extended-spectrum β-lactamase (ESBL) producing |
| Priority 2: High | *Enterococcus faecium* | Vancomycin resistance |
| - | *Staphylococcus aureus* | Methicillin resistance, Vancomycin intermediate and resistance |
| - | *Helicobacter pylori* | Clarithromycin resistance |
| - | *Campylobacter* spp. | Fluoroquinolone resistance |
| - | *Salmonellae* | Fluoroquinolone resistance |
| - | *Neisseria gonorrhoeae* | Cephalosporin resistance, Fluoroquinolone resistance |
| Priority 3: Medium | *Streptococcus pneumoniae* | Penicillin non-susceptible |
| - | *Haemophilus influenzae* | Ampicillin resistance |
| - | *Shigella* spp. | Fluoroquinolone resistance |

Additionally, many recent reports have supported the hypothesis that antimicrobial drug tolerance perpetrates treatment failure by facilitating the acquisition of antibiotic resistance [42, 43]. Multi-drug resistant bacterial strains account for more than two million cases of severe ailments and as well responsible for over twenty-three thousand annual deaths only in the United States [44]. These "super burgs" are estimated to be killing over seven hundred thousand people on yearly bases across continents and are projected to escalate into ten million deaths by the year 2050; that is above the expected death estimated for cancer-related illnesses at the moment; if efforts are not intensified to arrest the occurrence of resistance and develop new sets of antimicrobials [32].

In general, pattern of antibiotic consumption has contributed immensely to the spread of clinically important resistance genes within a community. Several studies have established a relationship between drug resistance within a community and antibiotic consumption, antibiotic prescription in primary healthcare units, and resistance to invasive infection [45 - 49]. There has ever been a very short timeline between the introduction of major antibiotics and the subsequent evolution of clinically significant resistance to the same antibiotics. For instance, methicillin-resistant *Staphylococcus aureus* (MRSA) evolved in 1961 after the methicillin antibiotic was introduced in 1959, and ever since, MRSA has been in circulation and rapidly spreading across the world, hence, potentially posing a threat on global public health [50].

Moreover, daptomycin was presumed to be a difficult drug to develop a resistance towards, partly due to its unique mechanism of action. It was highly potent against the most difficult-to-treat Gram positive bacteria such as MRSA, glycopeptide intermediate *Staphylococcus aureus* (GISA), and vancomycin resistant *Enterococci* (VRE) [51]. But on the contrary, there have been an increasing number of reports on the development of daptomycin resistance in patients under daptomycin treatment. More worrisome is the presence of a cross-resistance between vancomycin and daptomycin, while the underlying mechanism for the cross-resistance is yet to be substantially deciphered [52]. Acquisition of resistance genes is not the only mechanism adopted by bacterial pathogens in sustaining tolerance to antibiotic therapy; there has been an indication of pathogens that are genetically susceptible but could withstand treatment based on certain phenotypic traits; such strains equally play a critical role in propagating chronic and recurrent bacterial infections [53].

On a last note, it is now becoming increasingly obvious that access in terms of the availability and affordability of viable conventional antibiotics is a pressing global issue. Drug companies perceive investment in new antibiotics as a losing proposition; the new drugs would mostly be reserved to combat infections due to resistant strains, while the old drugs are given preference against susceptible strains [32]. This threatening situation demands urgent attention, which must be met with a prompt response to ensure victims of bacterial infection receive the best available therapy [54]. Because non-affordability or non-availability of drugs will definitely interfere with the treatment option and, in turn, affect the patient outcome. Intensive efforts on the bioactive compounds of natural origin as an alternative therapy against infectious diseases will be more decisive both in terms of availability and affordability, among other medical benefits.

## 3. WHAT BIOACTIVE COMPOUNDS DO DIFFERENTLY

Application of alternative therapy can help alleviate the resistance crisis. They can be used to manage infections that are no longer responsive to the conventional antibiotics and/or serve as complementary agents to the antibiotics with the aim to reduce the rate of antibiotic consumption and thereby step-down selection for drug resistance [49]. For instance, bioactive peptides are important sources of newly derived therapeutic agents. They have minimal likelihood of inducing unintended immune reactions, reduced level of toxicity, are structurally diverse in nature; and exhibit broad-spectrum therapeutic effects [14]. Antimicrobial peptides are short poly-cationic peptides that are expressed in different forms of organisms as innate immediate host defence against pathogens [55].

The mechanisms of action for various bioactive compounds as related to reducing the risk of diseases are not fully understood. Some act as antioxidants, while some others stimulate defence mechanisms, enhance response to oxidative stress, repair lost tissues, and prevent widespread damage to the body system [56]. Moreover, there is insufficient evidence for the prescribed intake, efficacy, and safety of these important agents. Although, it is generally agreed to have significant benefits when consumed in foods as part of a balanced diet [56]. Food sourced bioactive peptides are similar in structure compared to the endogenous peptides, hence, they interact with almost the same receptors and thus, play a significant role in immune regulation, growth induction system, and modification of food intake [57]. On a general note, the bioactivities and specificity of the bioactive peptides largely depend on the amino acid sequence of individual fragments, which may include antimicrobial, anti-inflammatory, antithrombotic, antioxidant, and antihypertensive, among others [20].

The entire world is experiencing growing interest in medicinal plants and other sources of natural products for their significant contribution to new drug discovery [18]. Medicinal plants may contain bioactive compounds that possess synergistic potential with conventional antimicrobial drugs or contain certain chemical groups which are devoid of antimicrobial potential but able to present the target pathogen in a more susceptible way to the previously ineffective antibiotics [29]. It is an established fact that the efficacy of antibiotics can be improved through combination with plant-based bioactive molecules and therefore reduces the minimum inhibitory concentrations (MICs) of the antibiotics against previously resistant strains [29, 58]. This form of combination therapy indicates an alternative approach in the treatment of infectious diseases and could open a wide gate toward the development of new and more efficacious agents.

Synergism is a significant factor in the low-dosage effectiveness of the active constituents in herbal products, based on the hypothesis that a consortium of the plant-based active principles often offers a timely and effective remedy over a single isolated ingredient. The inherent synergy could result from the interaction between different constituents in the plant extracts which subsequently leads to increased solubility, enhancing the active ingredients' bioavailability. And alternatively, it may be due to different components of the consortium targeting different sites of action [13, 59]. It is equally worthy of note that several plant-based bioactive principles are inhibitors of drug resistance mechanisms to enhance the effective delivery of the antibacterial compounds [13].

Microorganisms are another important source of bioactive natural molecules with enormous potential for drug discovery and industrial and agricultural applications [60]. Probiotic bacteria are known to produce antibacterial peptides as secondary metabolites, such as bacteriocin and short-chain fatty acids, functioning in the elimination of various pathogens within the gut system [61, 62]. Bacteriocins have a number of advantages compared to several other antimicrobial agents. They are safe to consume due to their ease and complete digestion in the alimentary canal, multiple folds more potent than many conventional antibiotics, and are heat tolerant [63]. Bacteriocins are specific in their bioactive role and operate distinctly away from the mechanisms applied by the synthetic antimicrobial agents. Taking advantage of their peptide nature, they are equally susceptible to genetic manipulation with a target at desired traits. This is coupled with the fact that the specificity of the bacteriocins paves the ways for a controlled target against a specific pathogen with little or no undesirable effects on the gut microbiota [64]. Most antimicrobial peptides employ the mechanism of cell membrane disruption, which directly compromises the integrity of the bacterial plasma membrane and cell wall, while others effectively form a trans-membrane channel through self-aggregation, which may lead to leakages in the cytoplasmic contents and eventual death of the cell [55].

Besides the therapeutic potential of the short-chain fatty acids against pathogens, 10% of the required daily calorie in human beings is supplied in the form of short-chain fatty acids produced in the large intestine [61]. The short-chain fatty acids also function *via* activation of the mammalian G protein-coupled receptors (GPCR), and the two major host receptors for the short-chain fatty acids are GPR41 and GPR43 [65]. The GPR43 receptor has been established through several studies to have a direct impact on induction of antimicrobial peptides production by the intestinal epithelial cells; enhancement of metabolic activities and immune system; maintenance of homeostasis in the host cells; reduction of obesity condition; and as well offers to protect against viral infections [65 - 68].

## 3.1. Efficiency of Bioactive Compounds against Bacterial Pathogens

Infectious and parasitic diseases account for almost half of the estimated yearly deaths across continents [69]. The increasing demands for improved health and prevention against diseases through dietary herbs and natural products, such as polyphenols, organic acids, minerals, vitamins, carotenoids, short-chain fatty acids, bioactive peptides, and dietary fibres among others, have led to an intensive investigation to further elucidate on their potential applications in the pharmaceuticals and functional foods [70, 71]. Medicinal plants have been used for centuries in providing folklore remedies, which has galvanized global attention lately [30]. Likewise, the aromatic herbs and spices, which form an integral part of the human diet, are being used as flavours, colorants and preservatives coupled with their antimicrobial and antioxidant functions [72].

Besides the therapeutic potentials of the medicinal and aromatic plants, they also serve as prophylactic agents for improving the health and wellbeing of human beings and livestock [73]. More equally, the natural products of microbial origin *viz*; bacteria, actinomycetes and fungi, are as well an established important source of bioactive compounds driving the discovery of new drugs and biomedical agents [19]. Natural products are relatively safe compared to their synthetic counterparts and are derived from inexpensive raw materials using relatively cheap technology. This makes them readily available in healthy functional foods and can also be added to foods [16]. Specific bioactivities of some of these active secondary metabolites, which substantiate their intervention in treating infectious diseases caused by bacterial pathogens, are highlighted below.

## 3.2. Phenols and Phenolic Compounds

The phenolic compounds isolated from the mume fruit (*Prunus mume*), a consumable fruit mostly by Chinese and Japanese, showed a very strong antimicrobial effect against all groups of the *enterobacteriacea* tested in a study conducted by Mitani *et al.* [74]. Polyphenols extracted from winery by-products of skins, seeds, and stems of Portuguese red grape varieties, Preto Martinho and Touriga Nacional, exhibit significant antimicrobial activity against a wider range of multi-drug resistant bacterial pathogens which are responsible for important clinical infections and foodborne diseases [75]. The shoot of *Salvia cadmica,* which was confirmed *via* UPLC-DAD-ESI-MS/MS analysis to contain a total of 14 phenolic compounds and 11 phenolic acid derivatives; and the root containing 10 phenolic acid derivatives both extracted in the hydro-methanol solvent, demonstrated commendable antimicrobial activity against different strains of pathogenic bacteria and fungi [76].

The genetically modified venus flytrap (*Dionaea muscipula*), with a focus on improving the synthesis of phenolic compounds indicated a remarkable increase in the 1,4-naphtoquinone derivative, plumbagin and phenolic acids (salicylic, caffeic and ellagic acid). This, in turn, markedly increased the antibacterial efficacy of the cloned carnivorous plant against multi-drug resistant pathogens of clinical importance such as *Enterococcus faecalis, Escherichia coli, Pseudomonas aeruginosa* and *Staphylococcus aureus* [77]. The Bracts of *Cynara cardunculus* (Cardoon) were collected at various maturation phases to investigate seasonal changes in its phenolic compound profiles. The bracts at the very early growth phase, which happened to have the highest content of the phenolic compounds; equally exhibited the highest and broad spectrum antibacterial and antifungal activities against different strains of pathogens, including *Listeria monocytogenes, E. coli, Enterobacter cloacae, Salmonella* Typhimurium, *Aspergillus fumigatus* and *A. niger* [78].

## 3.3. Alkaloids

Alkaloids are another important group of plant-based bioactive compounds with proven remarkable potential for drug discovery, and are believed to be responsible for innate chemical defence against pathogens and also serve as repellents against parasites and other herbivores [79]. The monoterpenoid indole alkaloids isolated from the fresh trunk of *Neolamarckia cadamba* reportedly induced an excellent anti-inflammatory response both in the *in vitro* and *in vivo* (ICR male mice) studies by Yuan and his team [80]. While the cage-like monoterpenoid indole alkaloids (scholarisines) isolated from *Alstonia scholaris* leaves were able to repress the growth of *E. coli* at a very low MIC value of 0.78 µg/ml [81]. Romeo and colleagues [82] profiled twenty-two different genotypes of *Lupinus* species (lupin): *Lupinus albus, Lupinus luteus,* and *Lupinus angustifolius,* for their alkaloids contents. The genotypes with the highest amounts of total alkaloid content showcased excellent pharmacological potential, with the extracted alkaloids exhibiting significant efficacy towards a number of clinical isolates, including *Klebsiella pneumoniae* and *P. aeruginosa.*

Moreover, 12 different alkaloids isolated from the aerial portion of the *Papaver rhoeas* L. (Papaveraceae) also exhibited strong activities against bacterial pathogens, while the fractions containing roemerine as the major alkaloid content expressed the most significant antibacterial activity [83]. A three unique subtipyrrolines, novel bioactive alkaloids, isolated from *Bacillus subtilis* SY2101 were also reported to have demonstrated moderate antibacterial and antifungal activities against *E. coli* and *Candida albicans,* respectively [84]. In another study, two monoterpenoid indole alkaloid erchinines, which possess unique 1,4-diazepine fused with oxazolidine architecture and three hemiaminals, isolated from *Ervatamia chinensis* equally expressed laudable antimicrobial effectiveness towards *Bacillus subtilis* and *Trichophyton rubrum* with the level of efficacy favourably compared with the first line drugs, cefotaxime and griseofulvin, respectively [85].

## 3.4. Tannins

Tannins are also among an important group of bioactive compounds, they are heterogeneous water-soluble polyphenolic compounds present in several vegetables and various parts of plants such as twigs, leaves, flowers, fruits, seeds and roots [86]. Tannins extracted from different grape peels were incorporated into gelatine and casein to form protein-based films. The tannin-protein interactions resulted in improved integrity of the films and commendable antimicrobial activities against *Listeria innocua* and *E. coli*. Thus, confirmed the effectiveness of tannin in the production of biocompatible and biodegradable films for use in food industries to prevent bacterial contamination and spoilage [24].

Additionally, encapsulated tannins sourced from *Acacia mearnsii* equally showed significant antimicrobial efficacy against *S. aureus*, *E. coli*, *A. niger* and *Candida* sp [86]. It was also revealed in a study conducted by Othman and cohort [87] that tannins extracted from the stem bark of *Phyllanthus columnaris* reportedly inhibit the growth of a number of tested pathogens that have been implicated in oral infections. Tannins have also been shown to reduce protein synthesis by methicillin-resistant *Staphylococcus aureus* through modulation of essential ribosomal pathways, which then causes a substantial decrease in the translation process and eventual death of the MRSA cells [88].

## 3.5. Terpenoids and Terpenes

Terpenoids and terpenes are aromatic bioactive secondary metabolites with diverse molecular structures and are found in several plant species and marine organisms. As natural products, terpenoids play an important role in the pharmaceuticals, food and cosmetics industries. In recent discoveries, a group of diterpene and sesquiterpene hydrocarbon olefins were modified by cytochromes P3.550 to produce non-volatile end-products such as β-costic acid, dolabralexins, zealexins and kauralexins which consequently provide effective direct defence towards attacking pathogens and pests in plants [89]. Terpenoids extracted from the leaves of endangered *Baliospermum montanum* and the contents identified as containing botulin, lanosterol, alpha-amyrin, olean-12-ene, 3 methoxy, and lap-20(29)-en-3-ol, significantly inhibit the growth of different strains of human bacterial pathogens [90].

A comprehensive study on a chemical-rich species of marine sponge, *Dendrilla antarctica*, resulted in a library of eleven diterpenoids including three novel dendrillins. Several of these sponge-derived diterpenoids exhibited remarkable bioactivity against the notorious and difficult-to-treat biofilm phase of MRSA, coupled with the expression of low mammalian cytotoxicity. And most importantly, the strong activity by one among the dendrillin and membranolide at the lowest test concentration [91]. In addition, another sponge-derived diterpene isolated from the antarctic dendroceratid sponge, *Dendrilla membranosa*, also reportedly had four-fold selectivity against the biofilm formed by MRSA [92]. These could represent an index developing an effective therapeutic agent against the notorious biofilm phase of the methicillin-resistant *Staphylococcus aureus* infection. Three new diterpenes, gersemiols; a new eunicellane diterpene and eunicellol were also isolated from the Arctic soft coral *Gersemia fruticosa*. Only one among the gersemiols and eunicellol demonstrated antibacterial effectiveness against a panel of test organisms which include MRSA, *Acinetobacter baumannii*, *E. coli*, *P. aeruginosa*, *C. albicans* and *A. fumigatus* [93].

## 3.6. Saponins

Saponins are an important group of active secondary metabolites widely distributed within the plant kingdom with a diverse range of applications and have been in use traditionally as natural detergents for ages [94, 95]. Plant-based natural saponins extracted from soap nuts, horse chestnuts and the bark of quillaja, significantly reduced the concentration of *Escherichia coli* attached to glass surfaces and exhibited greater efficacy when compared to the standard saponins used in the same experiment [96]. This will go a long way in reducing surface contaminations in the cosmetics and food production processing; thus, reducing the recurrent outbreak and spread of skin and foodborne pathogens with the less financial burden. In another *in vitro* and *in vivo* investigation conducted by Khan and cohorts [97], saponins isolated from the seeds of green tea plant exhibited remarkable antibacterial activity against *E. coli*, *Staphylococcus aureus* and different strains of *Salmonella* spp. with mechanism action confirmed as cell wall and cell membrane disruption. While the qRT-PCR analysis of the faecal and blood samples collected from the 5-week old chickens selected for the *in vivo* study only reveals the presence of the pathogens in the infected chickens and highly reduced expression level in the chickens treated with the isolated saponin.

Furthermore, the antibacterial potential and mechanism of biocidal action of the saponin extracted from *Sapindus mukorossi*, soap berry, was evaluated and exhibited significant effectiveness against *E. coli* through a reduction in the viability of the cells and increased permeability of the cell membrane due to loss of membrane polarity [98]. The saponins produced by two identified endophytic fungi, *Fusarium* sp. PN8 and *Aspergillus* sp. PN17, isolated from *Panax notoginseng*, a traditional Chinese medicinal herb, was also confirmed to be highly potent against test bacterial pathogens [99].

## 3.7. Flavonoids

Flavonoids belong to a group of polyphenols with low molecular weights; they are structurally diverse, easily obtained in nature, and have been used in traditional medicine for the treatment of bacterial infections of various kinds [100]. They have the basic skeletal structure of diphenylpropane, C6- C3-C6, and are well known for their antibacterial potency against a wider range of pathogens [101]. Wu *et al.* [102] investigated antibacterial activities of flavonoids, glabrol; licochalcone A; licochalcone C; and licochalcone E, isolated from *Glycyrrhiza glabra* (licorice or liquorice) against methicillin-resistant *Staphylococcus aureus* and *Escherichia coli* were investigated. The flavonoids showed excellent efficiency against test pathogens with very low toxicity toward human cells, and no apparent haemolytic reaction was displayed when evaluated for safety features. Moreover, seven different flavonoids isolated from the kino exuded from eucalyptus tree, *Corymbia torelliana*, were tested against *Pseudomonas aeruginosa* with remarkable antibacterial activities and no trace of cytotoxic effect. While one of the test flavonoids, 3,40,5,7-tetrahydroxyflavanone, was also found significantly reduce the adhesion of *P. aeruginosa* toward Vero cells [103].

## 3.8. Bioactive Peptides

Antimicrobial peptides have been mentioned to have advantages; of delayed or reduced emergence of resistance, wider range of anti-biofilm activity and modulation of host immunity; over the conventional antibiotics [104]. Bioactive peptides were produced using raw milk from bovine and goats through the proteolytic enzyme activities of *Aspergillus oryzae* and *Aspergillus flavipes* in the solid-state fermentation process. The milk-derived peptides therein demonstrated significant activity against selected human pathogens, including *S. aureus*, *E. coli*, *P. aeruginosa* and *Salmonella enterica Enteritidis*. This was concluded as a cost-effective approach valuable for the pharmaceutical and functional food industries [105]. A consortium of antibacterial peptides isolated from hydrolysed proteins that were extracted from the alga, *Macroalga Saccharina longicruris*, was also reported to have remarkably repressed the growth of *S. aureus* [106].

In an experiment conducted by Xu and colleagues [107], bacteriocin 1.0320 produced by *Lactobacillus rhamnosus* 1.0320 was purified and assessed for antibacterial potential. The purified peptide exhibited broad-spectrum antimicrobial effectiveness against a wider range of clinical isolates through increasing trans-membrane leakages of cellular contents due to the formation of pore spaces that, in turn, compromised selective permeability integrity of the membrane. A partially characterized bacteriocin KT11 synthesised by *Enterococcus faecalis* KT11 isolated from a traditional Turkish cheese showed a strong effect against a test panel of bacterial isolates, among which were vancomycin and methicillin resistant strains. Additionally, the peptide remains stable at both acidic and alkaline pH ranges; after 30 min of autoclaving at 121°C; and treatment with several surfactants and organic solvents [108].

Furthermore, an endophytic fungus, *Chaetomium globosum*, isolated from *Moringa oleifera* and optimised for improved bioactive metabolites *via* physicochemical parameters, showed commendable antimicrobial and anti-biofilm effectiveness against a wide array of pathogens, including eleven different strains of methicillin-resistant *Staphylococcus aureus* and as well confirmed to be bio-safe [109]. In another two separate studies, probiotic bacteria, *Lactobacillus reuteri* PNW1 and *Lactobacillus acidophilus* PNW3, synthesised bioactive secondary metabolite identified as bacteriocin, which was partially purified and was able to significantly suppress the growth of Shiga-toxin producing *E. coli* O177 [62, 64].

## CONCLUSION

There are increasing demands for manufacturing new antibiotics due to the continuous evolution of multi-drug resistant strains of pathogens. While on the other hand, multinational drug companies are reluctant to yield to these demands because investment in new antibiotics is perceived as a losing proposition. The new antimicrobial drugs would mostly be reserved by regulations and only allowed or encouraged to be used in the infections due to resistant strains, while the old drugs are given preference against susceptible ones. This tends to make viable antibiotics in relative situations unavailable or excessively expensive, thus, having a direct impact on the outcome of the concerned patient. Intensive efforts on bioactive natural products to provide alternative therapy against infectious diseases could represent a precise approach because they are readily available and susceptible to cheap technology.

## CONSENT FOR PUBLICATION

Not applicable.

## CONFLICT OF INTEREST

The authors declare no conflict of interest, financial or otherwise.

## ACKNOWLEDGEMENTS

Declared none.

## REFERENCES

[1]    Jackson Seukep A, Zhang Y-L, Xu Y-B, Guo M-Q. *In Vitro* Antibacterial and Antiproliferative Potential of *Echinops lanceolatus* Mattf. (Asteraceae) and Identification of Potential Bioactive Compounds. Pharmaceuticals (Basel) 2020; 13(4): 59.
[http://dx.doi.org/10.3390/ph13040059] [PMID: 32235626]

[2]    Alayande KA, Aiyegoro OA, Ateba CN. Probiotics in Animal Husbandry: Applicability and Associated Risk Factors. Sustainability 2020; 12(3): 1087.
[http://dx.doi.org/10.3390/su12031087]

[3]    AlSheikh HMA, Sultan I, Kumar V, *et al.* Plant-Based Phytochemicals as Possible Alternative to Antibiotics in Combating Bacterial Drug Resistance. Antibiotics (Basel) 2020; 9(8): 480.
[http://dx.doi.org/10.3390/antibiotics9080480] [PMID: 32759771]

[4]    Santos DI, Saraiva JMA, Vicente AA, Moldão-Martins M. Methods for determining bioavailability

and bioaccessibility of bioactive compounds and nutrients. Innovative thermal and non-thermal processing, bioaccessibility and bioavailability of nutrients and bioactive compounds. Elsevier 2019; pp. 23-54.
[http://dx.doi.org/10.1016/B978-0-12-814174-8.00002-0]

[5]     Segneanu AE, Velciov SM, Olariu S, Cziple F, Damian D, Grozescu I. Bioactive Molecules Profile from Natural Compounds.Amino acid—new insights and roles in plant and animal. IntechOpen 2017; pp. 209-28.
[http://dx.doi.org/10.5772/intechopen.68643]

[6]     Gry J, Black L, Eriksen FD, *et al.* EuroFIR-BASIS–a combined composition and biological activity database for bioactive compounds in plant-based foods. Trends in food science 2007; 18(8): 434-44.

[7]     Lai HTM, Threapleton DE, Day AJ, Williamson G, Cade JE, Burley VJ. Fruit intake and cardiovascular disease mortality in the UK Women's Cohort Study. Eur J Epidemiol 2015; 30(9): 1035-48.
[http://dx.doi.org/10.1007/s10654-015-0050-5] [PMID: 26076918]

[8]     Martín-Ortega A, Segura-Campos M. Bioactive Compounds as Therapeutic Alternatives. Bioactive Compounds. Elsevier Inc 2019; pp. 247-64.

[9]     Plumb J, Pigat S, Bompola F, *et al.* Ebasis (bioactive substances in food information systems) and bioactive intakes: Major updates of the bioactive compound composition and beneficial bioeffects database and the development of a probabilistic model to assess intakes in europe. Nutrients 2017; 9(4): 320.
[http://dx.doi.org/10.3390/nu9040320] [PMID: 28333085]

[10]    USDA Database for the Flavonoid Content of Selected Foods. Nutrient Data Laboratory, Beltsville Human Nutrition Research Center, ARS, USDA 2016.

[11]    Phenol-Explorer 3.6: a major update of the Phenol-Explorer database to incorporate data on the effects of food processing on polyphenol content and new content values for lignans. (cited 2020-11-25). 2015. Available from: http://phenol-explorer.eu/

[12]    The EuroFIR eBASIS (Bioactive Substances in Food Information Systems) [Internet] (cited 2020-11-25). Available from: https://www.eurofir.org/our-tools/ebasis/#

[13]    Borges A, Abreu AC, Dias C, Saavedra MJ, Borges F, Simões M. New perspectives on the use of phytochemicals as an emergent strategy to control bacterial infections including biofilms. Molecules 2016; 21(7): 877.
[http://dx.doi.org/10.3390/molecules21070877] [PMID: 27399652]

[14]    Agyei D, Ongkudon CM, Wei CY, Chan AS, Danquah MK. Bioprocess challenges to the isolation and purification of bioactive peptides. Food Bioprod Process 2016; 98: 244-56.
[http://dx.doi.org/10.1016/j.fbp.2016.02.003]

[15]    Galanakis CM. Nutraceutical and functional food components: Effects of innovative processing techniques. Academic Press 2017.

[16]    Pogorzelska-Nowicka E, Atanasov AG, Horbańczuk J, Wierzbicka A. Bioactive compounds in functional meat products. Molecules 2018; 23(2): 307.
[http://dx.doi.org/10.3390/molecules23020307] [PMID: 29385097]

[17]    Singh M, Kumar A, Singh R, Pandey K. Endophytic bacteria: a new source of bioactive compounds. 3 Biotech 2017; 7: 315.

[18]    Gopane B, Tchatchouang CK, Regnier T, Ateba C, Manganyi M. Community diversity and stress tolerance of culturable endophytic fungi from black seed (*Nigella sativa* L.). S Afr J Bot 137: 272-7.
[http://dx.doi.org/10.1016/j.sajb.2020.10.026]

[19]    Matsumoto A, Takahashi Y. Endophytic actinomycetes: promising source of novel bioactive compounds. J Antibiot (Tokyo) 2017; 70(5): 514-9.
[http://dx.doi.org/10.1038/ja.2017.20] [PMID: 28270688]

[20]   Pujiastuti DY, Ghoyatul Amin MN, Alamsjah MA, Hsu J-L. Marine organisms as potential sources of bioactive peptides that inhibit the activity of angiotensin I-converting enzyme: a review. Molecules 2019; 24(14): 2541.
[http://dx.doi.org/10.3390/molecules24142541] [PMID: 31336853]

[21]   Núñez-Pons L, Shilling A, Verde C, Baker BJ, Giordano D. Marine Terpenoids from Polar Latitudes and Their Potential Applications in Biotechnology. Mar Drugs 2020; 18(8): 401.
[http://dx.doi.org/10.3390/md18080401] [PMID: 32751369]

[22]   Takó M, Kerekes EB, Zambrano C, *et al.* Plant phenolics and phenolic-enriched extracts as antimicrobial agents against food-contaminating microorganisms. Antioxidants 2020; 9(2): 165.
[http://dx.doi.org/10.3390/antiox9020165] [PMID: 32085580]

[23]   Othman L, Sleiman A, Abdel-Massih RM. Antimicrobial activity of polyphenols and alkaloids in middle eastern plants. Front Microbiol 2019; 10: 911.
[http://dx.doi.org/10.3389/fmicb.2019.00911] [PMID: 31156565]

[24]   Cano A, Andres M, Chiralt A, González-Martinez C. Use of tannins to enhance the functional properties of protein based films. Food Hydrocoll 2020; 100: 105443.
[http://dx.doi.org/10.1016/j.foodhyd.2019.105443]

[25]   Yang W, Chen X, Li Y, Guo S, Wang Z, Yu X. Advances in pharmacological activities of terpenoids. Natural Product Communications 2020; 15: 3.
[http://dx.doi.org/10.1177/1934578X20903555]

[26]   Donga S, Yangc X, Zhaoa L, Zhanga F, Houd Z, Xuea P. Antibacterial activity and mechanism of action saponins from Chenopodium quinoa Willd. husks against foodborne pathogenic bacteria. Ind Crops Prod 2020; 149: 112350.
[http://dx.doi.org/10.1016/j.indcrop.2020.112350]

[27]   Fleck JD, Betti AH, da Silva FP, *et al.* Saponins from Quillaja saponaria and Quillaja brasiliensis: particular chemical characteristics and biological activities. Molecules 2019; 24(1): 171.
[http://dx.doi.org/10.3390/molecules24010171] [PMID: 30621160]

[28]   Frost I, Smith WPJ, Mitri S, *et al.* Cooperation, competition and antibiotic resistance in bacterial colonies. ISME J 2018; 12(6): 1582-93.
[http://dx.doi.org/10.1038/s41396-018-0090-4] [PMID: 29563570]

[29]   Alayande K, Pohl C, Ashafa A. Significance of combination therapy between Euclea crispa (Thunb.)(leaf and stem bark) extracts and standard antibiotics against drug resistant bacteria. S Afr J Bot 2018; 118: 203-8.
[http://dx.doi.org/10.1016/j.sajb.2018.07.025]

[30]   Alayande KA, Pohl CH, Ashafa AOT. Evaluations of biocidal potential of Euclea crispa stem bark extract and ability to compromise the integrity of microbial cell membrane. J Herb Med 2020; 21: 100304.
[http://dx.doi.org/10.1016/j.hermed.2019.100304]

[31]   WHO. WHO publishes list of bacteria for which new antibiotics are urgently needed Geneva 2017. Available from: https://www.who.int/news/item/27-02-2017-who-publishes-list-of-bacteria--or-which-new-antibiotics-are-urgently-needed

[32]   Willyard C. The drug-resistant bacteria that pose the greatest health threats. Nature 2017; 543(7643): 15.
[http://dx.doi.org/10.1038/nature.2017.21550] [PMID: 28252092]

[33]   Madaha EL, Mienie C, Gonsu HK, *et al.* Whole-genome sequence of multi-drug resistant Pseudomonas aeruginosa strains UY1PSABAL and UY1PSABAL2 isolated from human broncho-alveolar lavage, Yaoundé, Cameroon. PLoS One 2020; 15(9): e0238390.
[http://dx.doi.org/10.1371/journal.pone.0238390] [PMID: 32886694]

[34]   Grandjean T, Le Guern R, Duployez C, Faure K, Kipnis E, Dessein R. Draft Genome Sequences of

Two Pseudomonas aeruginosa Multidrug-Resistant Clinical Isolates, PAL0.1 and PAL1.1. Microbiol Resour Announc 2018; 7(17): e00940-18.
[http://dx.doi.org/10.1128/MRA.00940-18] [PMID: 30533763]

[35]   Hussain M, Suliman M, Ahmed A, Altayb H, Elneima E. Draft genome sequence of a multidrug-resistant *Pseudomonas aeruginosa* strain isolated from a patient with a urinary tract infection in Khartoum, Sudan. Genome Announc 2017; 5(16): e00203-17.
[http://dx.doi.org/10.1128/genomeA.00203-17] [PMID: 28428302]

[36]   Taiaroa G, Samuelsen Ø, Kristensen T, Økstad OAL, Heikal A. Complete Genome Sequence of *Pseudomonas aeruginosa* K34-7, a Carbapenem-Resistant Isolate of the High-Risk Sequence Type 233. Microbiol Resour Announc 2018; 7(4): e00886-18.
[http://dx.doi.org/10.1128/MRA.00886-18] [PMID: 30533874]

[37]   Poole K. Aminoglycoside resistance in *Pseudomonas aeruginosa*. Antimicrob Agents Chemother 2005; 49(2): 479-87.
[http://dx.doi.org/10.1128/AAC.49.2.479-487.2005] [PMID: 15673721]

[38]   Subedi D, Vijay AK, Kohli GS, Rice SA, Willcox M. Comparative genomics of clinical strains of *Pseudomonas aeruginosa* strains isolated from different geographic sites. Sci Rep 2018; 8(1): 15668.
[http://dx.doi.org/10.1038/s41598-018-34020-7] [PMID: 30353070]

[39]   Finch RG, Greenwood D, Whitley RJ, Norrby SR. Antibiotic and chemotherapy e-book: Elsevier Health Sciences. 2010.

[40]   Bassetti M, Vena A, Croxatto A, Righi E, Guery B. How to manage *Pseudomonas aeruginosa* infections. Drugs Context 2018; 7: 212527.
[http://dx.doi.org/10.7573/dic.212527] [PMID: 29872449]

[41]   Girlich D, Naas T, Nordmann P. Biochemical characterization of the naturally occurring oxacillinase OXA-50 of *Pseudomonas aeruginosa*. Antimicrob Agents Chemother 2004; 48(6): 2043-8.
[http://dx.doi.org/10.1128/AAC.48.6.2043-2048.2004] [PMID: 15155197]

[42]   Levin-Reisman I, Ronin I, Gefen O, Braniss I, Shoresh N, Balaban NQ. Antibiotic tolerance facilitates the evolution of resistance. Science 2017; 355(6327): 826-30.
[http://dx.doi.org/10.1126/science.aaj2191] [PMID: 28183996]

[43]   Cohen NR, Lobritz MA, Collins JJ. Microbial persistence and the road to drug resistance. Cell host 2013; 13(6): 632-42.

[44]   Gupta A, Mumtaz S, Li C-H, Hussain I, Rotello VM. Combatting antibiotic-resistant bacteria using nanomaterials. Chem Soc Rev 2019; 48(2): 415-27.
[http://dx.doi.org/10.1039/C7CS00748E] [PMID: 30462112]

[45]   Costelloe C, Metcalfe C, Lovering A, Mant D, Hay AD. Effect of antibiotic prescribing in primary care on antimicrobial resistance in individual patients: systematic review and meta-analysis. BMJ 2010; 340: c2096.
[http://dx.doi.org/10.1136/bmj.c2096] [PMID: 20483949]

[46]   Bell BG, Schellevis F, Stobberingh E, Goossens H, Pringle M. A systematic review and meta-analysis of the effects of antibiotic consumption on antibiotic resistance. BMC Infect Dis 2014; 14(1): 13.
[http://dx.doi.org/10.1186/1471-2334-14-13] [PMID: 24405683]

[47]   Goossens H, Ferech M, Vander Stichele R, Elseviers M. Outpatient antibiotic use in Europe and association with resistance: a cross-national database study. Lancet 2005; 365(9459): 579-87.
[http://dx.doi.org/10.1016/S0140-6736(05)17907-0] [PMID: 15708101]

[48]   Hicks LA, Chien Y-W, Taylor TH Jr, Haber M, Klugman KP. Outpatient antibiotic prescribing and nonsusceptible *Streptococcus pneumoniae* in the United States, 1996-2003. Clin Infect Dis 2011; 53(7): 631-9.
[http://dx.doi.org/10.1093/cid/cir443] [PMID: 21890767]

[49]   Wollein Waldetoft K, Brown SP. Alternative therapeutics for self-limiting infections-An indirect

approach to the antibiotic resistance challenge. PLoS Biol 2017; 15(12): e2003533.
[http://dx.doi.org/10.1371/journal.pbio.2003533] [PMID: 29283999]

[50]   Li B, Webster TJ. Bacteria antibiotic resistance: New challenges and opportunities for implant-associated orthopedic infections. J Orthop Res 2018; 36(1): 22-32.
[PMID: 28722231]

[51]   Rybak MJ, Hershberger E, Moldovan T, Grucz RG. *In vitro* activities of daptomycin, vancomycin, linezolid, and quinupristin-dalfopristin against Staphylococci and Enterococci, including vancomycin-intermediate and -resistant strains. Antimicrob Agents Chemother 2000; 44(4): 1062-6.
[http://dx.doi.org/10.1128/AAC.44.4.1062-1066.2000] [PMID: 10722513]

[52]   Zaffiri L, Gardner J, Toledo-Pereyra LH. History of antibiotics: from fluoroquinolones to daptomycin (Part 2). J Invest Surg 2013; 26(4): 167-79.
[http://dx.doi.org/10.3109/08941939.2013.808461] [PMID: 23869821]

[53]   Meylan S, Andrews IW, Collins JJ. Targeting antibiotic tolerance, pathogen by pathogen. Cell 2018; 172(6): 1228-38.
[http://dx.doi.org/10.1016/j.cell.2018.01.037] [PMID: 29522744]

[54]   Tängdén T, Pulcini C, Aagaard H, *et al.* Unavailability of old antibiotics threatens effective treatment for common bacterial infections. Lancet Infect Dis 2018; 18(3): 242-4.
[http://dx.doi.org/10.1016/S1473-3099(18)30075-6] [PMID: 29485082]

[55]   Le C-F, Fang C-M, Sekaran SD. Intracellular targeting mechanisms by antimicrobial peptides. Antimicrob Agents Chemother 2017; 61(4): e02340-16.
[http://dx.doi.org/10.1128/AAC.02340-16] [PMID: 28167546]

[56]   Astley S, Finglas P. Nutrition and health. Reference Module in Food Science 2016; pp. 1-6.

[57]   Sánchez-Rivera L, Martínez-Maqueda D, Cruz-Huerta E, Miralles B, Recio I. Peptidomics for discovery, bioavailability and monitoring of dairy bioactive peptides. Food Res Int 2014; 63: 170-81.
[http://dx.doi.org/10.1016/j.foodres.2014.01.069]

[58]   Aiyegoro O, Adewusi A, Oyedemi S, Akinpelu D, Okoh A. Interactions of antibiotics and methanolic crude extracts of Afzelia Africana (Smith.) against drug resistance bacterial isolates. Int J Mol Sci 2011; 12(7): 4477-503.
[http://dx.doi.org/10.3390/ijms12074477] [PMID: 21845091]

[59]   Aiyegoro O, Okoh A. Use of bioactive plant products in combination with standard antibiotics: implications in antimicrobial chemotherapy. J Med Plants Res 2009; 3(13): 1147-52.

[60]   Nwakanma C, Njoku E, Pharamat T. Antimicrobial activity of secondary metabolites of fungi isolated from leaves of bush mango. Journal of next generation sequencing applications 2016; 3(135): 2.

[61]   Indira M, Venkateswarulu T, Peele KA, Bobby MN, Krupanidhi S. Bioactive molecules of probiotic bacteria and their mechanism of action: a review. 3 Biotech 2019; 9(8): 306.

[62]   Alayande KA, Aiyegoro OA, Ateba CN. Distribution of Important Probiotic Genes and Identification of the Biogenic Amines Produced by *Lactobacillus acidophilus* PNW3. Foods 2020; 9(12): 1840.
[http://dx.doi.org/10.3390/foods9121840] [PMID: 33321968]

[63]   Bédard F, Hammami R, Zirah S, Rebuffat S, Fliss I, Biron E. Synthesis, antimicrobial activity and conformational analysis of the class IIa bacteriocin pediocin PA-1 and analogs thereof. Sci Rep 2018; 8(1): 9029.
[http://dx.doi.org/10.1038/s41598-018-27225-3] [PMID: 29899567]

[64]   Alayande KA, Aiyegoro OA, Nengwekhulu TM, Katata-Seru L, Ateba CN. Integrated genome-based probiotic relevance and safety evaluation of Lactobacillus reuteri PNW1. PLoS One 2020; 15(7): e0235873.
[http://dx.doi.org/10.1371/journal.pone.0235873] [PMID: 32687505]

[65]   Zhao Y, Chen F, Wu W, *et al.* GPR43 mediates microbiota metabolite SCFA regulation of

antimicrobial peptide expression in intestinal epithelial cells *via* activation of mTOR and STAT3. Mucosal Immunol 2018; 11(3): 752-62.
[http://dx.doi.org/10.1038/mi.2017.118] [PMID: 29411774]

[66]    Horiuchi H, Kamikado K, Aoki R, *et al.* Bifidobacterium animalis subsp. lactis GCL2505 modulates host energy metabolism *via* the short-chain fatty acid receptor GPR43. Sci Rep 2020; 10(1): 4158.
[http://dx.doi.org/10.1038/s41598-020-60984-6] [PMID: 32139755]

[67]    Kimura I, Ozawa K, Inoue D, *et al.* The gut microbiota suppresses insulin-mediated fat accumulation *via* the short-chain fatty acid receptor GPR43. Nat Commun 2013; 4(1): 1829.
[http://dx.doi.org/10.1038/ncomms2852] [PMID: 23652017]

[68]    Antunes KH, Fachi JL, de Paula R, *et al.* Microbiota-derived acetate protects against respiratory syncytial virus infection through a GPR43-type 1 interferon response. Nat Commun 2019; 10(1): 3273.
[http://dx.doi.org/10.1038/s41467-019-11152-6] [PMID: 31332169]

[69]    Gouda S, Das G, Sen SK, Shin H-S, Patra JK. Endophytes: a treasure house of bioactive compounds of medicinal importance. Front Microbiol 2016; 7: 1538.
[http://dx.doi.org/10.3389/fmicb.2016.01538] [PMID: 27746767]

[70]    Wen P, Zong M-H, Linhardt RJ, Feng K, Wu H. Electrospinning: A novel nano-encapsulation approach for bioactive compounds. Trends Food Sci Technol 2017; 70: 56-68.
[http://dx.doi.org/10.1016/j.tifs.2017.10.009]

[71]    Bai Z-Z, Ni J, Tang J-M, *et al.* Bioactive components, antioxidant and antimicrobial activities of Paeonia rockii fruit during development. Food Chem 2021; 343: 128444.
[http://dx.doi.org/10.1016/j.foodchem.2020.128444] [PMID: 33131958]

[72]    Puvača N. Bioactive compounds in selected hot spices and medicinal plants. J Agron 2018; 11(1): 8-17.

[73]    Puvača N, Kostadinović L, Popović S, *et al.* Proximate composition, cholesterol concentration and lipid oxidation of meat from chickens fed dietary spice addition (*Allium sativum, Piper nigrum, Capsicum annuum*). Anim Prod Sci 2016; 56(11): 1920-7.
[http://dx.doi.org/10.1071/AN15115]

[74]    Mitani T, Ota K, Inaba N, Kishida K, Koyama HA, Bulletin P. Antimicrobial activity of the phenolic compounds of Prunus mume against Enterobacteria. Biological 2018; 41(2): 208-12.
[http://dx.doi.org/10.1248/bpb.b17-00711] [PMID: 29386480]

[75]    Silva V, Igrejas G, Falco V, *et al.* Chemical composition, antioxidant and antimicrobial activity of phenolic compounds extracted from wine industry by-products. Food Control 2018; 92: 516-22.
[http://dx.doi.org/10.1016/j.foodcont.2018.05.031]

[76]    Piątczak E, Owczarek A, Lisiecki P, *et al.* Identification and quantification of phenolic compounds in Salvia cadmica Boiss. and their biological potential. Ind Crops Prod 2020.: 113113.

[77]    Makowski W, Królicka A, Nowicka A, *et al.* Transformed tissue of Dionaea muscipula J. Ellis as a source of biologically active phenolic compounds with bactericidal properties. Appl Microbiol Biotechnol 2021; 105(3): 1215-26.
[http://dx.doi.org/10.1007/s00253-021-11101-8] [PMID: 33447868]

[78]    Mandim F, Petropoulos SA, Dias MI, *et al.* Seasonal variation in bioactive properties and phenolic composition of cardoon (Cynara cardunculus var. altilis) bracts. Food Chem 2021; 336: 127744.
[http://dx.doi.org/10.1016/j.foodchem.2020.127744] [PMID: 32781352]

[79]    Naidoo D, Manning J, Slavětínská L, Van Staden J. Isolation of the antibacterial alkaloid distichamine from Crossyne Salisb.(Amaryllidaceae: Amaryllideae: Strumariinae). S Afr J Bot 2021; 137: 331-4.
[http://dx.doi.org/10.1016/j.sajb.2020.10.011]

[80]    Yuan H-L, Zhao Y-L, Qin X-J, *et al.* Anti-inflammatory and analgesic activities of Neolamarckia cadamba and its bioactive monoterpenoid indole alkaloids. J Ethnopharmacol 2020; 260: 113103.

[http://dx.doi.org/10.1016/j.jep.2020.113103] [PMID: 32569718]

[81]    Yu H-F, Huang W-Y, Ding C-F, *et al.* Cage-like monoterpenoid indole alkaloids with antimicrobial activity from Alstonia scholaris. Tetrahedron Lett 2018; 59(31): 2975-8.
[http://dx.doi.org/10.1016/j.tetlet.2018.06.047]

[82]    Romeo FV, Fabroni S, Ballistreri G, Muccilli S, Spina A, Rapisarda P. Characterization and Antimicrobial Activity of Alkaloid Extracts from Seeds of Different Genotypes of Lupinus spp. Sustainability 2018; 10(3): 788.
[http://dx.doi.org/10.3390/su10030788]

[83]    Çoban İ, Toplan GG, Özbek B, Gürer ÇU, Sarıyar G. Variation of alkaloid contents and antimicrobial activities of Papaver rhoeas L. growing in Turkey and northern Cyprus. Pharm Biol 2017; 55(1): 1894-8.
[http://dx.doi.org/10.1080/13880209.2017.1340964] [PMID: 28633584]

[84]    Qin L, Yi W, Lian X-Y, Wang N, Zhang ZJT. Subtipyrrolines A–C, novel bioactive alkaloids from the Mariana Trench-associated bacterium Bacillus subtilis SY2101 2020; 76(42): 131516.
[http://dx.doi.org/10.1016/j.tet.2020.131516]

[85]    Yu H-F, Qin X-J, Ding C-F, *et al.* Nepenthe-like indole alkaloids with antimicrobial activity from Ervatamia chinensis. Org Lett 2018; 20(13): 4116-20.
[http://dx.doi.org/10.1021/acs.orglett.8b01675] [PMID: 29927253]

[86]    Dos Santos C, Vargas Á, Fronza N, Dos Santos JHZ. Structural, textural and morphological characteristics of tannins from Acacia mearnsii encapsulated using sol-gel methods: Applications as antimicrobial agents. Colloids Surf B Biointerfaces 2017; 151: 26-33.
[http://dx.doi.org/10.1016/j.colsurfb.2016.11.041] [PMID: 27940166]

[87]    Othman T, Hanafiah RM, Nam NA, Mohd-Said S, Adnan SNA. Chemical composition and *in vitro* antimicrobial properties of phyllanthus columnaris stem bark tannins against oral pathogens. Int J Int Dent Med Res 2019; 12(3): 848-53.

[88]    Adnan SN, Ibrahim N, Yaacob WA. Disruption of methicillin-resistant *Staphylococcus aureus* protein synthesis by tannins. Germs 2017; 7(4): 186-92.
[http://dx.doi.org/10.18683/germs.2017.1125] [PMID: 29264356]

[89]    Block AK, Vaughan MM, Schmelz EA, Christensen SA. Biosynthesis and function of terpenoid defense compounds in maize (Zea mays). Planta 2019; 249(1): 21-30.
[http://dx.doi.org/10.1007/s00425-018-2999-2] [PMID: 30187155]

[90]    Radhakrishna S, Kumari S. GCMS Analysis of total terpenoids from Baliospermum montanum and its antimicrobial activity. J Adv Res Appl Sci 2018; 5(3): 94-101.

[91]    Bory A, Shilling AJ, Allen J, *et al.* Bioactivity of spongian diterpenoid scaffolds from the Antarctic sponge Dendrilla Antarctica. Mar Drugs 2020; 18(6): 327.
[http://dx.doi.org/10.3390/md18060327] [PMID: 32586020]

[92]    von Salm JL, Witowski CG, Fleeman RM, *et al.* Darwinolide, a new diterpene scaffold that inhibits methicillin-resistant *Staphylococcus aureus* biofilm from the Antarctic sponge Dendrilla membranosa. Org Lett 2016; 18(11): 2596-9.
[http://dx.doi.org/10.1021/acs.orglett.6b00979] [PMID: 27175857]

[93]    Angulo-Preckler C, Genta-Jouve G, Mahajan N, *et al.* Gersemiols A-C and Eunicellol A, Diterpenoids from the Arctic Soft Coral Gersemia fruticosa. J Nat Prod 2016; 79(4): 1132-6.
[http://dx.doi.org/10.1021/acs.jnatprod.6b00040] [PMID: 26894524]

[94]    Kregiel D, Berlowska J, Witonska I, *et al.* Saponin-based, biological-active surfactants from plants. Application characterization of surfactants 2017; 6(1): 184-205.
[http://dx.doi.org/10.5772/68062]

[95]    Nguyen LT, Fărcaş AC, Socaci SA, *et al.* An Overview of Saponins–A Bioactive Group. Bulletin UASVM Food Science Technology 2020; 77: 1.

[96]    Fink R, Potočnik A, Oder M. Plant-based natural saponins for *Escherichia coli* surface hygiene management. Lebensm Wiss Technol 2020; 122: 109018.
[http://dx.doi.org/10.1016/j.lwt.2020.109018]

[97]    Khan MI, Ahhmed A, Shin JH, Baek JS, Kim MY, Kim JD. Green tea seed isolated saponins exerts antibacterial effects against various strains of gram positive and gram negative bacteria, a comprehensive study *in vitro* and *in vivo*. Evidence-Based Complementary Alternative Medicine 2018; 2018
[http://dx.doi.org/10.1155/2018/3486106]

[98]    Faling L, Lei X, Chunyan Y, Zengli W. Antimicrobial Mechanism of Saponin from Sapindus mukorossi against *Escherichia coli*. Med Plant 2019; 10(6)

[99]    Jin Z, Gao L, Zhang L, *et al.* Antimicrobial activity of saponins produced by two novel endophytic fungi from Panax notoginseng. Nat Prod Res 2017; 31(22): 2700-3.
[http://dx.doi.org/10.1080/14786419.2017.1292265] [PMID: 28278662]

[100]   Farhadi F, Khameneh B, Iranshahi M, Iranshahy M. Antibacterial activity of flavonoids and their structure-activity relationship: An update review. Phytother Res 2019; 33(1): 13-40.
[http://dx.doi.org/10.1002/ptr.6208] [PMID: 30346068]

[101]   Xie Y, Yang W, Tang F, Chen X, Ren L. Antibacterial activities of flavonoids: structure-activity relationship and mechanism. Curr Med Chem 2015; 22(1): 132-49.
[http://dx.doi.org/10.2174/0929867321666140916113443] [PMID: 25245513]

[102]   Wu S-C, Yang Z-Q, Liu F, *et al.* Antibacterial effect and mode of action of flavonoids from licorice against methicillin-resistant *Staphylococcus aureus*. Front Microbiol 2019; 10: 2489.
[http://dx.doi.org/10.3389/fmicb.2019.02489] [PMID: 31749783]

[103]   Nobakht M, Trueman SJ, Wallace HM, Brooks PR, Streeter KJ, Katouli M. Antibacterial properties of flavonoids from kino of the eucalypt tree, Corymbia torelliana. Plants 2017; 6(3): 39.
[http://dx.doi.org/10.3390/plants6030039] [PMID: 28906457]

[104]   Magana M, Pushpanathan M, Santos AL, *et al.* The value of antimicrobial peptides in the age of resistance. Lancet Infect Dis 2020; 20(9): e216-30.
[http://dx.doi.org/10.1016/S1473-3099(20)30327-3] [PMID: 32653070]

[105]   Zanutto-Elgui MR, Vieira JCS, Prado DZD, *et al.* Production of milk peptides with antimicrobial and antioxidant properties through fungal proteases. Food Chem 2019; 278: 823 31.
[http://dx.doi.org/10.1016/j.foodchem.2018.11.119] [PMID: 30583449]

[106]   Beaulieu L, Bondu S, Doiron K, Rioux L-E, Turgeon SL. Characterization of antibacterial activity from protein hydrolysates of the macroalga Saccharina longicruris and identification of peptides implied in bioactivity. J Funct Foods 2015; 17: 685-97.
[http://dx.doi.org/10.1016/j.jff.2015.06.026]

[107]   Xu C, Fu Y, Liu F, *et al.* Purification and antimicrobial mechanism of a novel bacteriocin produced by *Lactobacillus rhamnosus* 1.0320. Lebensm Wiss Technol 2020; 137: 110338.
[http://dx.doi.org/10.1016/j.lwt.2020.110338]

[108]   Abanoz HS, Kunduhoglu B. Antimicrobial activity of a bacteriocin produced by Enterococcus faecalis KT11 against some pathogens and antibiotic-resistant bacteria. Han-gug Chugsan Sigpum Hag-hoeji 2018; 38(5): 1064-79.
[http://dx.doi.org/10.5851/kosfa.2018.e40] [PMID: 30479512]

[109]   Kaur N, Arora DS. Prospecting the antimicrobial and antibiofilm potential of Chaetomium globosum an endophytic fungus from Moringa oleifera. AMB Express 2020; 10(1): 206.
[http://dx.doi.org/10.1186/s13568-020-01143-y] [PMID: 33175340]

# CHAPTER 7

# The Use of Plant Secondary Metabolites in the Treatment of Bacterial Diseases

**Pillay Charlene[1,\*], Ramdhani Nishani[2] and Singh Seema[3]**

[1] *Department of Biotechnology and Food Science, Durban University of Technology, Durban, South Africa*

[2] *Council for Scientific and Industrial Research, Durban, South Africa*

[3] *Subinite (Pty) Ltd - Godrej Consumer Products South Africa, Durban, South Africa*

**Abstract:** Plants produce an array of secondary metabolites identified as possible anti-microbial agents that are used across the globe to treat numerous diseases and ailments. These secondary metabolites serve as unique commercial sources of various pharmaceuticals, food additives and flavouring agents, and possess diverse industrial applications. Alkaloids, flavonoids, and polyphenols are secondary metabolites shown to attack numerous gram-positive and gram negative bacteria in response to microbial infections. Secondary plant metabolites have a detrimental effect on microbial cells in several ways, such as alteration of the structure and function of the cytoplasmic membrane as well as DNA/RNA synthesis, interference with intermediary metabolism, interaction with membrane proteins, a disruption in the movement of protons leading to ion leakage, enzyme synthesis inhibition, the clotting of cytoplasmic components and interference in typical cell communication. This ultimately results in cell death. The focus of this chapter is to provide an overview of the function and benefits of plant secondary metabolites as therapeutic agents to combat pathogenic bacterial infections.

**Keywords:** Alkaloids, Anti-microbial agents, Bacteria, Infectious diseases, Medicinal plants, Secondary metabolites.

## 1. INTRODUCTION

Mankind has used several plants and their derivatives for medicinal purposes, since ancient times, especially for the treatment of infectious diseases. An excellent example of this is quinine, an alkaloid derived from the cinchona tree bark. Achan *et al.* [1] has reported on this alkaloid as a treatment for malaria and infectious diseases such as pneumonia and typhoid fever. Another wondrous anti-

---

\* **Corresponding author Pillay Charlene:** Department of Biotechnology and Food Science, Durban University of Technology, Durban, South Africa; Tel: 031 373 5324; E-mail: CharleneP@dut.ac.za

**Saheed Sabiu (Ed)**

microbial agent is cinnamon which is widely used in ancient Chinese medicine and has multipurpose applications due to its main biologically active agent, cinnamaldehyde [2]. There are several remedies that stem from traditional therapeutic practices which require the biological activity of various substances derived from plants to treat different diseases, including bacterial infections. Several of these traditional remedial practices are still extensively used currently. Several drugs that are currently used in medicine come from folk medicine [3].

Secondary plant metabolites, a group of biochemical substances produced by metabolic pathways of plant cells, have shown to promote the curative effects of plants. Contrary to primary metabolites, namely nucleic acids, amino acids, carbohydrates, and fats that are essential for survival, secondary metabolites are not crucial for plant growth but play a vital role in the competition between species and provide a defense against insects, herbivores, and microbes [4 - 11]. Kessler and Kalske [12] have reported that "approximately two-hundred thousand different secondary metabolites have been isolated and identified," which were grouped in accordance with the chemical structures and/or biosynthetic pathways [13].

These secondary metabolites have been simply classified into four main groups based on their chemical structures (Table **1**): terpenes (polymeric isoprene derivatives), phenolics (comprising of one or more hydroxylated aromatic ring), sulphur-containing compounds (lectins, defensins, phytoalexins and thionins) and compounds containing nitrogen (amino acids and alkaloids that lacks protein). In combination, these groups make up about 90% of all secondary metabolites [14, 15]. There are minority groups which are inclusive of saponins, lipids, essential oils, carbohydrates, and ketones [16]. Secondary metabolites are extensively used in many pharmaceutical and food industries in the production of perfumes, agrochemicals and cosmetics [3, 17]. The use of these secondary metabolites as anti-microbial agents targeting a number of pathogenic microbes is endless. Phytochemical screening of various plants has revealed several bioactive compounds such as alkaloids, flavonoids, terpenes, tannins, quinones and resins that possess antibacterial properties [18]. These could be used exclusively or as a combination to enhance the mechanism of action of conventional antibiotics. This is relevant due to the rapid emergence and dissemination of drug-resistant microorganisms [19, 20]. With the wide diversity of substances that are produced by a variety of plants, many have been discovered and studied. However, there are several that are yet to be discovered and some that are still not sufficiently studied. The antibacterial activities of many plants have been extensively researched, such as the crude extracts of basil, garlic, cinnamon, ginger, mustard and other herbs that exhibit anti-microbial properties against numerous gram-positive and gram-negative bacteria [21].

**Table 1. Types of secondary metabolites of plants (adapted from Ramirez-Gomez *et al.* [22]).**

| Classification | Types | Example |
|---|---|---|
| Terpenes | Monoterpene | Geraniol |
| | Sesquiterpenes | Humulene |
| | Diterpenes | Cafestol |
| | Sesterpenes | Geranylfarsol |
| | Triterpenes | Squalene |
| | Sesquarterpenes | Ferrugicadiol |
| | Tetraterpenes | Lycopenes |
| | Polyterpenes | Gutta-percha |
| Phenolics | Coumarin | Hydroxycoumarins |
| | Furano-coumarins | Psoralin |
| | Lignin | Resveratrol |
| | Flavonoids | Quercitin |
| | Isoflavonoids | Genistein |
| | Tanins | Tanins acid |
| N containing compounds | Alkaloids | Cocaine |
| | Cyanogenic glucosides | Dhurrin |
| | Non-protein amino acids | Canavanin |
| S containing compounds | Glutathione | - |
| | Glucosinolate | B-D-Glucopyrinose |
| | Thionins | - |
| | Defensins | - |
| | Allinin | - |

There is a good chance that some novel compounds will be found that demonstrate antibacterial activities. The reason for this is that several plants use secondary metabolites as a defense mechanism against microbial pathogens. Thus, plants can partially or completely mitigate the spread of microorganisms, animal, and human pathogens [23]. Advancement in high-performance screening methods allows for the detection of novel secondary metabolites, even those from well-studied plants. In addition, genetic engineering or chemically induced synthesis are used to produce vast quantities of bioactive substances [24].

Eukaryotic organelles, the mitochondria and chloroplasts evolved from bacteria through the process of endosymbiosis [25]. These processes of endosymbiosis involve the genetic transfer of material between bacteria and the host genome

[26]. Thus, for this to be successful, the import systems of proteins present in the proto-organelle membranes must be efficient to be able to re-introduce the gene products of those transported to the nuclear genome. Consequently, the genomes from the mitochondria and chloroplast can encode fewer than a hundred proteins, and the localized proteins are introduced into the organelle after translation within the cytosol [27].

Many nuclear-encoded proteins possess a targeting peptide (TP) and a N-terminal pre-sequence that functions as an address tag to determine the localization of these proteins within the endosymbiotic organelle [28]. These TPs can be identified by the translocation pathways within the mitochondria and chloroplasts [29] and are destroyed upon entry into organelles [27]. The development of TP-based importations is not clearly understood, although this revolutionary mechanism allows for endosymbiosis and eukaryotism [30]. Anti-microbial peptides (AMPs) form part of the innate immune system of Archaea, bacteria, and eukaryotes to eliminate microorganisms through the process of membrane permeabilization [31].

Previous studies have shown AMPs to be part of many symbiotic interactions [32, 33], depicting their primary host and endosymbiont association. Existing heterotrophic protists eliminate engulfed prey using AMPs, suggesting that the initial eukaryotes may have similarly used AMPs against cyanobacterial prey that then evolved into the chloroplast [34]. Likewise, the host cell (eukaryotic ancestor) that had a close association with modern archaea [5] will have used AMPs against the proteobacterial mitochondrial ancestor similar to Rickettsiales [35]. In addition, it is important to note that mutualism at the beginning of endosymbiosis may have been due to AMPs since existing hosts control the growth of symbionts and integrate metabolic processes through the exchange of nutrients by using non-toxic AMP concentrations [36].

Furthermore, a subgroup of targeting peptides and helical amphiphilic ribosomally-synthesized AMPs may demonstrate both antibacterial activities as well as those targeting the organelles. Work done with *Chlamydomonas reinhardtii*, a unicellular green alga, has shown that host bacterial resistance is responsible for the advent of eukaryotism. *C. reinhardtii* plays host to both the mitochondria and chloroplast and in addition, provides multicellularity to models of advanced plants [33].

In recent years, there seems to be a profound change from synthetic to herbal medicines. Several drugs derived from plants have been well-established within the healthcare sector. With a vast number of plant species globally, approximately 400 000 – 500 000 species, many have been identified for their beneficial medicinal purposes [37, 38]. In addition, according to WHO, medicinal plants are defined as any plant that possesses a substance with potential use for therapeutic purposes [6]. Medicinal plants have been used for the extraction, synthesis, and development of drugs [7]. Plants synthesize a heterogeneous group of small organic molecules known as secondary metabolites that are required for their reproduction and as a defence mechanism against many bacteria, fungi, viruses, and vertebrates [39, 40]. These secondary metabolites account for less than 10% of those accumulated in plants and have numerous biological effects [4, 8]. In 2019, WHO projected that 25% of plant-derived drugs are used in traditional therapeutic practices [WHO global report on traditional and complementary medicine, (9,10)].

Herbal products have displayed a broad spectrum of activity against both Gram-positive and Gram-negative bacteria and thus control various infectious bacterial diseases [11, 16]. Methanol and ethanol extraction from medicinal plants have been studied and proved to be effective in the treatment of biofilms and active against pathogens [7]. In this chapter, the focus is based on the antibacterial activities of the broad spectrum of secondary metabolites found in plants and their impact on several pathogenic microorganisms. Therefore, the primary aim of this review is to provide insight into the number of secondary metabolites found in plants and their activities against several bacterial pathogens.

## 2. GROUPS OF SECONDARY METABOLITES WITH ANTIBACTERIAL ACTIVITIES

### Terpenes

Previous studies have shown that terpenes are the major group of plant secondary metabolites comprising more than 30 000 identified structures [4, 41]. The number of isoprene units present in the molecule allows for the identification and classification of terpenes [4]. Cowan [8] stated that the chemical structure of terpenes ($C_{10}H_{16}$) occurs as hemiterpenes ($C_5$), monoterpenes ($C_{10}$), sesquiterpenes ($C_{15}$), diterpenes ($C_{20}$), triterpenes ($C_{30}$) and tetraterpenes ($C_{40}$) [8]. Terpenes or terpenoids (compounds with an additional element such as oxygen) are found to be active against a wide array of bacteria [8, 42]. The anti-microbial action of terpenes, terpenoids and essential oils involves the disruption of microbial membranes [43]. Essential oils consist of monoterpenes or sesquiterpenes [41]. Two common examples of monoterpenes obtained from *Thymus vulgaris* are the hydrophobic substances carvacrol and thymol that can disrupt the normal membrane functioning by integrating into the bacterial cell membranes, thus increasing the permeability for the release of [44]. Scanning electron microscopy conducted by Khan *et al*. [45] illustrated the interaction between the carvacrol and the lipid bilayer of *Escherichia coli*. Nearly 39% of the products derived from essential oils are shown to be inhibitory against bacteria [46]. Many food scientists have shown that terpenoids present in essential oils inhibited the growth of *Listeria monocytogenes* [47]. In addition, the seed oil of *Nigella sativa* Linn. (Ranunculaceae) was discovered to possess anti-microbial activity [48]. Pentacyclic triterpenes isolated from *Combretum imberbe* have shown to be novel glycosidic derivatives (hydroxyimberbic acid). In addition, imberbic acid has displayed potent anti-microbial activity against *Mycobacterium fortuitum* and *Staphylococcus aureus* [49]. In addition, ether extraction from the aerial parts of *Tinospora cordifolia* inhibited the growth of *M. tuberculosis* [50].

## Phenolics

Phenolics are widespread in plants and contribute to the largest group of plant secondary metabolites [4]. The characteristic properties of these phenolics are antioxidant, anti-inflammatory, and anti-carcinogenic, and they is protective against certain diseases and oxidative stress [51, 52]. In foods and beverages, they significantly contribute to colour, taste, and flavour [4].

Many traditional medicinal plants possess such compounds that are effective against bacteria [53, 54]. Catechol (2OH groups) and pyrogallol (3OH groups) are hydroxylated phenols that are lethal to many microorganisms [8]. The number of hydroxyl groups present in the phenol groups is a contributing factor to the level of toxicity to microorganisms. Urs and Dunleavy [55] have proven that the more oxidized phenols are, the greater is their inhibitory action. The mechanism of action contributing to the lethality of the phenolics to microorganisms includes the inhibition of the enzyme by the oxidized compounds through a possible interaction with the sulfhydryl groups on the proteins [8, 56]. Polyphenols interact with proteins by forming heavy soluble complexes bound to bacterial adhesions disrupting the accessibility of cell surface receptors [57]. These polyphenols affect the intestinal microbiota due to the lack of being absorbed as it passes the gastrointestinal system. There are two consequences of this process; whereby firstly, there is an alteration of polyphenols into a more active form which consequently changes the intestinal microbiota composition. This may lead to the inhibition of pathogenic bacteria and enrichment of beneficial bacteria, possibly impacting the human host health [58].

### *Flavonoids*

Hussein and El-Anssary [4]; Kabera *et al*. [51] have stated that flavonoids are a large group of naturally occurring phenols and are classified as the first class of polyphenols. The various classes of flavonoids, according to the oxidation level of the central ring, are anthocyanins, flavones and flavonols [51]. These flavonoids are known for their antioxidant, anti-inflammatory, anti-allergic, anti-cancer, anti-viral and antifungal properties [10, 41]. "Flavones are phenolic structures encompassing one carbonyl group" as stated by Samy and Gopalakrishnakone [57]. Flavones are vastly distributed in nature, but most are found in younger tissues occurring in the cell sap and higher plants such as Polygonaceae, Rutaceae, Leguminosae, Umbelliferae and Compositae [4]. A wide variety of flavonoids synthesized by plants, especially catechins, may also be useful as anti-microbial agents targeting a number of microorganisms [57, 59, 60]. The ability to complex with both the extracellular and soluble proteins, and the microbial cell wall allows flavonoids to possess anti-microbial characteristics. This will allow for microbial cell membrane disruption [8]. Flavonoids have been detected in various plants with anti-microbial activities against MRSA and *P. aeruginosa* [10]. Flavonoids are considered highly active against microorganisms when hydroxyl groups are absent on their β-rings, targeting the bacterial membrane with –OH groups [46, 57]. In response to microbially-induced infections, flavonoids synthesized by plants have generally sparked interest in these secondary metabolites due to their antibacterial characteristics and potential applications as therapeutics for human disease and infections [10].

The anti-microbial activity of flavonoids against Gram positive and Gram-negative bacteria has been extensively studied [10, 61]. Galangin (3,5,7-trihydroxyflavone) derived from *Helichyrsum aureonitens* (perennial herb) was shown to be inhibitory against many Gram-positive bacteria [62]. The interaction of flavonoids with the lipid bilayers involves two general mechanisms, which increase membrane permeability by disruption [63, 64]. The first mechanism partitions the non-polar compounds to the hydrophobic interior of the membrane and thereafter the second mechanism is associated with hydrogen bonding between the polar lipids and the hydrophilic flavonoids present at the interface of the membrane [63]. Various structural changes to the membrane properties, such as thickness and fluctuations, are induced by the non-specific interactions with phospholipids and flavonoids [65]. Catechins, a reduced form of the flavonoid compounds, were shown to bind to the lipid bilayer and inactivate or inhibit intracellular and extracellular enzyme synthesis leading to membrane rupture of bacteria [8, 66]. A previous study reported that catechin was responsible for membrane permeability and membrane damage stimulated by an oxidative burst generated by reactive oxygen species [67].

There have been numerous reports on other flavonoids having membrane permeability and disrupting activities. In one study, the compound 2,4,60-trihydroxy-30-methylchalcone stimulated *Streptococcus mutans* to generate intracellular leakage of proteins and ions [68]. In addition, natural flavones such as acacetin and apigenin, and flavonols such as morin and rhamnetin were shown to induce membrane destabilization by generating membrane lipid disorientation [69]. Bacterial cell aggregation influencing membrane integrity was induced by synthetic lipophilic 3-arylideneflavanones that target *S. aureus*, *S. epidermidis* and *Enterococcus faecalis* [70].

## Tannins

Tannins are phenolic compounds composed of a diverse group of oligomers and polymers involved in protein precipitation [51]. These compounds are mostly found in every plant structure, such as the bark, wood, leaves, fruits, and roots [71]. Tannins consist of two types such as the hydrolysable and condensed tannins. Hydrolysable tannins occur as multiple esters with D-glucose to phenolic acids such as gallic acids and hexahydroxydiphenic acids. Two major types of hydrolysable tannins are gallotannins and ellagitannins [4, 57]. Proanthocyanidins (condensed tannins) are mostly derived from flavonoid monomers and is the common type of tannin that are mostly found in forage legumes [57, 72].

Tannins have various biological activities, including antifungal, antiviral, and antibacterial [57, 73 - 75]. The anti-microbial efficacy of tannins is a result of the inactivation of cell envelope transport proteins by covalent and non-covalent interactions and microbial adhesions [41]. Both epicatechin and catechin (*Vaccinium vitis-idaea* L.) were shown to display great anti-microbial activity, and due to this, these components could serve as an alternative treatment for many periodontal diseases [76]. It has been previously discovered that the aqueous extraction from *Psidium guajava* (Myrtaceae) displayed potent antibacterial activities against a number of bacteria such as *S. aureus*, *S. faecalis*, *B. subtilis*, *E. coli* and *Salmonella* sp [18, 77]. In addition, tannic acid, and propyl gallate are shown to be inhibitory against both food-borne and aquatic microorganisms as well as microbes that produces off-flavours [57]. Within the species of Myrtaceae and Elaeagnaceae, the macrocyclic structures of both the bioactive and oligomeric ellagitannins were shown to possess antibacterial activities against *Helicobacter pylori* [78]. The anti-microbial properties of tannins are thought to be a result of an esterage linkage hydrolyzed between gallic acid and polyols hydrolysis upon maturation of some edible fruits. Therefore, the presence of tannins in many fruits aid as a naturally induced defence mechanism against many pathogenic microbial infections [57].

## Coumarins

Coumarins are phenolic substances consisting of fused benzene and α-pyrone rings [79]. Hussein and El-Anssary [4] have stated that "coumarins have been found in approximately 150 species belonging to more than 30 different families such as Solanaceae, Thymeliaceae, Umbrelliferae, Hippocastanaceae and some Rosaceae". According to Xu [80], "coumarins have been shown to possess many activities such as anti-inflammatory, anticoagulant, anticancer, and anti-Alzheimer's activities". Hydroxycinnamic acids associated with coumarins were found to inhibit the growth of Gram-positive bacteria [81].

## *Quinones*

Quinones are ubiquitous in nature and are present as aromatic rings with two ketone substitutions found in 20 plant families, including Plumbaginaceae, Ebanaceae and Boraginaceae [8, 18, 41]. There are approximately 400 quinones identified in plant organs [105]. The class naphthoquinones are a major group of secondary metabolites exhibiting a broad array of biological activities [18]. The anti-microbial activities of quinones stem from the capability to donate free radicals. These can also form irreversible complexes with the nucleophilic amino acids in proteins leading to the inactivation of microbial cells and loss of function. These properties enable the quinones to target the surface-exposed adhesions, cell wall polypeptides, and membrane-bound enzymes [8, 41]. One of the largest groups of secondary metabolites are the naphthoquinones that has a vast array of biological activities [41]. An example of a naphthoquinone is Vitamin K having antihemorrhagic activities related to its oxidation potential in body tissues [41]. Anthraquinones extracted from *Cassia italica* were found to be bacteriostatic against *Bacillus anthracis*, *Corynebacterium pseudodiphthericum* and *Pseudomonas aeruginosa* and bactericidal for *Pseudomonas pseudomalliae* [82].

## Nitrogen Containing Compounds

### *Alkaloids*

Heterocyclic nitrogen compounds called alkaloids are produced mainly by plants as secondary metabolites but also by various bacteria, fungi, and animals [51, 57]. These are a group of heterocyclic nitrogen compounds [4]. Gupta and Birdi [41] have categorised alkaloids into three classes, namely True alkaloids, Pseudoalkaloids and Protoalkaloids. Tadeusz [83] stated that "these can be further divided according to their basic chemical structure into the following types: acridones, aromatics, carbolines, ephedras, ergots, imidazoles, indoles, bisindoles, indolizidines, manzamines, oxindoles, quinolines, quinozolines, phenylisoquinolines, phenylethylamines, piperidines, purines, pyrrolidines pyrrolizidines, pyrroloindoles, pyridines and simple tetrahydroisoquinolines". Alkaloids could intercalate with DNA disrupting the processes of transcription and replication, inhibiting cell division, and ultimately resulting in cell death [41, 75].

The first alkaloid known to be medically useful was morphine which was isolated from *Paver somniferum* (opium poppy) in 1805 [84]. *Tamarindus indica* (Fabaceae) extract was found to possess a high concentration of alkaloids (4.32%) targeting *E. coli, S. aureus, S. typhi* and *P. aeruginosa* [18, 85]. Diterpenoid alkaloids extracted from the Ranunculaceae family of plants have been shown to possess anti-microbial properties [57, 86]. In a study conducted by Ahamd [42], it has been reported that "lanuginosine has weak inhibitory effects against fungi whereas liriodenine has shown anti-microbial activities against both bacteria and *Candida albicans*". Berberine is known to be an important representative of the alkaloid group [8]. A naturally occurring isoquinoline alkaloid, berberine shown to be present in several plants such as *Coptis chinensis, Berberis vulgaris, Hydrastis canadensis* and *Mahonia aquifolium* have exhibited good antibacterial activities [53, 57, 87]. The mechanism of action of berberine and most other alkaloids is the ability to intercalate with DNA resulting in impaired cell division and cell death [8, 41, 88]. Chi *et al.* [89] and Gentry *et al.* [90] had shown that berberine inhibited the growth of *S. aureus* with an MIC of 25.0 mg/ml. An outstanding example of an alkaloid is quinine, which has vast applications not only for malaria treatment but also effective against many infectious diseases such as pneumonia and typhoid fever [1]. Another example is cinnamon that is commonly used in many food dishes. Due to the presence of an active agent, cinnamaldehyde, cinnamon was vastly used as a remedy in Indian and Chinese medicinal practices that have depicted to be an effective anti-microbial [2].

## Sulphur Containing Compounds

There has been extensive research surrounding the antibacterial properties of plant-derived compounds containing sulphur [91, 92]. Ober *et al.* [93] discovered that members of the family Crucifereae and *Allium* genus are a rich source of sulphur containing compounds. Sulphur-containing secondary metabolites such as allicin, ajoene, dialkenyl, and dialkyl sulphides, S-allyl cysteine, S-ally-mercapto cysteine, and isothiocyanates have displayed anti-microbial activities targeting both Gram positive and Gram-negative bacteria [94, 95].

### *Allicin*

An organosulfur compound, allicin, known as diallyl thiosulfinate, is derived from garlic (*Allium sativum*), belonging to the family Alliaceae. Allicin has displayed antibacterial activity towards a number of microbes such as *S. epidermidis, P. aeruginosa, S. agalactiae*, and oral pathogens causing periodontitis [19, 96]. The inhibition of sulfhydryl-dependent enzymes such as alcohol dehydrogenase, thioredoxin reductase and RNA polymerase have been found to contribute to the anti-microbial activities of allicin [97]. In addition, it has been reported that allicin was shown to be partially inhibitory to the synthesis of DNA and proteins [19].

## *Ajoene*

Ajoene is an organosulfur compound present in garlic extracts. This compound has exhibited broad-spectrum anti-microbial activities against both Gram positive and Gram-negative microorganisms [19]. Rehman and Mairaj [98] have concluded that ajoene and allicin present the same antibacterial activity, which functions in accordance with different thiol-dependent enzymatic systems.

## *Sulforaphane*

Sulforaphane found in plants such as *Diplotaxis harra* is a compound existing within the Isothiocyanates (ITCs). This compound has been found to have strong anti-microbial activities targeting *Helicobacter pylori*, *S. aureus* and *Listeria monocytogenes* [99]. The cidal mechanism of action of ITCs against *H. pylori* is by urease inhibition and minimising inflammation caused by infection [100].

## 3. THE MODE OF ACTION OF SECONDARY METABOLITES ON MICROBIAL CELLS

Anti-microbial activities of secondary plant metabolites are exerted by eliminating microorganisms and also by disrupting an important event in the pathogenic process [41, 101]. Table **2** displays the secondary metabolites which were found to have anti-microbial activities against several pathogens.

**Table 2. Plant-derived secondary metabolites depicting anti-microbial activities against pathogens. Adapted from Gorlenko *et al.* [101].**

| Microorganism | Substance | Group | Plant Source | Minimal Inhibitory Concentration ($\mu g/mL$) | Mechanism of Action | Refs. |
|---|---|---|---|---|---|---|
| *Pseudomonas aeruginosa* | Thymol | Terpenoids | *Thymus vulgaris, Thymus capitatus* | 5 | Cell membrane disruption | [102] |
| - | Berberine | Alkaloids | *Berberis vulgaris* | 4 mM | Cell division protein FtsZ inhibitor | [103] |
| - | Allicin | Organosulphur compound | *Allium sp.* | 64 | Inhibition of DNA and protein synthesis | [96] |

(Table 2) cont.....

| Microorganism | Substance | Group | Plant Source | Minimal Inhibitory Concentration (µg/mL) | Mechanism of Action | Refs. |
|---|---|---|---|---|---|---|
| *Acinetobacter baummannii* | conessine | alkaloids | *Holarrhena floribunda, Holarrhena antidysenterica, Funtumia elastica* | 40 | Inhibition of the efflux pump | [104] |
| - | Allicin | Organosulphur compound | *Allium sativum* | 16 | Inhibition of DNA and protein synthesis | [96] |
| *Escherichia coli* | quercetin | flavonoids | *Capparis spinosa* | 300 | Inhibition of the efflux pump | [105] |
| - | Protocatechuic acid | Phenolic acids | *Scrophularia frutescens* | >2000 | Efflux pump inhibitor | [106] |
| - | hydroquinone | phenol | *Vaccinium myrtillus* | >2000 | Efflux pump inhibitor | |
| - | Thymol | Terpenoids | *Thymus capitatus, Thymus vulgaris* | 8,800 | Cell membrane disruption | [102, 106] |
| *Klebsiella pneumoniae* | Allicin | Organosulphur compound | *Allium sativum* | 128 | Inhibition of DNA and protein synthesis | [96] |
| - | osthole | coumarin | *Cnidium monnieri* | 125 | Inhibition of DNA gyrase | [107] |
| *Enterococcus faecalis* | Eriodictyol | flavonoids | *Eriodictyon californicum* | 256 | Efflux pump inhibitor | [108] |
| - | piperine | alkaloids | *Piper nigrum* | 100 | Efflux pump inhibitor | [109] |
| - | osthole | coumarin | *Cnidium monnieri, Angelica archangelica, Angelica pubescens* | 125 | Inhibition of DNA gyrase | [108] |
| - | Sophoraflavanone B | coumarin | *Desmodium caudatum* | 15.6-31.25 | Direct contact with peptidoglycan | [110] |
| *Staphylococcus aureus (including MRSA)* | Allicin | Organosulphur compounds | *Allium sativum* | 32,64 | Inhibition of DNA and protein synthesis | [96] |

*(Table 2) cont.....*

| Microorganism | Substance | Group | Plant Source | Minimal Inhibitory Concentration (μg/mL) | Mechanism of Action | Refs. |
|---|---|---|---|---|---|---|
| - | farnesol | terpenes | *Vachellia farnesiana* | 20 (Minimal Bactericidal Concentration) | Cell membrane disruption | [111] |
| - | thymol | terpenoids | *Thymus capitatus* | 6.5 | Cell membrane disruption | [102, 112] |
| - | plumbagin | naphthoquinone | *Plumbago zeylanica* | 4-8 | Disintegration of the outer membrane | [113] |
| - | cinnamaldehyde | coumarin | *Cinnamomum sp.* | 2 | Cell membrane disturbance | [114] |
| *Helicobacter pylori* | quercetin | flavonoids | *Capparis spinosa* | 100-200 | Efflux pump inhibitors | [105] |
| - | apigenin | flavonoids | *Polymnia fruticosa* | 92.5 μM | Inhibitor of enzymes involved in the pathway of type II fatty acid biosynthesis (FabZ) | [115] |
| - | eugenol | terpernoid | *Eugenia caryophillis and Syzygium aromaticum* | 2 | Cell membrane disturbance | [114] |
| *Salmonella typhii* | agasyllin | pyranocouramin | *Ferulago campestris* | 32 | Inhibition of DNA gyrase | [116] |
| *Mycobacterium tuberculosis* | Evocarpine, evodiamine | alkaloids | *Evodiae fructus* | 5-20,10-80 | Inhibitor of ATP-dependant MurE ligase that is required for peptidoglycan biosynthesis | [117] |

Plant-derived therapeutics play a role in the breakdown of the cell wall and cell membranes of bacteria leading to the release of intracellular components, enzyme inactivation and ultimately, cell death [11, 16]. Plant secondary metabolites affect microbial cells detrimentally in several ways such as disintegration of the function and structure of the cytoplasmic membrane, including the efflux system [118], interference with intermediary metabolism [119], interaction with membrane proteins such as ATPases, disruption of DNA/RNA synthesis and function [120], ion leakage promoted by the destabilization of the proton motive force, enzyme synthesis inhibition, initiation of cytoplasmic constituents coagulation [121], and disturbance of normal cell communication such as quorum sensing [16, 19, 101, 122].

A contributing factor to bacterial multi-drug resistance is efflux pump mediated resistance. Energy derived from $H^+$ and $Na^+$ is the driving forces of efflux systems. Many efflux pump inhibitors (EPIs) are derived from various plant families. Efflux pump inhibitors target $H^+/Na^+$ motive force or inhibit the binding of substrates. EPIs may also use other mechanisms like dissipation of the ionic gradient through the cell membrane, minimising the regulatory pathways of efflux pump genes, interference with ATP hydrolysis and structural variations of the efflux proteins [123]. Biofilms can cause persistent infections due to antibiotic resistance. Three *Carex* plant extracts at a specific concentration showed more than 80% inhibition of biofilms formed by *P. aeruginosa*. In *Carex pumila*, the main compound targeting *P. aeruginosa*-stimulates biofilm is the resveratrol dimer, ε-viniferin. ε-viniferin has also inhibited biofilm formation of enterohemorrhagic *Escherichia coli* O157:H7 by 98% [124]. Immunomodulators include immunostimulants and immunosuppressants, which increase and decrease immune responses, respectively. Various medicinal plants have demonstrated immunomodulatory effects [125]. Numerous plant therapies have shown anti-infectious properties by directly affecting the pathogen or provoking the host's natural and adaptive defence mechanisms [126]. Muthamilasaran and Prasad [127] found that plant immune systems can be divided into microbial-associated molecular-patterns-triggered immunity (MTI) conferring basal resistance and effector-triggered immunity (ETI) that confers durable resistance. Plants also possess systemic acquired resistance (SAR), which provides long-term defence against pathogens [127]. Pathogen- or microbe-associated molecular patterns (PAMPs or MAMPs) and the associated responses from plants are known as PAMP-triggered immunity (PTI). According to Boller and He [128], the contributing role of PTI to disease resistance is evaded by pathogen virulence effectors that have evolved to suppress it.

Studies on *Arabidopsis thaliana* have shown the molecular mechanisms involved in the biosynthesis and activation of secondary metabolites derived as a defence mechanism from pathogens. Evidence suggests that some plant compounds may control numerous immune responses that are evolutionarily conserved within the plant kingdom. For example, *in vitro* studies indicated that saponins and steroidal glycoalkaloids are involved in the lysis of both natural and artificial lipid membranes. The defensive function of some phenylpropanoid phytoalexins has been shown to disrupt membranes and can also have an indirect effect on some of the processes involved in membrane function [129].

# CONCLUSION

With an urgent need to continuously strive to find new anti-microbial agents that would enhance the effectiveness of anti-microbial drugs, plants have been extensively studied for their therapeutic uses. For hundreds of years, plants served as important base models for the development of drugs. Nowadays, medicinal plants are being extensively studied for their potential uses as anti-microbial agents. This is due to plants being readily available and demonstrating a broad spectrum of activity against pathogenic bacteria that may cause several infectious diseases. The relationship between plant and bacterial cells and the role of endosymbiosis has been well documented in evolutionary biology. Many years ago, an endosymbiosis relationship between a single-celled protist and a photosynthesizing cyanobacterium led to the evolvement of the chloroplast. The initial lineage of photosynthetic eukaryotes served as the ancestors of red and green algae, and land plants [130]. Thanks to advances made in genetic engineering, we now have a total genome sequence for a cyanobacterium. The chloroplast endosymbiont within the plant cell host retains clear hallmarks of its bacterial ancestry [131]. There is growing evidence that chloroplasts serve as integrators of environmental signals and key defence organelles. These organelles are important as initial biosynthesis sites and for the transmissibility of pro-defence signals stimulated as an immune response [132]. Chloroplasts are vital for the synthesis of secondary metabolites, defence compounds, and phytohormones. Defence molecules such as reactive oxygen species and nitric oxide are a result of chloroplast metabolism [133]. We can therefore conclude that there is immense and promising potential to continually research and develop anti-microbial agents from the vast array of available plant-derived secondary metabolites. The development of plant-based anti-microbial therapies could boost and improve drug development for specifically targeting pathogenic bacterial diseases.

## CONSENT FOR PUBLICATION

Not applicable.

## CONFLICT OF INTEREST

The authors declare no conflict of interest, financial or otherwise.

## ACKNOWLEDGEMENTS

Declared none.

## REFERENCES

[1]     Achan J, Talisuna AO, Erhart A, *et al.* Quinine, an old anti-malarial drug in a modern world: role in the treatment of malaria. Malar J 2011; 10: 144.

[http://dx.doi.org/10.1186/1475-2875-10-144] [PMID: 21609473]

[2]     Vasconcelos NG, Croda J, Simionatto S. Antibacterial mechanisms of cinnamon and its constituents: A review. Microb Pathog 2018; 120: 198-203.
[http://dx.doi.org/10.1016/j.micpath.2018.04.036] [PMID: 29702210]

[3]     Li Y, Kong D, Fu Y, Sussman MR, Wu H. The effect of developmental and environmental factors on secondary metabolites in medicinal plants. Plant Physiol Biochem 2020; 148: 80-9.
[http://dx.doi.org/10.1016/j.plaphy.2020.01.006] [PMID: 31951944]

[4]     Hussein RA, El-Anssary AA. Plant Secondary Metabolites: the key drivers of the pharmacological actions of medicinal plants. Intech Open 2018.
[http://dx.doi.org/10.5772/intechopen.76139]

[5]     Archibald JM. Endosymbiosis and Eukaryotic Cell Evolution. Curr Biol 2015; 25(19): R911-21.
[http://dx.doi.org/10.1016/j.cub.2015.07.055] [PMID: 26439354]

[6]     Jain C, Khatana S, Vijayvergia R. Bioactivity of secondary metabolites of various plants: A review. Int J Pharm Sci Res 2019; 10(2): 494-504.

[7]     Lee-Huang S, Zhang L, Huang PL, Chang YT, Huang PL. Anti-HIV activity of olive leaf extract (OLE) and modulation of host cell gene expression by HIV-1 infection and OLE treatment. Biochem Biophys Res Commun 2003; 307(4): 1029-37.
[http://dx.doi.org/10.1016/S0006-291X(03)01292-0] [PMID: 12878215]

[8]     Cowan MM. Plant products as antimicrobial agents. Clin Microbiol Rev 1999; 12(4): 564-82.
[http://dx.doi.org/10.1128/CMR.12.4.564] [PMID: 10515903]

[9]     Cushnie TP, Taylor PW, Nagaoka Y, Uesato S, Hara Y, Lamb AJ. Investigation of the antibacterial activity of 3-O-octanoyl-(-)-epicatechin. J Appl Microbiol 2008; 105(5): 1461-9.
[http://dx.doi.org/10.1111/j.1365-2672.2008.03881.x] [PMID: 18795977]

[10]    Gorniak I, Bartoszewski R, Kroliczewski J. Comprehensive review of anti-microbial activities of plant flavonoids. Phytochem Rev 2019; 18: 241-72.
[http://dx.doi.org/10.1007/s11101-018-9591-z]

[11]    Singh SB, Young K, Silver LL. What is an "ideal" antibiotic? Discovery challenges and path forward. Biochem Pharmacol 2017; 133: 63-73.
[http://dx.doi.org/10.1016/j.bcp.2017.01.003] [PMID: 28087253]

[12]    Kessler A, Kalske A. Plant secondary metabolite diversity and species interactions. Annu Rev Ecol Evol Syst 2018; 49: 115-38.
[http://dx.doi.org/10.1146/annurev-ecolsys-110617-062406]

[13]    Ashraf MA, Iqbal M, Rasheed R, Hussain I, Riaz M, Arif MS. Environmental stress and secondary metabolites in plants: An overview.Plant Metabolites and Regulation under Environmental Stress. Amsterdam, The Netherlands: Academic Press: Cambridge, MA, USA; Elsevier Inc. 2018; pp. 153-67.

[14]    De Filippis LF. Plant secondary metabolites: From molecular biology to health products.Plant-environment Interaction: Responses and Approaches to Mitigate Stress. 1st ed., Hoboken, NJ, USA: Wiley Blackwell 2016.
[http://dx.doi.org/10.1002/9781119081005.ch15]

[15]    Ahmed E, Arshad M, Khan MZ, *et al.* Secondary metabolites and their multidimensional prospective in plant life. J Pharmacogn Phytochem 2017; 6(2): 205-14.

[16]    Anand U, Jacobo-Herrera N, Altemimi A, Lakhssassi N. A comprehensive review on medicinal plants as anti-microbial therapeutics: Potential avenues of biocompatible drug discovery. Metabolites 2019; 9(11): 258.
[http://dx.doi.org/10.3390/metabo9110258] [PMID: 31683833]

[17]    Seca AML, Pinto DCGA. Plant secondary metabolites as anticancer agents: Successes in clinical trials and therapeutic application. Int J Mol Sci 2018; 19(1): 263.

[http://dx.doi.org/10.3390/ijms19010263] [PMID: 29337925]

[18]    Compean KL, Ynalvez RA. Anti-microbial activity of plant secondary metabolites: a review. Res J Med Plant 2014; 8(5): 204-13.
[http://dx.doi.org/10.3923/rjmp.2014.204.213]

[19]    Khameneh B, Iranshahy M, Soheili V, Fazly Bazzaz BS. Review on plant antimicrobials: a mechanistic viewpoint. Antimicrob Resist Infect Control 2019; 8: 118.
[http://dx.doi.org/10.1186/s13756-019-0559-6] [PMID: 31346459]

[20]    Yu Z, Tang J, Khare T, Kumar V. The alarming antimicrobial resistance in ESKAPEE pathogens: Can essential oils come to the rescue? Fitoterapia 2020; 140: 104433.
[http://dx.doi.org/10.1016/j.fitote.2019.104433] [PMID: 31760066]

[21]    Gonelimali FD, Lin J, Miao W, *et al*. Antimicrobial Properties and Mechanism of Action of Some Plant Extracts Against Food Pathogens and Spoilage Microorganisms. Front Microbiol 2018; 9(1639): 1639.
[http://dx.doi.org/10.3389/fmicb.2018.01639] [PMID: 30087662]

[22]    Ramírez-Gómez XS, Jiménez-García SN, Campos VB, Campos MLG. Plant metabolites in plant defense against pathogens.Plant Pathology and Management of Plant Diseases. IntechOpen 2019.

[23]    Kenny CR, Furey A, Lucey B. A post-antibiotic era looms: can plant natural product research fill the void? Br J Biomed Sci 2015; 72(4): 191-200.
[http://dx.doi.org/10.1080/09674845.2015.11665752] [PMID: 26738402]

[24]    Zhou M-L, Zhu X-M, Shao J-R, Tang Y-X, Wu Y-M. Production and metabolic engineering of bioactive substances in plant hairy root culture. Appl Microbiol Biotechnol 2011; 90(4): 1229-39.
[http://dx.doi.org/10.1007/s00253-011-3228-0] [PMID: 21468707]

[25]    Martin WF, Garg S, Zimorski V. Endosymbiotic theories for eukaryote origin. Philos Trans R Soc Lond B Biol Sci 2015; 370(1678): 20140330.
[http://dx.doi.org/10.1098/rstb.2014.0330] [PMID: 26323761]

[26]    Timmis JN, Ayliffe MA, Huang CY, Martin W. Endosymbiotic gene transfer: organelle genomes forge eukaryotic chromosomes. Nat Rev Genet 2004; 5(2): 123-35.
[http://dx.doi.org/10.1038/nrg1271] [PMID: 14735123]

[27]    Chotewutmontri P, Holbrook K, Bruce BD. Chapter Six-Plastid Protein Targeting: Preprotein Recognition and Translocation.Galluzzi L. International Review of Cell and Molecular Biology. Academic Press 2017; 330: pp. 227-94.

[28]    von Heijne G, Steppuhn J, Herrmann RG. Domain structure of mitochondrial and chloroplast targeting peptides. Eur J Biochem 1989; 180(3): 535-45.
[http://dx.doi.org/10.1111/j.1432-1033.1989.tb14679.x] [PMID: 2653818]

[29]    Nakai M. New Perspectives on Chloroplast Protein Import. Plant Cell Physiol 2018; 59(6): 1111-9.
[http://dx.doi.org/10.1093/pcp/pcy083] [PMID: 29684214]

[30]    Fukasawa Y, Oda T, Tomii K, Imai K. Origin and Evolutionary Alteration of the Mitochondrial Import System in Eukaryotic Lineages. Mol Biol Evol 2017; 34(7): 1574-86.
[http://dx.doi.org/10.1093/molbev/msx096] [PMID: 28369657]

[31]    Besse A, Peduzzi J, Rebuffat S, Carré-Mlouka A. Antimicrobial peptides and proteins in the face of extremes: Lessons from archaeocins. Biochimie 2015; 118: 344-55.
[http://dx.doi.org/10.1016/j.biochi.2015.06.004] [PMID: 26092421]

[32]    Mergaert P. Role of antimicrobial peptides in controlling symbiotic bacterial populations. Nat Prod Rep 2018; 35(4): 336-56.
[http://dx.doi.org/10.1039/C7NP00056A] [PMID: 29393944]

[33]    Garrido C, Caspari OD, Choquet Y, Wollman FA, Lafontaine I. Evidence Supporting an Antimicrobial Origin of Targeting Peptides to Endosymbiotic Organelles. Cells 2020; 9(8): 1795.

[http://dx.doi.org/10.3390/cells9081795] [PMID: 32731621]

[34]    Ball SG, Bhattacharya D, Weber APM. EVOLUTION. Pathogen to powerhouse. Science 2016; 351(6274): 659-60.
[http://dx.doi.org/10.1126/science.aad8864] [PMID: 26912842]

[35]    Zachar I, Szathmáry E. Breath-giving cooperation: critical review of origin of mitochondria hypotheses : Major unanswered questions point to the importance of early ecology. Biol Direct 2017; 12(1): 19.
[http://dx.doi.org/10.1186/s13062-017-0190-5] [PMID: 28806979]

[36]    Maróti G, Kereszt A, Kondorosi E, Mergaert P, Maro G. Natural roles of antimicrobial peptides in microbes, plants and animals. Res Microbiol 2011; 162(4): 363-74.
[http://dx.doi.org/10.1016/j.resmic.2011.02.005] [PMID: 21320593]

[37]    Othman L, Sleiman A, Abdel-Massih RM. Antimicrobial Activity of Polyphenols and Alkaloids in Middle Eastern Plants. Front Microbiol 2019; 10: 911.
[http://dx.doi.org/10.3389/fmicb.2019.00911] [PMID: 31156565]

[38]    Pan SY, Litscher G, Gao SH, *et al.* Historical perspective of traditional indigenous medical practices: the current renaissance and conservation of herbal resources. Evid Based Complement Alternat Med 2014; 2014: 525340.
[http://dx.doi.org/10.1155/2014/525340] [PMID: 24872833]

[39]    Boy HI, Rutilla AJ, Santos KA, *et al.* Recommended Medicinal Plants as Source of Natural Products: A Review Digit. Chin Med 2018; 1: 131-42.
[http://dx.doi.org/10.1016/S2589-3777(19)30018-7]

[40]    Mawalagedera SM, Symonds MR, Callahan DL, Gaskett AC, Rønsted N. Combining evolutionary inference and metabolomics to identify plants with medicinal potential. Front Ecol Evol 2019; 7: 267.
[http://dx.doi.org/10.3389/fevo.2019.00267]

[41]    Gupta PD, Birdi TJ. Development of botanicals to combat antibiotic resistance. J Ayurveda Integr Med 2017; 8(4): 266-75.
[http://dx.doi.org/10.1016/j.jaim.2017.05.004] [PMID: 28869082]

[42]    Ahmed AA, Mahmoud AA, Williams HJ, Scott AI, Reibenspies JH, Mabry TJ. New sesquiterpene α-methylene lactones from the Egyptian plant Jasonia candicans. J Nat Prod 1993; 56(8): 1276-80.
[http://dx.doi.org/10.1021/np50098a011] [PMID: 8229012]

[43]    Guimarães AC, Meireles LM, Lemos MF, *et al.* Antibacterial activity of terpenes and terpenoids present in essential oils. Molecules 2019; 24(13): 2471.
[http://dx.doi.org/10.3390/molecules24132471] [PMID: 31284397]

[44]    Kachur K, Suntres Z. The antibacterial properties of phenolic isomers, carvacrol and thymol. Crit Rev Food Sci Nutr 2019; 1-12.
[PMID: 31617738]

[45]    Khan I, Bahuguna A, Kumar P, Bajpai VK, Kang SC. Antimicrobial Potential of Carvacrol against Uropathogenic *Escherichia coli via* Membrane Disruption, Depolarization, and Reactive Oxygen Species Generation. Front Microbiol 2017; 8: 2421.
[http://dx.doi.org/10.3389/fmicb.2017.02421] [PMID: 29270161]

[46]    Chaurasia SC, Vyas KK. *In vitro* effect of some volatile oil against *Phytophtora parasitica* var. *piperina*. J Res Indian Med Yoga Homeopath 1997; 1: 24-6.

[47]    Aureli P, Costantini A, Zolea S. Antimicrobial activity of some plant essential oils against *Listeria monocytogenes*. J Food Prot 1992; 55(5): 344-8.
[http://dx.doi.org/10.4315/0362-028X-55.5.344] [PMID: 31071867]

[48]    Ali BH, Blunden G. Pharmacological and toxicological properties of *Nigella sativa.* Phytother Res 2003; 17(4): 299-305.
[http://dx.doi.org/10.1002/ptr.1309] [PMID: 12722128]

[49]    Katerere DR, Gray AI, Nash RJ, Waigh RD. Antimicrobial activity of pentacyclic triterpenes isolated from African *Combretaceae*. Phytochemistry 2003; 63(1): 81-8.
[http://dx.doi.org/10.1016/S0031-9422(02)00726-4] [PMID: 12657301]

[50]    Sampson JH, Raman A, Karlsen G, Navsaria H, Leigh IM. *In vitro* keratinocyte antiproliferant effect of *Centella asiatica* extract and triterpenoid saponins. Phytomedicine 2001; 8(3): 230-5.
[http://dx.doi.org/10.1078/0944-7113-00032] [PMID: 11417919]

[51]    Kabera JN, Semana E, Mussa AR, He X. Plant Secondary Metabolites: Biosynthesis, Classification, Function and Pharmacological Properties. J Pharm Pharmacol 2014; 2(7): 377-92.

[52]    Park ES, Moon WS, Song MJ, Kim MN, Chung KH, Yoon JS. Anti-microbial Activity of Phenol and Benzoic Acid Derivatives. Int Biodeterior Biodegradation 2001; 47(4): 209-14.
[http://dx.doi.org/10.1016/S0964-8305(01)00058-0]

[53]    Mahady GB. Medicinal plants for the prevention and treatment of bacterial infections. Curr Pharm Des 2005; 11(19): 2405-27.
[http://dx.doi.org/10.2174/1381612054367481] [PMID: 16026296]

[54]    Brantner A, Males Z, Pepeljnjak S, Antolić A. Antimicrobial activity of Paliurus spina-christi Mill. (Christ's thorn). J Ethnopharmacol 1996; 52(2): 119-22.
[http://dx.doi.org/10.1016/0378-8741(96)01408-0] [PMID: 8735457]

[55]    Urs NRR, Dunleavy JM. Enhancement of the bactericidal activity of a peroxidase system by phenolic compounds (*Xanthomonas phaseoli* var. sojensis, soybeans). Phytopathology 1975; 65: 686-90.
[http://dx.doi.org/10.1094/Phyto-65-686]

[56]    Mason TL, Wasserman BP. Inactivation of red beet beta-glucan synthase by native oxidized phenolic compounds. Phytochemistry 1987; 26: 2197-202.
[http://dx.doi.org/10.1016/S0031-9422(00)84683-X]

[57]    Samy RP, Gopalakrishnakone P. Therapeutic potential of plants as anti-microbials for drug discovery. eCAM 2010; 7(3): 283-94.

[58]    Abbas F, Ke Y, Yu R, *et al.* Volatile terpenoids: multiple functions, biosynthesis, modulation and manipulation by genetic engineering. Planta 2017; 246(5): 803-16.
[http://dx.doi.org/10.1007/s00425-017-2749-x] [PMID: 28803364]

[59]    Dixon RA, Dey PM, Lamb CJ. Phytoalexins: enzymology and molecular biology. Adv Enzymol Relat Areas Mol Biol 1983; 55: 1-136.
[PMID: 6353887]

[60]    Hu L, Chen Z. Sesquiterpenoid alcohols from *Chrysanthemum morifolium*. Phytochemistry 1997; 44: 1287-90.
[http://dx.doi.org/10.1016/S0031-9422(96)00690-5]

[61]    Tsuchiya H, Sato M, Miyazaki T, *et al.* Comparative study on the antibacterial activity of phytochemical flavanones against methicillin-resistant *Staphylococcus aureus*. J Ethnopharmacol 1996; 50(1): 27-34.
[http://dx.doi.org/10.1016/0378-8741(96)85514-0] [PMID: 8778504]

[62]    Afolayan AJ, Meyer JJM. The antimicrobial activity of 3,5,7-trihydroxyflavone isolated from the shoots of *Helichrysum aureonitens*. J Ethnopharmacol 1997; 57(3): 177-81.
[http://dx.doi.org/10.1016/S0378-8741(97)00065-2] [PMID: 9292410]

[63]    Tsuchiya H. Membrane interactions of phytochemicals as their molecular mechanism applicable to the discovery of drug leads from plants. Molecules 2015; 20(10): 18923-66.
[http://dx.doi.org/10.3390/molecules201018923] [PMID: 26501254]

[64]    Pandey AK, Kumar S. Perspective on plant products as anti-microbial agents: A review. Pharmacologia 2013; 4: 469-80.
[http://dx.doi.org/10.5567/pharmacologia.2013.469.480]

[65]   Arora A, Byrem TM, Nair MG, Strasburg GM. Modulation of liposomal membrane fluidity by flavonoids and isoflavonoids. Arch Biochem Biophys 2000; 373(1): 102-9.
[http://dx.doi.org/10.1006/abbi.1999.1525] [PMID: 10620328]

[66]   Reygaert WC. The antimicrobial possibilities of green tea. Front Microbiol 2014; 5: 434.
[http://dx.doi.org/10.3389/fmicb.2014.00434] [PMID: 25191312]

[67]   Fathima A, Rao JR. Selective toxicity of Catechin-a natural flavonoid towards bacteria. Appl Microbiol Biotechnol 2016; 100(14): 6395-402.
[http://dx.doi.org/10.1007/s00253-016-7492-x] [PMID: 27052380]

[68]   Sato M, Tsuchiya H, Akagiri M, Takagi N, Iinuma M. Growth inhibition of oral bacteria related to denture stomatitis by anti-candidal chalcones. Aust Dent J 1997; 42(5): 343-6.
[http://dx.doi.org/10.1111/j.1834-7819.1997.tb00141.x] [PMID: 9409052]

[69]   Ollila F, Halling K, Vuorela P, Vuorela H, Slotte JP. Characterization of flavonoid--biomembrane interactions. Arch Biochem Biophys 2002; 399(1): 103-8.
[http://dx.doi.org/10.1006/abbi.2001.2759] [PMID: 11883909]

[70]   Budzyńska A, Rózalski M, Karolczak W, Wieckowska-Szakiel M, Sadowska B, Rózalska B. Synthetic 3-arylideneflavanones as inhibitors of the initial stages of biofilm formation by *Staphylococcus aureus* and *Enterococcus faecalis*. Z Naturforsch C J Biosci 2011; 66(3-4): 104-14.
[http://dx.doi.org/10.1515/znc-2011-3-403] [PMID: 21630583]

[71]   Scalbert A. Antimicrobial properties of tannins. Phytochemistry 1991; 30: 3875-83.
[http://dx.doi.org/10.1016/0031-9422(91)83426-L]

[72]   Reed JD. Nutritional toxicology of tannins and related polyphenols in forage legumes. J Anim Sci 1995; 73(5): 1516-28.
[http://dx.doi.org/10.2527/1995.7351516x] [PMID: 7665384]

[73]   Ramawat KG. Secondary plant products in nature.Biotechnology: Secondary Metabolites; Plants and Microbes. Enfield, NH: Science Publishers 2007; pp. 21-57.

[74]   Carson CF, Hammer KA. Chemistry and bioactivity of essential oils.Lipids and Essential Oils as Anti-microbial Agents. New York, USA: John Wiley & Sons 2010; pp. 203-38.

[75]   Savoia D. Plant-derived antimicrobial compounds: alternatives to antibiotics. Future Microbiol 2012; 7(8): 979-90.
[http://dx.doi.org/10.2217/fmb.12.68] [PMID: 22913356]

[76]   Ho KY, Tsai CC, Huang JS, Chen CP, Lin TC, Lin CC. Antimicrobial activity of tannin components from *Vaccinium vitis-idaea* L. J Pharm Pharmacol 2001; 53(2): 187-91.
[http://dx.doi.org/10.1211/0022357011775389] [PMID: 11273014]

[77]   Abdulhamid A, Fakai IM, Sani I, Argungu AU, Bello F. Preliminary phytochemical and antibacterial activity of ethanolic and aqueous stem bark extracts of *Psidium guajava*. Am J Drug Discovery Dev 2014; 4: 85-9.
[http://dx.doi.org/10.3923/ajdd.2014.85.89]

[78]   Yoshida T, Hatano T, Ito H. Chemistry and function of vegetable polyphenols with high molecular weights. Biofactors 2000; 13(1-4): 121-5.
[http://dx.doi.org/10.1002/biof.5520130120] [PMID: 11237170]

[79]   O'Kennedy R, Thornes RD, Eds. Coumarins: biology, applications and mode of action. New York, N.Y.: John Wiley & Sons, Inc. 1997.

[80]   Xu L, Wu Y, Zhao X, Zhang W. The study on biological and pharmacological activity of coumarins.Asia-Pacific Energy Equipment Engineering Research Conference. 2015; pp. 135-8.
[http://dx.doi.org/10.2991/ap3er-15.2015.33]

[81]   Fernández MA, García MD, Sáenz MT. Antibacterial activity of the phenolic acids fractions of Scrophularia frutescens and Scrophularia sambucifolia. J Ethnopharmacol 1996; 53(1): 11-4.

[http://dx.doi.org/10.1016/0378-8741(96)01419-5] [PMID: 8807471]

[82]    Kazmi MH, Malik A, Hameed S, Akhtar N, Noor Ali S. An anthraquinone derivative from *Cassia italica*. Phytochemistry 1994; 36: 761-3.
[http://dx.doi.org/10.1016/S0031-9422(00)89812-X]

[83]    Tadeusz A. Alkaloids: Chemistry, Biology, Ecology, and Applications.Amsterdam, Netherlands: Elsevier 2015.

[84]    Fessenden RJ, Fessenden JS. Organic Chemistry. 2nd ed. Boston, MA: Willard Grant Press 1982; p. 139.

[85]    Abukakar MG, Ukwuani AN, Shehu RA. Phytochemical screening and antibacterial activity of *Tamarindus indica* pulp extract. Asian J Biochem 2008; 3(2): 134-8.
[http://dx.doi.org/10.3923/ajb.2008.134.138]

[86]    Faizi S, Khan RA, Azher S, Khan SA, Tauseef S, Ahmad A. New antimicrobial alkaloids from the roots of *Polyalthia longifolia* var. pendula. Planta Med 2003; 69(4): 350-5.
[http://dx.doi.org/10.1055/s-2003-38883] [PMID: 12709903]

[87]    Cernáková M, Kostálová D. Antimicrobial activity of berberine--a constituent of *Mahonia aquifolium*. Folia Microbiol (Praha) 2002; 47(4): 375-8.
[http://dx.doi.org/10.1007/BF02818693] [PMID: 12422513]

[88]    Phillipson JD, O'Neill MJ. New leads to the treatment of protozoal infections based on natural product molecules. Acta Pharm Nord 1987; 1: 131-44.

[89]    Chi HJ, Woo YS, Lee YJ. Effect of berberine and some antibiotics on the growth of microorganisms. Korean J Pharmacogn 1991; 22: 45-50.

[90]    Gentry EJ, Jampani HB, Keshavarz-Shokri A, *et al.* Antitubercular natural products: berberine from the roots of commercial Hydrastis canadensis powder. Isolation of inactive 8-oxotetrahydrothalifendine, canadine, beta-hydrastine, and two new quinic acid esters, hycandinic acid esters-1 and -2. J Nat Prod 1998; 61(10): 1187-93.
[http://dx.doi.org/10.1021/np9701889] [PMID: 9784149]

[91]    Kim S, Kubec R, Musah RA. Antibacterial and antifungal activity of sulfur-containing compounds from *Petiveria alliacea* L. J Ethnopharmacol 2006; 104(1-2): 188-92.
[http://dx.doi.org/10.1016/j.jep.2005.08.072] [PMID: 16229980]

[92]    Iranshahi M, Hassanzadeh-Khayat M, Bazzaz BSF, Sabeti Z, Enayati F. High content of polysulphides in the volatile oil of Ferula latisecta Rech. F. et Aell. Fruits and anti-microbial activity of the oil. J Essent Oil Res 2008; 20(2): 183-5.
[http://dx.doi.org/10.1080/10412905.2008.9699986]

[93]    Ober D, Harms R, Witte L, Hartmann T. Molecular evolution by change of function. Alkaloid-specific homospermidine synthase retained all properties of deoxyhypusine synthase except binding the eIF5A precursor protein. J Biol Chem 2003; 278(15): 12805-12.
[http://dx.doi.org/10.1074/jbc.M207112200] [PMID: 12562768]

[94]    Sobolewska D, Podolak I, Makowska-Wąs J. *Allium ursinum*: botanical, phytochemical and pharmacological overview. Phytochem Rev 2015; 14(1): 81-97.
[http://dx.doi.org/10.1007/s11101-013-9334-0] [PMID: 25774103]

[95]    Barbieri R, Coppo E, Marchese A, *et al.* Phytochemicals for human disease: An update on plant-derived compounds antibacterial activity. Microbiol Res 2017; 196: 44-68.
[http://dx.doi.org/10.1016/j.micres.2016.12.003] [PMID: 28164790]

[96]    Reiter J, Levina N, van der Linden M, Gruhlke M, Martin C, Slusarenko AJ. Diallylthiosulfinate (allicin), a volatile anti-microbial from garlic (*Allium sativum*), kills human lung pathogenic bacteria, including MDR strains, as a vapor. Molecules 2017; 22(10): 1711.
[http://dx.doi.org/10.3390/molecules22101711] [PMID: 29023413]

[97] Lanzotti V, Scala F, Bonanomi G. Compounds from allium species with cytotoxic and anti-microbial activity. Phytochem Rev 2014; 13(4): 769-91.
[http://dx.doi.org/10.1007/s11101-014-9366-0]

[98] Rehman F, Mairaj S. Antimicrobial studies of allicin and ajoene. Int J Pharm Bio Sci 2013; 4(2): 1095-105.

[99] Benzekri R, Bouslama L, Papetti A, Snoussi M, Benslimene I, Hamami M, *et al.* Isolation and identification of an antibacterial compound from *Diplotaxis harra* (Forssk.) Boiss. Ind Crops Prod 2016; 80: 228-34.
[http://dx.doi.org/10.1016/j.indcrop.2015.11.059]

[100] Fahey JW, Zalcmann AT, Talalay P. The chemical diversity and distribution of glucosinolates and isothiocyanates among plants. Phytochemistry 2001; 56(1): 5-51.
[http://dx.doi.org/10.1016/S0031-9422(00)00316-2] [PMID: 11198818]

[101] Gorlenko CL, Kiselev HY, Budanova EV, Zamyatnin AA Jr, Ikryannikova LN. Plant secondary metabolites in the battle of drugs and drug-resistant bacteria: New heroes or worst clone of antibiotics? Antibiotics (Basel) 2020; 9(4): 170.
[http://dx.doi.org/10.3390/antibiotics9040170] [PMID: 32290036]

[102] Althunibat OY, Qaralleh H, Al-Dalin SYA, *et al.* Effect of thymol and carvacrol, the major components of *Thymus capitatus* on the growth of *Pseudomonas aeruginosa*. J Pure Appl Microbiol 2016; 10: 367-74.

[103] Boberek JM, Stach J, Good L. Genetic evidence for inhibition of bacterial division protein FtsZ by berberine. PLoS One 2010; 5(10): e13745.
[http://dx.doi.org/10.1371/journal.pone.0013745] [PMID: 21060782]

[104] Siriyong T, Srimanote P, Chusri S, *et al.* Conessine as a novel inhibitor of multidrug efflux pump systems in *Pseudomonas aeruginosa*. BMC Complement Altern Med 2017; 17(1): 405.
[http://dx.doi.org/10.1186/s12906-017-1913-y] [PMID: 28806947]

[105] Wu D, Kong Y, Han C, *et al.* D-Alanine:D-alanine ligase as a new target for the flavonoids quercetin and apigenin. Int J Antimicrob Agents 2008; 32(5): 421-6.
[http://dx.doi.org/10.1016/j.ijantimicag.2008.06.010] [PMID: 18774266]

[106] Gutiérrez S, Morán A, Martínez-Blanco H, Ferrero MA, Rodríguez-Aparicio LB. The usefulness of non-toxic plant metabolites in the control of bacterial proliferation. Probiotics Antimicrob Proteins 2017; 9(3): 323-33.
[http://dx.doi.org/10.1007/s12602-017-9259-9] [PMID: 28357646]

[107] Tan N, Yazıcı-Tütüniş S, Bilgin M, Tan E, Miski M. Antibacterial activities of pyrenylated coumarins from the roots of *Prangos hulusii*. Molecules 2017; 22(7): 1098.
[http://dx.doi.org/10.3390/molecules22071098] [PMID: 28671568]

[108] Jeong KW, Lee JY, Kang DI, Lee JU, Shin SY, Kim Y. Screening of flavonoids as candidate antibiotics against *Enterococcus faecalis*. J Nat Prod 2009; 72(4): 719-24.
[http://dx.doi.org/10.1021/np800698d] [PMID: 19236029]

[109] Khameneh B, Iranshahy M, Ghandadi M, Ghoochi Atashbeyk D, Fazly Bazzaz BS, Iranshahi M. Investigation of the antibacterial activity and efflux pump inhibitory effect of co-loaded piperine and gentamicin nanoliposomes in methicillin-resistant *Staphylococcus aureus*. Drug Dev Ind Pharm 2015; 41(6): 989-94.
[http://dx.doi.org/10.3109/03639045.2014.920025] [PMID: 24842547]

[110] Mun SH, Joung DK, Kim SB, *et al.* The mechanism of antimicrobial activity of sophoraflavanone B against methicillin-resistant *Staphylococcus aureus*. Foodborne Pathog Dis 2014; 11(3): 234-9.
[http://dx.doi.org/10.1089/fpd.2013.1627] [PMID: 24601672]

[111] Togashi N, Hamashima H, Shiraishi A, Inoue Y, Takano A. Antibacterial activities against *Staphylococcus aureus* of terpene alcohols with aliphatic carbon chains. J Essent Oil Res 2010; 22:

263-9.
[http://dx.doi.org/10.1080/10412905.2010.9700321]

[112]  Qiu J, Feng H, Lu J, *et al.* Eugenol reduces the expression of virulence-related exoproteins in *Staphylococcus aureus.* Appl Environ Microbiol 2010; 76(17): 5846-51.
[http://dx.doi.org/10.1128/AEM.00704-10] [PMID: 20639367]

[113]  Periasamy H, Iswarya S, Pavithra N, Senthilnathan S, Gnanamani A. *In vitro* antibacterial activity of plumbagin isolated from *Plumbago zeylanica* L. against methicillin-resistant *Staphylococcus aureus.* Lett Appl Microbiol 2019; 69(1): 41-9.
[http://dx.doi.org/10.1111/lam.13160] [PMID: 31044446]

[114]  Ali SM, Khan AA, Ahmed I, *et al.* Antimicrobial activities of Eugenol and Cinnamaldehyde against the human gastric pathogen *Helicobacter pylori.* Ann Clin Microbiol Antimicrob 2005; 4: 20.
[http://dx.doi.org/10.1186/1476-0711-4-20] [PMID: 16371157]

[115]  Zhang L, Kong Y, Wu D, *et al.* Three flavonoids targeting the β-hydroxyacyl-acyl carrier protein dehydratase from *Helicobacter pylori*: crystal structure characterization with enzymatic inhibition assay. Protein Sci 2008; 17(11): 1971-8.
[http://dx.doi.org/10.1110/ps.036186.108] [PMID: 18780820]

[116]  Basile A, Sorbo S, Spadaro V, *et al.* Antimicrobial and antioxidant activities of coumarins from the roots of *Ferulago campestris* (Apiaceae). Molecules 2009; 14(3): 939-52.
[http://dx.doi.org/10.3390/molecules14030939] [PMID: 19255552]

[117]  Hochfellner C, Evangelopoulos D, Zloh M, *et al.* Antagonistic effects of indoloquinazoline alkaloids on antimycobacterial activity of evocarpine. J Appl Microbiol 2015; 118(4): 864-72.
[http://dx.doi.org/10.1111/jam.12753] [PMID: 25604161]

[118]  Chitemerere TA, Mukanganyama S. Evaluation of cell membrane integrity as a potential antimicrobial target for plant products. BMC Complement Altern Med 2014; 14: 278.
[http://dx.doi.org/10.1186/1472-6882-14-278] [PMID: 25078023]

[119]  Anandhi D, Srinivasan PT, Kumar G, Jagatheesh S. DNA fragmentation induced by the glycosides and flavonoids from *C. coriaria.* Int J Curr Microbiol Appl Sci 2014; 3: 666-73.

[120]  Zhao X, Zhao F, Zhong N. Quorum Sensing Inhibition and Anti-Biofilm Activity of Traditional Chinese Medicines.Food Safety-Some Global Trends. London, UK: IntechOpen 2018; p. 37.
[http://dx.doi.org/10.5772/intechopen.74658]

[121]  Mogosanu GD, Grumezescu AM, Huang KS, Bejenaru LE, Bejenaru C. Prevention of microbial communities: novel approaches based natural products. Curr Pharm Biotechnol 2015; 16(2): 94-111.
[http://dx.doi.org/10.2174/1389201016021501121459916] [PMID: 25594287]

[122]  Radulović NS, Blagojević PD, Stojanović-Radić ZZ, Stojanović NM. Antimicrobial plant metabolites: structural diversity and mechanism of action. Curr Med Chem 2013; 20(7): 932-52.
[PMID: 23210781]

[123]  Seukep AJ, Kuete V, Nahar L, Sarker SD, Guo M. Plant-derived secondary metabolites as the main source of efflux pump inhibitors and methods for identification. J Pharm Anal 2020; 10(4): 277-90.
[http://dx.doi.org/10.1016/j.jpha.2019.11.002] [PMID: 32923005]

[124]  Cho HS, Lee JH, Ryu SY, Joo SW, Cho MH, Lee J. Inhibition of *Pseudomonas aeruginosa* and *Escherichia coli* O157:H7 biofilm formation by plant metabolite ε-viniferin. J Agric Food Chem 2013; 61(29): 7120-6.
[http://dx.doi.org/10.1021/jf4009313] [PMID: 23819562]

[125]  Mukherjee PK, Neema NK, Bhadra S, Mukherjee D, Braga FC, Matsabisa MG. Immunomodulatory leads from medicinal plants. Indian J Tradit Knowl 2014; 13(2): 235-56.

[126]  Shukla S, Bajpai VK, Myunghee K. Plants as Potential Sources of Natural Immunomodulators. Rev Environ Sci Biotechnol 2014; 13(1): 17-33.
[http://dx.doi.org/10.1007/s11157-012-9303-x]

[127]   Muthamilarasan M, Prasad M. Plant innate immunity: an updated insight into defense mechanism. J Biosci 2013; 38(2): 433-49.
[http://dx.doi.org/10.1007/s12038-013-9302-2] [PMID: 23660678]

[128]   Boller T, He SY. Innate immunity in plants: an arms race between pattern recognition receptors in plants and effectors in microbial pathogens. Science 2009; 324(5928): 742-4.
[http://dx.doi.org/10.1126/science.1171647] [PMID: 19423812]

[129]   Piasecka A, Jedrzejczak-Rey N, Bednarek P. Secondary metabolites in plant innate immunity: conserved function of divergent chemicals. New Phytol 2015; 206(3): 948-64.
[http://dx.doi.org/10.1111/nph.13325] [PMID: 25659829]

[130]   Wernegreen JJ. Endosymbiosis. Curr Biol 2012; 22(14): R555-61.
[http://dx.doi.org/10.1016/j.cub.2012.06.010] [PMID: 22835786]

[131]   McFadden GI. Endosymbiosis and evolution of the plant cell. Curr Opin Plant Biol 1999; 2(6): 513-9.
[http://dx.doi.org/10.1016/S1369-5266(99)00025-4] [PMID: 10607659]

[132]   Serrano I, Audran C, Rivas S. Chloroplasts at work during plant innate immunity. J Exp Bot 2016; 67(13): 3845-54.
[http://dx.doi.org/10.1093/jxb/erw088] [PMID: 26994477]

[133]   Kretschmer M, Damoo D, Djamei A, Kronstad J. Chloroplasts and Plant Immunity: Where Are the Fungal Effectors? Pathogens 2019; 9(1): 19.
[http://dx.doi.org/10.3390/pathogens9010019] [PMID: 31878153]

# CHAPTER 8

# Plant Secondary Metabolites in the Management of Degenerative Diseases

**Judith N. Ohanaka[1,*], Uwazie C. Kenneth[2], Fatai O. Balogun[3] and Saheed Sabiu[3]**

[1] *Department of Biochemistry, Nile University of Nigeria, Abuja, Nigeria*

[2] *Department of Biochemistry, Ladoke Akintola University of Technology, Ogbomoso, Oyo State, Nigeria*

[3] *Department of Biotechnology and Food Science, Durban University of Technology, P.O.Box 1334, Durban 4000, South Africa*

**Abstract:** Medicinal plants have been indispensable in the development of lead compounds for the management of human health. However, herbal remedies have not been explored maximally in modern therapeutics for the management of drug-resistant diseases, re-emerging diseases, metabolic syndrome, *etc.*

Several secondary metabolites with proven efficacious pharmacological effects have been identified from plants, some isolated but unfortunately never developed into a marketable pharmaceutical product.

Thus, this chapter provides resourceful information on the secondary metabolites of herbal plants with great pharmacological potential. Databases such as JSTOR, Science Direct, Google, PubMed, and Medline were explored for relevant information on this concept.

A spectrum of plant secondary metabolites with potent antibactarial, antiviral, antimalarial, anticancer, antidiabetic activities in different plant species were collated, the class of these metabolites and mechanism of action was compiled.

An acquaintance with efficacious secondary metabolites used in the management of various diseases will serve as a basic tool for Ethnomedical Scientists in the integration of folkloric knowledge in contemporary medicine for the formulation of herbal remedies with superior pharmacological relevance than conventional medicine.

**Keywords:** Antibactarial, Anticancer, Antidiabetic, Antimalarial, Antiviral, Secondary metabolites.

---

* Corresponding author Ohanaka N. Judith: Department of Biochemistry, Nile University of Nigeria, Abuja, Nigeria; Tel: +2348068903076; E-mail: nkechinyere.uwazie@nileuniversity.edu.ng

Saheed Sabiu (Ed)

# 1. INTRODUCTION

In recent times, the improvement of health in the society has been a challenge in most countries in the world. The availability of limited resources has soft-pedaled the effectiveness, efficiency, and equity in health gains. However, the mobilization and management of societal resources to maximize success in health management are of paramount importance. Amongst the health care needs of the society; the provision of appropriate therapeutic treatment for different diseases is of paramount importance for the promotion of the well-being of the society.

Nature has been a source of medicinal agents since time immemorial. Globally, herbal drugs have been a part of the evolution of human, civilization and healthcare for thousands of years. Folklore medicine has documented the use of plants in herbal formulation for disease management. Herbal plants were prepared using common methods such as powders, poultices, tinctures, decoctions, teas, and other types of formulations [1] until the 18th century.

In the early 19th century, the evaluation of herbal plant's composition began with advances in chemical analysis and organic chemistry and this has led to the isolation/ purification and characterization of several bioactive principles. This giant stride in drug discovery led to a phenomenon of innovation in the medical field. The earliest quantum leap was the isolation of an alkaloid from the plant, *Papaver somniferum* (Opium Poppy), for the formulation of the drug, morphine, in 1805.

Later in the 19th century, several drugs were formulated from plant secondary metabolites. These include salicylic acid, the precursor of aspirin produced from *Salix alba* (Willow Bark), *Erythroxylum coca*, a primary source of cocaine- a local anaesthetic, Quinine, an antimalarial drug derived from *Cinchona officinalis*, digitoxin, a cardioactive glycoside drug synthesized from *Digitalis purpurea and Digitalis lanata*, and many others with clinical relevance [2].

Over the years and even in recent times, a larger number of approved drugs are originally from herbal plants and they serve as templates for synthetic modification, and pharmacological inquest and drug precursors [3]. Thus, it is imperative to state that the use of plant products for herbal drug formulation provides the bedrock to modern therapeutic sciences and validates the initiation of a verifiable system of medicine. Several benefits of using medicinal plants include its high therapeutic efficacy, little/absence of side effects, cost-effectiveness, availability, *etc* [4].

Currently, researchers continuously adopt approaches that explore plant for the development of new pharmaceuticals [5]. The high therapeutic value of medicinal plants has been accorded to the presence of several active principles referred to as secondary metabolites. Thus, in this chapter, several secondary metabolites, the plant sources and mechanism of actions were highlighted to serve as a repository of information for further research that will link nature to modern disease management, thereby proferring solutions to several ailments.

The literature used for this chapter was obtained through an in-depth search of scientific databases such as Science Direct, Google, PubMed and Medline. The reports mostly cover the use of plant secondary metabolites in ameliorating/ treatment of selected common aliments in folklore and modern medicine from the 19th century to date.

Seventy-nine (79) journal articles were retrieved using the keywords (Secondary metabolites, mechanism of action, anti-malarial, anti-diabetic, anti-bacterial, anti-viral, anti-cancer activities of plants) and utilized for the conceptualization of the chapter.

## 2. SECONDARY METABOLITES

Secondary metabolites are a group of chemical compounds produced by the plant cell through secondary metabolic pathways such as the shikimic acid and mevalonic acid pathways. These metabolites are not required for plant growth; they rather play a major role in plant interspecies competition, protection against herbivores, ultraviolet radiation, and microbes' response to abiotic and biotic stress [6]. It is also responsible for the colour, smell and flavour in plant products. Over the years, they have shown great pharmacological potential, served as sources of lead compounds with several biological activities utilized in disease management [7]. Plants' secondary metabolites could elicit therapeutic effects on humans by acting as neurotransmitters, hormones, endogenous metabolites, signalling molecules, ligands, *etc* [8]. Secondary metabolites include the diverse group of chemicals, which include alkaloids, glycosides, lipids amines, saponins, essential oils, steroids, flavonoids, carbohydrates *etc*. Currently, about two-hundred thousand different plant secondary metabolites have been isolated and identified [9].

## 2.1. Major Classifications of Secondary Metabolites

Secondary metabolites are simply classified into three main groups:

### 2.1.1. Terpenoids

Terpenoids are secondary metabolites with molecular structures made up of isoprene (2-methylbuta-1, 3-diene) units biosynthesized majorly *via* the mevalonic acid (MVA) and 2C-methyl-d-erythritol-4-phosphate (MEP) pathways. They are diverse chemical compounds that constitute one of the largest groups of secondary metabolites widely distributed in plant kingdom and microorganisms. Terpenes are classified as monoterpenes, diterpenes, triterpenes, tetraterpenes, and sesquiterpenes based on the number of isoprene units in the chemical structure (Fig. **1**). The major plant sources of terpenes include cannabis, tea, citrus fruits (*e.g.* grape, pomelos, lemon, orange, mandarin *etc.*) and Spanish sage thyme, *etc.* Terpenes are responsible for the fragrance, taste, and pigment of plants and also serve as thermoprotectant, signalling molecules, *etc* [10].

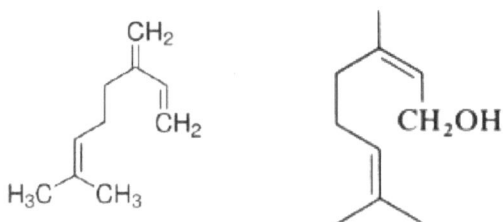

**(a) Myrcene (monoterpene) (b)    Nerol (monoterpene)**

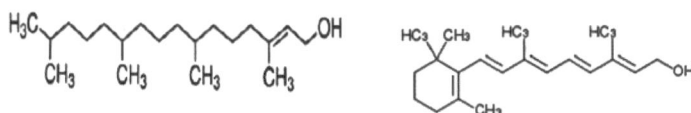

**(c) Phytol (Diterpene)**      d)Retinol (Diterpenes)

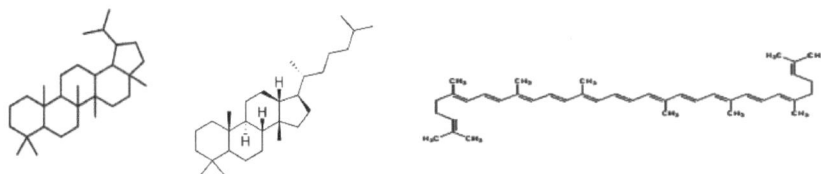

**(e)  Lupane (triterpenes) (f) Dammarane (triterpenes)  (g) Lycopene ((tetraterpenes)**

*(Fig. 1) contd.....*

**(h) Lutein (tetraterpenes)**          **(i) Farnesol (sesquiterpene)**

**(j) Humulene (sesquiterpene)**

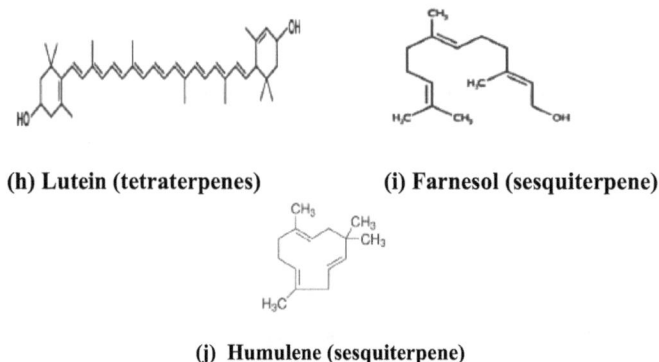

**Fig. (1).** Chemical structures of classes of terpenoid.

A broad spectrum of pharmacological and physiological activities have been recorded on terpenes; these include; antiplasmodial activities of quinine and artemisinin, anti-inflammatory, antioxidant, anticancer, antiseptic, astringent and diuretic activities of curcumin, antitumor activity of limonene and carvone, anti-inflammatory effect of chamazulene, antibacterial and anticancer activities of avarol and avarone, *etc.*

## 2.1.2. Phenolics

Phenolics are compounds containing one or more hydroxylated aromatic rings, biosynthesized mainly from L-phenylalanine and L-tyrosine through the shikimate pathway [11]. Flavonoids, tannins, and phenolic acids are the major dietary phenolic compounds; others include stilbenes, coumarins, catechin, ellagic acid, coumaric acid, gallic acid, lignans and lignins, *etc.* (Fig. (2)). Flavonoids are a pervasive group of naturally occurring polyphenolic compounds characterized by the flavan nucleus, and they are classified into sub-groups: isoflavones, flavonol, flavone, anthocyanidin, flavanone, flavan-3-ol. Phenolics are known to be present in the highest concentration in several plant foods, such as grains, seeds, fruits and leaves of vegetables, *etc.* They are strong natural antioxidants that inhibit diseases induced by oxidative stress and also possess a wide range of biological and pharmacological properties, such as antimicrobial, anti-allergic, antiviral, hepatoprotective, anti-inflammatory, anti-cancer, antithrombotic, *etc.*

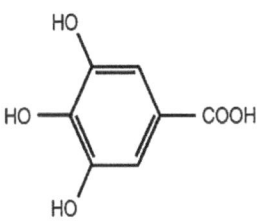

**(a) Gallic acid**

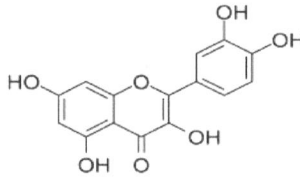

**(b) Flavonoid**

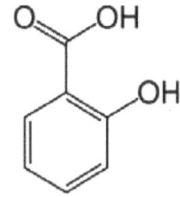

**(c) Phenolic acids**

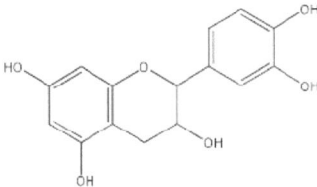

**(d) Catechin**

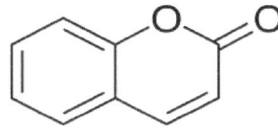

**(e) Coumarin**

**Fig. (2).** Chemical structures of some phenolic compounds.

## 2.1.3. Alkaloids

Alkaloids are non-protein nitrogen-containing compounds biosynthesized from amino acids. These compounds are classified as true alkaloids, protoalkaloids, and pseudoalkaloids according to their molecular structure and biosynthetic pathways. Typical examples of alkaloids include ephedrine, mescaline, adrenaline, xanthine, atropine, caffeine, coniine, nicotine, colchicine, sparteine, cocaine, theobromine, theophylline *etc.* (Fig. (**3**)). They are widely distributed in the plant kingdom and also found in some micro-organisms.

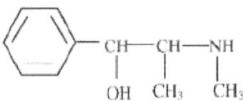

**(a) Ephedrine**

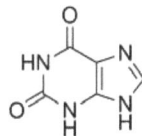

**(b) Xanthine**

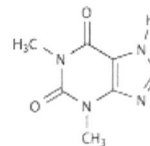

**(c) Theophylline**

*(Fig. 3) contd.....*

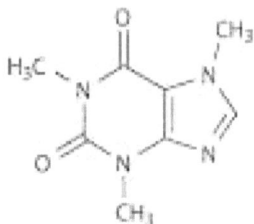

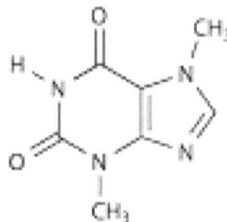

(d) Cafeine                    (e) Theobromine

**Fig. (3).** Chemical structures of some alkaloids.

Alkaloids isolated from different plant parts shows a quite diverse pharmacological effect and relevance in disease management. Examples include the soothing effect of ephedrine in asthmatic patients, anticancer effects of vinblastine, analgesic action of morphine, antioxidant and cytotoxic activity of berberine and anonaine, anti-paralytic activity of tubocurarine, anti-bacterial, antifungal, and antiplasmodial activities of cycleanine and cocsoline, anti-fungal activities of quinolones, *etc.* This chapter will focus on several secondary metabolites that have been scientifically validated for the management of different disease conditions, the medicinal plants from which it has been isolated and their roles in health management.

## 3. SECONDARY METABOLITES IN THE MANAGEMENT OF BACTERIAL INFECTIONS

The human tissues, organs, and systems are constantly exposed to invasion from the environment *via* microorganisms especially bacteria. The host immune systems resist these microbial pathological effects. However, bacterial infections result when natural immunity is submerged by invading pathogenic bacteria. Anti-bacterial drugs produced through chemical synthesis have been utilized as a therapeutic measure against microbial infections, but drug-resistant strains of microorganisms are increasingly arising from the extensive use of antibacterial drugs, and this has contributed to limited control of bacterial infections [12]. These microorganisms exhibit resistance to drugs through innate and/or acquired immunity.

In 2017, the World Health Organization listed *Staphylococcus aureus, Enterobacter, Acinetobacter baumannii, Klebsiella pneumoniae, Pseudomonasaeruginosa* species, and *Enterococcus faecium* as the highest life-threatening bacteria due to their rapid resistance to drugs [13]. Bacteria are unable to develop resistance to several chemically complex secondary metabolites found in plant extracts [14]. Thus, the plant kingdom has been a versatile resource for the search of anti-bacterial agents. The antibacterial agents obtained from plant secondary metabolites could act independently or synergistically to enhance the therapeutic efficacy of conventional antibiotics. Furthermore, these compounds are readily available, cost-effective, and possess high therapeutic efficacy against pathogens without severe side effects. The structure of these plant secondary metabolites with anti-bacteria activities are shown in Fig. (**4**).

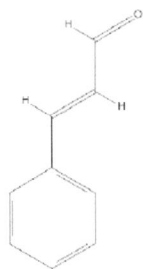
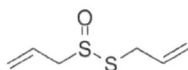
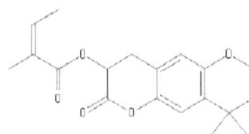

**Cinnamaldehyde**                    **Allicin**                    **Agasyllin**

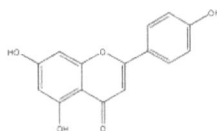
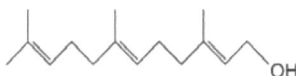

**Apigenin**                    **Farnesol**

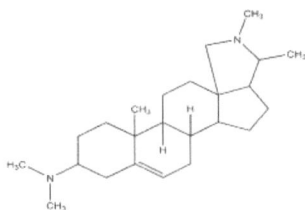
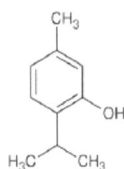
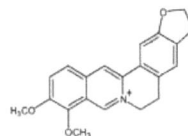

**Conessine**                    **Thymol**

**Berberine**

*(Fig. 4) contd.....*

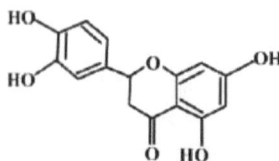

## Eridoctyol

**Fig. (4).** Structure of plant secondary metabolites with anti-bacteria activities.

Furthermore, the table below shows the examples of secondary metabolites obtained from plants that have been found to demonstrate significant bactericidal or bacteriostatic activities (Table **1**).

**Table 1. Plant secondary metabolites with anti-bacterial activities.**

| Plant Specie | Plants Secondary Metabolite | Classification of Secondary Metabolite | Bacteria Strain | MIC µg/mL | Mechanism of Anti-bacteria Activity | Reference |
|---|---|---|---|---|---|---|
| *Cinnamomum spp.* | Cinnamaldehyde | Coumarins | *Staphylococcus aureus* | 0.78–50 µl/ml | Disruption of bacteria cell membrane | [15] |
| *Allium sativa* | Allicin | Organosulfur compounds | *Staphylococcus aureus, Klebsiella pneumonia, Acinetobacter baumanii* | 32 | DNA and protein synthesis inhibition | [16] |
| *Ferulago asparagifolia* | Agasyllin | Coumarins | *Staphylococcus aureus* | 31.25 µg/mL | Inhibition of DNA gyrase | [17] |
| *Polymnia fruticosa* | Apigenin | Flavonoids | *Staphylococcus aureus* | 92.5µM | Efflux pump inhibitor | [18] |
| *Vachellia farnesiana* | Farnesol | Terpenes | *Staphylococcus aureus* | 20 MBC | Disruption of the cell membrane | [19] |
| *Pinus roxburghii* | taxifolin | Organosulfur compound | *Klebsiella pneumoniae* | 128 | DNA and protein synthesis inhibitor | [20] |
| *Holarrhena floribunda* | Conessine | Alkaloid | *Acinetobacter baumannii* | 40 | Efflux pump inhibitor | [21] |

*(Table 1) cont.....*

| Plant Specie | Plants Secondary Metabolite | Classification of Secondary Metabolite | Bacteria Strain | MIC µg/mL | Mechanism of Anti-bacteria Activity | Reference |
|---|---|---|---|---|---|---|
| *Thymus vulgaris* | Thymol | Terpenoids | *Pseudomonas aeaeruginosa* | 5 | Disintegration of the outer membrane | [22] |
| *Berberis vulgaris* | Berberine | Alkaloids | *Pseudomonas aeaeruginosa* | 4mM | Inhibition of protein FtsZ | [23] |
| *Eridictyon californicum* | Eridoctyol | Flavonoids | *Enterococcus faecium* | 256 | Inhibits protein and DNA synthesis | [24] |

## 4. SECONDARY METABOLITES IN THE MANAGEMENT OF VIRAL INFECTIONS

Viral infection has been a major cause of substantial morbidity and mortality globally. The most common viral infections include hepatitis virus, AIDS (Acquired Immunodeficiency Syndrome), influenza, SARS (Severe Acute Respiratory Syndrome), Ebola, herpes virus and the most recent, coronavirus. Different viral epidemics such as the severe acute respiratory syndrome coronavirus (SARS-CoV), H1N1 influenza, and the Middle East respiratory syndrome coronavirus (MERS-CoV) have been recorded in the last twenty years [25]. The re-emergence of viral diseases poses a serious public health concern; this could be attributed to its rapid transmission. Viral diseases are easily acquired with close personal contact in homes, indoor environments, offices, schools, and community, even in hospitals during blood transfusion, organ transplantations, and the use of hypodermic syringes. The death rate associated with the coronavirus has been the highest in the history of humans' infectious diseases globally. This disease killedmore than one thousand eight hundred individuals and infected over seventy thousand individuals within the first fifty days of the epidemic, owing to its rapid mode of transmission [26]. Viral infections are difficult to control due to the mutative nature of the viral genomes; thus, they pose a distressing threat to human health [27].

Antiviral drugs have been made available to treat a limited number of viral infections viruses such as HIV, HSV, hepatits, and influenza. These agents are expensive, associated with several side effects, and a long-term administration of such drugs has resulted into viral resistance.

This has prompted an extensive study of the antiviral activity of phytoconstituents derived from medicinal herbs as an alternative therapeutic cure with little/no side effects [28].

Secondary metabolites of plant products have been reported to inhibit viral replication and transcription by binding to cell receptors, inhibiting penetration of the virus into the host cell, regulating viral adsorption and competing for intracellular signals activation pathways [29].

About 25% of the anti-viral drugs have been derived from plant products [30]. Several studies of secondary metabolites exhibiting antiviral effects have been reported targeting viruses such as human papillomavirus, dengue virus, influenza virus, hepatitis virus, human immunodeficiency virus (HIV), coronavirus, chikungunya virus, rotavirus, herpes virus, Zika virus, *etc* [31].

Herein, we will focus on the secondary metabolites with antiviral properties (Fig. (**5**)) and the mechanism of their actions (Table **2**).

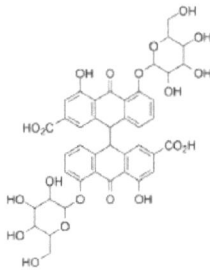

**Sennoside A**

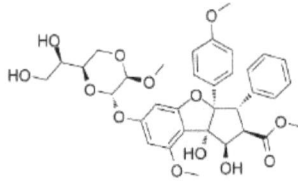

**Silvestrol**

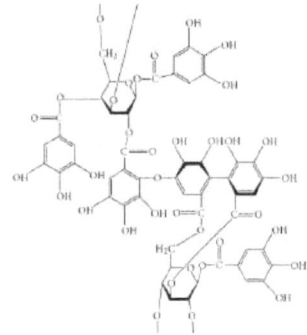

**Excoecarianin**

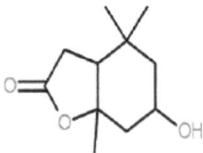

**Loliolide**

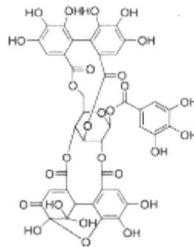

**Geraniin**

*(Fig. 5) contd.....*

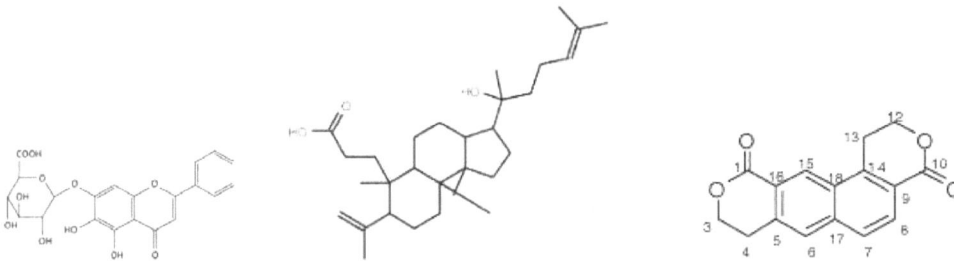

| Baicalin | Dammarenolic acid | Swerilactones |

**Fig. (5).** Structure of plant secondary metabolites with antiviral activities.

**Table 2. Plants' secondary metabolites with anti-viral activities.**

| Plants specie | Plant parts | Secondary metabolites | Classification of secondary metabolite | Antiviral activity | Mechanism of action | Reference |
|---|---|---|---|---|---|---|
| *Phyllanthus urinaria* | Whole plant | Excoecarianin, Loliolide | Tannin | HSV-2, HCV | Interferes with the early stage of HSV-2 replication and reduces HSV-2 infectivity, thereby inhibiting HSV-2 infection | [32] |
| *Sambucus nigra* | Whole plant | Geraniin and 1,3,4,6-TODG, excoecarianin, | Tannin | HSV-2 | Inactivation of HSV-2 virus particles | [33, 34] |
| *Polygonum cuspidatum* | Rhizome | Resveratrol, emodin | Stilbenes, hydroxyanthraquinones | Influenza virus | Attenuate influenza viral replication in A549 cells. | [35] |
| *Azadirachta indica* | **Leaves** | Baicalin | Flavonoids | Dengue fever | Inhibition of the Dengue virus type-2 virus replication | [36] |
| *Scutellaria baicalensis* | Root | Baicalin | Flavonoids | Dengue fever | Inhibit Dengue fever type-2 virus replication | [37] |
| *Aglaia* sp. | Bark | Dammarenolic acid | Triterpenoid | HIV-1 | Inhibit the proliferation of HIV 1 virus | [38] |
| *Rheum palmatum* | Root | Sennoside A | Glycoside | HIV-1 | Inhibition of HIV-1 IN activity and HIV-1 replication | [39] |

*(Table 2) cont.....*

| Plants specie | Plant parts | Secondary metabolites | Classification of secondary metabolite | Antiviral activity | Mechanism of action | Reference |
|---|---|---|---|---|---|---|
| *Aglaia foveolata* | Leaves, bark | Silvestrol | Benzofuran | Ebola virus | Inhibition of proto-oncoprotein PIM1 expression | [40] |
| *Schisandra micrantha* | Root | SJP-L-5 | Ligningomisin | HIV-1 | Inhibitor of HIV-1 infection by blocking viral DNA nuclear entry. | [41] |
| *Embelia ribes* | Seed | Quercetin | Flavonoid | Hepatitis C | Quercetin directly inhibits HCV NS3 protease | [42] |
| *Swertia mileensis* | Whole plant | Swerilactones | Lactones | HBV | Inhibition of HBV DNA replication | [43] |

## 5. SECONDARY METABOLITES IN THE MANAGEMENT OF MALARIA DISEASES

Malaria is an endemic disease in human caused by *Plasmodium* species such as *Plasmodium malariae, Plasmodium ovale*, *Plasmodium vivax*, *Plasmodium knowlesi,* and *Plasmodium falciparum*. Malarial infections are mostly caused by *Plasmodium falciparum* and *Plasmodium vivax*. However, *P. vivax* is less dangerous, while *P. falciparum* is lethal and foremost in Africa [44]. The disease affects poor populations in areas suitable for the development of vectors and parasites, mostly tropics and sub-tropics areas. Plant and their derivatives have been used traditionally for the treatment of malarial diseases. Several classes of secondary metabolites such as alkaloids, terpenes, steroids, and flavonoids have been explored in modern medicine for the treatment of malaria diseases. Quinine, isolated from the bark of *Cinchona* (Rubiaceae) species tree, is the oldest and the first antimalarial drug used to treat human malaria in 1632 and is currently an important therapeutic for malaria treatment [45]. Another clinically relevant anti-malaria drug is Artemisinin, a natural endoperoxide isolated from the wood plant *Artemisia annua,* a medicinal plant rediscovered in China in the seventies. However, the emanation and spread of multiple drug-resistant malaria parasites against many of these therapeutic drugs call for the development of novel antimalarial chemotherapeutic agents from natural sources, particularly medicinal plants [46]. Several anti-malarial compounds have not been tested for their cytotoxicity and this is a limitation to their potential as future antimalarial drugs. Some of the secondary metabolites identified in plants with promising anti-malarial activities are listed in Table **3** and the structures are provided in Fig. (**6**).

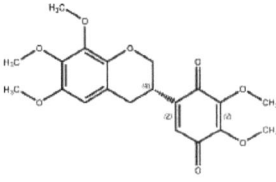

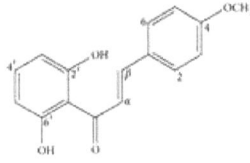

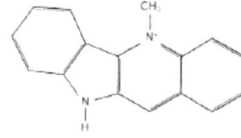

**Abruquinone B 1**               **Cajachalcone**                    **Cryptolepine**

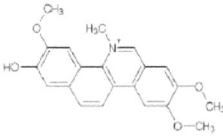

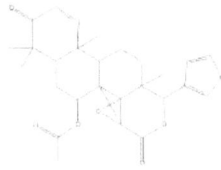

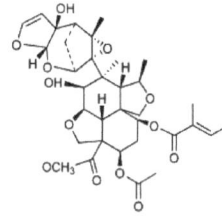

**Fagaronine**                    **Gedunin**                      **Azadirachtin**

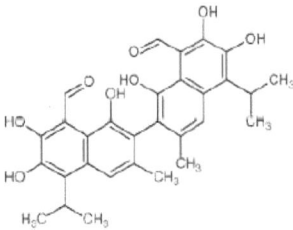

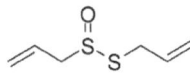

**Gossypol**                                **Allicin**

**Fig. (6).** Structures of some plant secondary metabolites with antimalarial activities.

**Table 3. Plants' secondary metabolites with anti-viral and anti-malarial activities.**

| Plant Specie | Plant Part(s) | Secondary Metabolite | Class | Anti-plasmodic Activity (Strain) | Mechanism of Action | References |
|---|---|---|---|---|---|---|
| *Azadirachta indica* | Leaves | Gedunin | Triterpenoid | (Pf D6) 0.039 µg/mL (Pf W2) 0.02 µg/mL | Alkylation | [47] |
| *Azadirachta indica* | Leaves | Azadirachtin | Triterpenoid | 2.40 (W2) 25. | Inhibits the formation of mobile micmrogametes by interference with the formation of mitotic spindles and the assembly of microtubules in gametes | [48] |
| *Friesodielsia discolor* | Leaves | 3′-formyl-2′,4′-dihydroxy-6′-methoxychalcone, 8-formyl-7-hydroxy-5-methoxyflava-none | Flavonoids | 9.2, 9.3 and 7.8 µM (K1) | - | [49] |
| *Allium sativum* | Bulb | Allicin, Ajoene | Organophosphorous compound | - | Prevents sporozoite invasion of host cells by inhibition of proteolytic processing of circumsporozoite | [50] |
| *Abrus precatorius* Stem bark | Stem bark | Abruquinone B 1 | Isoflavanquinone | 1.500 µg/mL (K1) | - | [51] |
| *Gossypium arboreum* | Leaves | Gossypol | Disesquiterpene | - | Inhibits plasmodium falciparum lactate dehydrogenase (pfLDH) | [52] |
| *Ficus fistulosa* | Leaves and stem bark | Verrucarin L acetate | Triterprnoid | 0.001 (D6); 0.001 (W2) | - | [53] |
| *Cajanus cajan* | Leaves | Cajachalcone | Chalcone | 2.0 µg/mL (K1) | Inhibition of cysteine protease | [54] |
| *Salvia radula* Benth. | Leaves | Salvigenin, betulafolientriol oxide | Flavonoid | 10.4µM and 75.0 µM (FCR-3) | - | [55] |
| *Cassia siamea* | Stem bark | Emodin Lupeol Cassiarin A | Triterpenoid, Anthraquinone, Alkaloid | 2.70 (K1) | - | [56] |
| *Sida acuta* | Stem | Cryptolepine | Alkaloids | *0.114 (K1) 0.050 (N.S.)* | Hemozoin polymerization inhibition in the parasite and intercalation with plasmodium DNA | [57, 58] |

(Table 3) cont.....

| Plant Specie | Plant Part(s) | Secondary Metabolite | Class | Anti-plasmodic Activity (Strain) | Mechanism of Action | References |
|---|---|---|---|---|---|---|
| *Fagara zanthoxyloide* | - | Fagaronine | Alkaloid | IC50 (0.018 g/ml) (Ka | - | [59] |

## 6. SECONDARY METABOLITES IN CANCER MANAGEMENT

Cancer is a devastating disease characterized by uncontrolled cell proliferation, resulting in genetic mutation, leading to malignancy. These genetic mutations include alteration in tumor suppressor genes (NF1, RB, p53, NF2), DNA repair genes (p27, p51, p22, p53 p21), oncogenes (Bcl-2, MYC, RAF, RAS), genes regulating cell growth metabolism, *etc* [60]. This disease has disrupted key cellular processes, such as immune response, apoptotic signaling, gene stability, growth signaling, and regulation of the stromal microenvironment. However, these cellular functions have been the major targets for the treatment of cancer diseases. Cancer has, over the years, been a severe metabolic syndrome and a leading cause of death regardless of the advancement in therapeutic modalities [61]. Cancer is one of the prevalent principal causes of mortality and morbidity around the globe, with a significantly increasing number of cases estimated to be 21 million by 2030. Several therapeutic treatments of cancer involve the combination of processes such as photodynamic therapy, surgery of tumor, stem cell transformation radiotherapy, immunotherapy, chemotherapy, cancer vaccinations, *etc.* However, these measures are often accompanied by severe side effects, including toxicity, limited bioavailability, non-specificity, restriction in metastasis, and fast clearance [62]. The advances in the knowledge of the molecular mechanisms underlying cancer progression have led to the evolution of many anticancer drugs.

Plants' secondary metabolites have been known to exhibit anti-cancer potential, are less cytotoxic, and serve as lead molecules for cancer therapy [63]. They act specifically on tumour cells without affecting normal cells. About 60% of clinically approved anticancer drugs used for chemotherapy are derivatives of these medicinal plants [64].

Secondary metabolites elicit their anti-cancer activity by inhibiting cancer activating enzymes, proteins, and cell signalling pathways such as CDK2 and CDK4 kinases, COX-2 (Cyclooxygenase), Bcl-2, MAPK/ERK, cytokines, PI3K, Akt, mechanistic target of rapamycin (mTOR), TNK, MMP, topoisomerase enzyme, Cdc2, or by activating DNA repair mechanism, Bax, Bid, Bak proteins, inducing antioxidant enzymes.

Typical examples of herbal drugs of plant origin include taxol analogs derived from *Taxus brevifolia*, vinca alkaloids from *Catharanthus roseus* (periwinkle plant), and vinblastine, vincristine, and podophyllotoxin analogs derived from *Podophyllum peltatumetc*. The specific mechanism of action of these compounds includes modulation of the immune system, inhibition of proliferation, induction of cell cycle arrest and apoptosis, increasing antioxidant status *etc.*

Approximately 50% of anticancer drugs approved by the FDA between the years 1940 to 2014 are derivatives of natural products [65]. Drugs such as homoharringtonine and paclitaxel are currently in clinical use; ingenol, mebutate, and curcumin are in clinical trials [66].

Thus, secondary metabolites offer promising results in the quest for new efficacious and safer anticancer agents. The structures of different secondary metabolites with anticancer activities are shown in Fig. (**7**). Futhermore, the table below shows different examples of secondary metabolites obtained from plants that have been found to demonstrate significant anti-cancer activities (Table **4**).

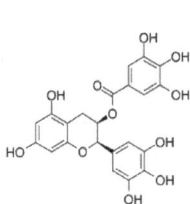

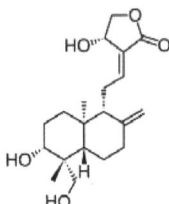

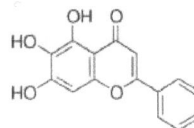

**Epigallocatechin**              **Andrographolide**              **Baicalein**

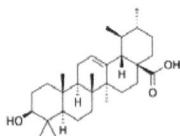

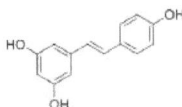

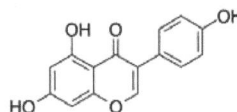

**Ursolic acid**                **Resveratrol**                **Genistein**

**Fig. (7).** Structures of plant secondary metabolites with anti-cancer activities.

**Table 4. Plants' secondary metabolites with anti-cancer activities.**

| Plant Specie And Family | Plant Part | Plants Secondary Metabolites | Class of Compound | Cancer | Mechanism of Anti-cancer Activity | References |
|---|---|---|---|---|---|---|
| *Allium sativum (Amaryllidaceae)* | Bulb | Allicin | Organosulfur | Colorectal cancer | STAT3 signaling pathway | [67, 68] |
| *Curcuma longa (Zingiberaceae)* | Root, Rhizome | Curcumin | Polylphenol | Breast cancer | Modulates cell signaling and gene expression regulatory pathways | [69] |
| *Camellia sinensis (Theaceae)* | Leaves | Epigallocatechin | Flavonoids | Colon cancer | Inhibits cell proliferation and apoptosis | [70, 71] |
| *Berberis lycium (Berberidaceae)* | Leaves | Berberine | Alkaloid | Colorectal cancer | Inactivation of Wnt/β-catenin signaling | [72] |
| *Brassica oleracea (Brassicaceae)* | Leaves | Sulforaphane | Isothiocyanate | Lung cancer | Cell cycle arrest and apoptosis. Targets caspase 8, p21, and hsp90 | [73] |
| *Scutellaria baicalensis (Lamiaceae)* | Root | Baicalein | Flavonoid | Breast cancer | Downregulation of MAPK and ERK and activating p38 signalling pathways | [74, 75] |
| *Andrographis paniculata (Acanthaceae)* | Leaves | Andrographolide | Diterpenoid | Colon cancer, Ovarian cancer, Breast cancer | HIF-1a, VEGF, and PI3K pathway | [76] |
| *Rheum palmatum (Polygonaceae)* | Root | Emodin | Hydroxyanthraquinones | Breast cancer, Human endometrial cancer | PI3K/AKT and MAPK signaling pathways | [77 - 79] |
| *Glycine max (Fabaceae)* | Seed | Genistein | Isoflavonoid | Postrate cancer | Suppresses WNT/b-catenin and Akt signaling pathway | [80, 81] |

*(Table 4) cont.....*

| Plant Specie And Family | Plant Part | Plants Secondary Metabolites | Class of Compound | Cancer | Mechanism of Anti-cancer Activity | References |
|---|---|---|---|---|---|---|
| *Polygonum cuspidatum (Polygonaceae)* | Root | Resveratrol | Phenol | Skin cancer | Regulating cell cycle and apoptosis pathways | [82] |
| *Oldenlandia diffusa (Rubiaceae)* | Aerial parts | Ursolic acid | Triterpenoids | Colorectal cancer | Ki-67, CD31, and miR-29a | [83, 84] |

## 7. SECONDARY METABOLITES IN DIABETES MELLITUS MANAGEMENT

Diabetes mellitus is considered a chronic metabolic disorder characterized by hyperglycemia resulting from a defect in insulin secretion, insulin action or both [85]. It is a global epidemic, with a worldwide prevalence estimate showing that in 2019, 465 million adults aged between 20 and 79, were living with diabetes mellitus. This figure is expected to rise by 2045 to about 700 million [86].

There are three major classifications of diabetes mellitus characterized by progressive β-cell death. Type I diabetes is an autoimmune disease characterized by the targeted destruction of the insulin secreting β-cells within the pancreatic islet [87]. Type II diabetes mellitus results from progressive insulin secretory defect along with insulin resistance [88]. Gestational diabetes is a form of glucose intolerance diagnosed in pregnant women and about five to ten percent (5-10%) of women with gestational diabetes become T2D patients after pregnancy [89]. Other less common causes of diabetes mellitus could result from genetic defects of the pancreatic ß-cell or in insulin action pathways, pancreatitis or cystic fibrosis, and excessive production of endocrinopathies producing insulin.

This condition distorts the metabolism of carbohydrates, fats, and proteins, resulting in hyperglycemia, glycosuria, hyperlipidemia *etc*. The classical features of diabetes mellitus include polydipsia, blurred vision, polyuria, polyphagia, and weight loss. The progression of this disease leads to physiological damage and failure of several organs in the body, such as the eyes, blood vessels, kidneys, nerves, and heart, thereby resulting in vascular complications [90] These complications are the major causes of mortality in diabetic patients and they include retinopathy, neuropathy, nephropathy cardiovascular complications, ulceration, *etc* [91]. Insulin injections and oral anti-diabetic agents (sulfonylureas, biguanides, α-glucosidase inhibitors, and troglitazones) have been the centrepiece in the management of diabetes, but none of these therapeutic modalities has given a long term glycaemic control without causing any adverse side effect such as worsening of hearing, obesity, hypoglycemia, oedema, diarrhoea, *etc* [92].

This has led to the increasing application of herbal options with proven high efficacy, mostly less expensive, readily available, and with little or no adverse side effects in managing and treating diabetes mellitus. In recent times, a large number of pharmaceuticals are structurally derived from the secondary metabolites found in traditional medicinal plants. Most plants contain secondary metabolites such as flavonoids, terpenoids, alkaloids, carotenoids, glycosides, anthraquinone, which are known to possess anti-diabetic activities [93].

Secondary metabolites used for the treatment/management of diabetes mellitus elicit their anti-diabetic activity through several mechanisms, which include; regulation of insulin signalling pathways, translocation of GLUT-4 receptor and/or activation of the PPARγ, regenerating/repair of pancreatic beta cells, reducing insulin resistance, retardation of renal glucose absorption by inhibiting intestinal α-amylase and α-glucosidase, stimulating glycogenesis and glycolysis, stimulation of insulin secretions from beta cells of the pancreatic islet of Langerhans *etc* [94].

The figure (Fig. **8**) and table (Table **5**) below shows different examples of secondary metabolites obtained from plants that have been found to demonstrate significant anti-diabetic activity.

**Table 5. Plants' secondary metabolites with anti-diabetic activity.**

| Plant Species | Plant Part | Secondary Metabolite | Class of Compound | Mechanism of Action | References |
|---|---|---|---|---|---|
| *Allium cepa* | Bulb | Allyl propyl disulfide | Organosulfur | Stimulation of insulin secretion in the pancreas | [95, 96] |
| *Allium sativum* | Bulb | Allicin | Organosulfur | Stimulation of insulin secretion in the pancreas | [97] |
| *Senna alata* | Flower | 1, 3, 8-trihydroxy-6-methylanthraquinone | Emodin | Inhibition of amylase and glucosidase activities | [98] |
| *Acacia arabica* | Flower | Robinetinidol and fisetinidol | Phenol | Enhances the expression of GLUT-4 transporter, lowers Tumor Necrosis Factor (TNF)-α secretion, and elevates adiponectin secretion | [99] |

(Table 5) cont.....

| Plant Species | Plant Part | Secondary Metabolite | Class of Compound | Mechanism of Action | References |
|---|---|---|---|---|---|
| *Camellia sinensis* | Leaves | Epigallocatechin gallate | Phenolics | Increases glucose uptake *via* GLUT1 | [100] |
| *Momordica charantia* | Fruits, seed | Charantin, vicine, polypeptide-p, Oleanolic acid glycosides, ginsenosides, 19-epoxy-3-β,25-dihydroxycucurbita-6,23(E)-diene and 3-β,7-β,25-trihydroxycucurbta-5,23(E)-dien19-al. | Alkaloids, Arenes, triterpenoid | Increasing AMPK activity in L6 myotubes and 3T3-L1 adipocytes and stimulation of GLUT4 translocation | [101] |
| *Coptis Chinensis* | Root, rhizome, stem, and bark | Berberine | Alkaloid | Increasing GLUT4 translocation in adipocytes and myotubes, AMPK activity increases, glucose-stimulated insulin secretion (GSIS) decreases | [102, 103] |

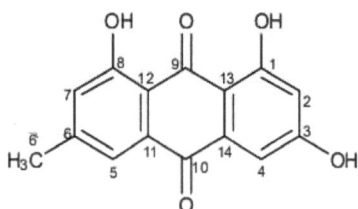

(a) 1, 3, 8-trihydroxy-6-methylanthraquinone

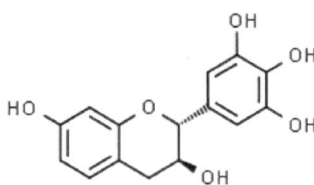

(b) Robinetinidol

(c) Allicin

(d) Allyl propyl disulfide

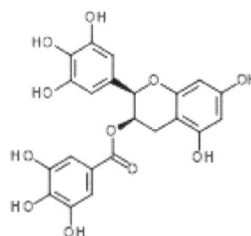

(e) Epigallocatechin gallate

**Fig. (8).** Selected secondary metabolites of anti-diabetic significance.

## CONCLUDING REMARKS

Several secondary metabolites have been isolated and evaluated for their pharmacological activities in proffering solutions to several ailments. Scientifically validated plant species, the secondary metabolites present and their mechanism of action against bacterial infections, viral diseases, malaria, cancer, and diabetes mellitus are herein discussed. Thus, this chapter is directed toward these potent secondary metabolites present in indigenous plants with the hope that they will be explored maximally to produce more efficacious and affordable lead compounds in the management of human health

## CONSENT FOR PUBLICATION

Not applicable.

## CONFLICT OF INTEREST

The authors declare no conflict of interest, financial or otherwise.

## ACKNOWLEDGEMENTS

Declared none.

## REFERENCES

[1]     Fridlender M, Kapulnik Y, Koltai H. Plant derived substances with anti-cancer activity: from folklore to practice. Front Plant Sci 2015; 6: 799.
        [http://dx.doi.org/10.3389/fpls.2015.00799] [PMID: 26483815]

[2]     Alamgir AN. Therapeutic Use of Medicinal Plants and Their Extracts. Springer International PU 2018; Vol. 1.
        [http://dx.doi.org/10.1007/978-3-319-92387-1]

[3]     Choudhari AS, Mandave PC, Deshpande M, Ranjekar P, Prakash O. Phytochemicals in cancer treatment: From preclinical studies to clinical practice. Front Pharmacol 2020; 10: 1614.
        [http://dx.doi.org/10.3389/fphar.2019.01614] [PMID: 32116665]

[4]     Calixto JB. Efficacy, safety, quality control, marketing and regulatory guidelines for herbal medicines (phytotherapeutic agents). Braz J Med Biol Res 2000; 33(2): 179-89.
        [http://dx.doi.org/10.1590/S0100-879X2000000200004] [PMID: 10657057]

[5]     Pan SY, Zhou SF, Gao SH, *et al.* New perspectives on how to discover drugs from herbal medicines: CAM's outstanding contribution to modern therapeutics. Evid Based Complement Alternat Med 2013; 2013: 627375.
        [http://dx.doi.org/10.1155/2013/627375] [PMID: 23634172]

[6]     Isah T. Stress and defense responses in plant secondary metabolites production. Biol Res 2019; 52(1): 39.
        [http://dx.doi.org/10.1186/s40659-019-0246-3] [PMID: 31358053]

[7]     Thirumurugan D, Cholarajan A, Raja SS, Vijayakumar R. An introductory chapter: secondary metabolites. Second metab—sources Appl 2018; 5: 1-21.
        [http://dx.doi.org/10.5772/intechopen.79766]

[8]     Bilal M, Rasheed T, Iqbal HMN, Hu H, Wang W, Zhang X. Macromolecular agents with antimicrobial potentialities: A drive to combat antimicrobial resistance. Int J Biol Macromol 2017; 103: 554-74.
[http://dx.doi.org/10.1016/j.ijbiomac.2017.05.071] [PMID: 28528940]

[9]     Kessler A, Kalske A. Plant secondary metabolite diversity and species interactions. Annu Rev Ecol Evol Syst 2018; 49: 115-38.
[http://dx.doi.org/10.1146/annurev-ecolsys-110617-062406]

[10]    Yang J, Xian M, Su S, *et al.* Enhancing production of bio-isoprene using hybrid MVA pathway and isoprene synthase in *E. coli.* PLoS One 2012; 7(4): e33509.
[http://dx.doi.org/10.1371/journal.pone.0033509] [PMID: 22558074]

[11]    Chirinos R, Betalleluz-Pallardel I, Huamán A, Arbizu C, Pedreschi R, Campos D. HPLC-DAD characterisation of phenolic compounds from Andean oca (Oxalis tuberosa Mol.) tubers and their contribution to the antioxidant capacity. Food Chem 2009; 113(4): 1243-51.
[http://dx.doi.org/10.1016/j.foodchem.2008.08.015]

[12]    Riffel A, Medina LF, Stefani V, Santos RC, Bizani D, Brandelli A. *In vitro* antimicrobial activity of a new series of 1,4-naphthoquinones. Braz J Med Biol Res 2002; 35(7): 811-8.
[http://dx.doi.org/10.1590/S0100-879X2002000700008] [PMID: 12131921]

[13]    Ramsamy Y, Essack SY, Sartorius B, Patel M, Mlisana KP. Antibiotic resistance trends of ESKAPE pathogens in Kwazulu-Natal, South Africa: A five-year retrospective analysis. Afr J Lab Med 2018; 7(2): 887.
[http://dx.doi.org/10.4102/ajlm.v7i2.887] [PMID: 30568908]

[14]    Ody P. The Complete Medicinal Herbal: A Practical Guide to the Healing Properties of Herbs. New York, NY, USA: Skyhorse Publishing Inc. 2017.

[15]    Ali SM, Khan AA, Ahmed I, *et al.* Antimicrobial activities of Eugenol and Cinnamaldehyde against the human gastric pathogen Helicobacter pylori. Ann Clin Microbiol Antimicrob 2005; 4: 20.
[http://dx.doi.org/10.1186/1476-0711-4-20] [PMID: 16371157]

[16]    Reiter J, Levina N, van der Linden M, Gruhlke M, Martin C, Slusarenko AJ. Diallylthiosulfinate (allicin), a volatile antimicrobial from garlic (*Allium sativum*), kills human lung pathogenic bacteria, including MDR strains, as a vapor. Molecules 2017; 22(10): 1711.
[http://dx.doi.org/10.3390/molecules22101711] [PMID: 29023413]

[17]    Karakaya S, Şimşek D, Özbek H, *et al.* Antimicrobial activities of extracts and isolated coumarins from the roots of four Ferulago species growing in Turkey. Iran J Pharm Res 2019; 18(3): 1516-29.
[PMID: 32641960]

[18]    Wu D, Kong Y, Han C, *et al.* D-Alanine:D-alanine ligase as a new target for the flavonoids quercetin and apigenin. Int J Antimicrob Agents 2008; 32(5): 421-6.
[http://dx.doi.org/10.1016/j.ijantimicag.2008.06.010] [PMID: 18774266]

[19]    Togashi N, Hamashima H, Shiraishi A, Inoue Y, Takano A. Antibacterial activities against Staphylococcus aureus of terpene alcohols with aliphatic carbon chains. J Essent Oil Res 2010; 22: 263-9.
[http://dx.doi.org/10.1080/10412905.2010.9700321]

[20]    Chaudhary AK, Ahmad S, Mazumder A. Study of antibacterial and antifungal activity of traditional Cedrus deodara and Pinus roxburghii Sarg. Cell Med 2012; 2(4): 37-41.

[21]    Siriyong T, Srimanote P, Chusri S, *et al.* Conessine as a novel inhibitor of multidrug efflux pump systems in *Pseudomonas aeruginosa.* BMC Complement Altern Med 2017; 17(1): 405.
[http://dx.doi.org/10.1186/s12906-017-1913-y] [PMID: 28806947]

[22]    Boberek JM, Stach J, Good L. Genetic evidence for inhibition of bacterial division protein FtsZ by berberine. PLoS One 2010; 5(10): e13745.
[http://dx.doi.org/10.1371/journal.pone.0013745] [PMID: 21060782]

[23]   Pinna R, Filigheddu E, Juliano C, *et al.* Antimicrobial Effect of *Thymus capitatus* and *Citrus limon* var. *pompia* as Raw Extracts and Nanovesicles. Pharmaceutics 2019; 11(5): 234.
[http://dx.doi.org/10.3390/pharmaceutics11050234] [PMID: 31091818]

[24]   Jeong KW, Lee JY, Kang DI, Lee JU, Shin SY, Kim Y. Screening of flavonoids as candidate antibiotics against Enterococcus faecalis. J Nat Prod 2009; 72(4): 719-24.
[http://dx.doi.org/10.1021/np800698d] [PMID: 19236029]

[25]   Rajnik M, Cascella M, Cuomo A, Dulebohn SC, Di Napoli R. Features, evaluation, and treatment of coronavirus (COVID-19).. Uniformed Services University of The Health Sciences 2020.

[26]   Shereen MA, Khan S, Kazmi A, Bashir N, Siddique R. COVID-19 infection: Origin, transmission, and characteristics of human coronaviruses. J Adv Res 2020; 24: 91-8.
[http://dx.doi.org/10.1016/j.jare.2020.03.005] [PMID: 32257431]

[27]   Yasuhara-Bell J, Lu Y. Marine compounds and their antiviral activities. Antiviral Res 2010; 86(3): 231-40.
[http://dx.doi.org/10.1016/j.antiviral.2010.03.009] [PMID: 20338196]

[28]   Kapoor R, Sharma B, Kanwar SS. Antiviral phytochemicals: an overview. J Physiol Biochem 2017; 6(2): 7.

[29]   Khan MT, Ather A, Thompson KD, Gambari R. Extracts and molecules from medicinal plants against herpes simplex viruses. Antiviral Res 2005; 67(2): 107-19.
[http://dx.doi.org/10.1016/j.antiviral.2005.05.002] [PMID: 16040137]

[30]   Hostettmann K, Marston A. Twenty years of research into medicinal plants: results and perspectives. Phytochem Rev 2002; 1(3): 275-85.
[http://dx.doi.org/10.1023/A:1026046026057]

[31]   Oliveira SG, Piva E, Lund RG. The possibility of interactions between medicinal herbs and allopathic medicines used by patients attended at basic care units of the brazilian unified health system. Nat Prod Chem Res 2015.

[32]   Yang CM, Cheng HY, Lin TC, Chiang LC, Lin CC. Acetone, ethanol and methanol extracts of Phyllanthus urinaria inhibit HSV-2 infection *in vitro*. Antiviral Res 2005; 67(1): 24-30.
[http://dx.doi.org/10.1016/j.antiviral.2005.02.008] [PMID: 15885815]

[33]   Cheng HY, Yang CM, Lin TC, Lin LT, Chiang LC, Lin CC. Excoecarianin, isolated from Phyllanthus urinaria Linnea, inhibits herpes simplex virus type 2 infection through inactivation of viral particles. Evid Based Complement Alternat Med 2011; 2011: 259103-10.
[http://dx.doi.org/10.1093/ecam/nep157] [PMID: 19808846]

[34]   Tan WC, Jaganath IB, Manikam R, Sekaran SD. Evaluation of antiviral activities of four local Malaysian Phyllanthus species against herpes simplex viruses and possible antiviral target. Int J Med Sci 2013; 10(13): 1817-29.
[http://dx.doi.org/10.7150/ijms.6902] [PMID: 24324358]

[35]   Lin CJ, Lin HJ, Chen TH, *et al.* Polygonum cuspidatum and its active components inhibit replication of the influenza virus through toll-like receptor 9-induced interferon beta expression. PLoS One 2015; 10(2): e0117602.
[http://dx.doi.org/10.1371/journal.pone.0117602] [PMID: 25658356]

[36]   Parida MM, Upadhyay C, Pandya G, Jana AM. Inhibitory potential of neem (Azadirachta indica Juss) leaves on dengue virus type-2 replication. J Ethnopharmacol 2002; 79(2): 273-8.
[http://dx.doi.org/10.1016/S0378-8741(01)00395-6] [PMID: 11801392]

[37]   Moghaddam E, Teoh BT, Sam SS, *et al.* Baicalin, a metabolite of baicalein with antiviral activity against dengue virus. Sci Rep 2014; 4: 5452.
[http://dx.doi.org/10.1038/srep05452] [PMID: 24965553]

[38]   Esimone CO, Eck G, Nworu CS, Hoffmann D, Überla K, Proksch P. Dammarenolic acid, a

secodammarane triterpenoid from Aglaia sp. shows potent anti-retroviral activity *in vitro*. Phytomedicine 2010; 17(7): 540-7.
[http://dx.doi.org/10.1016/j.phymed.2009.10.015] [PMID: 19962871]

[39]   Esposito F, Carli I, Del Vecchio C, *et al.* Sennoside A, derived from the traditional chinese medicine plant Rheum L., is a new dual HIV-1 inhibitor effective on HIV-1 replication. Phytomedicine 2016; 23(12): 1383-91.
[http://dx.doi.org/10.1016/j.phymed.2016.08.001] [PMID: 27765358]

[40]   Biedenkopf N, Lange-Grünweller K, Schulte FW, *et al.* The natural compound silvestrol is a potent inhibitor of Ebola virus replication. Antiviral Res 2017; 137: 76-81.
[http://dx.doi.org/10.1016/j.antiviral.2016.11.011] [PMID: 27864075]

[41]   Bai R, Zhang XJ, Li YL, *et al.* SJP-L-5, a novel small-molecule compound, inhibits HIV-1 infection by blocking viral DNA nuclear entry. BMC Microbiol 2015; 15(1): 274.
[http://dx.doi.org/10.1186/s12866-015-0605-3] [PMID: 26630969]

[42]   Bachmetov L, Gal-Tanamy M, Shapira A, *et al.* Suppression of hepatitis C virus by the flavonoid quercetin is mediated by inhibition of NS3 protease activity. J Viral Hepat 2012; 19(2): e81-8.
[http://dx.doi.org/10.1111/j.1365-2893.2011.01507.x] [PMID: 22239530]

[43]   Geng CA, Zhang XM, Ma YB, Luo J, Chen JJ. Swerilactones L-O, secoiridoids with $C_{12}$ and $C_{13}$ skeletons from Swertia mileensis. J Nat Prod 2011; 74(8): 1822-5.
[http://dx.doi.org/10.1021/np200256b] [PMID: 21823575]

[44]   Ashok P, Ganguly S, Murugesan S. Review on *in-vitro* anti-malarial activity of natural β-carboline alkaloids. Mini Rev Med Chem 2013; 13(12): 1778-91.
[http://dx.doi.org/10.2174/1389557511313120008] [PMID: 24059727]

[45]   Baird JK, Sustriayu Nalim MF, Basri H, *et al.* Survey of resistance to chloroquine by Plasmodium vivax in Indonesia. Trans R Soc Trop Med Hyg 1996; 90(4): 409-11.
[http://dx.doi.org/10.1016/S0035-9203(96)90526-X] [PMID: 8882190]

[46]   Amoa Onguéné P, Ntie-Kang F, Lifongo LL, Ndom JC, Sippl W, Mbaze LM. The potential of anti-malarial compounds derived from African medicinal plants, part I: a pharmacological evaluation of alkaloids and terpenoids. Malar J 2013; 12(1): 449.
[http://dx.doi.org/10.1186/1475-2875-12-449] [PMID: 24330395]

[47]   Khalid SA, Duddeck H, Gonzalez-Sierra M. Isolation and characterization of an antimalarial agent of the neem tree Azadirachta indica. J Nat Prod 1989; 52(5): 922-6.
[http://dx.doi.org/10.1021/np50065a002] [PMID: 2607354]

[48]   Billker O, Shaw MK, Jones IW, Ley SV, Mordue AJ, Sinden RE. Azadirachtin disrupts formation of organised microtubule arrays during microgametogenesis of Plasmodium berghei. J Eukaryot Microbiol 2002; 49(6): 489-97.
[http://dx.doi.org/10.1111/j.1550-7408.2002.tb00234.x] [PMID: 12503686]

[49]   Prawat U, Phupornprasert D, Butsuri A, Salae AW, Boonsri S, Tuntiwachwuttikul P. Flavonoids from *Friesodielsia discolor.* Phytochem Lett 2012; 5: 809-13.
[http://dx.doi.org/10.1016/j.phytol.2012.09.007]

[50]   Coppi A, Cabinian M, Mirelman D, Sinnis P. Antimalarial activity of allicin, a biologically active compound from garlic cloves. Antimicrob Agents Chemother 2006; 50(5): 1731-7.
[http://dx.doi.org/10.1128/AAC.50.5.1731-1737.2006] [PMID: 16641443]

[51]   Limmatvapirat C, Sirisopanaporn S, Kittakoop P. Antitubercular and antiplasmodial constituents of Abrus precatorius. Planta Med 2004; 70(3): 276-8.
[http://dx.doi.org/10.1055/s-2004-818924] [PMID: 15114511]

[52]   Gomez MS, Piper RC, Hunsaker LA, *et al.* Substrate and cofactor specificity and selective inhibition of lactate dehydrogenase from the malarial parasite P. falciparum. Mol Biochem Parasitol 1997; 90(1): 235-46.

[http://dx.doi.org/10.1016/S0166-6851(97)00140-0] [PMID: 9497046]

[53] Zhang HJ, Tamez PA, Aydogmus Z, *et al.* Antimalarial agents from plants. III. Trichothecenes from *Ficus fistulosa* and *Rhaphidophora decursiva.* Planta Med 2002; 68(12): 1088-91.
[http://dx.doi.org/10.1055/s-2002-36350] [PMID: 12494335]

[54] Ajaiyeoba EO, Ogbole OO, Abiodun OO, Ashidi JS, Houghton PJ, Wright CW. Cajachalcone: An antimalarial compound from *Cajanus cajan* leaf extract. J Parasitol Res 2013; 2013: 703781.
[http://dx.doi.org/10.1155/2013/703781] [PMID: 23970954]

[55] Kamatou GP, Van Zyl RL, Davids H, Van Heerden FR, Lourens AC, Viljoen AM. Antimalarial and anticancer activities of selected South African Salvia species and isolated compounds from S. radula. S Afr J Bot 2008; 74(2): 238-43.
[http://dx.doi.org/10.1016/j.sajb.2007.08.001]

[56] Ajaiyeoba EO, Abiodun OO, Falade MO, *et al.* In vitro cytotoxicity studies of 20 plants used in Nigerian antimalarial ethnomedicine. Phytomedicine 2006; 13(4): 295-8.
[http://dx.doi.org/10.1016/j.phymed.2005.01.015] [PMID: 16492535]

[57] Banzouzi JT, Prado R, Menan H, *et al.* Studies on medicinal plants of Ivory Coast: investigation of Sida acuta for *in vitro* antiplasmodial activities and identification of an active constituent. Phytomedicine 2004; 11(4): 338-41.
[http://dx.doi.org/10.1078/0944711041495245] [PMID: 15185848]

[58] Kirby GC, Paine A, Warhurst DC, Noamese BK, Phillipson JD. *In vitro* and *in vivo* antimalarial activity of cryptolepine, a plant-derived indoloquinoline. Phytother Res 1995; 9(5): 359-63.
[http://dx.doi.org/10.1002/ptr.2650090510]

[59] Kassim OO, Loyevsky M, Elliott B, Geall A, Amonoo H, Gordeuk VR. Effects of root extracts of Fagara zanthoxyloides on the *in vitro* growth and stage distribution of *Plasmodium falciparum.* Antimicrob Agents Chemother 2005; 49(1): 264-8.
[http://dx.doi.org/10.1128/AAC.49.1.264-268.2005] [PMID: 15616304]

[60] Yap YS, McPherson JR, Ong CK, *et al.* The NF1 gene revisited - from bench to bedside. Oncotarget 2014; 5(15): 5873-92.
[http://dx.doi.org/10.18632/oncotarget.2194] [PMID: 25026295]

[61] Quin JE, Devlin JR, Cameron D, Hannan KM, Pearson RB, Hannan RD. Targeting the nucleolus for cancer intervention. *Biochimica et Biophysica Acta (BBA)-.* Molecular Basis of Disease 2014; 1842(6): 802-16.
[http://dx.doi.org/10.1016/j.bbadis.2013.12.009]

[62] Mukherjee S, Manna A, Bhattacharjee P, *et al.* Non-migratory tumorigenic intrinsic cancer stem cells ensure breast cancer metastasis by generation of CXCR4(+) migrating cancer stem cells. Oncogene 2016; 35(37): 4937-48.
[http://dx.doi.org/10.1038/onc.2016.26] [PMID: 26923331]

[63] Chang JH, Cheng CW, Yang YC, *et al.* Downregulating CD26/DPPIV by apigenin modulates the interplay between Akt and Snail/Slug signaling to restrain metastasis of lung cancer with multiple EGFR statuses. J Exp Clin Cancer Res 2018; 37(1): 199.
[http://dx.doi.org/10.1186/s13046-018-0869-1] [PMID: 30134935]

[64] Cragg GM, Pezzuto JM. Natural products as a vital source for the discovery of cancer chemotherapeutic and chemopreventive agents. Med Princ Pract 2016; 25 (Suppl. 2): 41-59.
[http://dx.doi.org/10.1159/000443404] [PMID: 26679767]

[65] Newman DJ, Cragg GM. Natural products as sources of new drugs from 1981 to 2014. J Nat Prod 2016; 79(3): 629-61.
[http://dx.doi.org/10.1021/acs.jnatprod.5b01055] [PMID: 26852623]

[66] Seca AML, Pinto DCGA. Plant secondary metabolites as anticancer agents: successes in clinical trials and therapeutic application. Int J Mol Sci 2018; 19(1): 263.

[http://dx.doi.org/10.3390/ijms19010263] [PMID: 29337925]

[67]    Huang L, Song Y, Lian J, Wang Z. Allicin inhibits the invasion of lung adenocarcinoma cells by altering tissue inhibitor of metalloproteinase/matrix metalloproteinase balance *via* reducing the activity of phosphoinositide 3-kinase/AKT signaling. Oncol Lett 2017; 14(1): 468-74.
[http://dx.doi.org/10.3892/ol.2017.6129] [PMID: 28693193]

[68]    Chen H, Zhu B, Zhao L, *et al.* Allicin inhibits proliferation and invasion *in vitro* and *in vivo via* SHP-1-mediated STAT3 signaling in cholangiocarcinoma. Cell Physiol Biochem 2018; 47(2): 641-53.
[http://dx.doi.org/10.1159/000490019] [PMID: 29794468]

[69]    Kunnumakkara AB, Bordoloi D, Harsha C, Banik K, Gupta SC, Aggarwal BB. Curcumin mediates anticancer effects by modulating multiple cell signaling pathways. Clin Sci (Lond) 2017; 131(15): 1781-99.
[http://dx.doi.org/10.1042/CS20160935] [PMID: 28679846]

[70]    Xu Y, Ho CT, Amin SG, Han C, Chung FL. Inhibition of tobacco-specific nitrosamine-induced lung tumorigenesis in A/J mice by green tea and its major polyphenol as antioxidants. Cancer Res 1992; 52(14): 3875-9.
[PMID: 1617663]

[71]    Thangapazham RL, Singh AK, Sharma A, Warren J, Gaddipati JP, Maheshwari RK. Green tea polyphenols and its constituent epigallocatechin gallate inhibits proliferation of human breast cancer cells *in vitro* and *in vivo*. Cancer Lett 2007; 245(1-2): 232-41.
[http://dx.doi.org/10.1016/j.canlet.2006.01.027] [PMID: 16519995]

[72]    Wu K, Yang Q, Mu Y, *et al.* Berberine inhibits the proliferation of colon cancer cells by inactivating Wnt/β-catenin signaling. Int J Oncol 2012; 41(1): 292-8.
[PMID: 22469784]

[73]    Qazi A, Pal J, Maitah M, *et al.* Anticancer activity of a broccoli derivative, sulforaphane, in barrett adenocarcinoma: potential use in chemoprevention and as adjuvant in chemotherapy. Transl Oncol 2010; 3(6): 389-99.
[http://dx.doi.org/10.1593/tlo.10235] [PMID: 21151478]

[74]    Dou J, Wang Z, Ma L, *et al.* Baicalein and baicalin inhibit colon cancer using two distinct fashions of apoptosis and senescence. Oncotarget 2018; 9(28): 20089-102.
[http://dx.doi.org/10.18632/oncotarget.24015] [PMID: 29732005]

[75]    Tao Y, Zhan S, Wang Y, *et al.* Baicalin, the major component of traditional Chinese medicine Scutellaria baicalensis induces colon cancer cell apoptosis through inhibition of oncomiRNAs. Sci Rep 2018; 8(1): 14477.
[http://dx.doi.org/10.1038/s41598-018-32734-2] [PMID: 30262902]

[76]    Li J, Zhang C, Jiang H, Cheng J. Andrographolide inhibits hypoxia-inducible factor-1 through phosphatidylinositol 3-kinase/AKT pathway and suppresses breast cancer growth. OncoTargets Ther 2015; 8: 427-35.
[http://dx.doi.org/10.2147/OTT.S76116] [PMID: 25709476]

[77]    Iwanowycz S, Wang J, Hodge J, Wang Y, Yu F, Fan D. Emodin inhibits breast cancer growth by blocking the tumor-promoting feedforward loop between cancer cells and macrophages. Mol Cancer Ther 2016; 15(8): 1931-42.
[http://dx.doi.org/10.1158/1535-7163.MCT-15-0987] [PMID: 27196773]

[78]    Lin W, Zhong M, Yin H, *et al.* Emodin induces hepatocellular carcinoma cell apoptosis through MAPK and PI3K/AKT signaling pathways *in vitro* and *in vivo*. Oncol Rep 2016; 36(2): 961-7.
[http://dx.doi.org/10.3892/or.2016.4861] [PMID: 27278720]

[79]    Su J, Yan Y, Qu J, Xue X, Liu Z, Cai H. Emodin induces apoptosis of lung cancer cells through ER stress and the TRIB3/NF-κB pathway. Oncol Rep 2017; 37(3): 1565-72.
[http://dx.doi.org/10.3892/or.2017.5428] [PMID: 28184934]

[80]    Zhang Y, Li Q, Zhou D, Chen H. Genistein, a soya isoflavone, prevents azoxymethane-induced up-regulation of WNT/β-catenin signalling and reduces colon pre-neoplasia in rats. Br J Nutr 2013; 109(1): 33-42.
[http://dx.doi.org/10.1017/S0007114512000876] [PMID: 22716201]

[81]    Hsiao YC, Peng SF, Lai KC, *et al.* Genistein induces apoptosis *in vitro* and has antitumor activity against human leukemia HL-60 cancer cell xenograft growth *in vivo*. Environ Toxicol 2019; 34(4): 443-56.
[http://dx.doi.org/10.1002/tox.22698] [PMID: 30618158]

[82]    Banerjee S, Bueso-Ramos C, Aggarwal BB. Suppression of 7,12-dimethylbenz(a)anthracene-induced mammary carcinogenesis in rats by resveratrol: role of nuclear factor-kappaB, cyclooxygenase 2, and matrix metalloprotease 9. Cancer Res 2002; 62(17): 4945-54.
[PMID: 12208745]

[83]    Prasad S, Yadav VR, Sung B, *et al.* Ursolic acid inhibits growth and metastasis of human colorectal cancer in an orthotopic nude mouse model by targeting multiple cell signaling pathways: chemosensitization with capecitabine. Clin Cancer Res 2012; 18(18): 4942-53.
[http://dx.doi.org/10.1158/1078-0432.CCR-11-2805] [PMID: 22832932]

[84]    Zhang Y, Huang L, Shi H, *et al.* Ursolic acid enhances the therapeutic effects of oxaliplatin in colorectal cancer by inhibition of drug resistance. Cancer Sci 2018; 109(1): 94-102.
[http://dx.doi.org/10.1111/cas.13425] [PMID: 29034540]

[85]    Standards of medical care in diabetes--2010. Diabetes Care 2010; 33 (Suppl. 1): S11-61.
[http://dx.doi.org/10.2337/dc10-S011] [PMID: 20042772]

[86]    Saeedi P, Petersohn I, Salpea P, *et al.* Global and regional diabetes prevalence estimates for 2019 and projections for 2030 and 2045: Results from the International Diabetes Federation Diabetes Atlas, 9th edition. Diabetes Res Clin Pract 2019; 157: 107843.
[http://dx.doi.org/10.1016/j.diabres.2019.107843] [PMID: 31518657]

[87]    Baumann B, Salem HH, Boehm BO. Anti-inflammatory therapy in type 1 diabetes. Curr Diab Rep 2012; 12(5): 499-509.
[http://dx.doi.org/10.1007/s11892-012-0299-y] [PMID: 22791179]

[88]    Srinivasan K, Ramarao P. Animal models in type 2 diabetes research: an overview. Indian J Med Res 2007; 125(3): 451-72.
[PMID: 17496368]

[89]    Sivaraman SC, Vinnamala S, Jenkins D. Gestational diabetes and future risk of diabetes. J Clin Med Res 2013; 5(2): 92-6.
[http://dx.doi.org/10.4021/jocmr1201w] [PMID: 23519363]

[90]    Executive summary: Standards of medical care in diabetes--2013. Diabetes Care 2013; 36 (Suppl. 1): S4-S10.
[http://dx.doi.org/10.2337/dc13-S004] [PMID: 23264424]

[91]    Saely CH, Aczel S, Marte T, Langer P, Drexel H. Cardiovascular complications in Type 2 diabetes mellitus depend on the coronary angiographic state rather than on the diabetic state. Diabetologia 2004; 47(1): 145-6.
[http://dx.doi.org/10.1007/s00125-003-1274-6] [PMID: 14676943]

[92]    Krentz AJ, Bailey CJ. Oral antidiabetic agents: current role in type 2 diabetes mellitus. Drugs 2005; 65(3): 385-411.
[http://dx.doi.org/10.2165/00003495-200565030-00005] [PMID: 15669880]

[93]    Kooti W, Farokhipour M, Asadzadeh Z, Ashtary-Larky D, Asadi-Samani M. The role of medicinal plants in the treatment of diabetes: a systematic review. Electron Physician 2016; 8(1): 1832-42.
[http://dx.doi.org/10.19082/1832] [PMID: 26955456]

[94]    Ota A, Ulrih NP. An overview of herbal products and secondary metabolites used for management of

type two diabetes. Front Pharmacol 2017; 8: 436.
[http://dx.doi.org/10.3389/fphar.2017.00436] [PMID: 28729836]

[95]   Sabiu S, Madende M, Ajao AA, Aladodo RA, Nurain IO, Ahmad JB. Bioactive food as dietary interventions for diabetes: The genus Allium (Amaryllidaceae: Alloideae): Features, phytoconstituents, and mechanisms of antidiabetic potential of *Allium cepa* and *Allium sativum*. Watson RR and Preedy VR Ed. Academic Press, Elsevier, London 2019; 137-54.

[96]   Jevas C. Anti-diabetic effects of Allium cepa (onions) aqueous extracts on alloxan-induced diabetic Rattus novergicus. J Med Plants Res 2011; 5(7): 1134-9.

[97]   Patel DK, Prasad SK, Kumar R, Hemalatha S. An overview on antidiabetic medicinal plants having insulin mimetic property. Asian Pac J Trop Biomed 2012; 2(4): 320-30.
[http://dx.doi.org/10.1016/S2221-1691(12)60032-X] [PMID: 23569923]

[98]   Uwazie JN, Yakubu MT, Ashafa AOT, Ajiboye TO. Identification and characterization of anti-diabetic principle in Senna alata (Linn.) flower using alloxan-induced diabetic male Wistar rats. J Ethnopharmacol 2020; 261: 112997.
[http://dx.doi.org/10.1016/j.jep.2020.112997] [PMID: 32534114]

[99]   Ikarashi N, Toda T, Okaniwa T, Ito K, Ochiai W, Sugiyama K. Anti-obesity and anti-diabetic effects of acacia polyphenol in obese diabetic KKAy mice fed high-fat diet. Evid Based Complement Alternat Med 2011; 2011: 952031.
[http://dx.doi.org/10.1093/ecam/nep241] [PMID: 21799697]

[100]  Ku HC, Tsuei YW, Kao CC, *et al.* Green tea (-)-epigallocatechin gallate suppresses IGF-I and IGF-II stimulation of 3T3-L1 adipocyte glucose uptake *via* the glucose transporter 4, but not glucose transporter 1 pathway. Gen Comp Endocrinol 2014; 199: 46-55.
[http://dx.doi.org/10.1016/j.ygcen.2014.01.008] [PMID: 24486085]

[101]  Tan MJ, Ye JM, Turner N, *et al.* Antidiabetic activities of triterpenoids isolated from bitter melon associated with activation of the AMPK pathway. Chem Biol 2008; 15(3): 263-73.
[http://dx.doi.org/10.1016/j.chembiol.2008.01.013] [PMID: 18355726]

[102]  Lee YS, Kim WS, Kim KH, *et al.* Berberine, a natural plant product, activates AMP-activated protein kinase with beneficial metabolic effects in diabetic and insulin-resistant states. Diabetes 2006; 55(8): 2256-64.
[http://dx.doi.org/10.2337/db06-0006] [PMID: 16873688]

[103]  Zhou JY, Zhou SW, Zhang KB, *et al.* Chronic effects of berberine on blood, liver glucolipid metabolism and liver PPARs expression in diabetic hyperlipidemic rats. Biol Pharm Bull 2008; 31(6): 1169-76.
[http://dx.doi.org/10.1248/bpb.31.1169] [PMID: 18520050]

# CHAPTER 9

# Bioactive Compounds as Therapeutic Intervention in Neurodegenerative Diseases

**N. Suleiman[1,*], I. Bulama[2] and L.S. Bilbis[3]**

[1] *Department of Veterinary Physiology and Biochemistry, Faculty of Veterinary Medicine, Usmanu Danfodiyo University Sokoto, Nigeria*

[2] *Department of Veterinary Physiology and Biochemistry, University of Maiduguri, Maiduguri, Nigeria*

[3] *Department of Biochemistry, Usmanu Danfodiyo University Sokoto, Nigeria*

**Abstract:** Neurodegenerative disorders have been implicated as the cause of many devastating diseases that are characterized by gradual loss of susceptible neurons, that are increasingly rising the prevalence of neurodegenerative diseases globally; however, therapeutics for them are lacking. There is an urgent need to develop an effective therapy that can combat the menace caused by disorders of neurodegenerative origin such as Alzheimer's and Parkinson's diseases, stroke, and traumatic brain injury. Peer-reviewed articles were explored for the purpose of this review. Several natural products from medicinal plants have been reported to have phytochemical components with bioactive effects in addition to nutritional value. An appropriate bioactive component is essential for a healthy lifestyle as it plays a significant role in the modulation of neurodegenerative diseases. This review covers the mechanism of action of neurodegenerative disorders and highlights selected classes of bioactive compounds and their effects on neurodegenerative disorders. The use of bioactive compounds in the management of neurodegenerative diseases could solve the problem of the non-availability of therapy.

**Keywords:** Bioactive Compounds, Disease, Intervention, Neurodegenerative, Therapeutic.

## 1. INTRODUCTION

Among older people worldwide, neurodegenerative disorders are a major cause of disability and premature death [1]. Among the most common neurodegenerative diseases are Alzheimer's disease (AD), vascular dementia (VaD), frontotemporal

* **Corresponding author Suleiman N.:** Department of Veterinary Physiology and Biochemistry, Faculty of Veterinary Medicine, Usmanu Danfodiyo University Sokoto, Nigeria; Tel: +2348030411807; E-mail: suleiman.nasiru@udusok.edu.ng

**Saheed Sabiu (Ed)**

dementia (FTD), Parkinson's disease (PD), stroke, and Huntington's disease (HD) [2]. Neurodegeneration is a component of numerous growth-related, devastating, hopeless illnesses that influence the sensory system and have become a significant danger to the strength of the old. The prevalence of neurodegenerative disease has become a global public health problem due to the ongoing aging situation facing western societies [3].

The incidence and damage of oxidants are termed as oxidative stress, and are referred to as pathogenic or etiological agents for diseases such as cancer, Alzheimer's, diabetes and aging [3, 4]. Such illnesses and evidence stimulated by oxidative stress have called for concern among scientists in finding antioxidants to prevent and treat such diseases [5]. Aging-related diseases have long been associated with oxidative stress. Continued dysfunction and death of neurons are characterized by neurodegenerative diseases. Oxidative stress is linked to mitochondrial dysfunction and endoplasmic reticulum, which causes apoptosis and disruption of protein synthesis in neurons. In neurodegenerative conditions, decreased activity of antioxidant enzymes such as catalase, SOD, glutathione, glutathione peroxidase means a decrease in the role of an antioxidant in neurodegeneration [6].

There is growing interest in antioxidants, especially, the naturally occurring type. Natural products are derived from the food, cosmetics, and pharmaceutical industries to include man-made antioxidants that are often limited owing to their carcinogenic potentials [1, 4]. Plants are a source of various secondary metabolites, many of which are natural antioxidants that can be considered sources of these substances, such as polyphenols, flavonoids, and essential oils [5].

The aim of this chapter is to report the beneficial role of bioactive compounds as the therapeutic intervention of neurodegenerative diseases. In this review, the discussion introduces bioactive compounds and its roles, separation and synthesis of bioactive compounds, applications of bioactive compounds, and pathophysiology of neurodegenerative diseases.

## 2. BIOACTIVE CHEMICALS

Currently, the use of medicinal plants in ancient times reflects the history of living particles. 'Bioactive chemicals' are additional nutrients commonly found in foods in small amounts [7]. Humans had no knowledge of bioactive molecules in the past, nonetheless, the use of these substances differs significantly in various ways. Natural plant chemicals are often synthesized as secondary metabolites [6]. Everyone, from a single cell to a million plant cells, makes a wide variety of survival and survival chemicals.

It is possible to break all the chemical elements of the biological system into two broad spheres. One of the main metabolites, such as amino acids, carbohydrates, lipids and proteins, are chemical substances aimed at growth and development. Other secondary metabolites, a class of chemicals that are not basic metabolites are thought to help plants improve their overall survival potential and solve environmental challenges by enabling them to interact with their environment [3].

## 2.1. Role and Types of Bioactive Compounds

An appropriate diet is an essential influence in a nourishing lifestyle and also plays a vital role in the inhibition of neurodegenerative diseases, including AD. The threat of dementia can be decreased by consuming a balanced diet abundant in respiratory chemicals [8]. Regardless of whether these compounds use entirely the neuro-protective impacts seen in *in-vitro* and investigations on animal species, and people under physical situations remain uncertain due to the lack of human intervention studies. There is also a lack of awareness as to whether the prices and types of chemicals contained in food make them readily available. However, their positive results have been largely confirmed by experimental studies of the epidemiological group and laboratory studies detailing the successful biological mechanisms of compound action in the mitigation of AD. Such significant improvements in selected bioactive chemicals are listed in the study. Several of these substances are in any one of the subsequent chemical categories: fat-soluble vitamins, phenolic compounds, essential fatty acids, carotenoids or isothiocyanates.

### 2.1.1. Phenolic Compounds

Phenolic components are present in common vegetable diets and olive oil comprising oleuropein, their most significant sources are hydroxytyrosol and oleocanthal. Oleuropein is a glycosylated seco-iridoid with several advantageous characteristics that has an important antioxidant prospect and protects nerve cells from apoptosis induced by neurotoxin [9]. It can likewise lessen the degree of Aβ and inhibit its production, and at the same time decrease the expression of glutaminylcyclase and the enzyme involved in the synthesis of Aβ. Additionally, oleuropein has a metabolic effect. Escherichia coli cell culture *in vitro* experiment showed that Oleuropein has been shown to be immune to mutant synthesis, which rapidly binds tau protein by 67% compared to the control group [3, 7].

The efficacy of wild-type tau was 79%, whereas methylene blue, the comparison tau aggregation resistor, was 75% effective. These results propose that oleuropein can evade the production of toxic tau collections, likely owing to the combination of aldehyde groups in the forms of tautomeric of its aglycone metabolite.

Oleuropein is hydrolyzed in the digestive system to some other phenolic compound, hydroxytyrosol. In the digestive system, oleuropein is hydrolyzed to some other phenolic compound, hydroxytyrosol, Hydroxytyrosol is a strong antioxidant and reactive oxygen species scavenger that can contribute to the triggering of phase II detoxification enzymes eg glutathione-S- tranferase, UDP-glucuronosyltransferase [10]. *In vitro* analysis of St-Laurent- Sperling *et al*. [11], revealed that it helps protect nerve cells from Aβ-induced toxicity.

The study offered that hydroxytyrosol acts as an agent of anti-inflammatory which reduces the action of the nuclear factor-kappa B (NF-£B) triggering certain neurotoxic conditions induced by the amyloid plaque. Oleocanthal is also a phenolic compound that possesses the bitter taste of olive oil and decreases inflammation by blocking the enzyme cyclooxygenase (COX) that assists in the development of pro-inflammatory prostaglandins.

A study by Rodríguez-Morató *et al*. [12] illustrated its capacity to lessen the production of Aβ and to calculate its brain sensitivity. *In-vitro* studies on tau protein found in *E. Coli*, Li *et al*. [3] found that oleocanthal prevented protein aggregation relative to the control group. Additional study has indicated that the molecule forms a covalent bond with amino acid lysine contained in the PHF6 peptide C-terminus, which is part of the tau protein required for its polymerization [13]. These findings show that oleocanthal can enhance the processes of the disease responsible for the development of AD. Epidemiological studies have partially verified the neuroprotective effects of olive oil. Scarmeas *et al*. [14] have shown that MD, which contains a significant amount of fat, is associated with a lower risk of AD.

The researchers evaluated dietary questions collected in respondents in 1984, aged 76, and found that high compliance with MD vaccines with low risk of AD, With the exception of other variables such as sex, schooling, the BMI or the APOE allele gene.

Psaltopoulou *et al*. [15] reported related inferences, who described that a meta-analysis of 22 studies shows that MD is related to a little risk of AD development and that inadequate devotion to these nutritional instructions reduces the loss of mental function. Authors have explored that this immune response outcome could be a result of the anti-inflammatory activity of MD constituents.

They additionally argued that this sort of diet can be powerful in forestalling CNS degeneration. The previously mentioned advantages of olive oil were additionally affirmed in a preliminary study of a randomized controlled led by Valls-Pedret *et al*. [14]. AD high risk group comprising of 447 aged participants who received dietary supplementation, which were classified into three different groups which include: MD with 1 L / week of olive oil, MD with 30 g of nuts per day, and a low-fat diet. Variations in memory and brain abilities were evaluated with 6 different tests performed at the start and end of the project.

The group that receives MD supplemented with olive oil demonstrated enhanced retention and performance and showed a better Mini-Mental State Assessment (MMSE) test to assess the degree of dementia. Anthocyanins are other neuroprotective phenolic substances that are flavonoids and are characterized in making many fruits and vegetables get either red, purple and blue color. Li *et al.* [15], opined that anthocyanins reduce oxidative stress by reducing the development of free radicals and lipid peroxidation.

Another phenolic compound with an attractive neuroprotective property is curcumin, a natural element of turmeric. It is an effective antioxidant, that lessens oxidation of protein products, overwhelms inflammation by averting both lipoxygenase enzymes and COX and decreases the action of microglia.

### 2.1.2. Omega-3 Fatty Acids and Fat-Soluble Vitamins

Potentially useful medicinal plants used for the treatment of AD can also be found in vitamins and some vital fatty acids, which are extracellular chemicals essential for the effective running of the individual body system. Amongst these numerous body tissues, the central nervous system is mainly susceptible to oxidative stress owing to its heavy oxygen consumption and excessive polyunsaturated fat content.

One of the useful approaches to reduce the risk of AD is to employ the removal of oxidative stress by lipophilic antioxidants and vitamins. Docosahexaenoic acid (DHA) which is the most concentrated fatty acid in the brain [4, 8], a polyunsaturated fatty acid found primarily in fish is one of the compounds, it belongs to the long chain family of omega-3s, and this also includes EPA (eicosapentaenoic acid) and DPA (n-3 docosapentaenoic acid).

Compared to EPA, the content of DHA in the brain is significantly greater. As an important part of the phospholipide membrane formation of brain cells, DHA is present in the cerebral cortex and synaptic membrane. Furthermore, Δ4 activity of desaturase, an enzyme involved in the synthesis of DHA, decreases with age, leading to a decrease in DHA synthesis in the elderly. These factors make DHA omega-3 fatty acid very promising in CNS-related diseases. The concentration of DHA in the brain depends on diet and the conversion of the liver from its temporary precursors.

PHA precursors for DHA essential for nutrition: EPA and α-linolenic acid (ALA) were available in limited amounts in the brain [13]. Except for DHA, with a brain concentration of about 10,000 nmol/g, EPA is generally reported to be of relatively low dose (less than 250 nmol/g) in both human brains and mice attributable to its fast and thorough β pooling. Brain EPA concentrations are controlled by fast metabolism and β-oxidation, not by the absorption of neurons and glial cells [17]. DHA rivals with arachidonic acid, a complement to prostaglandins, by being integrated further into cellular membranes. It may also reduce inflammation of the brain by lowering the concentration of these eicosanoids. Moreover, docosahexaenoic acid leads to the conversion of APP by increasing the level of researchers involved in the compilation of APP and inhibiting the production of Aβ. DHA can protect the nervous system by increasing the combination of neuroprotectin D1 and neurotrophic factor (BDNF) found in the brain, they both prevent neuronal damage and contribute to neurogenesis [9, 14]. In addition, DHA leads to the merger of Aβ and Tau, as established by Green *et al.* [16].

The researchers performed an *in vivo* study with knockout mice containing both Aβ marker and pumpkin. Animals have been distributed to the control category or to one of three treatment groups that have received DHA, arachidonic acid and DHA or DHA and n-6 docosapentaenoic acid for the different duration [3, 6, 9]. The researchers observed that nutritional supplementation with DHA reduces Aβ production and protein concentrations declined three months later. Nine months later, this impact was substantially greater, especially in the DHA group alone, which also recorded a decrease in tau phosphorylate levels [17].

### 2.1.3. Isothiocyanates

Isothiocyanates are the next group of bioactive compounds that can help prevent AD. It is the release of glucosinolates found mainly in concentrated vegetables. In view of the presence of sulfur atom in their constituents, isothiocyanates function as antioxidants, particularly those containing an odor ring that is closely connected to the thiocyanate group. They are also strong regulators of COX and have anti-inflammatory impact. In addition, certain isothiocyanates effectively inhibit the action of acetylcholinesterase, thus extending the half-life of acetylcholine, a neurotransmitter that focuses on its concentration in patients with AD [14]. Sulforaphane, a compound derived from glucoraphanin during plant tissue repair, is one of the most studied isothiocyanates. It raises the concentrations of antioxidant enzymes including glutathion peroxidase and glutaredoxine. Neuron and glial cells improve the production of sulfiredoxin, which activates some antioxidant enzymes. In addition, sulforaphane modifies the action of proteasomes in nerve cells, which are complex enzymatic compounds with elevated levels of protease but may lead to the synthesis of Aβ [17]. It has been shown by epidemiological data that isothiocyanates may have neuroprotective effects. Nurk *et al.* [16] investigated the nutrition and mental health of 2031 participants ranging between 70 and 74 years of age. The researchers have demonstrated that a lot of vegetables, such as cabbage, cauliflower, broccoli and Brussels sprouts, have been cognitively tested. There were also good results from the experiments.

## 2.1.4. Carotenoids

Carotenoids are plant fragments found in several vegetables and fruits in their yellow, orange and red colors. Microalgae, a marine food source, that also makes these organisms an extra food source for these molecules, can also be produced. Carotenoids have a favorable impact on photosynthetic activity and defend against photooxidation. Astaxanthin is a free radical scavenger, reducing oxidative stress, protein and lipid peroxidation. It also enhances the volume of antioxidant enzymes such as catalase and superoxide dismutase.

Katagiri *et al* have reported neuroprotective properties of astaxanthin [17]. Astaxanthin have been reported to decrease the activity of caspase-3 and increasing neurogenesis by enhancing kinase-activated kinase [15]. In a controlled placebo study involving people from 45 to 64 years, who obtained astaxanthin rich extract (6 or 12 mg astaxanthin/day) for 12 weeks. The researchers established that these two intervention groups had higher comprehension and learning scores compared to the placebo group [3, 15]. Two other compounds in this category may also have psychological benefits: lutein and zeaxanthin. The pilot research conducted by Christensen *et al.* [14], that involved 2796 participants above the age of 60, showed a correlation between high intake of these carotenoids and enhanced cognitive functioning. The incorporation of lutein and zeaxanthin was assessed by 24-hour memory and three tests were taken by the participants to determine their memory, oral communication and perception. The investigators found that the optimum production of carotenoids from both foods and nutrients was strongly associated with enhanced cognitive performance. Similar promising findings have been replicated in a controlled p study conducted by Power *et al.* [18]. The research engaged 91 people aged 45 years and older, the participants received supplements that included lutein (10 mg), zeaxanthin (2 mg) and masozeaxanthin (10 mg) or placebo for 12 months.

Numerous neuropsychological studies have shown that people who have added extra carotenoids have improved brain and episodic memory activity more than the placebo group. Researchers have reported that such findings could be attributed to the antioxidant properties of lutein and zeaxanthin and their significant impact on the reliability of the neuronal membrane.

### 2.1.5. Mind Food

Even though the exact relationship for both nutrition and Alzheimer's disease development is not well understood and further experimental research is needed, the disease results appear to be encouraging. Both the MD and DASH diets have been shown to support mental well-being, but interventions that include their selective neuroprotective properties may be more efficient [8, 9]. This form of balanced diet plan, termed the MIND diet, is documented by Morris *et al*. [8, 9] which centers on whole foods rich in bioactive chemicals. In any event whole grains should be served 3 times per day, raw vegetables are expected to be served 6 times per week, some vegetables are to be served once per day, berries are to be served twice per week according to the feed formulation. Fish and chicken are to be served once and twice per week respectively, so also, legumes and nuts are to be served 3 and 5 times per week respectively. The key constituent of the diets is olive oil and it is the main source of fat and oil. Dietary efficacy of MIND was established in a 4.5-year study to evaluate 923 people between the ages of 58 and 98, which showed a 53 percent reduction in AD risk in participants who followed this diet plan [18, 9]. Although, more clinical research is needed on the efficacy of MIND diet, current information suggests that foods rich in bioactive chemicals may help prevent AD [16].

## 2.2. Application of Some of the Bioactive Compounds in the Treatment of Neurodegenerative Diseases

### a. Phytochemicals

Polyphenols are among the most widely studied phytochemicals and form a large family of molecules that contain one or more phenolic rings and are found in many food sources such as wine, green tea, grapes, vegetables, red fruits and coffee [18]. Many types of phytochemicals have been shown to provide significant health benefits. Carotenoids and flavonoids play an important role in the prevention, control, and management of chronic diseases [19]. For instance, due to their characteristic structure, carotenoids have bioactive properties, such as antioxidant, anti-inflammatory, and autophagy-modulatory activities. Given the protective function of carotenoids, their levels in the human body have been significantly associated with the treatment and prevention of various diseases, including neurodegenerative diseases [18].

## b. Vitamins

Vitamins are the main ingredients of food and fruit, which are fat-soluble or soluble in water, and are high in other foods. They have an important role to play in the fight against various diseases. They are needed in small quantities and are found in a balanced diet [3]. Various therapeutic effects have been demonstrated, for example; vitamin E A fat-soluble vitamin with high antioxidant properties. As it dissolves in fat, vitamin E (especially α-tocopherol) protects the cell membrane from damage by free radicals. Its antioxidant role is closely related to preventing lipid peroxidation [7]. Food sources of vitamin E include vegetable oil, germ oil, whole grains, nuts, cereals, fruits, eggs, poultry, meat [18].

Vitamin E deficiency is associated with many neurological problems. Although the mechanisms of vitamin E action in neurodegenerative diseases are not clear, there are many possible mechanisms. Examples of such mechanisms are the protective effects of vitamin E against oxidative stress damage and its suppressive role in the expression of many genes involved in the development of neurodegeneration [7]. Many studies have evaluated the relationship between vitamin E intake or vitamin E levels in body fluids and neurodegenerative diseases. Some studies concluded that vitamin E can play a protective role in neurodegeneration with respect to diseases such as Alzheimer's disease (AD), Parkinson's disease (PD), stroke and amyotrophic lateral sclerosis (ALS).

a. Dietary minerals: Selenium (Se) is a residual mineral, water, vegetable (garlic, onion, wheat, nuts, bean), fish, meat, liver and yeast. At low prices, Se has health benefits of antioxidant, anti-carcinogenic and immunomodulator [11]. Calcium is one of the most effective minerals that aid in the prevention and treatment of diseases such as osteoporosis, colorectal cancer, kidney stones, preeclampsia, and lead poisoning [16].

Specifically, selenium is an essential micronutrient, imparting a biological function as a key component of the $21^{st}$ amino acid, selenocysteine. To date, 25 selenoproteins have been discovered within the human proteome, which can be classified according to a range of functions. Although these proteins are in low abundance in the brain, studies have reported their relevance to normal neurological function, primarily due to antioxidant activity and mechanisms that modulate mitochondrial function. Selenium has also been identified as playing a role in several neurodegenerative disorders, including Alzheimer's and Parkinson's disease, and recent research has suggested possible association with other diseases as multiple sclerosis, amyotrophic lateral sclerosis, and Huntington's disease [16].

a. Essential fatty acids: Omega-3 fatty acids are important long chain polyunsaturated fatty acids because they cannot be produced by humans. Omega-3 fatty acids can be found in fish such as salmon, sardines and tuna, and can be found in walnut and linseed. Omega-3 fatty acids prevent chronic diseases such as heart disease, dementia, depression, arthritis, stroke, cataract, cancer and other neurological diseases.

There is accumulating scientific evidence on the possible efficacy of PUFAs supplementation in neurodegenerative disorders, such as Parkinson's (PD) and Alzheimer's disease (AD). Although dietary recommendations are far from being a treatment for PD or AD, they may be able to alleviate some of the symptoms or slow the cognitive and physical decline.

a. Active sugar: Trehalose, a natural sugar, is usually made from non-male animals such as fungi, yeast and similar species. It can maintain cell integrity by preventing the release of proteins [7, 13]. Active fibers such as inulin, cellulose and maltodextran extracted from foods from which they naturally occur are often used in processed foods to enhance its healthy food profile. Consumption of fiber has many health advantages which include inhibition of chronic sicknesses [14].

Trehalose, known as the "sugar of life," is found in many plants, insects, and microorganisms and acts as an important autophagy modulator and antioxidant. The neuroprotective effects of trehalose have been demonstrated in various neurodegeneration models, and the general hypothesis is that trehalose promotes the elimination of protein aggregates by inducing autophagy.

## 2.3. Constituents of Bioactive compounds

### 2.3.1. Flavonoids

Flavonoids make the biggest class of bioactive compounds identified as phytochemicals or phytonutrients which are the main components of polyphenols that can be regarded as flavanes, flavanols, isoflavones, flavanes, anthocyanins, flavanonols and flavors (proanthocyanidins and carrots) [17]. Each subclass with its own flavonoids type has a dissimilar collection of health benefits and functions of plant resources. This series of dietary compounds is considered to be of immense benefit to people's health due to their anti-inflammatory effects [16]. Flavonoids are derived from all fruits and vegetables, and in combination with carotenoids are accountable for their distinctive colors. Research has shown that there are higher than 6,000 diverse classes of flavonoids known to benefit the human diet.

Chemical structure: Flavonoids usually soluble in water and mature in cell vacuoles. The basic molecular structure of flavonoids comprises of two benzene rings attached to a chain of three carbon forms forming a closed pyran ring.

Sources: Flavonoids are found in many vegetables and fruits. Its main sources consist of leeks, berries, grapes, ginger, carrots, broccoli, apples, onions, cabbage, kale, tomatoes, buckwheat, lemons, and legumes, parsley. Coffee, tea, chocolate, many spices, herbs and red wine are all full of flavonoids.

- Health benefits: Numerous researches have revealed that foods that are rich in phytonutrients are beneficial to human wellbeing and health. The flavonoids are very useful as they act as powerful antioxidants which reduce free radicals and decrease cellular damage and that of other tissues [19]. Moreover, flavonoids have anti-aging and anti-inflammatory effects [12, 19]. Numerous studies have revealed that there is a connection between these polyphenols and their defensive properties on diseases that can help in reducing 'oxidative stress' (e.g. tissue, cardiovascular and neurodegenerative diseases). Their capability to increase the stability of walls of the blood vessel has also been proven in many laboratory studies. Flavonoids have also been found to have positive effect on the nervous system. These substances can also control the activities of some cell receptors and enzymes. Some studies have shown that flavonoids are effective in the regulation of flow of the blood to the brain, which can help improve brain function [14].

### 2.3.2. Anthocyanins

Anthocyanins are compounds that are commonly found in body fluids that can easily dissolve in water. These substances are accountable for the colors of fruits, vegetables and flowers such as red, blue and purple.

- Chemical structure: By nature, anthocyanin is a phenolic molecule of fifteen carbon atoms appeared as two rings of benzene linked by a chain of three (3) carbons. The existence of a flavylium nucleus renders it extremely efficient.

Sources: Although anthocyanins are available in numerous plants, they are mostly found in acai, blueberry, blackcurrant, bilberry, red grape, cherry and purple corn.

- Health benefits: While anthocyanins are antioxidants that work well *In vitro*, their biological activity is usually low owing to their good absorption and low stability. Numerous researches have revealed the several health benefits associated with anthocyanins, with emphasis on their useful effects on the health of the heart, anti-cancer functions and anti-inflammatory properties [11].

## *2.3.3. Tannins*

Tannins belong to the class of astringent, a polyphenolic biomolecule which binds and decreases proteins and other macromolecules and organic compounds.

- Chemical structure: Tannins are complex combination of gallic acid and polymeric polyphenols, as the base unit (commonly refer to as gallotanic acid). Oak tree walnuts produce 50-70 percent tannins. Tannins are categorized into two classes, namely: water-based tannins and condensed tannins. The condensed tannins contain chemicals whose nucleus is composed of 'carbon-carbon' or ether, whereas the water-based tannins consist of chemicals that resemble 'Ester', which are polymers of ellagic acid and gallic acid. The color of the tannin varies from yellow to brown. Tannins contribute to the diet of astringency and enzymatic browning reaction.

Sources: The tannins are usually sourced primarily from tea beans, coffee, pomegranates, persimmon, many berries (blueberries, strawberries, cranberries,), red wine, grapes, chocolate (with a content of 70% or more) and spices (cloves, vanilla, cinnamon, thyme) [18].

- Health Benefits: Tannins is known to reduce growth rate, feed intake, feed quality, net energy metabolism, and protein digestion in laboratory animals. High-fat diets are also less important in nutrition. However, studies in recent time have shown that the main tannins effects may be due to reduced activity in the transmission of nutrients to body tissues that are new rather than to inhibit digestion or food use [12]. Recently, there has been a great deal of attention in seeing different tannins as organisms due to their ability to produce good results in the body system when introduced into the diet over a long duration. This is mainly due to their characteristics as antioxidant which defends body tissues from the activity of free radicals as a result of aging of cells and other developments in the body [15]. Tannins have been proven to have health beneficial which includes increased in blood pressure, lowering blood pressure, lowering levels of serum lipid, and regulation of immune reactions; the form of tannins and the quantity are important for the effects mentioned [17].

## *2.3.4. Betalins*

These pigs are yellow and red, and look like anthocyanins and flavonoids. However, unlike them, betalain contains nitrogen.

- Chemical Composition: Betalain is an indole-colored betalain that can be classified into yellow betaxanthins and the red-violet betacyanins, the colors of which are given to the two-bond betalain structures. They dissolve in water and can therefore be incorporated into the aqueous diet [15].

Sources: the major sources of betalains are the beetroot (yellow and red) colored swiss beetroot, leafy grainy or amaranth, red pitahaya, prickly pear and other cacti.

- Health benefits: Due to its anti-cancer, antioxidant, anti-lipid and anti-microbial properties, betalain has lasting health effects. They are non-toxic to food and can therefore be used as an effective food and a good alternative to the treatment of inflammation, oxidative stress, and diseases associated with dyslipidemia such as arterial stenosis, atherosclerosis, high blood pressure and cancer, among others [16, 19].

Because of their toxic protection, accessibility, low cost, biological decay and potentially beneficial health effects, the use of betalains in diet making and interrelated industries can pave the system for overcoming existing worries about the medical threats with artificial colors [19]. However, there is a need for longitudinal studies to determine the precise mechanism of these organic substances and their application practically to human health.

### 2.3.5. Carotenoids

It is commonly referred to as carotenes - members of the lipid-soluble hydrocarbon group; and their oxygen-producing products are referred to as xanthophylls. The word 'carotenes' comes from the red color of carrot; however, they are still widely distributed in a variety of other floras as they are present in green leaves, many roots many red and yellow fruits. The color of the yolk in egg and some fish similarly refers to carotenoids.

Chemical structure: Carotenoid comprises eight (8) isoprenoid units that are fused together in such a way that the structure of the isoprenoid units is secreted between molecules. Carotenoids with wavelengths of 400-550 nanometers (from violet to light green) are related to their composition and cause the substance to have a strong orange, yellow or red color.

Sources: Other rich sources of carotenoids include cabbage, plums, apricots, mango, cantaloupe, sweet potatoes, kale, spinach, cilantro (coriander), collard greens, fresh thyme, turnip greens and winter squash.

• Health Benefits: Carotenoids have numerous health benefits apart from the benefits on skin and vision; they have defensive effects on many types of cancer. Importantly, β-carotene is a precursor to vitamin A that is essential for strong immune systems, mucous membranes and healthy skin, and eye health (good vision). Numerous researches have proved that carotenoids are linked to an increased risk of various cancers, including lung cancer, breast cancer, and neck and head cancer [3, 7, 16]. Consequently, it has been revealed that there is a relationship between levels of serum β-carotene and reduced cancer risk (e.g. lung cancer). Though, most studies with β-carotene interventions as a supplement did not show any cancer effects; The interaction of β-carotene with other chemicals, be it carotenoids or other food substances, may play a part. Studies have proposed that among risk-related biological circumstances, the pro-oxidant effects of β-carotene are involved in lung cancer development.

### 2.3.6. Plant Sterols

The natural components of all plants are commonly referred to as plant sterols or phytosterols. Some of these substances are considered organic foods.

• Chemical structure of Plant sterols: these comprise phytostanols, phytosterols, and esters of fatty acids. Naturally, it's things like cholesterol; they can be used in a similar way to attract the absorption and formation of cholesterol in humans and animals.

Sources: The major sources of Plant sterols are vegetable oil available in small quantities in ginger, legumes, nuts, cereals, grains, and leaves. In many countries, other food products for instance yoghurt, margarine, breakfast cereals, milk, soybean and high-fat (pine) are stimulated with plant sterols to boost their level or sterol content [18].

• Health benefits: Factors such as plant sterol cholesterol can affect the absorption of cholesterol in the gut. Preferred absorption of plant sterols over LDL (low-density lipoprotein) cholesterol, which is the bad cholesterol that occurs when added to food or as a dietary supplement, which naturally lowers the LDL cholesterol level in the blood system. Studies have made known that when given a certain amount of plant sterols (such as 1.5-3 grams per day), can lower LDL cholesterol levels in the blood by a certain percentage (7.5-12%) [12].

## 2.3.7. Glucosinolates

Glucosinolates are the natural ingredients of many spicy plants such as cabbage, horseradish and mustard, and their secondary metabolites contain nitrogen and sulfur. Once such plant material is cut, or chewed, or damaged, its glucosinolates create mustard oil that gives the plants or its products a unique pungency.

- Chemical composition: Glucosinolates have nitrogen and sulfur that are found in glucose and amino acids. Each glucosinolate contains a medium carbon atom bound to the thioglucose group by the sulfur atom and the sulphate group by the nitrogen atom (sulphatealdoxime). Furthermore, the carbon at the center is linked to the side group. Diverse glucosinolates side groups have differed and this difference in the side group is owing to the differences in the biological functions of these plant substances [12].

Sources: Essential glucosinolate sources include cruciferous vegetables, such as broccoli, wasabi (Wasabia japonica), kale, cabbage, garden cress and watercress. Isothiocyanates are the main active products of glucosinolate. The cruciferous vegetables contain various glucosinolates, each producing a unique isothiocyanate with its own cellular material or body-matched.

- Health benefits: Many studies have revealed that other glucosinolates and biologically active metabolites, especially isothiocyanates, play a role in cancer prevention and dementia [17, 19]. These specific chemical compounds that are rarely present in most other vegetables are identified to be highly effective in destroying different cancerous cells with less damaging effect on the normal body cells. They reduce the risk of dementia and reduce the incidence of dementia among the aged people.

## 3. NEURODEGENERATIVE DISEASES

Neurodegenerative diseases are categorized by complicated and intensely related factors such as neuro-infigueatory, oxidative damage and synaptic failure. It is reported by the authors that some of the chemicals described in the review may indicate other efficient mechanisms for the management of neurodegenerative ailments such as the Parkinson's and Alzheimer's [14].

Anti-inflammatory compounds have been reported to delay the progression of the disease in the neuro-infigueatory concept of non-neurodegenerative diseases. fucoidan, Dieckol, floridoside, epitaondiol, caulerpin, pacifenol, fucoxanthin, pheophytin A, Δ-carrageenan, stypotriol triacetate and PUFAs have been revealed to overwhelm reactions of inflammation mainly with antioxidant effects and by controlling various signaling pathways [14].

Various studies have shown that differences between antioxidant and pro-oxidant homeostasis might be related to the pathophysiology of neurodegenerative disorders. Phlorotannins, sulphate carotenoids, polysaccharides, and sterols derived from various macroalgae species possess high antioxidant activity. The most effective tool, however, is still the use of ChE inhibitors in the treatment of non-neurodegenerative diseases. Numerous phlorotannines, just as sargachromenol, sargaquinoic acid and PUFAs, have been appeared to restrain the action of Throb and/or BuChE. CHE inhibitors are regularly connected with many results; subsequently, it very well may be proposed that the utilization of synthetic substances removed from macroalgae rather than engineered fixings may lessen the danger of poison in the body and keep certain unwanted impacts from happening [17].

## 3.1. Most Common Neurodegenerative Diseases

### 3.1.1. Alzheimer's disease (AD)

Alzheimer's disease is the most common cause of dementia worldwide, with the prevalence continuing to grow in part because of the aging world population. This neurodegenerative disease process is characterized classically by two hallmark pathologies: β-amyloid plaque deposition and neurofibrillary tangles of hyperphosphorylated tau. Diagnosis is based upon clinical presentation fulfilling several criteria as well as fluid and imaging biomarkers. Treatment is currently targeted toward symptomatic therapy, although trials are underway that aim to reduce the production and overall burden of pathology within the brain [20].

Although the prevalence of dementia continues to increase worldwide, incidence in the western world might have decreased as a result of better vascular care and improved brain health. Alzheimer's disease, the most prevalent cause of dementia, is still defined by the combined presence of amyloid and tau, but researchers are gradually moving away from the simple assumption of linear causality as proposed in the original amyloid hypothesis. Age-related, protective, and disease-promoting factors probably interact with the core mechanisms of the disease [21]. Alzheimer's disease (AD) is a multifactorial neurodegenerative disease which is mainly characterized by progressive impairment in cognition, emotion, language and memory in older population [22]. Fig. (**1**) shows a description of a normal and

Alzheimer diseased brain.

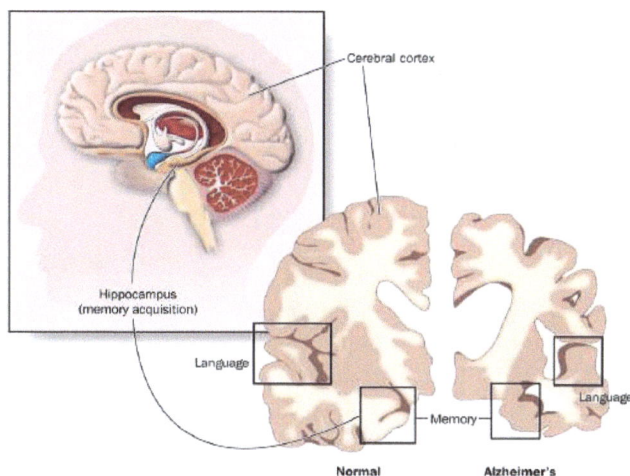

**Fig. (1).** Showing normal and abnormal cerebral cortex, Hippocampus for memory acquisition in Alzheimer's disease [23].

### *3.1.2. Parkinson disease (PD)*

Parkinson disease (PD) is the most common neurodegenerative movement disorder. Risk factors include age, male gender and some environmental factors. The aetiology of the disease in most patients is unknown, but different genetic causes have been identified. Although familial forms of PD account for only 5%–15% of cases, studies on these families provided interesting insight on the genetics and the pathogenesis of the disease allowing the identification of genes implicated in its pathogenesis and offering critical insights into the mechanisms of the disease [24].

The symptomatology of Parkinson's disease is now recognized as heterogeneous, with clinically significant non-motor features. The cause of Parkinson's disease remains unknown, but risk of developing Parkinson's disease is no longer viewed as primarily due to environmental factors. Instead, Parkinson's disease seems to result from a complicated interplay of genetic and environmental factors affecting numerous fundamental cellular processes [25]. Studies of large numbers of patients with PD have suggested that PD is a multifactorial illness with likely genetic and environmental determinants [24]. Fig. (**2**) shows a normal neurotransmitter and abnormal neurotransmitter of a Parkinson disease.

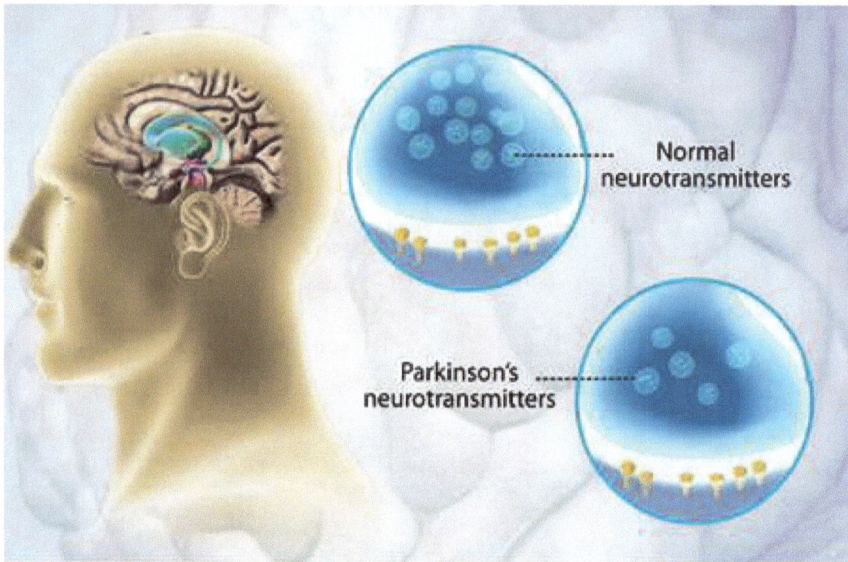

**Fig. (2).** Normal neurotransmitter compared to Parkinson's disease neurotransmitter [26].

### 3.1.3. Huntington's Disease (HD)

Huntington's disease (HD) is a fully penetrant neurodegenerative disease caused by a dominantly inherited CAG trinucleotide repeat expansion in the huntingtin gene on chromosome 4. In Western populations HD has a prevalence of 10.6-13.7 individuals per 100 000. It is characterized by cognitive, motor and psychiatric disturbance [27]. At the cellular level mutant huntingtin results in neuronal dysfunction and death through a number of mechanisms, including disruption of proteostasis, transcription and mitochondrial function and direct toxicity of the mutant protein. Early macroscopic changes are seen in the striatum with involvement of the cortex as the disease progresses [28].

Huntington's disease (HD) is an autosomal dominantly inherited neurodegenerative disease characterized by progressive motor, behavioral, and cognitive decline, ending in death. Despite the discovery of the underlying genetic mutation more than 20 years ago, treatment remains focused on symptomatic management [27]. Fig. (3) shows a normal brain section and Hutington's disease section of a brain.

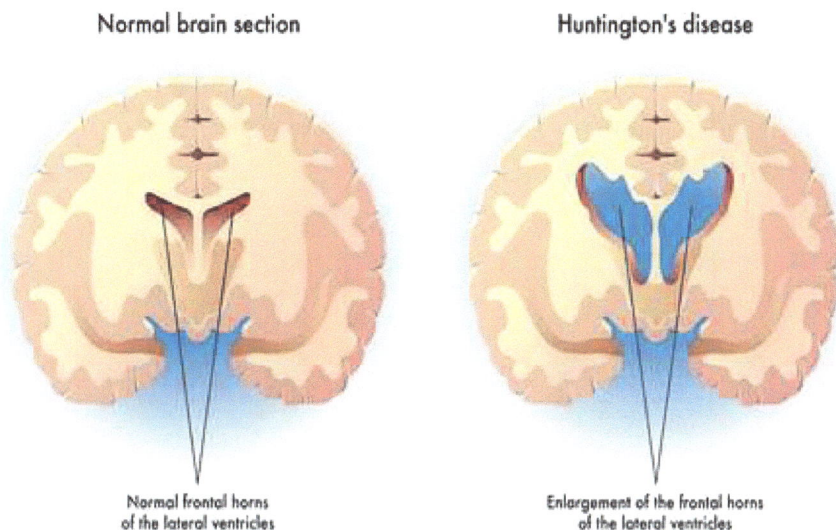

**Fig. (3).** Illustration showing the difference in structure of a normal brain and one with Huntington's disease [29].

### 3.1.4. Stroke

Stroke is the second leading cause of death and the third leading cause of disability worldwide and its burden is increasing rapidly in low-income and middle-income countries, many of which are unable to face the challenges it imposes [27].

The burden of stroke is a huge public health issue of growing importance. In 2019, stroke was the second leading cause of death (6·6 million people) and disability (143 million disability-adjusted life years lost [DALYs]) worldwide [26]. During the past three decades, in absolute terms, global stroke incidence increased by 70%, its prevalence increased by 85%, its mortality increased by 43%, and DALYs due to stroke increased by 32%, with a greater increase in stroke burden in low-income and middle-income countries than in high-income countries [28]. Fig. (4) shows common types of stroke in human brain.

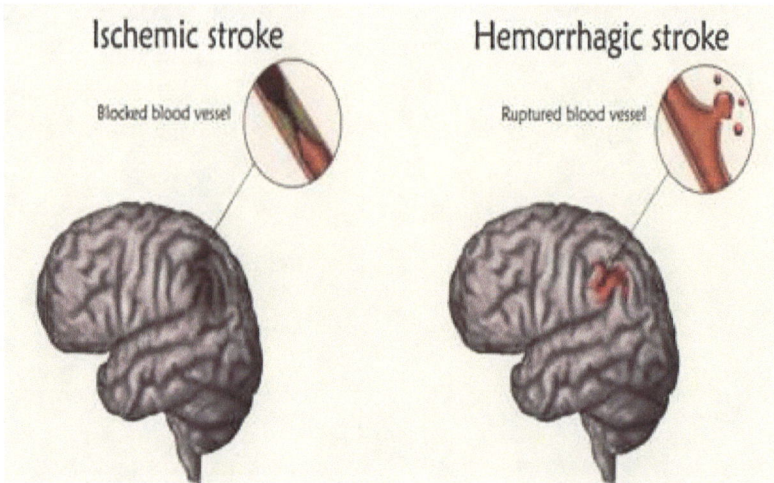

**Fig. (4).** Hemorrhagic stroke compared to ischemic stroke: Shown are the two broad categories of stroke. On the right, a ruptured blood vessel is visible causing damage to the surrounding brain tissues. On the left, a blood clot is interrupting the blood flow to the brain [30 - 32].

## 3.2. Pathophysiology of Neurodegenerative Diseases

### a. Neurodegeneration

Neurodegeneration is an element of many incapacitating, hopeless infections that influence the sensory system and represent a genuine danger to the strength of the older individuals. Because of the progress in the maturing of the circumstance confronting western social orders, the pervasiveness of neurodegenerative illnesses has become a general medical issue around the world [19]. Neurodegenerative illnesses are related with an assortment of complex conditions, for example, neuro-infigueation, serious oxidative harm brought about by dynamic nitrogen and oxygen species (RNS and ROS), synaptic misfortune and different types of neuronal cell passing [13, 16, 19].

### b. Neuro-inflammation

Ongoing investigations have indicated that the formation of microglia cells, which are found in the central nervous system (CNS) and causes the development of provocative and neurotoxic components, for example, prostaglandin E2 (PGE2), nitric oxide (NO), ROS, IL-6 and tumor rot factor (TNF) – III, interleukin (IL) - 1β can cause neurodegeneration [11, 18]. Expanded degrees of microglia-pr--inflammatory mediators were recognized during PD and AD pathogenesis. Subsequently, microglial initiation instruments can lessen neuronal harm or demise of neurodegenerative infections [18]. Without a doubt, epidemiological examinations have just indicated that drawn-out management with non-inflammatory drugs (NSAIDs) diminishes the danger of AD, eases back the beginning of the sickness, improves side effects and eases back despondency [14]. However, extensive use of NSAIDs raises the threat of acquiring kidney and kidney disorders. These health threats have increased the pursuit of other anti-inflammatory medications from the safer dietary origins, for instance, macroalgae. It is also reported in other findings that marine compounds can quantify sensing mechanisms such as mitogen-activated protein kinase (MAPK) and C-Jun N-terminal kinase (JNK) act/protein kinase B (PKB) mechanisms linked to neuro-infigeatory response.

## c. Oxidative stress

Various investigations have shown that the irregularity between pro-oxidant and antioxidant homeostasis resulting in the formation of noxious RNS and ROS can be identified with the pathogenesis of various neurodegenerative conditions [18]. The collection of RNS and ROS and the collaborations among these dynamic types can prompt protein oxidation, lipid peroxidation, DNA harm, and, at last, neuronal cell demise [19]. Numerous antioxidants may have favorable impacts on the elimination or reduction of ROS/RNS generation, mitigating neuronal cell loss. A significant amount of antioxidant molecules has also been found in various macroalgae, including phlorotannines, sulfate polysaccharides, carotenoids and sterols, rendering these marine species a significant origin of neuroprotective chemicals [11, 17]. Emerging literature indicates that antioxidant activity may not be a particular mechanism by which exercise is integrated, but perhaps its capacity to alter the signaling pathways involved in cell survival processes [4].

## d. Synaptic Loss

Loss of certain subsets of neurons is a common complication of various neurodegenerative diseases. While cholinergic depletion is considered a symptom of AD disease, *in vivo* neuroimaging research has indicated that the depletion of cerebral cholinergic markers in parkinsondemin is equivalent to or worse than prototypic AD [18]. Decreased levels of ACh are also apparent in both neurodegenerative diseases. There are two forms of cholinesterase (ChE) in the SNC: the butyrylcholinesterase (BuChE) and acetylcholinesterase (AChE). The AChE is a membrane enzyme that lowers ACh to cholinergic synapses, whereas BuChE is an unidentified enzyme found in neuroglia and located in the intestines, liver, kidneys, heart, lungs and serum. These two enzymes can bind up to higher than 10,000 ACh molecules per second of essential neurodegenerative agents [12]. CHE inhibitors invert ACh dysfunction after synaptic delivery, which is one of the best and compelling treatment modalities for neurodegenerative infections [16]. Studies have just demonstrated that CHE inhibitors increase ACh levels in the mind, yet in addition diminish and repress the advancement of β-amyloid (Aβ) stores, which shield neurons from neurodegeneration [15].

## CONCLUSION

The pathophysiology of neurodegenerative disorders is known to be complex and is characterized by phenomena such as neurodegeneration, neuro-inflammation, oxidative stress and synaptic loss. Some of the bioactive compounds described in this chapter can be an alternative in the management of neurodegenerative disorders such as stroke, Alzheimer's and Parkinson's. However, additional study is required in order to explore their maximum therapeutic ability.

## CONSENT FOR PUBLICATION

Not applicable.

## CONFLICT OF INTEREST

The authors declare no conflict of interest, financial or otherwise.

## ACKNOWLEDGEMENTS

Declared none.

## REFERENCES

[1]     Huang Y, Todd N, Thathiah A. The role of GPCRs in neurodegenerative diseases: avenues for therapeutic intervention. Curr Opin Pharmacol 2017; 32: 96-110.
        [http://dx.doi.org/10.1016/j.coph.2017.02.001] [PMID: 28288370]

[2]     Arlt S. Non-Alzheimer's disease-related memory impairment and dementia. Dialogues Clin Neurosci 2013; 15(4): 465-73.
        [http://dx.doi.org/10.31887/DCNS.2013.15.4/sarlt] [PMID: 24459413]

[3]     Grodzicki W, Dziendzikowska K. The Role of Selected Bioactive Compounds in the Prevention of Alzheimer ' s Disease. Antioxidants Rev. 2020; pp. 1-18.

[4]     Ghosh N, Ghosh R, Mandal SC. Antioxidant protection: A promising therapeutic intervention in neurodegenerative disease. Free Radic Res 2011; 45(8): 888-905.
        [http://dx.doi.org/10.3109/10715762.2011.574290] [PMID: 21615270]

[5]     Rojas J, Buitrago A. Antioxidant Activity of Phenolic Compounds Biosynthesized by Plants and Its Relationship With Prevention of Neurodegenerative Diseases.Bioactive Compounds: Health Benefits and Potential Applications. Elsevier Inc. 2018; pp. 3-31.
        [http://dx.doi.org/10.1016/B978-0-12-814774-0.00001-3]

[6]     Kris-Etherton PM, Hecker KD, Bonanome A, *et al.* Bioactive compounds in foods: their role in the prevention of cardiovascular disease and cancer. Am J Med 2002; 113(9) (Suppl. 9B): 71S-88S.
        [http://dx.doi.org/10.1016/S0002-9343(01)00995-0] [PMID: 12566142]

[7]     Azmir J, Zaidul ISM, Rahman MM, Sharif KM, Mohamed A, Sahena F, *et al.* Techniques for extraction of bioactive compounds from plant materials: A review. J Food Eng 2013; 117(4): 426-36.
[http://dx.doi.org/10.1016/j.jfoodeng.2013.01.014]

[8]     Cacciatore I, Ciulla M, Fornasari E, Marinelli L, Di A. Expert Opinion on Drug Delivery Solid lipid nanoparticles as a drug delivery system for the treatment of neurodegenerative diseases. Expert Opin Drug Deliv 2016; 5247: April.

[9]     Barbosa M, Andrade PB. marine drugs. Mar Drugs 2014; 12: 4934-72.
[http://dx.doi.org/10.3390/md12094934] [PMID: 25257784]

[10]    Caruso A, Nicoletti F, Mango D, Saidi A, Orlando R, Scaccianoce S. Stress as risk factor for Alzheimer's disease. Pharmacol Res 2018; 132: 130-4.
[http://dx.doi.org/10.1016/j.phrs.2018.04.017] [PMID: 29689315]

[11]    Sivanandam TM, Thakur MK. Traumatic brain injury: a risk factor for Alzheimer's disease. Neurosci Biobehav Rev 2012; 36(5): 1376-81.
[http://dx.doi.org/10.1016/j.neubiorev.2012.02.013] [PMID: 22390915]

[12]    Kivimäki M, Kawachi I. Work Stress as a Risk Factor for Cardiovascular Disease. Curr Cardiol Rep 2015; 17(9): 630.
[http://dx.doi.org/10.1007/s11886-015-0630-8] [PMID: 26238744]

[13]    Sperling RA, Aisen PS, Beckett LA, *et al.* Toward defining the preclinical stages of Alzheimer's disease: recommendations from the National Institute on Aging-Alzheimer's Association workgroups on diagnostic guidelines for Alzheimer's disease. Alzheimers Dement 2011; 7(3): 280-92.
[http://dx.doi.org/10.1016/j.jalz.2011.03.003] [PMID: 21514248]

[14]    Fu H, Hardy J, Duff KE. Selective vulnerability in neurodegenerative diseases. Nat Neurosci 2018; 21(10): 1350-8.
[http://dx.doi.org/10.1038/s41593-018-0221-2] [PMID: 30250262]

[15]    Vellas B, Carrie I, Gillette-Guyonnet S, *et al.* Alzheimer's Disease : Design and Baseline Data. J Prev Alzheimers Dis 2014; 1(1): 13-22.
[PMID: 26594639]

[16]    Niedzielska E, Smaga I, Gawlik M, *et al.* Oxidative Stress in Neurodegenerative Diseases. Mol Neurobiol 2016; 53(6): 4094-125.
[http://dx.doi.org/10.1007/s12035-015-9337-5] [PMID: 26198567]

[17]    Barnham KJ, Masters CL, Bush AI. Neurodegenerative diseases and oxidative stress. Nat Rev Drug Discov 2004; 3(3): 205-14.
[http://dx.doi.org/10.1038/nrd1330] [PMID: 15031734]

[18]    Rodríguez-Morató J, Xicota L, Fitó M, Farré M, Dierssen M, de la Torre R. Potential role of olive oil phenolic compounds in the prevention of neurodegenerative diseases. Molecules 2015; 20(3): 4655-80.
[http://dx.doi.org/10.3390/molecules20034655] [PMID: 25781069]

[19]    Reboredo-Rodríguez P, Varela-López A, Forbes-Hernández TY, *et al.* Phenolic compounds isolated from olive oil as nutraceutical tools for the prevention and management of cancer and cardiovascular diseases. Int J Mol Sci 2018; 19(8): E2305.
[http://dx.doi.org/10.3390/ijms19082305] [PMID: 30082650]

[20]    Weller J, Budson A. Current understanding of Alzheimer's disease diagnosis and treatment. F1000Res 2018; 7.
[http://dx.doi.org/10.12688/f1000research.14506.1]

[21]    Scheltens P, Blennow K, Breteler MM, *et al.* Alzheimer's disease. Lancet 2016; 388(10043): 505-17.
[http://dx.doi.org/10.1016/S0140-6736(15)01124-1] [PMID: 26921134]

[22]    Saeedi M, Rashidy-Pour A. Association between chronic stress and Alzheimer's disease: Therapeutic

effects of Saffron. Biomed Pharmacother 2021; 133: 110995.
[http://dx.doi.org/10.1016/j.biopha.2020.110995] [PMID: 33232931]

[23]   The Silverbirds. Alzheimer's Disease: Symptoms, Causes & Treatment of Alzheimer's Disease 2018. Available from: www.thesilverbirds.com

[24]   Balestrino R, Schapira AHV. Parkinson disease. Eur J Neurol 2020; 27(1): 27-42.
[http://dx.doi.org/10.1111/ene.14108] [PMID: 31631455]

[25]   Kalia LV, Lang AE. Parkinson's disease. Lancet 2015; 386(9996): 896-912.
[http://dx.doi.org/10.1016/S0140-6736(14)61393-3]

[26]   Mayoclinic. Parkinsons Disease condition Available from: https://www.mayoclinic.org/diseases-conditions/parkinsons-disease

[27]   McColgan P, Tabrizi SJ. Huntington's disease: a clinical review. Eur J Neurol 2018; 25(1): 24-34.
[http://dx.doi.org/10.1111/ene.13413] [PMID: 28817209]

[28]   Wyant KJ, Ridder AJ, Dayalu P. Huntington's Disease-Update on Treatments. Curr Neurol Neurosci Rep 2017; 17(4): 33.
[http://dx.doi.org/10.1007/s11910-017-0739-9] [PMID: 28324302]

[29]   Neuroepic. Demystifying the Search for a Cure: the Epigenetics of Huntington's Disease 2020. Available from: www.neuroepic.mcdb.lsa.umich.edu/wp/33

[30]   WHO. Global Action Plan for the prevention and control of noncommunicable diseases 2013–2020. Geneva: World Health Organization 2013.

[31]   Zhao W, Xiao ZJ, Zhao SP. The Benefits and Risk of Satin Therapy in Ischemic Stroke: A Review of the Literature. Neurol India 2020; 76-92.

[32]   MD Nutrition. Stroke: Types, Symptoms and Long-term Outlook 2020 2020. Available from: www.1md.org/health-guide/heart/disorder/stroke

# CHAPTER 10

# Green Synthesis Application in Diabetes Therapy

## Fatai O. Balogun[1,*] and Saheed Sabiu[1]

[1] *Department of Biotechnology and Food Science, Durban University of Technology, P.O. Box 1334, Durban 4000, South Africa*

**Abstract:** The use of medicinal plants and or medicinal plants-aided nanoparticles (NPs) in the management of diabetes mellitus has progressively received wider acceptance over the years due to the accompanying side effects with conventional therapy. The review explores the application of green-synthesized nanostructures in the control or management of diabetes as well as probable mechanism of NPs formation and possible toxicity. Information sourced from scientific databases including Science Direct, Google Scholar, PubMed, Web of Science, SciFinder, JSTOR revealed 58 medicinal plants explored in the synthesis of four (4) NS such as gold, silver, zinc oxide and platinum with established antidiabetic potential. The NS is characterized by varying microscopic and or spectroscopic instruments such as UV-Vis, SEM, EDS, FTIR and XRD commonly are stable, smaller-sized and mostly crystalline in nature. The functional groups responsible for the reduction and stabilization of the nanoparticles are predominantly C-O, C-H, COOH, N-H found in phenols, flavonoids, alkaloids, proteins and so on. The review identified and revealed 45% studies with less than 5% (mostly from India) conducted on animal models for antidiabetic and toxicity determinations, respectively with none for clinical studies, indicating the need for intensified efforts on research on these identified plants and unidentified species for drug development.

**Keywords:** Diabetes management, Characterization techniques, Functional groups, Green application, Nanoparticles, Reducing and/or stabilizing agents.

## INTRODUCTION

Nanotechnology is an aspect of science involving the synthesis of materials or substances in nanometer range (between 1- 100 nm) [1] or molecular level [2]. Nanoparticles (NPs), sometimes referred to as nanostructures (NS) is an evolved field whose substantial contribution to other scientific endeavours, including pharmaceutical, medicine, bioengineering, agriculture *etc.*, is far-reaching [3] and multidisciplinary. In fact, a number of applications such as micro-optoelectronic

---
* **Corresponding author Fatai O. Balogun:** Department of Biotechnology and Food Science, Durban University of Technology, P.O. Box 1334, Durban 4000, South Africa; Tel: +27834820022; E-mail: balogunfo@yahoo.co.uk

devices, solar cells, magnetic devices, electro and photocatalytic devices, drug (gene) delivery, textile, cosmetics, x-ray imaging, biosensors, *etc.* from these domains have been generated on NPs [1, 3, 4]. Nanostructures characterized into natural or artificial are synthesized in the form of metals such as gold, silver, platinum, zinc, copper, palladium, magnetite, silicon, nickel, cobalt and or their metallic oxides and or dioxides (semiconductors), including indium oxide, ZnO, CuO, $TiO_2$, MgO, CaO, FeO, $ZnO_2$ [1, 2, 5] and or carbon, *etc.*, and they are (sometimes) ascribed to different groups based on their unique properties, hence, partly the reason for the individually exhibited unique characters and well-endowed applications. Few of the features of prominent or selected nanostructures are summarized below:

Gold (Au), among other inorganic NPs was adjudged the most effective NP [6]. This could be attributed to numerous innate properties, which include but are not limited to the ease of synthesis, biocompatibility, light-scattering ability in cellular imaging, moderate susceptibility of the chemical surface functional groups, resistance to oxidation and plasma resonance, *etc.* [7, 8]. Its relevance as antidiabetic, antioxidant, anti-inflammatory and anticancer agents have been reported [6, 9 - 11].

Silver (Au) is another metal NP that has found its importance in many fields (medical, food, healthcare *etc.*) owing to its distinct features, including electrical, thermal, high electrical conductivity *etc.* [12, 13], which are linked to a number of applications such as antioxidative, antibacterial agents, drug delivery, antidiabetic, anticancer agents, *etc.* [14 - 16].

Platinum is one of the noble metals with high importance. It has been explored in nanotechnology and endowed with wide application in numerous scientific fields such as biological, medicine, chemical, electronics, *etc.* [17]. The antibacterial, antioxidant, anticancer and safety concerns of platinum nanoparticles have been reported [17].

Zinc oxide (ZnO), grouped with the like of graphene based on its unique importance and application is a metal oxide that has taken a prominent place in nanomedicine. ZnO, recognised to be the most important inorganic NP [18] due to the usefulness in biomedical, gas censors, cosmetics, agriculture *etc.* [18], is reported to possess semi conducting, piezoelectric and optical properties [19] with low toxicity and biodegradable ability, *etc.* [20]. Its relevance in nano-optical devices, nanosensors, energy storage, *etc.*, has been studied by many authors [11, 19, 21].

The low toxicity and unique biological potentials exhibited by selenium (Se) placed it in the group of NPs of significance [22]. Besides, it also possesses good absorptive capability as a result of its interactions between SeNPs and functional groups (*e.g.*, amino, carbonyl, carboxylic, cyano) of proteins [23]. It is a good antioxidative and antihyperglycaemic agent [24].

## Nano-synthesis Methods

Nanoparticles have continued to be developed either by top down or bottom up approaches through physical, chemical, and biological methods. While the 'top down' approach involves the breaking down of bulk material into smaller particles geared at size reduction and achieved greatly through physical processes such as milling, grinding, sputtering, evaporation *etc.*, 'bottom up' approach is brought-about by the aggregation of the atoms or particles into nuclei and the eventual NS is achieved *via* chemical and biological processes including laser pyrolysis, sol gel process, supercritical synthesis, chemical vapour deposition, atomic condensation, co-precipitation, green synthesis, and so on [2]. The choice of a particular method in the synthesis of NPs is determined by the extent of toxicity, cost of manufacture, energy requirement, treatment necessity in terms of regulated pressure, temperature and pH, *etc.* Notwithstanding the above, the type or methods used in synthesizing these NPs and the adopted characterization techniques may partly determine the size, shape, and eventual characteristics and/or their pharmacological and/or biological potentials.

## Characterization of Nanoparticles

The synthesis of the nanoparticles is accompanied by arrays of spectrometric and microscopic techniques such as ultraviolet-visible (UV-Vis), fourier-transform infrared (FTIR), transmission electron (TEM) or scanning electron (SEM) or fields emission scanning electron (FE-SEM), x-ray diffraction (XRD), dynamic light scattering (DLS), energy dispersive (EDS), differential centrifugal sedimentation (DCS), *etc.*, which determines the point of maximum absorption and or the band gap energy, depicts the type of size (from as small as 5 nm to as big as >500 nm), shapes (cubical, spherical, triangular, irregular, pyramidal, hexagonal, octahedral, decahedral *etc.*), morphology (crystalline, amorphous, *etc.*), stability, homogeneity, surface area, and so on. The characterization aspect is germane to afford information on the system and control of the NPs [1].

## Green Synthesis of Nanoparticles

Green nanotechnology is an evolving application that combines green chemistry and engineering [25] fields focusing on the reduction of energy consumption and the use of cost effective materials to produce ecofriendly materials. This type of synthesis falls into the biological method of NP synthesis using various biological substances, including enzymes, microorganisms (fungi, bacteria, algae), yeast, plants *etc.*, as precursors. Asides, from the possibility of modification of certain reaction conditions (pressure, temperature, pH, *etc.*) during the synthesis, the method is generally simple, the raw materials (and solvents) used are not toxic, and the whole system or process is cost effective, and the end result or product is ecofriendly, which makes green biological synthesis (technology) preferable. The use of plants for NS synthesis is advantageous compared to other biological materials (particularly on a commercial or larger scale) owing to their reliability, sustainability, renewability (can convert three-quarter of light energy to chemical energy), *etc.* Notwithstanding the above, each of these precursors has been studied on both noble metals and metal oxides alike by different researchers and found to establish astonishing pharmacological applications.

The use of the plant is considered a novel approach for NP synthesis, owing to their ability to prevent destructive effects (whether in the use of toxic solvents or harmful chemicals) obtainable in physical and chemical methods [26]. Additionally, plants are embraced for this purpose due to the presence of phytochemicals or secondary metabolite (SM) from virtually all parts of the plant, particularly leaves (mostly), roots, flower, stem, bud, seed, *etc.* [4]. The SM contains functional groups such as flavonoids, phenols, terpenoids, alkaloids, amines, amides, *etc.* [27], that act to reduce the metal ions resulting in the formation and stabilization of the NPs. It must be noted that the success or nature or the effectiveness of a synthesized NS is partly dependent on other reaction parameters, including but not limited to solvents (mostly water, organic polar solvents), pH (acidic, neutral, basic), temperature, pressure, *etc.*, all geared towards producing a small-sized and stable NPs with effective pharmacological applications. Typically, there are reports on the importance of high concentration and temperature [28] as well as distilled water (aqueous) as the preferred medium [27, 29], among others. Fig. (**1**) provides pictorial information on the major steps involved in NPs synthesis using plants.

**Interplay between Diabetes Mellitus, Medicinal Plants, and Nanotechnology**

Diabetes mellitus is one of the leading chronic non communicable diseases (NCD) in the world, with a tendency to cause disability and death [30]. The menace came into being due to derangement in the carbohydrate, lipids, and protein metabolism resulting in a state of hyperglycaemia (high level of glucose in the blood) due to the inability of the pancreatic beta cells to secrete insulin (a hormone concerned with the regulation of the blood sugar level) or ineffective insulin (secreted but unused) or both [31]. The implication is an excess of glucose in the systemic circulation that is not absorbed into body tissues. Additionally, the report indicates that many NCDs, particularly diabetes is linked to oxidative stress due to the influence or over production of free radicals [32].

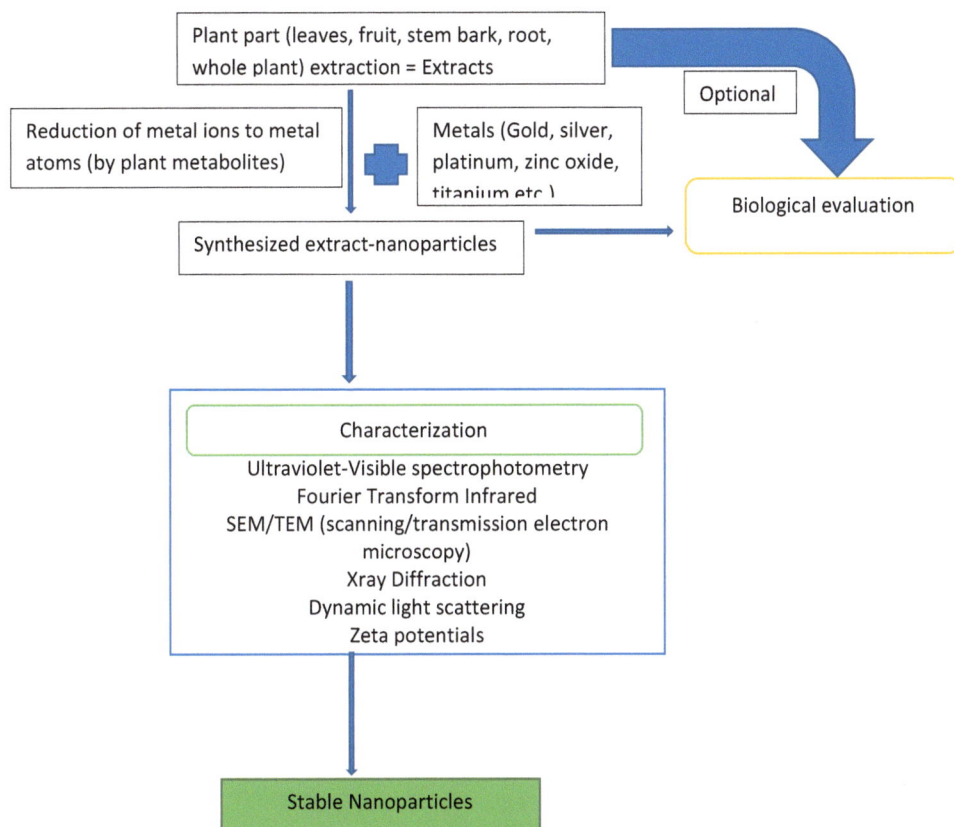

**Fig. (1).** Pictorial or stepwise procedure for green synthesized nanoparticles.

Diabetes prevalence continues to multiply as the global population increases [33]. Aside the fact that it manifested into a number of complications and or other diseases, including damage to the eyes (retinopathy), kidney (nephropathy), ulcer (foot), heart ailment *etc.*, it is mostly observed in the working population (age 20-69), particularly those from low and middle income countries. According to International Diabetic Federation [33], about 463 million people globally are living with the disease and a projected 700 million increase translating to 9.9% by 2045 has been reported as against 4.4% in 2014 [34].

The hallmark of diabetes therapy is to control the glucose level. The treatment option could be pharmacological and non-pharmacological despite the fact that it requires huge financial implications. The latter therapy option involves diet modification (eating less carbohydrates and more proteinous foods as well as consuming a diet rich in fibres, *etc.*) and increased physical exercise (to prevent overweight). The former involves the use of conventional drugs, *i.e.*, oral hypoglycaemic agents (OHAs), such as insulin, biguanides, sulphonyureas, acarbose *etc.* (Table **1**). However, these orthodox drugs come with various side effects such as obesity and gastrointestinal disturbances (*e.g.*, bloating, diarrhea *etc.*), hence, the need for an alternative form of therapy from nature (medicinal plants) with the ability to control diabetes with little or no side effects. In fact, medicinal plants, as compared with synthetic counterparts, tend to show comparative or better potential in the management of diabetes (and other diseased conditions), as determined through a number of assays, *i.e.*, *in vitro* (*via* alpha-amylase inhibition, alpha-glucosidase inhibition, glucose uptake determination *etc.*) and *in vivo* (through the evaluation of glucose level, glycogen content, oral glucose tolerance, hexokinase, glucose-6-phophatase, fructose 1,6-biphosphatase, glycogen phosphorylase, haemoglobin level and glycosylated haemoglobin level, lipid profiles, *etc.*) assays following streptozotocin or alloxan induction of experimental animals [35].

**Table 1. Classes of antidiabetic drugs and mechanism of antidiabetic action.**

| S/N | Class | Example(s) | Side Effects | Mechanism of Action | Reference(s) |
|---|---|---|---|---|---|
| 1 | Suphonyl ureas | Glibenclamide, gliclazide | Not suitable during pregnancy, GIT troubles *etc.* | Facilitate the secretion of insulin | [53] |
| 2 | Biguanides | Metformin | GIT disturbances, reduces plasma level of Vit. $B_{12}$ and folic acid *etc.* | Increases (hepatic) glucose uptake (into cells) | [53] |
| 3 | Thiazolidinediones | Rosiglitazone | Headache, dizziness, GIT troubles, oodema, eight gain *etc.* | Enhances the sensitivity of body cells to insulin | [53] |
| 4 | Dipeptidyl peptidase (DPP)-4 inhibitor | Gliptin: sitagliptin *etc.* | Headache, infection of the upper respiratory tract *etc.* | Stimulate insulin secretion and suppresses glucagon production | [53] |
| 5 | Sodium glucose cotransporter inhibitor (SGLT)-2 | Glifozin: Dapaglifozin, Canaglifozin | Urinary tract infection, nausea, vomiting | Inhibit glucose reabsorption and facilitate urine excretion | [53] |
| 6 | Meglitinides | Repaglinide | - | Short acting insulin secretagogues with similar action as sulphonyl ureas | [53] |

Alloxan and or streptozotocin are diabetogenic agents mostly used for diabetes evaluation in animal model studies. The latter acts by unwinding or breaking the

DNA strands of the beta cells of the islets in order to induce oxidative damage [36]. It must be noted that preference is given to the use of streptozotocin over alloxan based on the fact that there is the possibility of beta cells' recovery over a short period with the latter. Alpha-amylase is a pancreatic enzyme involved in the persistent carbohydrate breakdown into disaccharides and or oligosaccharide. Alpha-glucosidase is an important enzyme in diabetes management. It is the end stage of starch digestion to glucose and is responsible for the conversion of disaccharides to glucose (monosaccharide). The inhibition of the enzyme during postprandial hyperglycaemia is germane and promotes glucose control in the blood [37]. Hexokinase is a key regulatory and/or sensitive enzyme of the glycolytic (glucose breakdown) pathway whose level or activity would be reduced in diabetic status due to low mRNA synthesis coding for the enzyme and insulin secretion. On the other hand, fructose 1, 6-biphosphatase, is an important enzyme involved in gluconeogenesis (glucose formation). The enzyme's activity is enhanced as a result of excessive glucose production arising from triggered activation of the enzyme. It is important to mention the significance of glycolysis and gluconeogenesis (as complimentary episodes) in ensuring glucose balance in the liver (major site of metabolism) of the body.

The world is endowed with avalanches of plant species (more than 85 000) with medicinal properties [38]. The use of medicinal plants for disease control is an age long tradition. Interestingly, their usage, particularly against diabetes (and other ailments such as hypertension, cancer and so on), has been promoted by the leading health institution, World Health Organization [35, 39 - 41], based on their availability, little or no side effects, cost effectiveness, among others. It is worthy to mention that over 800 medicinal plants are available for ethnobotanical use and the evaluation of therapeutic potentials (pharmacological) for a number of them, such as *Dicomala anomala, Gazania krebsiana, Artemisia afra, Lessertia montana, Aloe vera, Moringa oleifera, Elephantina elephantorrhiza, Allium sativum, Casia fistulaetc.*, on diabetes reported in a number of reports [35, 38, 40, 42 - 45], is attributed to the various embedded phytoconstituents (flavonoids, phenolics, alkaloids *etc.*) and or compounds, which control the glucose level, protects against its complications, and thus provides an overall general healthy being. In fact, more than 80% of the global populace uses medicinal plants in one form or the other (as traditional medicine).

As indicated above, the use of medicinal plants in the synthesis of nanoparticles is a laudable alternative and, in particular, diabetes management, partly attributed to poor solubility and low bioavailability of lipid-containing plant extracts [46]. In order to overcome these step-backs, nano-delivery may come handy in delivering these products to the side of action, aside from the fact that it (phytonanoparticle) is simple (to develop), economical, and ecofriendly. Nanostructures including gold, silver, copper, platinum, and titanium synthesized from various parts (leaves, bark, fruits, flower, seeds, tubers, whole plant) of various medicinal plants have been established with a number of pharmacological effects such as antihyperglycaemic [4, 46]. Interestingly, a literature search revealed more than fifty-eight of these plants (at the time of compiling the report) employed in the synthesis of metallic and metallic oxides nanoparticles (Table **2**) embraced as potential antidiabetic agents, though fifteen of them are for the first time compiled or reported in this chapter (Table **3**).

**Table 2. Reported characteristic features of green-synthesized nanoparticles with established antidiabetic potential.**

| | Plant Name / Family | Part(s) or Substance Used | Nanoparticles | Medium of Synthesis | Characterization Techniques Used | Functional Groups Involved in Stabilization (Bands or Peaks in $cm^{-1}$) | Phytochemicals Responsible for Possible Capping and or Reduction | NPs Morphology/ Nature | Region/ Country of the Study | References |
|---|---|---|---|---|---|---|---|---|---|---|
| 1 | *Aegle marmelos* (L.) Corr. Rutaceae | Leaf | Silver | Aqueous | UV-Vis, SEM, AFS, TEM, SAED | NI | NI | NI | India | [54] |
| 2 | *Aloe vera* Liliaceae | Leaf | Silver | Aqueous | UV-Vis | NI | NI | NI | Chennai, India | [55] |
| 3 | *Ananas cosmos* (L.) Merr. Bromeliaceae | Fruit (Peel) | Silver | Aqueous | UV-Vis, SEM, EDS, FTIR, XRD | O-H stretching (3295.01), N-H (1634.03), C-O (1059.01), C-H (683.83) | Proteins, flavonoids, phenolics | Crystalline | Republic of Korea | [56] |
| 4 | *Andrographis paniculata* Acanthaceae | Leaf | Zinc oxide | Aqueous | UV–Vis, XRD, FTIR, SEM, TEM and SAED | O-H (peak at 3441), C-H (bands at 3002 and 2850), amide I and amide II regions (1731, 1601), C-N, C-O (1404, 1274 etc.) | Proteins, polyphenols, alkaloids, carboxylic acid, flavonoids | Crystalline | India | [29] |
| 5 | *Argyreia nervosa* (Burm. f.)** Convolvulaceae | Leaf | Silver | Aqueous | UV, HRTEM, SAED | Peaks at 3300-3490 due to O-H stretching, N-H (2390), C=O (1925, 1646), C-OH (1056) | NI | Crystalline | India | [57] |
| 6 | *Azadirachta indica* A. Juss.* Meliaceae | Leaf Leaf | Zinc oxide **Silver** | Aqueous Aqueous | UV-Vis, TEM, SEM, XRD, FTIR, SAED UV-Vis | O-H stretching (3413–3475), H-O-H (1509–1577), C-H (2920–2936), C-C (1414–1454) and Zn-O (454–481) NI | Carbohydrates, flavonoids, glycosides, phenolic compounds, saponins, tanins NI | Crystalline NI | Chennai, India India | [58] [55] |
| 7 | *Bauhinia variegata** Fabaceae | Flower | Silver | Aqueous | UV-Vis, FTIR, Zeta potential | O-H (3318) due to phenols, while other peaks are represented as 2921 (C-H), 1627 (N-H), 1508 (benzene), 1415 (C-H), 1376 (C-N) and 1046 (S=O) | Phenols, flavonoids, benzophenones, nitro compounds, aromatics and aliphatic amines | Crystalline | Tamil Nadu, India | [59] |
| 8 | *Calophyllum tomentosum** Callophyllaceae | Leaf | Silver | Aqueous | UV, FTIR, XRD, EDX, SEM | O-H (3401), N-H (2916), C-H (2844), C-O (1618), C-H (1381) while 1042 is due reported to be to aromatic group | Flavonoids, tannins, alkaloids, glycosides, phenols, terpenoids | Crystalline | Karnataka | [60] |

*(Table 2) cont.....*

| | Plant Name / Family | Part(s) or Substance Used | Nanoparticles | Medium of Synthesis | Characterization Techniques Used | Functional Groups Involved in Stabilization (Bands or Peaks in cm$^{-1}$) | Phytochemicals Responsible for Possible Capping and or Reduction | NPs Morphology/ Nature | Region/ Country of the Study | References |
|---|---|---|---|---|---|---|---|---|---|---|
| 9 | *Cassia auriculata** Caesalpiniaceae | Leaf | Gold | Aqueous | XRD, TEM, SEM-EDAX, FT-IR | O-H (3635), C-N stretching (1387), while peaks at 2884, 1600,1507,1074 and 1335 were unidentified | NI | Crystalline | India | [61] |
| 10 | *Cassia fistula* L. Leguminoceae | Stem bark | Gold | Aqueous | UV, FTIR SEM | O-H (3430.49), N-H (1627.15, N-O (1517.72), C-C (1455.61), C-H (2850–3000), C-N (1248.11 and 1113.35) | NI | NR | India | [62] |
| 11 | *Chamaecostus cuspidatus* (Nees &Mart.) C.D.Specht & D.W.Stev.* Costaceae | Leaf | Gold | Aqueous | UV, SEM, XRD, TGA, TEM | NI | NI | Crystalline | India | [63] |
| 12 | *Costus pictus* (D.) Don Costaceae | Leaf | Silver | Methanol | UV-Vis, SEM, zeta potential, polydispersity index, | NI | NI | NI | India | [64] |
| 13 | *Couroupita guianensis** Lecythidaceae | Leaf | Gold | Aqueous | DLS, Zeta potential, TEM, FTIR | O-H stretching (3290.56), C-H stretching and bending of alkanes (2927.94 and 1366.60), C-N (1282.66, 110.36 and 1205.51) stretching of aliphatic and aromatic amines | Polyphenols | Crystalline | India | [65] |
| 14 | *Cucuma longa* Zingiberaceae | Leaf | Silver | Aqueous | UV-Vis, SEM, EDAX, AFM, XRD, FTIR, DLS, Zeta potential | NI | NI | Crystalline | India | [66] |
| 15 | *Cymbopogon citratus* Poaceae | Leaf | Silver | Aqueous | UV-Vis, SEM, EDAX, AFM, XRD, FTIR, TEM | O-H stretching (peaks at 3312, 2920), C-H (2849), C=O (1705), C=C stretching (1603, 1333) of unsaturated ketone, | Phenol, ketones | Crystalline | India | [67] |
| 16 | *Dicoma anomala* (Sond.) Asteraceae | Root | Zinc oxide | Aqueous | UV-Vis, FTIR, EDS-SEM, XRD | O-H stretching (3799, 3528 and 3370), N-H stretching (2970), O=C=O (2328) while N=C=S stretching was 2087 | Alkaloids, flavonoids, tannins | Crystalline | South Africa | [50] |
| 17 | *Dioscorea bulbifera** Discoreaceae | Tuber | Copper | Aqueous | UV, TEM, EDS, DLS, XRD | NR | NR | Crystalline | India | [68] |
| 18 | *Equisetum arvense* Equisetaceae | Whole | Silver | Aqueous | UV-Vis, SEM, XRD, FTIR, Zeta potential | Peaks at 3302.55, 2120.45, 1632.15, 1064.6 and 685.71 are assigned to O-H stretch, H- bonds (alcohols, phenols), nitriles,–C=C–stretch (alkenes), C-O stretch (alcohols, carboxylic acids, esters, ethers), and CeBr stretch (alkyl halides) | flavonoids, terpenoids, and coumarins etc | Crystalline | Korea | [69] |

(Table 2) cont.....

| | Plant Name / Family | Part(s) or Substance Used | Nanoparticles | Medium of Synthesis | Characterization Techniques Used | Functional Groups Involved in Stabilization (Bands or Peaks in cm$^{-1}$) | Phytochemicals Responsible for Possible Capping and or Reduction | NPs Morphology/ Nature | Region/ Country of the Study | References |
|---|---|---|---|---|---|---|---|---|---|---|
| 19 | *Eysenhardtia polystachya* (Sarg.)[#] Leguminoceae | Bark | Silver | Aqueous | UV-Vis, TEM, FTIR, Zeta potential | O-H (3,456) due to phenols, C-H (2,816 and 2,844) due to alkanes, C-C (1,512) due to aromatic compounds, C=C (1,493) due to aromatic rings and C-H (1,436) bending. Peaks at 1,741, 1,071, 803, and 566 are due to C-H groups while C-O (1,248 and 1,042) due aryl alkyl esters. | Chalcones, dihydrochalcones, and flavonoids Arylnaphthalenes | NI | Mexico | [70] |
| 20 | *Ficus glomerata*[*] Moraceae | Gum | Silver | Aqueous | UV-Vis, SEM | IAI | IAI | IAI | IAI | [71] |
| 21 | *Gracilaria edulis*[*] Gracilariaceae | Leaf | Silver | Aqueous | UV-Vis, SEM, FTIR, XRD and EDX | C-O, H-Bonded (3418), C-H (2852, 2922), N-H (1650), N-O asymmetric bending (1539), C-C (1417), C-N stretching (1239, 1035), C-H (875) | NI | NI | India | [72] |
| 22 | *Gymnema sylvestre* (Retz.) R. Br. ex Sm.*[*] Asclepiadaceae | Leaf Whole plant | Gold, silver Starch | Aqueous Methanol | UV, HRTEM SEM, TEM, XRD, EDAX GCMS, FTIR, SEM, PSA, EDS, XRD | NI O-H stretching of amylopectin (band at 3348), asymmetric stretching of C-H (bands at 2938 and 2887), C-H (bands at 1421and 1348), C-O alcohol bond (1015), N-C=O (2260), NH bonds(1600 and 3400), C=O (1726) | NI alkaloids, flavonoids, saponins, proteins, Amylose, amylopectin | Crystalline Amorphous | India Namakkal, India | [73, 74] |
| 23 | *Halymenia poryphyroides*[*] Halymeniaceae | NI | Silver | Aqueous | UV-Nano, SEM, FTIR, XRD | O-H stretching (3662.45, 3703.80, 3690.50, 3884.34), free OH (3632.45), N-H (3393.63), =C-H (3276.53), H-NH (3183.09) | NI | Crystalline | India | [75] |
| 24 | *Heritiera fomes*[*] Malvaceae | Bark and Leaf | Zinc oxide and silver | Aqueous | UV, DLS, FTIR, PCS | C=O (1604.66), N-H bending (1512.52), C-N bending of amide II (1243.86), N-H bending of amide III (3597.54) | Oxime | Dispersed | India | [76] |
| 25 | *Hibiscus rosa-sinensi* L. Malvaceae | Leaf | Zinc oxide | Aqueous | UV-Vis, TEM, SEM, XRD, FTIR, SAED | O-H stretching (3413–3475), H-O-H (1509–1577), C-H (2920–2936), C-C (1414–1454) and Zn-O (454–481) | Carbohydrates, flavonoids, glycosides, phenolic compounds, saponins, tanins | Crystalline | Chennai, India | [58] |
| 26 | *Hibiscus subdariffa* L. calyx Malvaceae | Leaf | Zinc oxide | Aqueous | UV, FTIR, FESEM, HRTEM, XRD | O-H stretching of water (3441, 3478, 3450), C=C (1381), aromatic C-H (2289), C=C-C (1474), -C-OH (1102), NH2 (1629), -C=O (1422), C-O-C (1565) | Proteins, alkaloids, phenols, flavonoids | Amorphous | India | [77] |

*(Table 2) cont.....*

| | Plant Name / Family | Part(s) or Substance Used | Nanoparticles | Medium of Synthesis | Characterization Techniques Used | Functional Groups Involved in Stabilization (Bands or Peaks in $cm^{-1}$) | Phytochemicals Responsible for Possible Capping and or Reduction | NPs Morphology/ Nature | Region/ Country of the Study | References |
|---|---|---|---|---|---|---|---|---|---|---|
| 27 | *Ipomoea batatas* (L.) Lam Convolvulaceae | Tuber (peel) (Two varieties; Ib1 and Ib2) | Zinc oxide | Aqueous | UV-Vis, SEM-EDX, XRD, FTIR | Peaks at 3285.56 (Ib1) and 3275.54 (Ib2) due to O-H and H-bonded stretching. Peaks at 1620.66 (Ib1) and 1630.42 (Ib2) correspond to N-H due to amines while peaks at 1017.54 (Ib1) and 1018.51 (Ib2) is due to C-O stretching | Proteins, flavonoids | Crystalline | Korea | [56] |
| 28 | *Leucosidea sericea* Rosaceae | Leaf | Gold | Aqueous | UV-Vis, HRTEM, EDS, XRD, DLS | NI | Polyphenols | Poly(crystalline) | South Africa | [78] |
| 29 | *Lessertia montana* Fabaceae | Leaf | Zinc oxide | Aqueous | UV, FTIR, SEM-EDS, XRD | O-H bond (3365), C-H (2945), C-C (1412) CO-O-CO (1046), N-H (1596) and C=C (699) | alkaloids, flavonoids, phenolics, tannins, triterpenes, phytosterols, and cardiac 30glycosides | Crystalline | South Africa | [51] |
| 30 | *Lonicera japonica** Caprifoliacia | Leaf | silver | Aqueous | UV, TEM, FTIR DLS, zeta potentials | C-O stretching (1385), C-N stretching (1263), N=H (1458), C-H (2920), O-H stretching (3400) | NI3 | Crystalline | China | [16] |
| 31 | *Moricandia nitens* (Viv.)* Brassicaceae | Aerial part | Gold | Aqueous | UV, FTIR, TEM, XRD | O-H (3406.4), C-H (2922.3, 2852.0) and C=O (1738.5) | NI | Crystalline | Ageba area, Egypt | [79] |
| 32 | *Moringa oleifera* Lam." Moringaceae | Leaf | Zinc oxide | Aqueous | UV-Vis, TEM, SEM, XRD, FTIR, SAED | O-H stretching (3413–3475), H-O-H (1509–1577), C-H (2920–2936), C-C (1414–1454), N-H (1630, 1641) and Zn-O (454–481) | Carbohydrates, flavonoids, glycosides, phenolic compounds, saponins, tannins, amino acids, proteins | Crystalline | Chennai, India | [58] |
| 33 | *Morus alba"* Moraceae | Leaf | Gold | Aqueous | HR-TEM, UV–Vis, XRD and FT-IR. EDS, XRD and TEM | 1640, 2086, 3452 and 638 attributed to C-C bond, O-H stretch and C-H stretchings | NI | Crystalline | China | [80] |
| 34 | *Murraya Koenigii* L. Rutaceae | Leaf | Zinc oxide | Aqueous | UV-Vis, TEM, SEM, XRD, FTIR, SAED | O-H stretching (3413–3475), H-O-H (1509–1577), C-H (2920–2936), C-C (1414–1454) and Zn-O (454–481) | Carbohydrates, flavonoids, glycosides, phenolic compounds, saponins, tanins | Crystalline | Chennai, India | [58] |
| 35 | *Musa paradisiaca* (L.)" Musaceae | Stem | Silver | Aqueous | UV-Vis, TEM, SEM, XRD, FTIR | Peaks are at 464.74, 675.61, 797.07, 1059.42, 1402.58 (N-H), 1639.69 (C=O), 2115.61 and 3445.75 (N-H) | Proteins | Crystalline | India | [81] |
| 36 | *Nasturtium officinale"* Brassicaceae | Leaf | Zinc oxide | Aqueous | SEM, TEM, XRD, EDX, BET, FTIR, TGA, and UV-Vis DRS | Cyanide, azide (2100 to 2300), C=C (1652), O-H (3400) | NI | Crystalline | Iran | [82] |
| 37 | *Ocimum basilicum** Lamiaceae | Leaf | Silver | Aqueous | UV, DLS, Zeta potentials, SEM, EDX, FTIR | OH stretching (3300.21, 3297.12), C=O (1634.78, 1635.37) | Proteins, phenolic compounds | NI | South Africa | [83] |
| 38 | *Ocimum sanctum* (L.)* Lamiaceae | Leaf | Silver | Aqueous | UV, DLS, Zeta potentials, SEM, EDX, FTIR | OH stretching (3300.21, 3297.12) | Proteins, phenolic compounds | NI | South Africa | [83] |

*(Table 2) cont.....*

| | Plant Name / Family | Part(s) or Substance Used | Nanoparticles | Medium of Synthesis | Characterization Techniques Used | Functional Groups Involved in Stabilization (Bands or Peaks in cm⁻¹) | Phytochemicals Responsible for Possible Capping and or Reduction | NPs Morphology/ Nature | Region/ Country of the Study | References |
|---|---|---|---|---|---|---|---|---|---|---|
| 39 | *Olea europeae** Oleaceae | Leaf | Gold | Aqueous | UV-Vis, AFM, TEM, SEM, XRD, AFM | NR | NR | Crystalline | Baghdad | [84] |
| 40 | *Pouteria sapota* (Jacq.) Sapotaceae | Leaf | Silver | Aqueous | SEM, XRD | NR | NR | Crystalline | India | [85] |
| 41 | *Punica granatum*# Punicaceae | Leaf | Silver | Aqueous | UV-Vis, FESEM, HRTEM, Zeta potential, FTIR, XPS | Peaks at 3400 (O-H) and 3384 (C=O) due to phenols. Peaks at 2940 and 2933 due to C-H stretching while 1640 and 1632 are due to –C-C-. The peaks at 1070 and 1058 are assigned to C–OH stretching | Flavonoids, aromatic acids | Crystalline | Korea, Vietnam | [86] |
| 42 | *Pterocarpus marsupium* Roxb* Leguminoseae | Bark, wood | Silver | Aqueous | UV, FTIR, Zeta potential, SEM | Peaks (at 3618) due to OH stretching, C-H stretching (2789.53) due to aldehyde, C=O stretching (1771.53) due to carboxylic acids, 1541 to nitrogenous compounds | Carboxyl and hydroxyl groups, phenols | NI | Chennai, India | [87] |
| 43 | *Sambucus nigra* (L.)* Caprifoliaceae | Fruit | Gold | Aqueous | UV, TEM, zeta potentials | NR | NR | NR | Cluj-Napoca, Romania | [88] |
| 44 | *Saraca asoca** Leguminoceae | Leaf | Gold | Aqueous | UV, SEM, TEM, FTIR, XRD | C–H (3400), –C=O (2927), –C–H/C–O–H (1612), –C–O and –C–O–C- (1400) | NI | Crystalline | India | [89] |
| 45 | *Sargassum swartzii** Sargassaceae | NI (Seaweeds) | Gold | Aqueous | UV, HRTEM, FTIR, XRD | NR | NR | NR | India | [90] |
| 46 | *Silybum marianum* (L.)# Asteracecae | Seed | Zinc oxide | Aqueous | UV, SEM, TEM, XRD, EDS, FTIR, HRTEM, BET | O-H stretching (3400 and 1650) of water molecules, C=C (1376) and Zn-O (570). | NR | Crystalline | Iran | [91] |
| 47 | *Smilax glabra*# Smilacaceae | Rhizome | Gold | Aqueous | UV, SEM, TEM, XRD, EDS, FTIR | O-H stretching (3465), C-H (2719), C-O (1723), S (1457), C-N (1298) | Carbohydrates, amino acids, lipids, proteins | Crystalline | China | [92] |
| 48 | *Sonneratia apetala** Lythraceae | Bark and Leaf | Zinc oxide and silver | Aqueous | UV, DLS, FTIR, PCS | C=O stretching (1606.36), C-N and NH (1515.26), C-H (1515.26) | NI | Dispersed | Odisha coast, India | [76] |
| 50 | *Syringodium isoetifolium** Cymodoceaceae | Leaf | Silver | Aqueous | UV-Vis, SEM, FTIR, XRD and EDX | O-H (3418), C-H (2922), C-C (1600), C-N (1092), C-Br (597) | NI | NI | India | [72] |
| 51 | *Syzygium cumini* (Lam.) Skeels# Myrtaceae | Seeds | Silver | Methanol | UV, SEM, XRD, FTIR, Zeta potential | Peaks at 1700 for COOH, 1090 for C–O stretch of alcohols, 3737 and 3658 (free O-H) | Polyphenols | Crystalline | India | [93] |
| 52 | *Tamarindus indica* L.# Fabaceae | Leaf | Zinc oxide | Aqueous | UV-Vis, TEM, SEM, XRD, FTIR, SAED | O-H stretching (3413–3475), H-O-H (1509–1577), C-H (2920–2936), C-C (1414–1454), N-H (1630, 1641) and Zn-O (454–481) | Carbohydrates, flavonoids, glycosides, phenolic compounds, saponins, tanins, proteins, amino acids | Crystalline | Chennai, India | [58] |

*(Table 2) cont.....*

| | Plant Name / Family | Part(s) or Substance Used | Nanoparticles | Medium of Synthesis | Characterization Techniques Used | Functional Groups Involved in Stabilization (Bands or Peaks in cm⁻¹) | Phytochemicals Responsible for Possible Capping and or Reduction | NPs Morphology/ Nature | Region/ Country of the Study | References |
|---|---|---|---|---|---|---|---|---|---|---|
| 53 | *Tephrosia tinctoria**<br>Fabaceae | Leaf | Silver | Aqueous | UV, SEM, TEM, EDAX,, FTIR, XRD | O-H (3442), carboxylic (2923), alkyne (2141) and ether (1019) | Phenols, flavonoids, | Crystalline | India | [94] |
| 54 | *Trigonella foenum graecum* (L.)* Fabaceae | Seed | Silver, Gold | Aqueous | UV, SEM, TEM, EDAX, EDS | NI | Flavonoids, polyphenols, proteins | NI | Saudi Arabia | [95] |
| 55 | *Urtica dioica*<br>Urticaceae | Leaf | Zinc oxide | Aqueous | SEM, TEM, XRD, UV-Vis DRS, TGA, FTIR, BET, GCMS | C-O stretching (3000), Zn-O (555), C-H (2900), C=C (1650) and C=O (1250) | NI | Crystalline | Ardabil, Iran | [96] |
| 56 | *Vaccinium arctostaphylos* (L.)*<br>Ericaceae | Fruits | Zinc oxide | Ethanol (96%) | XRD, SEM, TEM, EDX, FT-IR, UV-vis DRS and TGA | Bond of O-H (3400) stretching of water molecules, C-H stretching (2930 and 2855), C-O (1250) C=C (1620), C=O (1735) and Zn-O stretching (570) | Anthocyanins, flavonoids, polyphenols and vitamins | Crystalline | Ardabil, Iran | [97] |
| 57 | *Withania somnifera**<br>Solanaceae | Leaf | Platinum | Aqueous | UV, TEM, XRD, Zeta potentials | Peaks at 3418, 1611, 1406, 1065, 629 are attributed to C=O, C-H and N-H functional groups of aliphatic, carbonyl amines and terpenoids | Terpenoids | Crystalline | China | [98] |
| 58 | *Zingiber officinale*<br>Zingiberaceae | Rhizome | Silver | Aqueous | AFM, XRD, FTIR | NO₃ (1384), O-H (2923) due to carboxylic acids, O-H stretching of H-bonded (3419) alcohols and phenols, N-H (1648), C-N (1163) | Alkaloids, flavonoids, phenols | Crystalline | India | [99] |

EDAX: Energy dispersion analysis of X-ray; AFM: Atomic force microscopy; XRD: X-ray diffractometer; TEM: Transmission electron microscopy; FTIR: Fourier transform infrared spectroscopy; SEM: Scanning electron microscopy; HRTEM: High Resolution Transmission Electron Microscopy; XPS: X-ray photoelectron spectroscopy; PCS: Photon correlation spectroscopy; TGA: Thermogravimetric analysis; UV–vis DRS: Ultraviolet–visible diffuse reflectance spectroscopy; GCMS: Gas chromatography-mass spectrometry; EDAX: Energy dispersive analysis of X-ray; SAED: Selected area electron diffraction; EDS: Energy dispersive spectroscopy; FESEM: Field emission scanning electron microscope; BET: Brunauer-Emmett-Teller

NI: Not indicated; NR: Not reported; IAI: Inability to Access Information
*#Reported in the work of Ashwini and Mahalinga [4] and Nouri *et al.* [46] respectively as green synthesized nanoparticles of antidiabetic importance

## Safety Concerns

The toxicity of a substance is germane, particularly when the synthesized molecules have to do with the safety of an individual (when ingested or exposed through the skin) and the environment. Hence, studying the impact of toxicity of nanoparticles in the organisms must therefore be fully elucidated, it is until this is achieved that efforts on clinical trials or application can be given a thought. Nano-based particles or substances are prone or much more likely to be toxic based on some metrics such as their reduced (nanometer) size, chemical reactivity, concentration, morphology, *etc.*, when compared to bulkier materials [47, 48] even at low levels. Interestingly, nanoparticles synthesized by physical and chemical means tend to elicit more toxic effect, attributed to the chemicals (organic solvent, biodegradable stabilizing and/or reducing agents *etc.*) involved in the synthesis methods. These responses are sometimes dependent on solubility and binding capability. It is worthy of mention that quite a number of them, when passed through different protective routes of the body, may accumulate at the potential site of action, thus causing dilapidating effects on the organs and body entirely. Hence, modifying the synthesis procedure or finding an alternative precursor or biocompatible stabilizing agent that could go a long way in averting the toxicity would be commendable. However, reports on the toxicity of nanoparticles associated with biological methods, particularly plants, are sometimes few or rather rare [48], most especially if ingested at low concentration. The reason for the likely non-toxic nature of the green method or plant-synthesized nanostructures may be associated with compounds or functional groups inherent in the precursor (plant), which reduces the metal ions and, in the process, stabilize the NPs [49]. Although, it must be noted that despite numerous studies determining the pharmacological impact of NPs, very few studies evaluated the toxic effect of the synthesized NPs (Table **4**), and without the toxicity evaluation, it would be difficult to give a general or plain assertion on the safety implication of green synthesized nanoparticles.

**Table 3. Updated list of green-synthesized nanoparticles with antidiabetic activity.**

| S/N | Plant Name | NPs Precursor | Assay & Concentrations Used | Particle Size: SEM (nm) | Shape | Antidiabetic Activity | Reference |
|---|---|---|---|---|---|---|---|
| 1 | *Aegle marmelos* | Ag | *In vitro* (25, 50, 75, 100, 125 µg/mL) | 20-60 | Spherical, irregular | Good α-amylase inhibition | [54] |
| 2 | *Aloe vera* | Ag | *In vitro* (50, 100, 150 µL) | NI | NI | Good α-amylase inhibition | [55] |
| 3 | *Ananas cosmos* | Ag | *In vitro* (10 µg/mL) | NI | Spherical | α-glucosidase is 100% inhibited | [56] |
| 4 | *Andrographis paniculata* | ZnO | *In vitro* | 96-115, 57 | Spherical, hexagonal | Excellent α-amylase inhibition with $IC_{50}$ value of 121.42 µg/mL | [29] |
| 5 | *Azadirachta indica* | Ag | *In vitro* (50, 100, 150 µL) | NI | NI | Good α-amylase inhibition | [55] |
| 6 | *Costus pictus* | Ag | ND | 100 | Spherical | ND | [64] |

(Table 3) cont.....

| S/N | Plant Name | NPs Precursor | Assay & Concentrations Used | Particle Size: SEM (nm) | Shape | Antidiabetic Activity | Reference |
|-----|-----------|---------------|-----------------------------|-------------------------|-------|----------------------|-----------|
| 7 | *Cucuma longa* | Ag | *In vitro* (20–100 µg/mL) | 90-111 nm | Spherical | Considerable α-amylase inhibition | [66] |
| 8 | *Cymbopogon citratus* | Ag | *In vitro* (20, 40, 60, 80, 100 µL) | 65.74 | Spherical, irregular | α-amylase, glucose diffusion retardation | [67] |
| 9 | *Dicoma anomala* | ZnO | *In vitro* (0.062-1.000 mg/mL) | 168.79 – 479.47 | Spherical, cubical | Excellent α-amylase inhibition with $IC_{50}$ value of 104.34 µg/mL while alpha-glucosidase was moderately inhibited. Kinetics of both enzymes were non-competitive | [50] |
| 10 | *Equisetum arvense* | Ag | *In vitro* | NI | Spherical | Showed a promising antidiabetic effect with $IC_{50}$ value of 1.73 microgram/mL against alpha-glucosidase | [69] |
| 11 | *Hibiscus rosa-sinensi* | ZnO | *In vitro* (1.52-100 µg/mL) | 25 - 32 | Spherical, hexagonal | Resulted in delayed carbohydrate ingestion with the inhibition of alpha-amylase and alpha-glucosidase above 80% | [58] |
| 12 | *Ipomoea batatas* (Two varieties; Ib1 and Ib2) | Ag | *In vitro* (10 µg/mL) | NI | NI | α-glucosidase is 97.73% and 64.81% inhibited at 1 µg/mL for Ib1 and Ib2 respectively | [56] |
| 13 | *Leucosidea sericea* | Au | *In vitro* | 21-27 | Spherical | Demonstrated high alpha-glucosidase and amylase inhibitory activities | [78] |

| S/N | Plant Name | NPs Precursor | Assay & Concentrations Used | Particle Size: SEM (nm) | Shape | Antidiabetic Activity | Reference |
|---|---|---|---|---|---|---|---|
| 14 | *Lessertia montana* | ZnO | *In vitro* (0.062-1.000 mg/mL) | 154.78 - 521.47 | Spherical, cubical | Excellent α-glucosidase inhibition with $IC_{50}$ value 37 μg/mL while alpha-amylase was moderately inhibited. Kinetics of alpha-amylase was competitive while alpha-glucosidase was non-competitive | [51] |
| 15 | *Urtica dioica* | ZnO | In *vivo* (200, 250 mg/kg body weight) | Average crystallite size of 19, 20 | Spherical | Reduces blood glucose (FBS) level in alloxan-induced diabetic rats. Insulin levels was improved and comparable to control | [96] |
| 16 | *Sphaeranthus amaranthoides* | Ag | *In vitro* | NI | NI | A dose-response inhibitory activity on α-amylase and an $IC_{50}$ result significantly lower than acarbose | [100] |

ND: Not determined; NI: not indicated; NPs: Nanoparticles

**Table 4. Reported mechanism of actions and potential toxicity and/ or safety of green-synthesized antihyperglycemic nanoparticles.**

| S/N | Plant Name | NP Type | Mechanism of Action | Toxicity | References |
|---|---|---|---|---|---|
| 1 | *Ananas comosus* | Ag | Carboxyl, ketones, aldehydes, and carboxyl groups reduces silver ion to $Ag^0$ in the conversion of the extract to AgNPs | Cytotoxic evaluation of the NPs through HepG2 cancer cell lines revealed the inhibition of cell growth particularly at lower concentration indicating cytotoxic potential | [56] |

*(Table 4) cont.....*

| S/N | Plant Name | NP Type | Mechanism of Action | Toxicity | References |
|---|---|---|---|---|---|
| 2 | *Andrographis paniculata* | ZnO | Free amino and carboxylic groups responsible for the conversion of metal ions to ZnONPs | - | [29] |
| 3 | *Cassia auriculata* | Au | Polysaccharides and flavoniods was assumed to have influenced the formation of gold nanoparticles and the antidiabetic potential while carbonyl groups from amino acid residues and peptides of proteins acting as encapsulating agent thus prevent the agglomeration of NPs | - | [61] |
| 4 | *Chamaecostus Cuspidatus* | Au | - | Non-toxic accompanied with protective action of organs when an higher dose of 1.5 mg/kg b.w. was orally administered for 10 days in a toxicity testing according to OECD guidelines–423 showed no mortality nor symptoms such as fatigue, weight loss *etc.* was witnessed. Blood chemistry examination and histologic analysis were also conducted. | [63] |
| 5 | *Couroupita guianensis* | Au | - | Restoration of the hepatocytes indicating potential amelioration of the liver cells in streptozotocin induced diabetic female rats | [101] |
| 6 | *Deverra tortuosa* | - | - | Cytotoxic potential investigated against two cancer cell lines (human colon adenocarcinoma "Caco-2" and human lung adenocarcinoma "A549".in an MTT assay and this revealed appreciable lower cytotoxic activity | [10] |
| 7 | *Dicoma anomala* | ZnO | $Zn^{2+}$ reacted with the functional groups like amide nitrile which resulted in the reduction of the $Zn^{2+}$ to ZnO | - | [50] |

*(Table 4) cont.....*

| S/N | Plant Name | NP Type | Mechanism of Action | Toxicity | References |
|-----|-----------|---------|--------------------|----------|-----------|
| 8 | *Discorea bulifera* | Cu | Probable role of amines, alcohols, ketones, aldehydes, and carboxylic acids in reduction of copper ions and stabilization of synthesized CuNPs | - | [68] |
| 9 | *Equisetum arvense* | Ag | - | Revealed a reduction in cell viability with increasing AgNPs concentration when assessed through HepG2 cancer cells | [69] |
| 10 | *Eysenhardtia polystachya* | Ag | Arylnaphthalenes responsible for the reduction of Ag metals | - | [70] |
| 11 | *Heritiera fomes* and *Sonneratia apetala* | Ag ZnO | Oxime and heterocyclic compound through bio-reduction process convert ZnO and Ag ions to ZnONP and AgNP | - | [76] |
| 12 | *Hibiscus subdariffa* | ZnO | Free amino and carboxylic groups of proteins, alkaloids, phenolics present bind to the surface of zinc ($Zn^{2+}$) and trigger the formation of ZnO NPs. | - | [77] |
| 13 | *Ipomoea batatas* (Two varieties; Ib1 and Ib2) | Ag | - | In the validation of cytotoxic potential against HepG2 cancer cells, it was reported that both species of AgNPs displayed a high level of cytotoxic potential against the cells, but the AgNPs of Ib2 were more active than the Ib1 at low concentrations | [56] |
| 14 | *Lessertia montana* | ZnO | $Zn^{2+}$ in the solution react with the polyphenols (flavonoids, alkaloids, phenols) in the extract resulting in the reduction of the $Zn^{2+}$ to ZnO, which on complexation will form ZnONPs | - | [51] |
| 15 | *Momordica charantia* | Ag | OH phenolic compound is majorly responsible for bioreduction of Ag ions | - | [102] |

*(Table 4) cont.....*

| S/N | Plant Name | NP Type | Mechanism of Action | Toxicity | References |
|---|---|---|---|---|---|
| 16 | *Ocimum sanctum* and *Ocimum basilicum* | Ag | Polyols, amines, phenolics, flavonoids, and water-soluble heterocyclic compounds as well as other factors such as reducing sugars, proteins and other oxido-reductive labile metabolites responsible for the reduction Ag metal ions to Ag° | - | [83] |
| 17 | *Punica granatum* | Ag | Polyphenol, amide, carbonyl and carboxylate groups convert the ionic form of Ag to the metallic nanoform | Cytotoxicity potential was determined by the MTT (3-(4,5-dimethyl thiazol-2yl-2,5-diphenyl tetrazolium bromide) assay using HepG2 cells revealed a dose-dependent response against human liver cancer cells (IC50; 70 µg/mL) indicating its greater efficacy in killing cancer cells | [86] |
| 18 | *Olea europeae* | Au | By insulin-stimulating effect on pancreatic beta cells | - | [84] |
| 19 | *Sambucus nigra* | Au | The involvement in the liver injury of NS in context of diabetes has not been completely elucidated | No observed morphological destruction of the liver cells when indicating acute liver toxicity was infirmed hence, suggesting that a safe dose of 0.3 mg/kg b.w. AuNPS | [88] |
| 20 | *Saraca asoca* | Ag/Au | N–H or O–H are involved in the reduction of Ag and Au ions forming a complexation hydroxylamine and carboxyl groups | - | [89, 103] |
| 21 | *Sargassum swartzii* | Au | The possible mechanism was reported to be attributed to insulin potentiation effect of plasma by AuNPs with enhanced pancreatic insulin secretion of the beta cells | At an administered oral dose levels from 0.5 mg to 5 mg/kg of body weight to rats for 7 days based on OECD guidelines–423 revealed no signs of gross behavioral, neurology, autonomic and general toxic signs or deaths. Hence, considered safe | [90] |
| 22 | *Sphaeranthus amaranthoides* | Ag | Hydroxyl groups of flavonoids/polyphenols mediated reduction of Ag metal ions | - | [100] |

| S/N | Plant Name | NP Type | Mechanism of Action | Toxicity | References |
|-----|------------|---------|---------------------|----------|------------|
| 23 | *Sygyzium cumini* | Ag | carbonyl groups and amines act as reductant to react with silver ions and thus employed as scaffolds to direct the formation of AgNP | - | [93] |
| 24 | *Tephrosia tinctoria* | Au | Hydroxyl/carboxylic groups responsible for the reduction of Au metal ions | - | [94] |
| 25 | *Trigonella foenum Graecum* | Au/Ag | Flavonoids is responsible for the reduction of chloroauric acid while the carboxylate group in proteins can act as surfactant which attach on the surface of Au/Ag NPs and this further stabilizes NPs through electrostatic stabilization. | - | [95] |
| 26 | *Vaccinium arctostaphylus* | ZnO | Hydroxyl groups of phenolic compounds form complexes through chelating with $Zn^{2+}$ ions, forming a p-track conjugation effect | - | [96] |

## Mechanism of Action (MOA)

The MOA of green synthesized NPs, particularly as it relates to antidiabetic activity, has not been fully elucidated, but it is believed that functional (especially amino and carboxylic) groups such as C=O, COOH, C-O, C-O-C *etc.*, in the phytochemicals (including carbohydrates, proteins *etc.*) of the concerned plants are responsible for the reduction of metal ion through two or more chemical processes (reduction, nucleation, complexation *etc.*) leading to the formation of the stable NS [5]. Studies that were submitted suggested that these plants, which can be found in Table **4**, were involved in some way in the synthesis of the particles. To summarize, oxygen produced (from plant extract or atmosphere) react with the metals to form metal oxides in a reduction process, followed by nucleation of the reduced metal ion by activation to form nanoparticles, which the phytochemicals would afterward stabilize.

## MATERIALS AND METHODOLOGY

Extensive literature search was done and obtained through typing keywords like metallic nanoparticles, metal ions, nanostructures, medicinal plants, green synthesis, antidiabetes, antihyperglycaemic, hypoglycaemic, green-synthesized nanoparticles on Google Scholar and scientific databases including PubMed, Medicine, Science direct, JSTOR. One hundred and five informative articles were retrieved and covered between 2000 and 2020. Antidiabetic applications of green-synthesized nanostructures were obtained from 63 peer-reviewed articles, as depicted in Tables **2 - 4**.

## DISCUSSION

Diabetes mellitus is a metabolic disorder whose prevalence has continued to increase with the growing population. Its existence has been attributed to the inability of the beta cells of the pancreas to produce insulin, leading to increased glucose levels in the systemic circulation. The adverse effects accompanying the management of pharmacological diabetes therapy necessitated the need for alternative therapy in nature (plants). World Health Organization, the highest global health body, supported the use of medicinal plants for the cure of diseases (communicable and non-communicable), most especially diabetes mellitus owing to their availability, eco-friendliness, and lesser or no side effects. Additionally, the usage of phytomedicine in different countries and/or continents is growing in popularity and is being accepted more widely than traditional treatments. In fact, typically, more than 80% of Africa, approximately 50% of the Asian populace, particularly China and close to 50-60% of Americans (translating to 158 million) make use of herbal therapy or formulations for disease management and attaining health [38].

Since the physical and chemical methods of forming these NS necessitate the use of expensive and harmful substances that result in the discharge of toxic compounds into the environment, the use of medicinal plants for nanoparticle synthesis is a promising area of research.Notwithstanding the above, research on nanoparticles mediated or aided green plant (Phytonanotherapy) over the bulk extract in disease management in recent times is receiving overwhelming preference [50] due to weak bioavailability and poor solubility of some herbal bioactives (lipophilic) [46]. Hence, a biological approach like the use of plants is germane to subdue or prevent these harmful results attributed to the simplicity of the process, safety, cost effectiveness, stability, ecofriendliness, *etc.*

Phytonanotherapy studies have established that various parts of a plants have the potential to produce nano-sized particles with good pharmacological potentials [27, 28, 50, 51]. These reports are in consonance with revelation from this review where thirty-five of the fifty-eight medicinal plants used leaves in the synthesis of the NPs, indicating a wider preference for the part. The reason for this could partly be attributed to its richness in functional groups (phenols, terpenoids, ketones, amide, carboxylic, *etc.*) and or phytochemicals [26] compared to other parts. Additionally, botanist or (medicinal) plant researchers advocated the use of the leaf or aerial parts for research to promote conservation and/or biodiversity aside from the most used part in traditional medicine in the preparation of formulations. Interestingly, the part tends to produce smaller size-NPs compared to other parts [4]. The medium between precursor and the metal ions during green synthesis was another point of focus as the majority of the studies considered the use of water for preparation or synthesis as established in the review (Table **2**), which was not only due to its use (mostly) in indigenous medicine practice or availability in nature but because of its desirability in nanotechnology [52], though the use of water was sometimes responsible for the agglomeration of some NPs such as ZnO [27, 50, 51].

The use of different metal/ metal ions has been explored in a number of phytonanotherapy research based on reasons or justification for the selection of the concerned metals ranging from availability or ease of purchase to their usefulness or application in scientific fields *etc.* while a number of plants vis-à-vis different metal ions have been explored as established in the work of Iravani [2] among other reviews for a range of pharmacological and or biological potentials not limited to antimicrobial, anticancer, antioxidant, antidiabetic, antihypertensive, and so on. This review, while updating on the works of Ashwini and Mahanligam [4] and Nouri *et al.* [46], revealed the use and green-synthesis of four nanoparticles (silver, gold, zinc oxide and platinum) with established antihyperglycaemic effects. The highest prevalence was observed with silver, followed by gold, zinc oxide, and platinum appearing once. The widest acceptance or utilization of these two nanoparticles (silver and gold) may not be unconnected to the fact that they were the first metal ions explored when consideration of nanostructure synthesis research using plants began [26].

The presence of phytochemicals and/or functional groups in medicinal plants had been established to be responsible for their various pharmacological potentials. Additionally, the investigation into the green synthesis of nanoparticles and their potential to produce an ecofriendly product, among others and which the probable mechanism was assumed to be due to the reduction of metal ions to form the nanoparticles and its stability (depending on surrounding affinity or aggregation) are attributed to these phytoconstituents (phenolic, flavonoids, terpenoids, proteins *etc.*) and corresponding functional groups. Most of these established antidiabetic green mediated nanoparticles from this report featured phenolics, flavonoids (to a larger extent), proteins, carbohydrates, saponins, *etc.* The prominent functional groups are hydroxyl group (OH), carbonyl (C=O), carboxyl (COOH), C-O, C=O, amino (NH$_2$), *etc.*, which are contained in phenols, alkaloids, flavonoids, and so on [5, 26, 28].

The antidiabetic activities of potential substances or compounds are principally assessed *in vitro* by the inhibition of alpha-amylase and alpha-glucosidase enzymes as well as glucose uptake determination. Besides, it should be noted that the activity of a substance *in vitro* does not necessarily signify its potency until tested in an animal model. In fact, it is necessary to determine the toxicity (cancer cell lines, acute, subacute, chronic and subchronic) level of the substance once it is found to be active in the aforementioned determinations in order to present or give an idea of the safety concerns of the substance and whether or not clinical trials can be signaled for possible drug development. The goal of any antidiabetic therapy is to be able to control blood glucose levels during postprandial hyperglycaemia or glucose overload. Interestingly twenty-six (26) of the fifty-eight established medicinal plants were said to ameliorate or reduce elevated glucose levels in alloxan or streptozotoxin –induced hyperglycaemia in an animal model, indicative of a positive step towards being employed for diabetic therapy. In terms of toxicity evaluation, three out of the nine (9) reports were conducted in animal models and they were found to be non-toxic at tested concentrations, suggesting the possible safety of green-synthesized nanoparticles in humans.

## CONCLUSION

The review provided updates on previous authors' works on the subject matter by identifying additional green synthesized nanoparticles whose effects were studied and established for possible diabetic therapy. The review differs to some extent from earlier studies by probing the safety concerns and probable mechanism of nanoparticle formation. Above all, the review established the prospect and application of 58 phytonanoparticles in diabetes therapy. Although most of these antidiabetic phytonanoparticles have not been evaluated in animal models, it does not rule out their possibility as potential and/ or alternative candidates in the management of diabetes mellitus. It is therefore encouraged that more research be conducted on yet-to-be identified antidiabetic plants vis-a-vis other metal (or metal oxides) ions (such as copper, palladium, magnetite, silicon, nickel, cobalt, CuO, $TiO_2$, MgO, CaO, FeO, $ZnO_2$ *etc.*) while efforts on the *in vivo* determination of the antihyperglycaemic potentials of already established *in vitro* antidiabetic NPs as well as toxicity testing be intensified.

## CONSENT FOR PUBLICATION

Not applicable.

## CONFLICT OF INTEREST

The authors declare no conflict of interest, financial or otherwise.

## ACKNOWLEDGEMENTS

The authors appreciate the National Research Foundation (NRF) of South Africa for the full funding of the project through the Innovation Postdoctoral Fellowship awarded to Dr. FO Balogun (UID: 129494) tenable at the Department of Biotechnology and Food Science, Durban University of Technology, Durban, South Africa. The authors also acknowledge the support from Directorate of Research and Development, DUT.

## REFERENCES

[1]  Salem SS, Fouda A. Green synthesis of metallic nanoparticles and their prospective biotechnological applications: an overview. Biol Trace Elem Res 2021; 199(1): 344-70.
[http://dx.doi.org/10.1007/s12011-020-02138-3] [PMID: 32377944]

[2]  Iravani S. Green synthesis of metal nanoparticles using plants. Green Chem 2011; 13: 2638.
[http://dx.doi.org/10.1039/c1gc15386b]

[3]  Gour A, Jain NK. Advances in green synthesis of nanoparticles. Artif Cells Nanomed Biotechnol 2019; 47(1): 844-51.
[http://dx.doi.org/10.1080/21691401.2019.1577878] [PMID: 30879351]

[4]  Ashwini D, Mahalingam G. Green synthesized metal nanoparticles, characterization and its antidiabetic activities- A review. Res J Pharm Tech 2020; 13: 468-74.
[http://dx.doi.org/10.5958/0974-360X.2020.00091.8]

[5]  El Shafey AM. Green synthesis of metal and metal oxide nanoparticles from plant leaf extracts and their applications: A review. Green Process Synthesis 2020; 9: 304-39.
[http://dx.doi.org/10.1515/gps-2020-0031]

[6]  Lazarus GG, Singh M. *In vitro* cytotoxic activity and transfection efficiency of polyethyleneimine functionalized gold nanoparticles. Colloids Surf B Biointerfaces 2016; 145: 906-11.
[http://dx.doi.org/10.1016/j.colsurfb.2016.05.072] [PMID: 27341304]

[7]  Ghosh PS, Kim CK, Han G, Forbes NS, Rotello VM. Efficient gene delivery vectors by tuning the surface charge density of amino acid-functionalized gold nanoparticles. ACS Nano 2008; 2(11): 2213-8.
[http://dx.doi.org/10.1021/nn800507t] [PMID: 19206385]

[8]  Krishna SA, Amarehwar P. Preparation of chitosan coated nanoparticles by emulsion polymerization technique. Asian J Pharm Clin Res 2011; 4.

[9]  BarathManiKanth S. Kalishwaralal K, Sriram M, Pandian SRK, Youn H, Eom S, Gurunathan S. Anti-oxidant effect of gold nanoparticles restrains hyperglycemic conditions in diabetic mice. J Nanobiotechnology 2010; 8: 16.
[http://dx.doi.org/10.1186/1477-3155-8-16]

[10]  Yasser AS, Maha AA, Islam R, Mohamed HMA. Green synthesis of zinc oxide nanoparticles using aqueous extract of Deverra tortuosa and their cytotoxic activities. 2020; 3445.
[http://dx.doi.org/10.1038/s41598-020-60541-1]

[11]  Hurtado RB, Calderon-Ayala G, Cortez-Valadez M, Ramírez-Rodríguez PL, Flores-Acosta M. Green synthesis of metallic and carbon nanostructures.Nanomechanics.
[http://dx.doi.org/10.5772/intechopen.68483]

[12]  Li WR, Xie XB, Shi QS, Zeng HY, Ou-Yang YS, Chen YB. Antibacterial activity and mechanism of silver nanoparticles on *Escherichia coli*. Appl Microbiol Biotechnol 2010; 85(4): 1115-22.
[http://dx.doi.org/10.1007/s00253-009-2159-5] [PMID: 19669753]

[13]   Gurunathan S, Jeong JK, Han JW, Zhang XF, Park JH, Kim JH. Multidimensional effects of biologically synthesized silver nanoparticles in *Helicobacter pylori*, Helicobacter felis, and human lung (L132) and lung carcinoma A549 cells. Nanoscale Res Lett 2015; 10: 35.
[http://dx.doi.org/10.1186/s11671-015-0747-0] [PMID: 25852332]

[14]   Banerjee P, Nath D. A phytochemical approach to synthesize silver nanoparticles for non-toxic biomedical application and study on their antibacterial efficacy. Nanosci Technol 2015; 2: 1-14.

[15]   Alkaladi A, Abdelazim AM, Afifi M. Antidiabetic activity of zinc oxide and silver nanoparticles on streptozotocin-induced diabetic rats. Int J Mol Sci 2014; 15(2): 2015-23.
[http://dx.doi.org/10.3390/ijms15022015] [PMID: 24477262]

[16]   Balan K, Qing W, Wang Y, *et al.* Antidiabetic activity of silver nanoparticles from green synthesis using Lonicera japonica leaf extract. RSC Advances 2016; 6: 40162.
[http://dx.doi.org/10.1039/C5RA24391B]

[17]   Niranjan T, Rajasekar C, Gan GR. Green synthesis of platinum nanoparticles and their biomedical applications.Green metals nanoparticles. Scrivener Publishing LLC 2018; pp. 603-27.

[18]   Bedi PS, Kaur A. An overview on uses of zinc oxide nanoparticles. World J Pharm Pharm Sci 2015; 4: 1177-96.

[19]   Yang P, Yan R, Fardy M. Semiconductor nanowire: what's next? Nano Lett 2010; 10(5): 1529-36.
[http://dx.doi.org/10.1021/nl100665r] [PMID: 20394412]

[20]   Zheng YF, Gu ZN, Witte F. Biodegradable metals. Mater Sci Eng Rep 2014; 77: 1-34.
[http://dx.doi.org/10.1016/j.mser.2014.01.001]

[21]   Yakimova R, Selegard L, Khranovskyy V, Pearce R, Spetz AL, Uvdal K. ZnO materials and surface tailoring for biosensing. Front Biosci (Elite Ed) 2012; 4(1): 254-78.
[http://dx.doi.org/10.2741/e374] [PMID: 22201869]

[22]   Srivastava P, Braganca JM, Kowshik M. *In vivo* synthesis of selenium nanoparticles by *Halococcus salifodinae* BK18 and their anti-proliferative properties against HeLa cell line. Biotechnol Prog 2014; 30(6): 1480-7.
[http://dx.doi.org/10.1002/btpr.1992] [PMID: 25219897]

[23]   Hassanin KMA, Abd El-Kawi SH, Hashem KS. The prospective protective effect of selenium nanoparticles against chromium-induced oxidative and cellular damage in rat thyroid. Int J Nanomedicine 2013; 8: 1713-20.
[PMID: 23658489]

[24]   Al-Quraishy S, Dkhil MA, Abdel Moneim AE. Anti-hyperglycemic activity of selenium nanoparticles in streptozotocin-induced diabetic rats. Int J Nanomedicine 2015; 10: 6741-56.
[PMID: 26604749]

[25]   Priyom B. The recent developments in the green synthesis of nanoparticles (Accessed Oct 2, 2020). Available from: https://www.azonano.com/article.aspx?ArticleID=5553

[26]   Singh J, Dutta T, Kim KH, Rawat M, Samddar P, Kumar P. 'Green' synthesis of metals and their oxide nanoparticles: applications for environmental remediation. J Nanobiotechnology 2018; 16(1): 84.
[http://dx.doi.org/10.1186/s12951-018-0408-4] [PMID: 30373622]

[27]   Ogunyemi SO, Abdallah Y, Zhang M, *et al.* Green synthesis of zinc oxide nanoparticles using different plant extracts and their antibacterial activity against *Xanthomonas oryzae* pv. oryzae. Artif Cells Nanomed Biotechnol 2019; 47(1): 341-52.
[http://dx.doi.org/10.1080/21691401.2018.1557671] [PMID: 30691311]

[28]   Vishnukumar P, Vivekanandhan S, Misra M, Mohanty AK. Recent advances and emerging opportunities in phytochemical synthesis of ZnO nanostructures. Mater Sci Semicond Process 2019; 80: 143-61.

[http://dx.doi.org/10.1016/j.mssp.2018.01.026]

[29]    Rajakumar G, Thiruvengadam M, Mydhili G, Gomathi T, Chung IM. Green approach for synthesis of zinc oxide nanoparticles from *Andrographis paniculata* leaf extract and evaluation of their antioxidant, anti-diabetic, and anti-inflammatory activities. Bioprocess Biosyst Eng 2018; 41(1): 21-30.
        [http://dx.doi.org/10.1007/s00449-017-1840-9] [PMID: 28916855]

[30]    Nasef NA, Mehta S, Ferguson LR. Susceptibility to chronic inflammation: an update. Arch Toxicol 2017; 91(3): 1131-41.
        [http://dx.doi.org/10.1007/s00204-016-1914-5] [PMID: 28130581]

[31]    Rani V, Deep G, Singh RK, Palle K, Yadav UCS. Oxidative stress and metabolic disorders: Pathogenesis and therapeutic strategies. Life Sci 2016; 148: 183-93.
        [http://dx.doi.org/10.1016/j.lfs.2016.02.002] [PMID: 26851532]

[32]    Etoundi CBO, Kuaté D, Ngondi JL, Oben JE. Effects of extracts of *Hypodaphnis zenkeri* and *Xylopia aethiopica* on blood lipids: glycemia and body weight of Triton WR-1339 and insulin resistant rats. Int J Res Ayurveda Pharm 2013; 4: 736-41.
        [http://dx.doi.org/10.7897/2277-4343.04523]

[33]    IDF Diabetes Atlas. International Diabetes Federation 9th., 2019.(Accessed November, 15, 2020). Available from: https://www.diabetesatlas.org/en/sections/worldwide-toll-of-diabetes.html

[34]    IDF Diabetes Atlas. International Diabetes Federation 8th. 2017; 1-150. Available from: http://www.diabetesatlas.org

[35]    Balogun FO, Ashafa AOT. Aqueous root extract of *Dicoma anomala* (Sond.) extenuates postprandial hyperglycaemia *in vitro* and its modulation on the activities of carbohydrate-metabolism enzymes in streptozotocin –induced diabetic Wistar rats. S Afr J Bot 2017; 112: 102-12.
        [http://dx.doi.org/10.1016/j.sajb.2017.05.014]

[36]    Gandhi GR, Sasikumar P. Antidiabetic effect of *Merremia emarginata* Burm. F. in streptozotocin induced diabetic rats. Asian Pac J Trop Biomed 2012; 2(4): 281-6.
        [http://dx.doi.org/10.1016/S2221-1691(12)60023-9] [PMID: 23569914]

[37]    Ouassou H, Zahidi T, Bouknana S, *et al.* Inhibition of α-glucosidase, intestinal glucose absorption and antidiabetic properties by Caralluma europaea. Evidence-Based Complement Altern Med 2018.
        [http://dx.doi.org/10.1155/2018/9589472]

[38]    Anand K, Tiloke C, Naidoo P, Chuturgoon AA. Phytonanotherapy for management of diabetes using green synthesis nanoparticles. J Photochem Photobiol B 2017; 173: 626-39.
        [http://dx.doi.org/10.1016/j.jphotobiol.2017.06.028] [PMID: 28709077]

[39]    Sarkhail P, Rahmanipour S, Fadyevatan S, *et al.* Antidiabetic effect of *Phlomis anisodonta*: effects on hepatic cells lipid peroxidation and antioxidant enzymes in experimental diabetes. Pharmacol Res 2007; 56(3): 261-6.
        [http://dx.doi.org/10.1016/j.phrs.2007.07.003] [PMID: 17714953]

[40]    Balogun FO, Tshabalala NT, Ashafa AOT. Antidiabetic medicinal plants used by the Basotho tribe of Eastern Free State: A review. J Diab Res 2016.

[41]    Balogun FO, Ashafa AOT. A review of plants in South African traditional medicine used in the prevention and management of hypertension. Planta Med 2019; 85: 312-34.
        [http://dx.doi.org/10.1055/a-0801-8771] [PMID: 30477041]

[42]    J Afolayan A, O Sunmonu T. *In vivo* studies on antidiabetic plants used in South African herbal medicine. J Clin Biochem Nutr 2010; 47(2): 98-106.
        [http://dx.doi.org/10.3164/jcbn.09-126R] [PMID: 20838564]

[43]    Oyagbemi AA, Salihu M, Oguntibeju OO, Esterhuyse AJ, Farombi EO. Some selected medicinal plants with antidiabetic potentials.Antioxidant antidiabetic agents and human health. Intechopen 2014.
        [http://dx.doi.org/10.5772/57230]

[44]     Balogun FO. Antioxidant, Antidiabetic and Cardioprotective Activities of Dicoma Anomala (Sond.) Used in the Basotho Traditional Medicine. 2016; 270. Available from: https://books.google.com.ng/books/about/Antioxidant_Antidiabetic_and_Cardioprote.html?id=lExztA EACAAJ&redir_esc=y

[45]     Mukhopadyay N, Sampath V, Pai S, Babu UV, Lobo R. Antidiabetic medicinal plants: A review. Int Res J Pharm 2019; 10: 31-7.
[http://dx.doi.org/10.7897/2230-8407.100237]

[46]     Nouri Z, Hajialyani M, Izadi Z, Bahramsoltani R, Farzaei MH, Abdollahi M. Nanophytomedicines for the prevention of metabolic syndrome: A pharmacological and biopharmaceutical review. Front Bioeng Biotechnol 2020; 8: 425.
[http://dx.doi.org/10.3389/fbioe.2020.00425] [PMID: 32478050]

[47]     Rana S, Kalaichelvan PT. Ecotoxicity of nanoparticles.Toxicology. Hindawi Publishing Corporation 2013; 2013: p. 11.
[http://dx.doi.org/10.1155/2013/574648]

[48]     Narendhran S, Reshma KN. Nanoparticles and their toxicology studies: A green chemistry approach. Res Dev Material Sci 2017; 2.
[http://dx.doi.org/10.31031/RDMS.2017.02.000539]

[49]     Saif S, Tahir A, Chen Y. Green synthesis of iron nanoparticles and their environmental applications and implications. Nanomaterials (Basel) 2016; 6(11): 209.
[http://dx.doi.org/10.3390/nano6110209] [PMID: 28335338]

[50]     Balogun FO, Ashafa AOT. Green synthesized zinc oxide nanoparticles using *Dicoma anomala* (Sond.) aqueous root extract mitigates free radicals and diabetes-linked Enzymes. Nanosci Nanotechnol Asia In Press.
[http://dx.doi.org/10.2174/2210681210666200117150727]

[51]     Balogun FO, Ashafa AOT. Potentials of synthesised *Lessertia montana* zinc oxide nanoparticles on free radicals-mediated oxidative stress and carbohydrate-hydrolysing enzymes. Acta Biol Szeged In Press
[http://dx.doi.org/10.14232/abs.2020.2.239-249]

[52]     Shanker U, Jassal V, Rani M, Kaith BS. Towards green synthesis of nanoparticles: from bio-assisted sources to benign solvents. A review. Int J Environ Anal Chem 2016; 96: 801-35.

[53]     Chaudhury A, Duvoor C, Reddy Dendi VS, *et al.* Clinical review of antidiabetic drugs: Implications for type 2 diabetes mellitus management. Front Endocrinol (Lausanne) 2017; 8: 6.
[http://dx.doi.org/10.3389/fendo.2017.00006] [PMID: 28167928]

[54]     Bhavani R, Sivakumar V, Prabakaran D. *In-vitro* antidiabetic and anti-microbial activity of silver nanoparticles synthesized using medicinal plant - *Aegle marmelos*. Int Res J Pharm Biosci 2018; 4: 1-12.

[55]     Sathvika K, Rajeshkumar S, Lakshmi T, Roy A. Antidiabetic activity of silver nanoparticles synthesized using neem and *Aloe vera* plant formulation. Drug Invention Today 2019; 12: 2026-9.

[56]     Das G, Patra JK, Debnath T, Ansari A, Shin H-S. Investigation of antioxidant, antibacterial, antidiabetic, and cytotoxicity potential of silver nanoparticles synthesized using the outer peel extract of Ananas comosus (L.). PLoS ONE 2019; 14: 0220950.

[57]     Saratale GD, Saratale RG, Benelli G, Kumar G, Pugazhendhi A, Kim DS, *et al.* Anti-diabetic potential of silver nanoparticles synthesized with *Argyreia nervosa* leaf extract high synergistic antibacterial activity with standard antibiotics against foodborne bacteria. J Cluster Sci 2017; 28: 1709-27.
[http://dx.doi.org/10.1007/s10876-017-1179-z]

[58]     Rehana D, Mahendiran D, Kumar RS, Rahiman AK. *In vitro* antioxidant and antidiabetic activities of zinc oxide nanoparticles synthesized using different plant extracts. Bioprocess Biosyst Eng 2017; 40(6): 943-57.

[http://dx.doi.org/10.1007/s00449-017-1758-2] [PMID: 28361361]

[59]　Johnson P, Krishnan V, Loganathan C, *et al.* Rapid biosynthesis of Bauhinia variegata flower extract-mediated silver nanoparticles: an effective antioxidant scavenger and α-amylase inhibitor. Artif Cells Nanomed Biotechnol 2018; 46(7): 1488-94.
　　　[http://dx.doi.org/10.1080/21691401.2017.1374283] [PMID: 28885044]

[60]　Govindappa M, Hemashekhar B, Arthikala MK, Ravishankar Rai V, Ramachandra YL. Characterization, antibacterial, antioxidant, antidiabetic, anti-inflammatory and antityrosinase activity of green synthesized silver nanoparticles using *Calophyllum tomentosum* leaves extract. Results Phys 2018; 9: 400-8.
　　　[http://dx.doi.org/10.1016/j.rinp.2018.02.049]

[61]　Kumar VG, Gokavarapu SD, Rajeswari A, *et al.* Facile green synthesis of gold nanoparticles using leaf extract of antidiabetic potent *Cassia auriculata.* Colloids Surf B Biointerfaces 2011; 87(1): 159-63.
　　　[http://dx.doi.org/10.1016/j.colsurfb.2011.05.016] [PMID: 21640563]

[62]　Daisy P, Saipriya K. Biochemical analysis of *Cassia fistula* aqueous extract and phytochemically synthesized gold nanoparticles as hypoglycemic treatment for diabetes mellitus. Int J Nanomedicine 2012; 7: 1189-202.
　　　[http://dx.doi.org/10.2147/IJN.S26650] [PMID: 22419867]

[63]　Ponnanikajamideen M, Rajeshkumar S, Vanaja M, Annadurai G. *In vivo* type-2 diabetes and wound-healing effects of antioxidant Gold nanoparticles synthesized using the insulin plant *Chamaecostus cuspidatus* in albino rats. Can J Diabetes 2018; 1-8.
　　　[PMID: 30413371]

[64]　Aruna A, Nandhini R, Karthikeyan V, Bose P. Synthesis and characterization of silver nanoparticles of insulin plant (*Costus pictus* D. Don) Leaves. Asian J Biomed Pharm Sci 2014; 04: 1-6.
　　　[http://dx.doi.org/10.15272/ajbps.v4i34.523]

[65]　Sengani M, Grumezescu AM, Devi Rajeswari V. Recent trends and methodologies in gold nanoparticle synthesis - a prospective review on drug delivery aspect. OpenNano 2017; 2: 37-46.
　　　[http://dx.doi.org/10.1016/j.onano.2017.07.001]

[66]　Guru Kumar D, Ninganna D, Kantharaju RM, Krishnegowda CS, Yogananda M. Antioxidant, antibacterial, antidiabetic potential and genotoxicity of silver nanoparticles using leaf extract of *Curcuma longa*: a novel green approach. Int Res J Pharm 2019; 10: 127-36.
　　　[http://dx.doi.org/10.7897/2230-8407.100391]

[67]　Agarwal H, Venkat Kumar S, Rajeshkumar S. Antidiabetic effect of silver nanoparticles synthesized using lemongrass (*Cymbopogon citratus*) through conventional heating and microwave irradiation approach. J Microbiol Biotechnol Food Sci 2018; 7: 371-6.
　　　[http://dx.doi.org/10.15414/jmbfs.2018.7.4.371-376]

[68]　Ghosh S, More P, Nitnavare R, Jagtap S, Chippalkatti R, *et al.* Antidiabetic and antioxidant properties of copper nanoparticles synthesized by medicinal plant Dioscorea bulbifera. J Nanomed Nanotechnol 2015; 6: 007.
　　　[http://dx.doi.org/10.4172/2157-7439.S6-007]

[69]　Das G, Patra JK, Shin HS. Biosynthesis, and potential effect of fern mediated biocompatible silver nanoparticles by cytotoxicity, antidiabetic, antioxidant and antibacterial, studies. Mater Sci Eng C 2020; 114: 111011.
　　　[http://dx.doi.org/10.1016/j.msec.2020.111011] [PMID: 32993988]

[70]　Garcia Campoy AH, Perez Gutierrez RM, Manriquez-Alvirde G, Muñiz Ramirez A. Protection of silver nanoparticles using *Eysenhardtia polystachya* in peroxide-induced pancreatic β-Cell damage and their antidiabetic properties in zebrafish. Int J Nanomedicine 2018; 13: 2601-12.
　　　[http://dx.doi.org/10.2147/IJN.S163714] [PMID: 29750032]

[71]    Das MP, Rebecca LJ, Das MP. Characterization of antidiabetic activity of silver nanoparticles using aqueous solution of *Ficus glomerata* (Fig.) gum. Int J Pharm Bio Sci 2017; 8: 424-9.

[72]    Abideen S, Sankar MV. *In-vitro* screening of antidiabetic and antimicrobial activity against green synthesized AgNO$_3$ using seaweeds. J Nanomed Nanotechnol 2015; S6-S001.
        [http://dx.doi.org/10.4172/2157-7439.S6-001]

[73]    Shanker K, Krishna Mohan G, Mayasa V, Pravallika L. Antihyperglycemic and anti-hyperlipidemic effect of biologically synthesized silver nanoparticles and *G. sylvestre* extract on streptozotocin induced diabetic rats-an *in vivo* approach. Mater Lett 2017; 195: 240-4.
        [http://dx.doi.org/10.1016/j.matlet.2017.02.137]

[74]    Varadharaj V, Ramaswamy A, Sakthivel R, *et al.* Antidiabetic and antioxidant activity of green synthesized starch nanoparticles: An *in vitro* study. J Cluster Sci 2019; 31: 1257-66.

[75]    Vishnu Kiran M, Murugesan S. Biogenic silver nanoparticles by *Halymenia poryphyroides* and its *in vitro* anti-diabetic efficacy. J Chem Pharm Res 2013; 5: 1001-8.

[76]    Thatoi P, Kerry RG, Gouda S, *et al.* Photo-mediated green synthesis of silver and zinc oxide nanoparticles using aqueous extracts of two mangrove plant species, *Heritiera fomes* and *Sonneratia apetala* and investigation of their biomedical applications. J Photochem Photobiol B 2016; 163: 311-8.
        [http://dx.doi.org/10.1016/j.jphotobiol.2016.07.029] [PMID: 27611454]

[77]    Bala N, Saha S, Chakraborty M, *et al.* Green synthesis of zinc oxide nanoparticles using *Hibiscus subdariffa* leaf extract: effect of temperature on synthesis, antibacterial activity and anti-diabetic activity. RSC Advances 2015; 5: 4993-5003.
        [http://dx.doi.org/10.1039/C4RA12784F]

[78]    Badeggi UM, Ismail E, Adeloye AO, *et al.* Green synthesis of gold nanoparticles capped with Procyanidins from *Leucosidea sericea* as potential antidiabetic and antioxidant agents. Biomolecules 2020; 10(3): 452.
        [http://dx.doi.org/10.3390/biom10030452] [PMID: 32183213]

[79]    Soliman N, Khalil M. Abdel- Moaty H, Ismael E, Sabry D. Anti-Helicobacter pylori, anti-diabetic and cytotoxicity activity of biosynthesized gold nanoparticles using *Moricandia nitens* water extract. Egypt J Chem 2018; 61: 691-703.

[80]    Xu L, Li W, Shi Q, *et al.* Synthesis of mulberry leaf extract mediated gold nanoparticles and their ameliorative effect on Aluminium intoxicated and diabetic retinopathy in rats during perinatal life. J Photochem Photobiol B 2019; 196: 111502.
        [http://dx.doi.org/10.1016/j.jphotobiol.2019.04.011] [PMID: 31129511]

[81]    Anbazhagan P, Murugan K, Jaganathan A, Sujitha V, Samidoss CM, Jayashanthani S, *et al.* Mosquitocidal, antimalarial and antidiabetic potential of *Musa paradisiaca*-synthesized silver nanoparticles: *in vivo* and *in vitro* approaches. J Cluster Sci 2017; 28: 91-107.
        [http://dx.doi.org/10.1007/s10876-016-1047-2]

[82]    Bayrami A, Ghorbani E, Rahim Pouran S, Habibi-Yangjeh A, Khataee A, Bayrami M. Enriched zinc oxide nanoparticles by *Nasturtium officinale* leaf extract: Joint ultrasound-microwave-facilitated synthesis, characterization, and implementation for diabetes control and bacterial inhibition. Ultrason Sonochem 2019; 58: 104613.
        [http://dx.doi.org/10.1016/j.ultsonch.2019.104613] [PMID: 31450359]

[83]    Malapermal V, Botha I, Krishna SBN, Mbatha JN. Enhancing antidiabetic and antimicrobial performance of *Ocimum basilicum*, and *Ocimum sanctum* (L.) using silver nanoparticles. Saudi J Biol Sci 2015; 24(6): 1294-305.
        [http://dx.doi.org/10.1016/j.sjbs.2015.06.026] [PMID: 28855825]

[84]    Hasan FA, Laith AY. Hoglycemic and antioxidant effect of gold nanoparticles in alloxan-induced diabetic rats. Int J Res Biotechnol Biochem 2016; 6: 12-20.

[85]    Prabhu S, Vinodhini S, Elanchezhiyan C, Rajeswari D. Evaluation of antidiabetic activity of

biologically synthesized silver nanoparticles using *Pouteria sapota* in streptozotocin-induced diabetic rats. J Diabetes 2018; 10(1): 28-42.
[http://dx.doi.org/10.1111/1753-0407.12554] [PMID: 28323393]

[86]   Saratale RG, Shin HS, Kumar G, Benelli G, Kim DS, Saratale GD. Exploiting antidiabetic activity of silver nanoparticles synthesized using *Punica granatum* leaves and anticancer potential against human liver cancer cells (HepG2). Artif Cells Nanomed Biotechnol 2018; 46(1): 211-22.
[http://dx.doi.org/10.1080/21691401.2017.1337031] [PMID: 28612655]

[87]   Bagyalakshmi J, Haritha H. Green synthesis and characterization of silver nanoparticles using *Pterocarpus marsupium* and assessment of its *in vitro* antidiabetic activity. Am J Adv Drug Deliv 2017; 118-30.
[http://dx.doi.org/10.21767/2321-547X.1000019]

[88]   Opris R, Tatomir C, Olteanu D, *et al.* The effect of Sambucus nigra L. extract and phytosinthezied gold nanoparticles on diabetic rats. Colloids Surf B Biointerfaces 2017; 150: 192-200.
[http://dx.doi.org/10.1016/j.colsurfb.2016.11.033] [PMID: 27914256]

[89]   Patra N, Kar D, Pal A, Behera A. Antibacterial, anticancer, anti-diabetic and catalytic activity of bio-conjugated metal nanoparticles. Adv Nat Sci Nanosci Nanotechnol 2018; 9: 1-6.
[http://dx.doi.org/10.1088/2043-6254/aad12d]

[90]   Dhas TS, Kumar VG, Karthick V, Vasanth K, Singaravelu G, Govindaraju K. Effect of biosynthesized gold nanoparticles by *Sargassum swartzii* in alloxan induced diabetic rats. Enzyme Microb Technol 2016; 95: 100-6.
[http://dx.doi.org/10.1016/j.enzmictec.2016.09.003] [PMID: 27866603]

[91]   Mohammadi Arvanag F, Bayrami A, Habibi-Yangjeh A, Rahim Pouran S. A comprehensive study on antidiabetic and antibacterial activities of ZnO nanoparticles biosynthesized using *Silybum marianum* L seed extract. Mater Sci Eng C 2019; 97: 397-405.
[http://dx.doi.org/10.1016/j.msec.2018.12.058] [PMID: 30678925]

[92]   Ansari S, Bari A, Ullah R, Mathanmohun M, Veeraraghavan VP, Sun Z. Gold nanoparticles synthesized with *Smilax glabra* rhizome modulates the anti-obesity parameters in high-fat diet and streptozotocin induced obese diabetes rat model. J Photochem Photobiol B 2019; 201: 111643.
[http://dx.doi.org/10.1016/j.jphotobiol.2019.111643] [PMID: 31698218]

[93]   Atale N, Saxena S, Nirmala JG, Narendhirakannan RT, Mohanty S, Rani V. Synthesis and characterization of *Sygyzium cumini* nanoparticles for its protective potential in high glucose-induced cardiac stress: a green approach. Appl Biochem Biotechnol 2017; 181(3): 1140-54.
[http://dx.doi.org/10.1007/s12010-016-2274-6] [PMID: 27734287]

[94]   Rajaram K, Aiswarya DC, Sureshkumar P. Green synthesis of silver nanoparticle using *Tephrosia tinctoria* and its antidiabetic activity. Mater Lett 2015; 138: 251-4.
[http://dx.doi.org/10.1016/j.matlet.2014.10.017]

[95]   Virk P. Antidiabetic activity of green gold-silver nanocomposite with *Trigonella foenum graecum* L. seeds extract on streptozotocin induced diabetic rats. Pak J Zool 2018; 50: 711-8.
[http://dx.doi.org/10.17582/journal.pjz/2018.2.711.718]

[96]   Bayrami A, Haghgooie S, Pouran SR, Arvanag FM, Habibi-Yangjeh A. Synergistic antidiabetic activity of ZnO nanoparticles encompassed by *Urtica dioica* extract. Adv Powder Technol 2020; 31: 2110-8.
[http://dx.doi.org/10.1016/j.apt.2020.03.004]

[97]   Bayrami A, Parvinroo S, Habibi-Yangjeh A, Rahim Pouran S. Bio-extract-mediated ZnO nanoparticles: microwave-assisted synthesis, characterization and antidiabetic activity evaluation. Artif Cells Nanomed Biotechnol 2018; 46(4): 730-9.
[http://dx.doi.org/10.1080/21691401.2017.1337025] [PMID: 28617629]

[98]   Li Y, Zhang J, Gu J, Chen S, Wang C, Jia W. Biosynthesis of polyphenol-stabilised nanoparticles and assessment of anti-diabetic activity. J Photochem Photobiol B 2017; 169: 96-100.

[http://dx.doi.org/10.1016/j.jphotobiol.2017.02.017] [PMID: 28314182]

[99]    Garg A, Pandey P, Sharma P, Shukla AK. Synthesis and characterization of silver nanoparticle of ginger rhizome (*Zingiber officinale*) extract: synthesis, characterization and antidiabetic activity in streptozotocin induced diabetic rats. Eur J Biomed Pharm Sci 2016; 3: 605-11.

[100]   Swarnalatha L, Rachela C, Ranjanb S, Baradwaj P. Evaluation of *in vitro* antidiabetic activity of *Sphaeranthus amaranthoides* silver nanoparticles. Int J Nano Biomater 2012; 2: 25-9.

[101]   Sengani M, v DR. Identification of potential antioxidant indices by biogenic gold nanoparticles in hyperglycemic Wistar rats. Environ Toxicol Pharmacol 2017; 50: 11-9.
[http://dx.doi.org/10.1016/j.etap.2017.01.007] [PMID: 28110133]

[102]   Dhivya G, Rajasimman M. Synthesis of silver nanoparticles using *Momordica charantia* and its applications. J Chem Pharm Res 2015; 7: 107-13.

[103]   Ajani EO, Afolayan JS, Sabiu S. Characterization of *Blighia sapida* synthesized-copper nanoparticle and its application in periodic pharmaceutical effluent treatment. J Environ Sci Health Part A Tox Hazard Subst Environ Eng 2021; 56(5): 508-15.
[http://dx.doi.org/10.1080/10934529.2021.1890497] [PMID: 33656407]

# CHAPTER 11

# An Update on Green Synthesis Application in Cancer Therapy

**Karishma Singh**[1] and **Saheed Sabiu**[1,*]

[1] *Department of Biotechnology and Food Science, Faculty of Applied Sciences, Durban University of Technology, P.O. Box 1334, Durban, 4000, South Africa*

**Abstract:** Cancer is one of the most common health problems affecting the human population globally. One of the major focus areas that bio-nanotechnology is taking nowadays relates to nanomedicine and the use of nanomaterials in cancer therapy. Furthermore, the green synthesis of nanoparticles has been described as an effective, inexpensive, and environmentally friendly procedure. Biological organisms such as bacteria, fungi, cyanobacteria, algae, plant extracts, and enzymes and biomolecules have been reported to successfully synthesize metal nanoparticles. This review describes the types of green synthesized nanoparticles, the different green synthesis methods of nanoparticles, and their application against various cancer cell lines. Although the plant-mediated silver nanoparticle synthesis appeared to be the most common green synthesis approach used in cancer therapy, gold nanoparticles are postulated to be a better, more efficient alternative, whilst the use of zinc oxide nanoparticles is becoming an emerging trend. This review concludes that metal nanoparticles can be used as potential anticancer agents.

**Keywords:** Biomolecules, Cancer therapy, Drug-delivery, Metal nanoparticles, Microorganisms, Plant extracts.

## 1. INTRODUCTION

Nanotechnology has become a fast-growing field in the world of science and technology in recent times due to its multiple applications [1, 2]. It can be applied across a variety of fields such as optics, electronics, catalysis, biomedicine, energy science, mechanics, and the cosmetology and pharmacology industry [1, 3]. The word "nano" is of the Greek-origin, meaning extremely small; hence, nanoparticles are characterized as being relatively small in size (1-100 nm) and having an increased surface area to volume ratio [3, 4]. Generally, nanoparticles

---

* **Corresponding author Saheed Sabiu:** Department of Biotechnology and Food Science, Faculty of Applied Sciences, Durban University of Technology, P.O. Box 1334, Durban, 4000, South Africa; Tel: +2731 373 5330; E-mail: sabius@dut.ac.za

differ greatly in shapes (spherical, rod, and triangular) and sizes, and for the metal nanoparticles, for instance, their shapes have been reported to significantly influence their optical and electronic properties [5, 6]. The size of nanoparticles varies according to the field of application. For instance, in medicine and pharmaceutical sciences, nanoparticles synthesized for therapeutic drug delivery are often larger than 100 nm to accommodate an adequate quantity of drugs to be delivered to target tissues or organs [7, 8]. Specifically, for cancer therapy, the desired size of the nanoparticles ranges between 70 –150 nm as the arrangements in the endothelium in a developing tumour is about 100–780 nm [6]. To date, the metal nanoparticles for cancer therapy have remained a viable alternative to the conventional anticancer drugs (chemotherapy) and treatments (laser therapy, and surgery targeting tumour cells) due to several side effects such as weight loss, anemia, hair loss, fatigue, bleeding and bruising, appetite loss, diarrhea, blurred vision [7, 9]. Comparatively, cancer nanoparticle therapies, particularly those from biological sources, have been reported to be less toxic, more reliable, economical, environmentally friendly, and effective [1, 6]. Consequently, the bio-nanoscience has been employed as a potential weapon in cancer therapy.

The ultimate goal of nanoparticles is to diagnose cancer at an early stage and deliver the therapeutic agents (drugs) at an optimum dose to the right target to kill the cancerous cells. Conventional methods such as chemotherapy and radiotherapy are known for their harsh side effects and often target cells that are not specifically cancerous, resulting in the elimination of healthy cells [9]. Moreover, numerous problems in toxicity, inactivity, and limited bioassay are inferred from the weak pharmacokinetic effects of cancer medications resulting from lower solubility, stability, and metabolism. Therefore, effective formulations must be established that can address these difficulties and selectively target tumor sites without compromising the viability of healthy cells and tissues. Understanding the precise mechanism of metal nanoparticles as potential anticancer agents is also imperative. Here, various metal nanoparticles, as well as green synthesis and characterization methods, are discussed to offer an innovative possibility to examine biological units for nanoparticle synthesis and to evaluate their possible effects on cancer therapy.

## 2. GREEN SYNTHESIZED NANOPARTICLES IN CANCER THERAPY

Nanoparticles are desired for biomedical applications because they are essentially a bridge the gap between bulk materials and atomic or molecular structures with unique mechanistic, optic, and biology-related attributes [10, 11]. Each nanoparticle has a significant contribution to green synthesis applications. Nevertheless, metal nanoparticles are emerging as a preferred choice over conventional therapy and are being widely used in therapeutics [7, 12, 13]. Of the metals (silver, gold, zinc, nickel, iron, selenium, palladium, copper, and platinum, *etc.*) used in nanoparticle synthesis, those from silver, gold, and zinc have extensive and promising applications in cancer therapy. Hence, this section briefly highlights silver, gold, and zinc nanoparticles in both effective cancer diagnosis and therapy [8].

## 2.1. Silver

Silver is the most desired metal for nanoparticle synthesis due to its unique morphologies, stability, and controlled geometry [4, 14]. Silver nanoparticles (AgNPs) can be synthesized using either plant extracts or various microorganisms [6] and are being designated as most effective in the biomedical field because of their numerous applications [2, 15]. Besides their effective anti-cancer applications, studies have also implicated AgNPs as anti-parasitic, anti-septic, antimicrobial, anti-inflammatory, anti-diabetic, anticancer, and antioxidant agents [3, 5, 15 - 17]. The anticancer activities of AgNPs have been analyzed and reported against a range of cancer cells such as breast cancer, lung cancer, ovarian cancer, and human hepatoma cells *in vitro* [7]. Rattan *et al.* [18] have also reported the anticancer activity of 23 plant extracts used to synthesize AgNPs and lent credence to their being potent anticancer drug-delivery systems.

## 2.2. Gold

Gold is another metal that is also known to be compatible with biological material. Gold nanoparticles (AuNPs) are some of the most widely studied nanoparticles because of their surface plasmon resonance (SPR) and optical properties [15]. AuNPs can easily be synthesized, have high chemical and thermal stability, low cytotoxicity and show intense surface SPR, and can be used as drug carriers [15]. Gold nanoparticles can be prepared in a varying range of core sizes (1 to 150 nm), making it easier to control their dispersion [19]. They have a broad application range in biomedicine, such as biomolecular immobilization, leukemia therapy, antimalarial and anti-arthritic treatment, and biosensor design [20]. Furthermore, the ability of AuNPs to bind ligands (antibodies, peptides, and nucleotides) by interacting with their amine and thiols groups provides a suitable means of producing specified biomarkers and conjugating therapeutic agents [21].

The biocompatibility of soft bases like thiols and their strong interactions make it possible for AuNPs to be essential in cancer therapy [2, 21]. Due to the capability of AuNPs to inhibit proliferation induced by vascular endothelial growth factor (VEGF), they have been used to treat ovarian cancer and metastasis attributable to VEGF [22]. This submission has been substantiated *in vivo* by Bhattacharya and Mukherjee [23] in a Mouse Ovarian Tumour Model (MOT). The study found that in the peritoneal cavities of C3H female mice, the tumour cells are main-locked by serial passage. This is a highly aggressive type of tumor and all animals die from large ascites and metastases 3-4 weeks after the tumor cell is inserted. Consequently, the intraperitoneal injection of AuNPs decreased the accumulation of ascites in the treated mice compared with untreated tumour-bearing animals. The function of growth factors such as VEGF165, bFGF secreted by MOT cells was inhibited by AuNPs, thus reducing permeability and thereby decreasing the accumulation of ascites. Furthermore, as outlined by Tikariha *et al.* [3], for multiple myeloma (MM), plasma cell cancer, AuNPs inhibit VEGF activity causing cell proliferation. This inhibition of VEGF also contributes to the up-regulation of proteins such as p21 and p27, which inhibit proliferation. AuNPs have been reported to inhibit the function of the heparin-based growth factor and can also influence the function of factors that are isolated *via* chronic lymphocytic leukemia (CLL) [3]. Again, AuNPs can be applied to amplify the biorecognition of the commonly used anticancer drugs dacarbazine [5-(3, 3-dimethyl-1-triazolyl) imidazole-4-carboxamide] [24]. Gold nanoparticles are not produced only for the detection, target, and killing of cancer cells, but also carry the drug to delay cancer cell growth or destroy cancer cells. Moreover, as soon as AuNPs surround cancer cells, the gold particles are heated by infrared light or lasers, after which, the dendrimers release the different organic molecules to destroy cancer cells [6]. Just recently, Singh *et al.* [19] provided an overview of the role of AuNPs in diagnostics and therapeutics for human cancer, postulating that the AuNPs may be the future of nanotechnology.

## 2.3. Zinc Oxide

Zinc is an essential mineral for improved metabolism, catalysis, and the overall wellbeing and health of humans. The nanoparticles made from Zn in the form of ZnO (ZnONPs) are now receiving much attention in the field of nano-biotechnology for their desirable antimicrobial and anticancer properties [25]. The use of ZnONPs is considered to be highly efficient, a more affordable alternative, less toxic, and soluble making it easier to reach the targeted sites in comparison to copper and gold [26, 27]. Presently, ZnONPs has become an emerging trend for the treatment of cancer because they exhibit cytotoxicity in various cancer cell lines [26]. A report by Kalpana and Rajeshwari [27], provided a summary of the green synthesis, biomedical applications, and toxicity of ZnONPs. Their findings reported on various green synthesis methods to provide an overview of the role of ZnONPs in various biomedical practices such as drug delivery, bioimaging, biosensors, and gene delivery. They further elaborated that transferrin-conjugated green fluorescent ZnONPs were utilized with the least cytotoxicity for cancer cell imaging. ZnONPs can penetrate the cell nucleus and exhibit low toxicity [25, 27].

## 2.4. Mechanism of Action of AgNPs, AuNPs, and ZnONPs Against Cancer Cells

The mechanisms of action of nanoparticles in cancer therapy have been well studied. For instance, both silver and gold nanoparticles elicit their anti-cancer effect in similar mechanistic manners [7]. The impact of these nanoparticles on cancerous cells is the decreasing mitochondrial function, reactive oxygen species (ROS) induction, lactate dehydrogenase (LDH) release, deregulation of the cell cycle, and apoptotic genes such as Bax, micronuclei formation, aberration, and deoxyribonucleic acid (DNA) damage. The ingestion of nanoparticles into macrophages' is where the inflammatory response is initiated. Reactive oxygen species (ROS), Tumour necrosis factor-alpha TNF-a, inflammatory cytokines, and interleukins are released by these activated macrophages interleukin-6 (IL-6). Small-sized nanoparticles were more poisonous and more effective in the development of ROS [3, 7]. Besides these cell pathways, nanoparticles also have anti-angiogenic and anti-proliferative effects. Vascular endothelial growth factor (VEGF) binds to its receptor on endothelial cells in normal tissue cells to induce angiogenesis through Phosphatidylinositol 3-kinase (PI3K) and Akt/Protein Kinase B. (PI3K/Akt) signaling pathway activation [7]. Nanoparticles inhibit the phosphorylation of Akt by PI3K, hence, they are anti-angiogenic since the signaling phase cannot be effectively completed thus ending angiogenesis, starving the cell, depriving oxygen, and destroying the cancer cell. The nanoparticle-mediated anti-proliferative capacity of cancer cells is due to their ability to destroy DNA, inhibit chromosome-producing genomic instability, calcium ($Ca^{2+}$) homeostasis disorder that caused apoptosis, cell injury and cytoskeletal instability, cytoskeletal injury prevents cell cycle and division, and promotes cancer cell antiproliferative activity [1]. The AuNPs' mechanism is similar to AgNPs, but other studies have shown that AuNPs are directly targeting the tumour cells, once in the cells and AuNPs are targeting the tumour suppressor genes (p53) and oncogenes (c-myc), which is a caspase-9-initiator involving apoptosis [3, 6]. Unlike AgNPs, AuNPs are less cytotoxic and display an increased plasmonic activity.

On the other hand, the ZnONPs elicit their action by weakening mitochondria which produce increased ROS, lipid peroxides, and DNA damage when interacting with the cancerous cell [26, 27]. When the ZnONPs interact with the tumour cells, it disrupts the protein equilibrium and affects other essential cellular processes such as DNA replication, apoptosis, DNA damage, the activity of electron transport chain, and cellular homeostasis thus increasing the cytotoxicity against tumour cells [26].

# 3. GREEN SYNTHESIS AND CHARACTERIZATION OF NANOPARTICLES

Three methods (physical, chemical, and biological) can be used to synthesize nanoparticles [7]. The physical approach involves dividing the appropriate bulk material into fine particles by size reduction using different techniques. such as evaporation-condensation, direct metal sputtering, Arc discharge, and laser ablation [1, 28], while the chemical approach makes use of techniques such as direct chemical reduction, electrolysis, UV-initiated photoreduction, microwave irradiation, pyrolysis, and cryo-chemical synthesis [3, 12, 29]. These two approaches are a non-conventional way of synthesizing nanoparticles and are time-consuming, highly toxic, expensive, and often not eligible for medical applications [5, 30]. On the other hand, the biological approach, which largely constitutes mainly green synthesis, is a more conventional method as it is eco-friendly, less toxic, and has various improved applications relative to the non-conventional ones [5, 31]. The green synthesis has developed a popular trend over the years and can be described as either utilization of (1) microorganisms such as bacteria, fungi, cyanobacteria, algae, (2) plant extracts, or (3) enzymes, and biomolecules to synthesize metal nanoparticles for biomedical and agricultural applications (Fig. **1**) [28, 29]. Also, as compared with the crude extracts, nanoparticles have different properties [30].

## 3.1. The Biological Approaches

It has been documented that microbes such as bacteria, fungi, yeast, and algae are capable of absorbing and accumulating metals, and as such make them suitable and viable agents in green synthesis [20]. Similarly, the ability of plants and plant extracts as reducing and capping agents of metals have received considerable attention in a way that makes them attractive in exhibiting a wide range of therapeutic uses [32]. The use of biomolecules and enzymes has also been explored in metal nanoparticle synthesis [33]. Boa and Lan [28], further elaborated on the production of green-mediated metal nanoparticles and their various applications. Their review presents the use of plants and microalgae to synthesize AgNPs and AuNPs. Furthermore, the anticancer properties of biomaterials highlighted in their study (AuNPs in particular) are of relevance to our review as it further describes the beneficial properties of AuNPs.

**Microorganisms**          **Plant extracts**          **Enzymes and biomolecules**

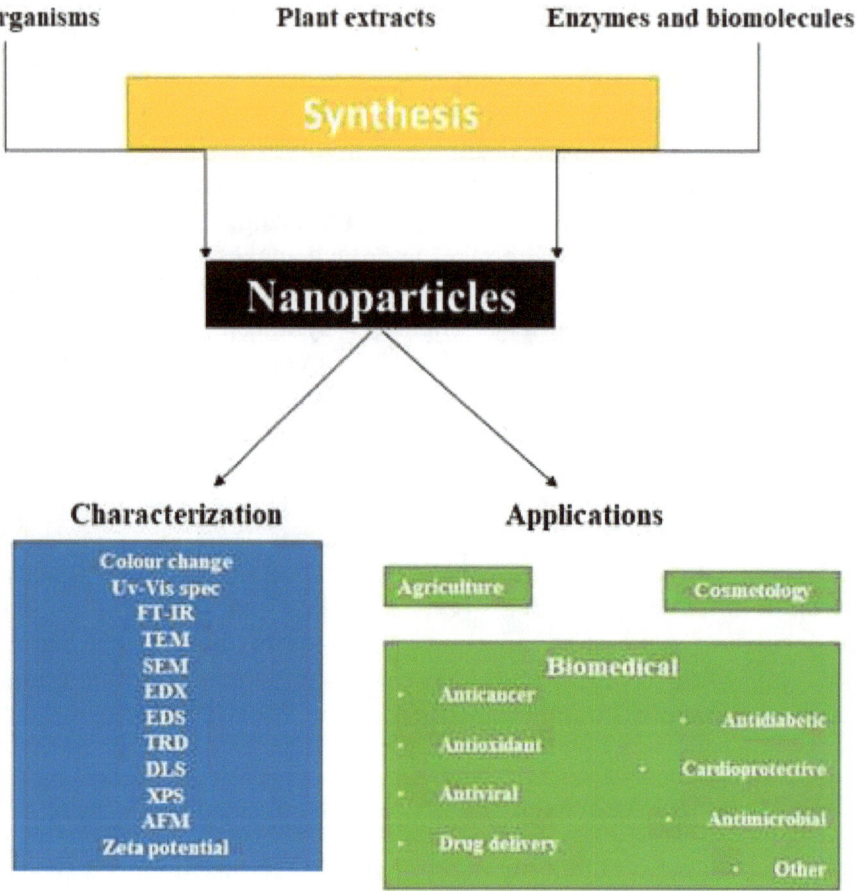

**Fig. (1).** Green synthesis characterization and application of metal nanoparticles.

## 3.2. Synthesis Using Microorganisms

### 3.2.1. Bacteria

Bacteria render inorganic materials either extracellularly or intracellularly depending on the site of synthesis. Their ability to manufacture these inorganic materials has turned them into potential biofactories for AgNPs and AuNPs [6, 31]. The basic steps to the green synthesis of metal nanoparticles used in bacterial cultures include 1) growth of bacteria in culture media, 2) biomass production from a medium, and 3) incubation of biomass with the sub-inhibitory concentration of metal salts [6, 18]. During the various phases of bacterial growth, intercellular or extracellular biologically reducing agents may be used to reduce the metal. Optimization of the reaction conditions can be achieved by controlling the experimental factors such as light regulation, incubation period, pH, temperature, and the composition of the culture medium [6]. Hence, improving the chemical composition, size, and shape of the particles synthesized.

Several studies using bacteria for synthesis revealed that the synthesis rate was much faster, supple, rational, and a better suitable protocol for large-scale nanoparticle synthesis compared to chemical and physical synthesis methods [31, 34, 35]. However, this method of synthesis is time-consuming, at risk of culture contamination, and minimal control over nanoparticle size.

Despite the known biocompatibility of AgNPs, some bacteria are known to be silver resistant by aggregating silver on their cell walls [31]. Hence, for effective synthesis in such an instance, AgNPs have been synthesized using silver-resistant bacterial strains (*Pseudomonas stulzeri, Escherichia coli, Vibrio cholera, Pseudomonas aeruginosa, Salmonella typhus,* and *Staphylococcus currens*). There are only a few reported bacteria such as *Pseudomonas aeruginosa, Staphylococcus aureus, Streptomyces sp., Lactobacillus sp.,* and *Bacillus megaterium* for the use of ZnONPs synthesis. Green synthesis of ZnONPs by utilizing bacteria could represent a novel source of key advancements in the biomedical industry. The use of thermophilic bacteria to synthesize gold nanoparticles has shown to be an excellent tool for extracellular synthesis [27]. Tikariha *et al.* [3] presented in their study a range of bacterial strains used to synthesize gold nanoparticles such as; *Bacillus cereus, Bacillus flexus, Enterococcus sp, Halococcus salifodinae* BK18, and *Klebsiella pneumoniae* (KACC 11402).

### 3.2.2. Fungi

The use of fungi is an extremely good and viable candidate for the synthesis of metal nanoparticles due to their economically large production capacity [3, 36]. As a result of their metal bioaccumulation and higher tolerance characteristic fungal strains are often the preferred choice over bacterial strains [18]. The synthesis process using fungi is less labour intensive, can be carried out at room temperature, and requires the use of a lesser amount of chemicals [3]. Green synthesis using fungi such as *Colletotrichum sp-, Trichothecium sp., Trichoderma asperellum, Cladosporium cladosporioides, Phaenerochaete chryso sporium, Fusarium semitectum, Aspergillus fumigates, Coriolus versicolor, Phoma glomerata, F. oxysporum, Penicillium brevicompactum, Penicillium fellutanum,* and *Volvariella volvacea.* have been reported, and the steps involved are similar to that highlighted for bacterial strains [15]. However, fungi are reported to produce larger amounts of AgNPs in comparison to bacteria because of their ability to efficiently secrete a protein [18].

### 3.2.3. Cyanobacteria

In this method of synthesis, an enzyme called nitrate reductase is involved in the synthesis of metal nanoparticles [5]. This is due to the biomass used in the synthesis process is simpler to handle, biodegradable, and also the downstream processing of the biomass is much easier to manage [6]. The commonly reported strains of cyanobacteria used for green synthesis are *Plectonema boryanum* and *Plectonema terebrans*. However, the utilization of cyanobacteria to synthesize nanoparticles is not a popular research area as opposed to other microbes (bacteria and fungi). The use of cyanobacteria-mediated metal nanoparticles in cancer therapy remains unexplored.

### 3.2.4. Algae

Nanoparticle synthesis using algae has proved to be more beneficial in comparison to synthesis using other microbes (bacterial and fungi) because It removes the process of maintaining cell culture and is much more suitable for large-scale nanoparticle processing [22, 37]. Algae have been reported to contain a variety of valuable compounds possessing antimicrobial, antiviral, anticancer, and cytotoxic activities [28]. Many studies have reported on algae being used as a "biofactory" for the green synthesis of metal nanoparticles. Gahlawat and Choudhury [20], reported on the microalga, *Chlorella vulgaris* for the green synthesis of AgNPs within the range of $9.8 \pm 5.7$ nm. The spherical nanoparticles have demonstrated their use as a strong green alternative to fight cancer [7]. Vijayaraghavan and Ashokkumar [6] presented in their review the use of *Padina gymnospora* with an average size of 14-15 nm, spherical shaped gold nanoparticles. Their study also mentioned the use of *Sargassum muticum* to synthesize silver, gold, and zinc oxide nanoparticles. The size and shape of each algae-mediated nanoparticle varied such that: AgNPs (30 nm, cubical), AuNPs (5-10 nm, spherical), and ZnONPs (50-100 nm, hexagonal).

### 3.3. Plant Extracts

In general, plant biomass can either be whole plants or in extract or powdered form. Various plant parts such as leaves, roots, latex, seed coats, stems, flowers, and fruits are being used to synthesize metal nanoparticles [32]. Although whole plants can act as factories for synthesizing nanoparticles, many drawbacks have been identified with this technology especially when expanding industrial applications [6]. It is of interest to use plants/plant extracts in nanoparticle synthesis because plants are readily accessible making this technique cost-effective, environmentally friendly, and less toxic [4, 18]. One of the most extensively used approaches for the green synthesis of nanoparticles is employing the use of plant extracts. Over the past decade, researchers have investigated the potential use of plants to synthesize metal nanoparticles as an alternative source for drug production [6, 38]. Plants are well recognized for their metal accumulation properties and these accumulated metals are later reduced to nanomaterials intracellularly [8]. Although the precise mechanism of nanoparticles synthesized by different plant extracts is unclear, the bioactive compounds in plants have been shown to play an important role in the stabilization, reduction, and capping of metal ions [18, 39]. Numerous phytochemical classes such as alkaloids, phenols, terpenes, flavonoids, terpenoids, tannins, polysaccharides, and saponins have been identified as capable of producing metal nanoparticles [40]. The utilization of plant extracts to synthesize metal nanoparticles was introduced by Shankar *et al.* [41]. Their study focused on the extraction of phytocompounds responsible for the reduction of metal ions which was further used in a synthetic reaction medium to extracellularly produce nanoparticles [12]. This protocol offers several advantages compared to using whole plants. For example, the formation of nanoparticles occurs considerably faster compared to whole plants that require the diffusion of metal ions throughout the plant body. Despite this, the use of plant extracts in nanoparticle formation still appears to be cheaper due to the ease of purification in comparison to microbe-mediated synthesis. Generally, compared to green synthesis using bacteria and fungi, the plant options are often a preferred method because plants are readily available, less toxic, their stability can be controlled, are safer to handle, and can reduce metal ions much faster [4]. Karmous *et al.* [9] addressed the utilization of plant extracts to produce silver, gold, and zinc oxide nanoparticles for cancer therapy over the past 5 years on the plant-mediated synthesis of metal nanoparticles and their anticancer activity in different cell lines.

## 3.4. Enzymes and Biomolecules

The use of biomolecules as a template to synthesize metal nanoparticles has recently emerged in the field of nanotechnology showing significant potential for application in biomedicine [42]. In the method of bioreduction, development, and stabilization of metal nanoparticles, plant biomolecules such as alkaloids, amino acids, proteins/enzymes, alcoholic compounds, polysaccharides, and vitamins are used [8, 43]. The ion reduction potential of medicinal plants dependable on the presence of enzymes, polyphenols, and other metal-binding chemical compounds present in plants have critical effects on the amounts of nanoparticles produced [13, 43, 44]. Furthermore, naturally occurring molecules such as vitamins D, B12, C, and E have also been used to produce nanoparticles of platinum, silver, and gold [2, 44]. Up to now, several types of proteins have been used as templates for the production of various nanostructured materials. Proteins and peptides such as apopheritin, bovine serum albumine (BSA), lysozyme, and tryptophan-based peptides have also been used to synthesize metal nanoparticles [2, 43]. The use of proteins as bio-templates appears to be a promising method for the synthesis of nanoparticles. Certain proteins such as ferritin, ferritin-like protein (FLP), sapronin, and chlorotic cowpea virus (CCMV), have cavities in the medium. The protein cavity can be used as a growth template for nanoparticles. Proteins provide excellent scaffolds for the template-driven arrangement of specially formed nanostructured materials. In addition, the biologically designated nanomaterial can be easily changed to adjust its normal functions and properties [45]. In addition, nanotechnology has recently pushed DNA to be used as a reducing agent due to the strong affinity of the DNA bases for silver salts, making it a template stabilizer [3, 17, 42]. These biotemplates are often used not only to create nanoparticles but also to obtain clusters, superlattices, or hierarchical structures of various structures [45]. In biomedical applications, however, the use of biotemplates to synthesize nanoparticles is not widely used because biotemplate methods are superior in selectivity and sensitivity over the existing techniques.

## 3.5. Characterization of Nanoparticles

Newly synthesized metal nanoparticles are often characterized using the following techniques as presented in Fig. (**1**).

### • Colour Change

A colour change in the reaction mixture is the first step which indicates that the nanoparticles were synthesized [16]. This colour change following bioreduction is a result of the excitation of the surface plasmon resonance (SPR) in the newly synthesized nanoparticles, thus confirming the bioreduction of metal ions in the reaction between the biological extract and metallic solution [9]. The colour change observed is a clear to light yellow solution to a dark brown to red solution for AgNPs [36]. In AuNPs colour change observed was pink-ruby red [6]. This colour change seems to be consistent for metal nanoparticles. ZnONPs are characterized by the formation of a white precipitate in the reaction medium [37].

### • UV-visible Spectrophotometry

A UV-Vis spectrophotometer is used to track the reduction of pure metal ions [6]. This technique is to determine the formation and stability of metallic nanoparticles [6, 46]. The SPRs that shifts to longer wavelengths with growing particle size is reported to be the optical absorption spectrum of metallic nanoparticles [5]. The presence of SPR peaks provides a functional signature for the creation of nanoparticles. In a range between 300 to 700 nm, the absorption spectrum of the metal nanoparticles is formed. The SPR phenomenon is responsible for the high absorption of AgNP, AuNP, and ZnONP in the visible region, with a maximum range of 400 to 550 nm [5, 47].

### • Fourier Transform Infrared Spectroscopy (FT-IR)

Measurements of Fourier infrared transformers (FT-IR) define possible biomolecules responsible for reducing, covering, and stabilizing nanoparticles from metals and for the local molecular environment of nanoparticle blockers [4]. FT-IR spectroscopy also recognizes surface residues, such as functional groups (carbonyls and hydroxyl moieties), during metal nanoparticle synthesis [12, 21]. Reported absorbance bands of metal nanoparticles are in the range 1000-1700 cm$^{-1}$, 2100-2900 cm$^{-1}$, and 3000-3350cm$^{-1}$ [5, 17]. These absorbance bands are known to be linked with stretching vibrations for –C–O–C–, ether linkages, –C–O–, terminal methyls, –C–C– groups or from aromatic rings and alkyne bonds, respectively [12, 17]. At 1500-1650 cm$^{-1}$, the peak range is similar to that recorded for proteins indicating that proteins interacted with nanoparticles [1, 27]. Absorption peaks between 3200–3700 cm$^{-1}$ are potential alcohols (O–H bands) derived from proteins and carbohydrates [1]. The overall regions of 3300 cm – 1 showed an effective spectrum of carboxylic bands from oxygen and hydrogen (O–H) [1, 6]. FT-IR analyses of ZnONPs revealed the formation of nanoparticles through the involvement of alcohol, amide, carboxylic acid, carbonate groups, alkane, and amine [27].

### • X-ray Diffraction (XRD)

X-ray diffraction is one of the most used nanoparticle characterization techniques [34, 47]. Typically, XRD provides information regarding crystal structure, phase nature, lattice parameters, and crystal grain size. The benefit of XRD techniques, usually conducted on samples in powder form, is that these contribute to statistically representative average volume values, usually after their respective colloidal solutions have been dried [40]. XRD patterns for AuNPs in cancer therapy under optimum conditions usually peaks at angles at 20.32 °. 38. 32 °, 46.16 °, 57.50 °, and 76.81° [3, 11]. The XRD patterns for AgNPs showed diffraction peaks at about 38.183°, 46.287 °, 64.530 ° and 77.43 ° [11]. XRD patterns for ZnONPs were 21.52 °, 48. 34 °, 29, 46.13 °, 59.42 °, and 78.61° [27]. The XRD of the above-mentioned patterns reveals that the metal nanoparticles are crystalline due to their strong and narrow diffraction peaks [11, 27].

## • Scanning Electron Microscopy (SEM)

SEM is used to identify the shape and morphology of the nanoparticle cluster [19, 46]. This technique of surface imaging uses the electron beam to scan the nanoparticle surface to generate images as signals that correspond to the atomic composition and other topographical information [1]. The resolution of SEM is equivalent to or below 1 nm. Based on research findings, the morphology of AgNPs and AuNPs are mainly spherical with few triangular and cubic shapes, whilst ZnONPs are mainly spherical and hexagonal [3, 9, 27].

## • Transmission Electron Microscopy (TEM)

The size and shape of newly synthesized metal nanoparticles are characterized with TEM [5, 46]. Whilst TEM produces similar results as SEM, TEM is often the preferred choice as it provides better spatial resolution, hence analytic measurements can be obtained [7]. TEM micrographs show that AuNPs primarily have spherical shapes and the nanoparticles' typical size can be found in the range of 40-100 nm, whilst AgNPs are in the size range of 10-100 nm [1, 11]. The average size for ZnONPs is within the range of 50-100 nm [27]. As previously mentioned in cancer therapy the desired size of metal nanoparticles ranges between 70 –150 nm [6].

## • Energy-dispersive X-ray Spectroscopy (EDX/EDS)

In EDX analyses, the composition is determined and the presence of metal ions in the synthesized nanoparticle reaction media is confirmed [3]. Also, the basic composition of nanoparticles can be calculated through EDS mapping [21, 48].

## • Dynamic Light Scattering (DLS)

DLS spectroscopy can be used to measure the distribution and quantification of the surface charges of the metal nanoparticles suspended in a solution [21, 49]. Nanoparticle size in DLS differs from TEM possibly due to the agglomeration and stability of the particles. DLS for AuNPs demonstrated a mean size range of 154 nm [3]. The typical size range of AgNPs was 176.5 nm [11], whilst ZnONPs revealed a size range of 184 nm [27].

UV-Vis spec: Ultraviolet-Visible Spectrophotometry; FT-IR: Fourier Transform Infrared Spectroscopy; TEM: Transmission Electron Microscopy; SEM: Scanning Electron Microscopy; EDX/EDS: Energy-Dispersive X-Ray Spectroscopy; XRD: X-Ray Diffraction; DLS: Dynamic Light Scattering; XPS: X-ray photoelectron spectroscopy; AFM: Atomic Force Microscopy.

## 4. Application of Green Synthesized Nanoparticles in Cancer Therapy

Cancer is one of the most life-threatening human health problems and was responsible for an estimated 9.6 million deaths worldwide in 2018 [1, 13, 50]. Based on a global report, it has been speculated that cancer diagnosis and deaths will rise by 44% by 2030 if the incidence of the disease continues at the current rate [13]. The most common cancers are those affecting the lungs, breast, prostate, colorectal, skin, and stomach [13]. By avoiding risk factors such as obesity, alcohol consumption, smoking, harsh chemicals, excessive radiation exposure; embracing early diagnosis and adopting existing evidence-based preventive and appropriate treatment options, about 30-50 percent of currently known cancers and their burden can be avoided or greatly reduced [8, 13]. In addition to chemotherapy and other orthodox treatment options for the control and prevention of cancer, novel technologies and new therapeutic agents including the use of bio-nanoparticles are being explored. The utilization of nanoparticles for early diagnosis and treatment of cancer has recently gained momentum and fast-evolving into a focused research area in nanotechnology [8, 31, 50]. Specifically, the metal-green synthesized nanoparticles are being studied and can act under laser irradiation as effective photothermal transducers for triggering localized hyperthermia of cancer cells [22]. Adeola *et al.* [50] presented in their review a good understanding of the role of nanoparticles in cancer therapy.

**Table 1. Updated list of green synthesized nanoparticles with anticancer activity.**

| Nanomaterial | Type of Biological Approach | Species Name | Part (s)Substance Used | Cancer Cell Line (s) | Proposed Mechanism(s) | Reference |
|---|---|---|---|---|---|---|
| Silver | Biomolecules | *Matricaria chamomilla* L. | Leaves | A549 lung cancer cells | *In vitro* down-regulation of an anti-apoptotic gene (Bcl-2) and up-regulation of the pro-apoptotic members (Bax, caspase-3, and caspase-7) | [53] |
| Zinc oxide | Plant extract | *Mangifera indica* L. | Leaves | A549 lung cancer cells | *In vitro*, nanoparticle penetrates the cell membrane resulting in DNA degeneration | [37] |

*(Table 1) cont.....*

| Nanomaterial | Type of Biological Approach | Species Name | Part (s)Substance Used | Cancer Cell Line (s) | Proposed Mechanism(s) | Reference |
|---|---|---|---|---|---|---|
| Silver | Plant extract | *Cleome viscosa* L. | Fruits | A549 lung cancer cells and PAI ovarian cancer cells | *in vitro*, inhibition of tumour cells with the lowest $IC_{50}$ concentration of 28 mg/ml. | [54] |
| Silver & gold | Plant extract | *Dendropanax morbifera* Leveille. | Leaves | A549 lung cancer cells | Induced *in vitro* cell death *via* necrosis | [12] |
| Silver | Plant extract | *Dodonaea viscosa* Jacq. | Leaves | A549 lung cancer cells | Induced cell death *via* apoptosis | [55] |
| Silver | Plant extract | *Centella asiatica* L. | Leaves | MCF-7 breast cancer | Induced *in vitro* cell death *via* apoptosis | [56] |
| Silver | Plant extract | *Phoenix dactylifera* L. | Root hairs | MCF7 human breast cancer | *In vitro*, cell viability of MCF7 cell lines is reduced with $IC_{50}$ concentration of 29.6 µg/ml. | [57] |
| Zinc oxide | Plant extract | *Albizia lebbeck* (L) Benth. | Stem bark | MCF-7 breast cancer cells | In MC F-7 breast cancer cell ZNONPs showed significant *in vitro* cytotoxic effects based on concentration. ($P< 0.001$, $n \geq 3$) | [58] |

*(Table 1) cont.....*

| Nanomaterial | Type of Biological Approach | Species Name | Part (s)Substance Used | Cancer Cell Line (s) | Proposed Mechanism(s) | Reference |
|---|---|---|---|---|---|---|
| Gold | Plant extract and Biomolecues | *Curcuma longa* L. | Leaves | MCF-7 human breast cancer | *In vitro* studies showed that conjugates of AuNPs-Cur, AuNPs-Tur, AuNPs-Qu and AuNPs-Pacli were effective in inhibiting cell proliferation, apoptosis, angiogenesis, colony formation, and spheroid formation | [59] |
| Gold | Plant extract | *Anacardium occidentale* L. | Leaves | MCF-7 human breast cancer | Cell viability of 71.5% on MCF-7 cells at a concentration of 100ng was observed. The IC50 values were found to be 6 mg/ml. *in vitro.* | [60] |
| Silver | Plant extract | *Ficus krishnae* C.DC. | Stem bark | SKOV-3 ovarian cancer cells | *In vitro* studies showed that AgNPs induce cytotoxicity in the SKOV-3 cells in a dose-dependent manner. | [25] |
| Silver | Plant extract | *Artemisia turcomanica* Gand. | Leaves | AGS (Human Gastric Adenocarcinoma IBRC C10071 | *In vitro* studies revealed AgNPs induced apoptosis in a dose and time-dependent manner. | [61] |
| Silver | Biomolecules | Chitosan-curcumin | - | HeLa cells | CSCurNPs induced apoptosis *in vitro* on cancer cells. | [62] |

*(Table 1) cont.....*

| Nanomaterial | Type of Biological Approach | Species Name | Part (s)Substance Used | Cancer Cell Line (s) | Proposed Mechanism(s) | Reference |
|---|---|---|---|---|---|---|
| Zinc Oxide | Algae extract | *Sargassum muticum* (Yendo) Fensholt. | Thallus | Human liver (HepG2) cancer cells | Triggers cell cycle arrest | [63] |
| Silver | Plant extract | *Taraxacum officinale* (L.) Weber ex F.H.Wigg. | Leaves | Liver Hepato cellular Carcinoma HepG2 | Showed high cytotoxic effect. | [64] |
| Silver and gold | Plant extract | *Indigofera tinctoria* Mill. | Leaves | A549 lung cancer cells | Cell viability decreases with increasing NP concentration | [65] |
| Silver | Plant extract biomolecules | *Beta vulgaris* L. | Roots | HuH-7 Human Hepatic Cells | Induce apoptosis *in vitro* | [66] |
| Silver | Plant extract | *Clinacanthus nutans (Burm.f.) Lindau* | Leaves | NSC-4Oral squamous cell carcinoma | Induce apoptosis *in vitro* | [67] |
| Silver | Fungal extract | *Rhodotorula mucilaginosa Rhodotorula glutinis* (T. Haseg. & I. Banno) Fell, J.P. Samp. & Gadanho | Leaves | HK-2 (human kidney cells) | Induced cytotoxicity at a concentration of 0.08–2.5 µg/ml, *in vitro* | [68] |
| Gold | Algae extract | *Gracilaria verrucosa* (Hudson) Papenfuss | Thallus | HEK-293 Kidney cells | Induced apoptosis at an IC50 concentration of 43.09 ± 1.6 µg/ml. | [69] |
| Zinc oxide | Plant extract | *Rehmannia glutinosa* (Gaertn.) DC. | Roots | MG-63 bone cancer cells | Initiated increased generation of ROS and decreased MMP | [40] |
| Silver | Plant extract | *Scutellaria barbata* L. | Leaves | Pancreatic cancer cell (PANC☐1) | Induces apoptosis in a time and concentration dependent manner. | [70] |

Barabadi *et al.* [51] recently reviewed the anticancer activity of metal nanoparticles against different cancer cell lines using plant extracts and microbes and highlighted that *in vivo* mechanisms are crucial to the delivery of metal nanoparticles into the cancer cells. Similarly, Goel and Bhatia [52] also reported the effectiveness of green synthesized metal nanoparticles in cancer therapy by using a variety of medicinal plant extracts. Their study highlighted the *in vitro* mechanisms against various cancer cell lines. However, their review was not as extensive as Barabadi *et al.* [51] as their literature survey focused on studies before 2017. In the latest development in 2020, Alphandéry [8] appraised both the *in vitro* and *in vivo* anticancer efficacies of gold and silver nanoparticles using plant extracts and microbes. Despite these reports on the activity of NPs in cancer therapy, there are still several uncaptured data. Therefore, the findings of our review focusing on unreported literature from 2018-2020 are enumerated in Table **1** with citations.

Literature searches have uncovered studies of plant extracts, biomolecules, and microbes used for metal NPs preparation. Nanoparticles synthesized with the contribution of biological sources showed significant inhibitory activities against the viability of certain cancer cell lines. Many of these NPs were either toxic to the cancer cell lines or inhibited their growth. Moreover, some research outcomes showed that the half-maximal inhibitory concentration ($IC_{50}$) of NPs was dependent upon the dosage of concentration and incubation time. In 2018, Dadaspour *et al.* [53], demonstrated that the plant-mediated synthesized AgNPs exert *in vitro* cytotoxic effects of A549 lung cancer cells through an anti-apoptotic gene (Bcl-2) down-regulation and proapoptotic (Bax, Caspase-3, and Caspase-7) up-regulation of the pro-apoptotic members after exposing to AgNPs 63 μM for 24 hours and 42.5 μM for 48 hours respectively. However, they found that further research is required to provide insight into the mechanisms of the stimulated cancer effects of the AgNPs studied. Another study by Rajeskumar *et al.* [37], found that the anticancer activity of ZnONPs on A549 lung cancer cells increased with increasing concentration (1-100 mg/ml) of nanoparticles, which was comparable to cyclophosphamide cytotoxic effects at low doses. The concentration of the nanoparticles administered plays an important part in anti-cancer activity since the nanoparticles can reach the cell membrane *via* cell membranes' ion channels and interact with DNA and intracellular nitrogenous base proteins. However, this warrants further investigation to determine the desired dosage concentration. Furthermore, Lakshmanan *et al.* [54], reported a substantial *in vitro* anticancer activity against lung cancer (A549) and ovarian cancer (PAI) cell lines with minimum $IC_{50}$ concentration at 28 and 30 mg/ml respectively when administered with AgNPs synthesized using the fruit extract of *Cleome viscosa*. The nanoparticles ranged from 20 to 50 nm in size. Wang *et al.* [12] also synthesized AgNPs and AuNPs using *Dendropanax morbifera* leaf extract. The results indicated the AgNPs to be potently cytotoxic to the lung cancer cells at 100 μg/ml after 48 hours' exposure period, whereas AuNPs displayed no cytotoxicity at the same concentration in the cell lines. However, the cytotoxicity was increased after 48 hours in both AgNPs and AuNPs at 50 µg/ml. In a more recent 2019 *in vitro* study, the AgNPs synthesized using *Dodonaea viscosa* aqueous leaf extracts elicited a potential therapeutic effect against lung cancer (A549) cell lines [55]. After 24-hour treatments with AgNPs synthesized using methanol, acetone, acetonitrile, and water extracts, cells have been induced to death at slightly lower concentration levels: 49.11, 52.30, 51.23, and 49.98 µg/ml, respectively. The $IC_{50}$ values for the AgNPs were 14 µg/ml, 3 µg/ml, 80 µg/ml and 4 µg/ml.

The leaf extracts of *Centella asiatica* effectively synthesized silver nanoparticles and revealed that AgNPs were effective against human breast cancer (MCF-7) cell lines *via* apoptosis [56]. Similarly, *Phoenix dactylifera* extract mediated green silver nanoparticle synthesis was also reported to exhibit anticancer properties on MCF-7 cell lines *via* apoptosis [57]. In another study, Umar *et al.* [58], used *Albizia lebbeck* mediated ZnONPs against MCF-7 cancer cell lines and found increased cytotoxic effects in a concentration-dependent manner at a concentration of 5 µg/ml dose of 0.05 M ZnONPs showing less than 50% cancerous cell viability after 24 hours. In more recent studies, Vemuri *et al.* [59], used molecular modeling studies for the synthesis and evaluation of gold nanoparticles using *Curcuma longa*. Their findings revealed that the nanoconjugates (AuNPs-Cur 79.1 ug/cell; AuNPs-Tur 88.1 ug/cell; AuNPs-Qu 79.2 ug/cell, and AuNPs-Pacli 144.1 ug/cell) effectively prevented cell proliferation, apoptosis, angiogenesis, colony formation, and spheroid formation. Compared to a single treatment for MCF-7 breast cell lines, the synergistic effect of the conjugate was more successful. Similarly, Sunderam *et al.* [60] also reported *in vitro* cytotoxicity of AgNPs using *Anacardium occidentale* leaf extract. Their findings revealed cell viability of 71.5% on MCF-7 cells at a concentration of 100 ng and an $IC_{50}$ value of 6 mg/ml. Kanjikar *et al.* [25] reported that SKOV-3 cancer cell lines have shown notable *in-vitro* cytotoxicity at a concentration of 22,85 mg/ml when administered with *Ficus krishnae* stem bark synthesized ANPs. The findings of Mousavi *et al.* [61], showed that plant-mediated AgNPs induced apoptosis on AGS gastric cancer cells *in vitro* in a dose and time-dependent manner. The highest activity against AGS cells (95% and 84%) was observed at 100 µg/ml, and the $IC_{50}$ value of the AgNPs was 4.88l g/ml. Yadav *et al.* [62], investigated the enhancement of anticancer activity and drug delivery of chitosan-curcumin nanoparticles through molecular docking and *in vivo* simulation analysis. DNA injury, cell-cycle blockage, and elevated ROS levels were concluded in their analysis, confirming the CSCurNPs' anticancer activity following apoptotic pathways.

In recent works, Sanaeimehr *et al.* [63], synthesized ZnONPs using *Sargassum muticum* extract and evaluated its potential against human liver cancer (HepG2) cell lines *in vitro*. In their research it has been shown that cell cycle arrest is the preliminary event of cell death triggered by ZnONPs in all cells, resulting in cell death of HepG2 cell line following 48 hours of incubation. More than half of the cells (55.5%) still survived at the lowest concentration (175 µg/ml) of ZnONPs. Cell viability of the cells was reduced to less than 40% at concentrations (350, 700, 1400 µg/ml). More than 95% of the cells were dead at the maximum concentration (2800 µg/ml) of ZnONPs, and the survival rate of HepG2 cells was 4.5% at incubation periods of 24, 48, and 72 hours, respectively. The $IC_{50}$ values were calculated as 150 µg/ml at 48 hours of ZnONPS exposure time. In another, *in vitro* study, Saratale *et al.* [64], reported the biosynthesized AgNPs using *Taraxacum officinale* exhibited a high cytotoxic effect in HepG2 cancer cell lines. Their findings showed that the required concentration for 50% inhibition of cell viability ($IC_{50}$) was approximately 60 µg/ml and, at a higher concentration of 200 µg/ml, AgNPs showed significant inhibition of cell growth of approximately 95%. Similarly, Vijayan *et al.* [65] reported an enhanced antioxidant activity and more cytotoxic effect on lung cancer cells for AuNPs ($IC_{50}$ $59.33 \pm 0.57$ µg/ml) in comparison to AgNPs ($IC_{50}$ $56.62 \pm 0.86$ µg/ml) using *Indigofera tinctoria* for nanoparticle synthesis. However, both types of nanoparticles showed remarkable anticancer activity. Bin-jumah *et al.* [66], also evaluated the *in vitro* effects of AgNPs synthesized using *Beta vulgaris* root extracts on oxidative stress and apoptosis on cancerous human hepatic cells. Their findings suggested that AgNPs induced more ROS in the Human Hepatic cells causing DNA damage and apoptosis. They also concluded that the apoptosis induced by AgNPs was initiated by the activation of caspase-3, which was observed at 20 and 40 µg/ml; but higher concentrations of AgNPs were needed to bring about sufficient cytotoxic effect.

Yakop *et al.* [67] reported apoptotic effects observed at the G1 phase and $IC_{50}$ (1.61 µg/ml) when AgNPs (highest concentration- 3 µg/ml) synthesized from *Clinacanthus nutans* leaf extract and administered towards HSC-4 cell lines (oral squamous cell carcinoma cell lines). Cunha *et al.* [68], used fungal strains (*Rhodotorula glutinis* and *Rhodotorula mucilaginosa*) to synthesize AgNPs resulting in reasonable *in vitro* cytotoxicity to the cells of the renal glomerular system at high concentrations above 10 µg/ml. Chellapandian *et al.* [69], explored the use of red algae synthesized AuNPs against normal human embryonic kidney (HEK-293) cells, showing the non-toxic and biocompatibility nature of newly synthesized AuNPs at high concentrations (100 µg/ml). A slight cell death (< 10%) was noticed after a 24-hour exposure of the HEK-293 cells to the highest concentration (100 µg/ml) of the AuNPs. In a current study by Cheng *et al.* [26], ZnONPs have also been shown to initiate increased ROS generation and decreased mitochondrial membrane potential (MMP). Reduced MMP resulted in higher levels of the apoptotic proteins Bax, caspase-9, and caspase-3, and apoptosis induction was corroborated by Western blot analysis. The results of their work proposed that Rehmanniae Radix (RR) ZnONPs exhibit an effective anticancer action and apoptosis is induced on the MG-63 cells by stimulating higher ROS generation. Thus, RR ZnONPs could be employed as a promising drug target against various cancer cell lines. The use of *Scutellaria barbata* leaf extract to effectively synthesize AuNPs as an anticancer agent against pancreatic cancer cells (PANC-1) was investigated by Wang *et al* [70]. The AuNPS showed a significant ($p < 0.001$) cytotoxic activity against the pancreatic cancer cell lines and cell viability was gradually reduced in a time and dose-dependent manner. Twenty-five (25) ug/ml resulted in a 50% viability and 100 ug/ml resulted in a 25% viability of cancerous cells after 72 hours.

## 5. The Pros and Cons of Green Synthesized Nanoparticles in Cancer Therapy

The significance of nanoparticles in cancer therapy has been well documented. Nanoparticles provide a more targeted approach to cancer therapy, thus, preventing adverse effects such as fluctuating weight issues, hair loss, anemia, appetite loss, fertility issues in men and women, nausea and vomiting, insomnia, low sex drive in men and women, body aches and pains, delirium, peripheral neuropathy, fatigue, edema, bleeding and bruising, constipation, and skin discolouration, normally experienced with conventional chemotherapies [3, 6, 13]. Whilst there are many benefits in using green synthesized metal nanoparticles in cancer therapy, they do have their limitations ranging from toxic at higher doses, limited clinical trials to support research findings, time-consuming, environmental concerns resulting in over-harvesting of plant material, and low adsorption in certain serum proteins thus rendering it ineffective (Fig. **2**) [29].

Furthermore, Adeola *et al.* [50] reported the possibility that nanoparticles are transported through body fluids and are thus absorbed into other tissues/organisms in addition to the target cell, where their preventive or therapeutic effect originally was intended. This is due to the high nanoparticle volume-to-surface ratio.

Consequent to the available data in this review, it is clear that much attention has been focused on metal (silver, gold, and zinc) nanoparticles, with those of silver being the most commonly explored for cancer therapy [3, 6, 8, 18]. Despite this, the use of AgNPs has some toxicities and drawbacks. Therefore, the criteria for secure use of AgNPs in biological and clinical applications, including cancer therapy, should always be established. Generally, green synthesized AgNPs exhibited significant anticancer activity with little to no toxic effect but are dependent on the agents used to reduce and convert silver nitrate into silver. However, there is still a lack of authenticated information regarding the exposure of humans to AgNPs and the potential risks concerning their short-term and long-term harmful toxic effects. Besides, information on other metal/metal-oxide nanoparticles is scarce and this could form a basis for studies aimed at finding new nanotechnological approaches to successfully combatting cancer using other metals [8].

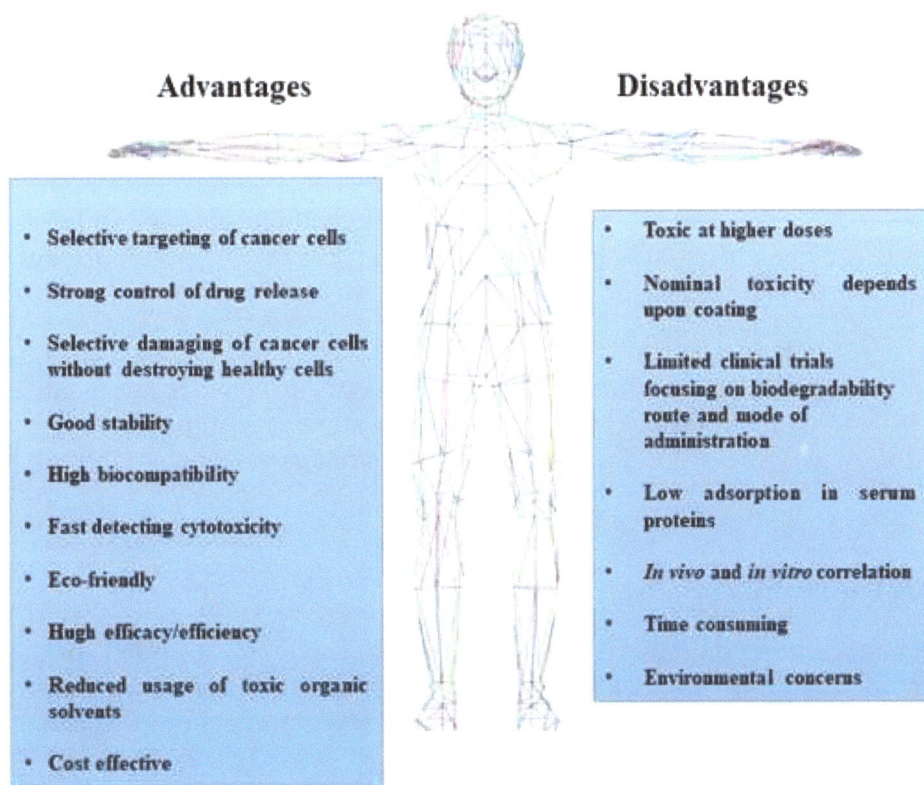

**Advantages**

- Selective targeting of cancer cells
- Strong control of drug release
- Selective damaging of cancer cells without destroying healthy cells
- Good stability
- High biocompatibility
- Fast detecting cytotoxicity
- Eco-friendly
- Hugh efficacy/efficiency
- Reduced usage of toxic organic solvents
- Cost effective

**Disadvantages**

- Toxic at higher doses
- Nominal toxicity depends upon coating
- Limited clinical trials focusing on biodegradability route and mode of administration
- Low adsorption in serum proteins
- *In vivo* and *in vitro* correlation
- Time consuming
- Environmental concerns

**Fig. (2).** The advantages and disadvantages of green synthesized metal nanoparticles in cancer therapy.

Green synthesis using plant extracts has received more attention as a suitable alternative to other biological processes [31, 40]. Many authors proposed reaction mechanisms based on their experimental results, although many of these submissions are characterized by a lack of conclusive evidence. The literature indicates that researchers are now exploring marine organisms for metallic nanoparticle synthesis as seaweeds contain various biologically active compounds, which enables them to act as "nanofactories" [45, 67, 71]. These macroalgae are inferred to have great potential as anticancer agents. Therefore, it is necessary to explore its role in green synthesis on a larger scale. Overall, there is a high potential for metallic nanoparticles to cross the regulatory barrier in clinical use as effective therapies in treating cancer. However, the majority of the substances used to synthesize these nanoparticles have yet to be approved by the main supervising agencies, such as the Food and Drug Administration (FDA) and the European Medicines Agency (EMA). The ultimate goal of using nanoparticles in therapeutics is to utilize the minimum dose of the nanoparticle to achieve the desired effect in the shortest time. However, these parameters have not yet been defined by research experts. Green synthesized metal nanoparticles have proved to be effective tools against various cancer cell lines [9, 18, 39], but, further investigation is needed to improve nanoparticle selectivity on cancer cells, and to evaluate biocompatibility and side effect with the use of animal models. Another limitation is the large production and marketing of biocompatible nanostructures with regulated sizes and shapes. Recently, researchers have been concentrating on large-scale culture techniques for synthesizing nanoparticles that are scalable and replicable with a narrow size distribution [3, 71]. However, these bulk culture techniques need to be improved for bio nanoparticles and downstream processing.

It was significant to note that most researchers explore *in vitro* mechanisms in cancer therapy. Whilst it is important to note that *in vitro* studies are required to begin *in vivo* studies, consequently, *in vivo* studies may reveal different findings in the future as some of the *in vivo* conditions may not be simulated through *in vitro* studies [51].

## CONCLUDING REMARKS AND PERSPECTIVES

Green nanoparticle synthesis is currently being exploited, and the study has become a priority of researchers in developing effective and environmentally friendly nanoparticles synthesis methods. The production of metallic nanoparticles with bio-organisms is one of the most desired methods. Plants seem to be the favoured approach amongst these organisms, as they are suitable for large-scale nanoparticle synthesis, are more stable, the synthesis speed is faster, low-cost, safer to handle, and they are readily available compared to the use of microorganisms. Plants are also known to possess bioactive compounds that yield many biological activities against a variety of human ailments. However, considering the plant's diversity and chemistry, more attempts should be made to explain the process through experimental techniques. Our literature findings suggest that metal nanoparticles have great potential as anticancer agents and drug delivery systems as they can be used to directly target cancer cells and optimize the biodistribution of drugs. Silver nanoparticles seemed to be the most commonly used metal of choice for synthesis, but over the years, the use of gold and zinc oxide nanoparticles has become quite interesting. Also, the anticancer potential of green synthesized metal nanoparticles could play an important role in the development of a new therapeutic agent for the treatment of targeted cancer cells, and it is hoped that this review will assist future findings in developing novel metal-based nanoparticles using green technology.

## CONSENT FOR PUBLICATION

Not applicable.

## CONFLICT OF INTEREST

The authors declare no conflict of interest, financial or otherwise.

## ACKNOWLEDGEMENTS

Declared none.

## REFERENCES

[1]   Erjaee H, Rajan H, Nazifi S. Synthesis and characterization of novel silver nanoparticles using Chamaemelum nobile extract for antibacterial application. Adv Nat Sci: Nanosci Nanotechnol 2017; 8(9pp): 025004.

[2]   Mittal J, Batra A, Singh A, Sharma MM. Phytofabrication of nanoparticles through plants as nanofactories. Adv Nat Sci Nanosci Nanotech 2014; 8: 5-15.
[http://dx.doi.org/10.1088/2043-6262/5/4/043002]

[3]   Tikariha S, Singh S, Banerjee S, Vidyarthi AS. Biosynthesis of gold nanoparticles, scope, and application: A review. Int J Pharm Sci Res 2012; 3: 1603-313.

[4]   Devi SR, Selvan SAC. Greener synthesis and characterization of silver nanoparticles using *Murraya koenigii* leaf extract and its antibacterial activity. Int J Pharm Bio. Sci 2017; 8: 292-303.

[5]   Singh K, Naidoo Y, Mocktar C, Baijnath H. Biosynthesis of silver nanoparticles using Plumbago auriculata leaf and calyx extracts and evaluation of their antimicrobial activities. Adv Nat Sci Nanosci Nanotech 2018; 9: 1-9.
[http://dx.doi.org/10.1088/2043-6254/aad1a3]

[6]   Vijayaraghavan K, Ashokkumar T. Plant-mediated biosynthesis of metallic nanoparticles: A review of literature, factors affecting synthesis, characterization techniques, and applications. J Environ Chem Eng 2017; 5: 4866-83.
[http://dx.doi.org/10.1016/j.jece.2017.09.026]

[7]   Cunha FA, Cunha MDCSO, da Frota SM, *et al.* Biogenic synthesis of multifunctional silver nanoparticles from Rhodotorula glutinis and Rhodotorula mucilaginosa: antifungal, catalytic and cytotoxicity activities. World J Microbiol Biotechnol 2018; 34(9): 127-42.
[http://dx.doi.org/10.1007/s11274-018-2514-8] [PMID: 30084085]

[8]   Alphandéry E. Natural metallic nanoparticles for application in nano-oncology. Int J Mol Sci 2020; 21(12): 4412-30.
[http://dx.doi.org/10.3390/ijms21124412] [PMID: 32575884]

[9]   Karmous I, Pandey A, Haj KB, Chaoui A. Efficiency of the green synthesized nanoparticles as new tools in cancer therapy: insights on plant-based bioengineered nanoparticles, biophysical properties, and anticancer roles. Biol Trace Elem Res 2020; 196(1): 330-42.
[http://dx.doi.org/10.1007/s12011-019-01895-0] [PMID: 31512171]

[10]  Rajkuberan C, Prabukumar S, Sathishkumar G, Wilson A, *et al.* Facile synthesis of silver nanoparticles using *Euphorbia antiquorum* L. latex extract and evaluation of their biomedical perspectives as anticancer agents'. J Saudi Chem Soc 2017; 8: 911-9.
[http://dx.doi.org/10.1016/j.jscs.2016.01.002]

[11]  Wang C, Mathiyalagan R, Kim YJ, *et al.* Rapid green synthesis of silver and gold nanoparticles using Dendropanax morbifera leaf extract and their anticancer activities. Int J Nanomedicine 2016; 11:

3691-701.
[http://dx.doi.org/10.2147/IJN.S97181] [PMID: 27570451]

[12] Mittal AK, Chisti Y, Banerjee UC. Synthesis of metallic nanoparticles using plant extracts. Biotechnol Adv 2013; 31(2): 346-56.
[http://dx.doi.org/10.1016/j.biotechadv.2013.01.003] [PMID: 23318667]

[13] World Health Organization (WHO). Cancer: key facts 2020. Available from: https://www.who.int/news-room/fact-sheets/detail/cancer

[14] Shaik RM, Khan M, Kuniyil M, *et al.* Al-Warthan, A. Plant-Extract-Assisted Green Synthesis of Silver Nanoparticles Using *Origanum vulgare* L. Extract and Their Microbicidal Activities. Sustain 2018; 10: 913-25.
[http://dx.doi.org/10.3390/su10040913]

[15] Teimuri-Mofrad R, Hadi R, Tahmasebi B, *et al.* Green synthesis of gold nanoparticles using plant extract: Mini-review. Nanochem Res 2017; 2: 8-19.

[16] Iravani S, Korbekandi H, Mirmohammadi SV, Zolfaghari B. Synthesis of silver nanoparticles: chemical, physical and biological methods. Res Pharm Sci 2014; 9(6): 385-406.
[PMID: 26339255]

[17] Dickerson MB, Sandhage KH, Naik RR. Protein- and peptide-directed syntheses of inorganic materials. Chem Rev 2008; 108(11): 4935-78.
[http://dx.doi.org/10.1021/cr8002328] [PMID: 18973389]

[18] Ratan ZA, Haidere MF, Nurunnabi M, *et al.* Green chemistry synthesis of silver nanoparticles and their potential anticancer effects: A review. Cancers (Basel) 2020; 12(4): 855.
[http://dx.doi.org/10.3390/cancers12040855] [PMID: 32244822]

[19] Singh P, Pandit S, Mokkapati VRSS, Garg A, Ravikumar V, Mijakovic I. Gold nanoparticles in diagnostics and therapeutics for human cancer. Int J Mol Sci 2018; 19(7): 1979-95.
[http://dx.doi.org/10.3390/ijms19071979] [PMID: 29986450]

[20] Gahlawat G, Choudhury AR. A review on the biosynthesis of metal and metal salt nanoparticles by microbes. RSC Advances 2019; 9(23): 12944-67.
[http://dx.doi.org/10.1039/C8RA10483B] [PMID: 35520790]

[21] Ben Tahar I, Fickers P, Dziedzic A, Płoch D, Skóra B, Kus-Liśkiewicz M. Green pyomelanin-mediated synthesis of gold nanoparticles: modelling and design, physico-chemical and biological characteristics. Microb Cell Fact 2019; 18(1): 210-22.
[http://dx.doi.org/10.1186/s12934-019-1254-2] [PMID: 31796078]

[22] Bhattacharya R, Patra CR, Verma R, Griepp PR, Mukherjee P. Gold nanoparticles inhibit the proliferation of multiple myeloma cells. Adv Mater 2007; 19: 711-6.
[http://dx.doi.org/10.1002/adma.200602098]

[23] Bhattacharya R, Mukherjee P. Biological properties of "naked" metal nanoparticles. Adv Drug Deliv Rev 2008; 60(11): 1289-306.
[http://dx.doi.org/10.1016/j.addr.2008.03.013] [PMID: 18501989]

[24] Shen Q, Wang X, Fu D. The amplification effect of functionalized gold nanoparticles on the binding of cancer drug dacarbazine to DNA and DNA bases. Appl Surf Sci 2008; 255: 577-80.
[http://dx.doi.org/10.1016/j.apsusc.2008.06.132]

[25] Kanjikar AP, Hugar AL, Londonkar RL. Characterization of Phyto-nanoparticles from Ficus krishnae for their antibacterial and anticancer activities. Drug Dev Ind Pharm 2018; 44(3): 377-84.
[http://dx.doi.org/10.1080/03639045.2017.1386205]

[26] Cheng J, Wang X, Qiu L, Li Y, *et al.* Green synthesized zinc oxide nanoparticles regulate the apoptotic expression in bone cancer cells MG-63 cells. J Phytochem Phytobio B: Biol 2020; 202: 1011-34.
[http://dx.doi.org/10.1016/j.jphotobiol.2019.111644]

[27]    Kalpana VN, Devi Rajeswari V. A review on green synthesis, biomedical applications, and toxicity studies of ZNONPs. Bioinorg Chem Appl 2018; 2018: 3569758.
[http://dx.doi.org/10.1155/2018/3569758] [PMID: 30154832]

[28]    Boa Z, Lan CQ. Advances in the biosynthesis of noble metal nanoparticles mediated by photosynthetic organisms—A review. Coll Surf B: Biointer 2019; 184: 1-8.

[29]    Tiwary M, Jha AK. Biosynthesis of silver nanoparticles using plant extracts: New approach in agriculture and pharmaceuticals: A Review. Int J Inno Res Multidisc Field 2017; 3: 101-11.

[30]    Vadivu BS, Sivasankari R, Santhoshkumar K, Aswini V. A phytochemical synthesis of silver nanoparticles using *Curcuma longa* and their applications in antibacterial and dye degradation studies. Glo J Eng Sci Res Manage 2017; 4: 26-32.

[31]    Rafique M, Sadaf I, Rafique MS, Tahir MB. A review on green synthesis of silver nanoparticles and their applications. Artif Cells Nanomed Biotechnol 2017; 45(7): 1272-91.
[http://dx.doi.org/10.1080/21691401.2016.1241792] [PMID: 27825269]

[32]    Savithramma N, Linga Rao M, Rukmini K, Suvarnalatha Devi P. Antimicrobial activity of silver nanoparticles synthesized by using medicinal plants. Int J Chemtech Res 2011; 3: 1394-402.

[33]    Lee HJ, Lee G, Jang NR, *et al.* Biological synthesis of copper nanoparticles using plant extract. NSTI-Nanotech 2011; 1: 371-4.

[34]    Samadi N, Golkaran D, Eslamifar A, Jamalifar H, Fazeli MR, Mohseni FA. Intra/extracellular biosynthesis of silver nanoparticles by an autochthonous strain of *Proteus mirabilis* isolated from photographic waste. J Biomed Nanotechnol 2009; 5(3): 247-53.
[http://dx.doi.org/10.1166/jbn.2009.1029] [PMID: 20055006]

[35]    Shivaji S, Madhu S, Singh S. Extracellular synthesis of antibacterial silver nanoparticles using psychrophilic bacteria. Process Biochem 2011; 46: 1800-7.
[http://dx.doi.org/10.1016/j.procbio.2011.06.008]

[36]    Ahmad S, Munir S, Zeb N, *et al.* Green nanotechnology: a review on green synthesis of silver nanoparticles - an ecofriendly approach. Int J Nanomedicine 2019; 14: 5087-107.
[http://dx.doi.org/10.2147/IJN.S200254] [PMID: 31371949]

[37]    Rajeshkumar S, Kumar SV, Ramaiah A, Agarwal H, Lakshmi T, Roopan SM. Biosynthesis of zinc oxide nanoparticles usingMangifera indica leaves and evaluation of their antioxidant and cytotoxic properties in lung cancer (A549) cells. Microb Techn 2018; 117: 91-5.
[http://dx.doi.org/10.1016/j.enzmictec.2018.06.009] [PMID: 30037558]

[38]    Ahmed S, Ahmad SM, Swami BL, Ikram S. Green synthesis of silver nanoparticles using *Az4dirachta indica* aqueous leaf extract. J Rad Res App Sci 2016; 9: 1-7.

[39]    Khatoon N, Mazumder JA, Sardar M. Biotechnological applications of green synthesized silver nanoparticles J Nanosci. Curr Res 2017; 2: 107-16.

[40]    Chinnasamy C, Tamilselvan P, Karthik V, Karthik B. Optimization and characterization studies on green synthesis of silver nanoparticles using response surface methodology. Adv Nat App Sci 2017; 11: 214-21.

[41]    Shankar SS, Ahmad A, Sastry M. Geranium leaf assisted biosynthesis of silver nanoparticles. Biotechnol Prog 2003; 19(6): 1627-31.
[http://dx.doi.org/10.1021/bp034070w] [PMID: 14656132]

[42]    Lu R, Yang D, Cui D, Wang Z. Guo Egg white-mediated green synthesis of silver nanoparticles with excellent biocompatibility and enhanced radiation effects on cancer cells. Int J Nanomedicine 2012; 7: 2107-7.

[43]    Nasrollahzadeh M, Atarod M, Sajjadi M, Sajadi SM, Issaabadi Z. Plant-Mediated Green Synthesis of Nanostructures: Mechanisms, Characterization, and Applications.Interf Sci Tech. 2019; 28: pp. 199-322.

[44]    Iravani S. Green synthesis of metal nanoparticles using plants. Green Chem 2011; 13: 2638-51.
        [http://dx.doi.org/10.1039/c1gc15386b]

[45]    Arulmani S, Anandan S, Ashokkumar M. Introduction to Advanced Nanomaterials. Nanomaterials for
        green energy.Micro and Nano Technologies. 2018; pp. 1-53.

[46]    Shah M, Fawcett D, Sharma S, Tripathy SK, Poinern GEJ. Green synthesis of metallic nanoparticles
        *via* biological entities. Materials (Basel) 2015; 8(11): 7278-308.
        [http://dx.doi.org/10.3390/ma8115377] [PMID: 28793638]

[47]    Mourdikoudis S, Pallares RM, Thanh NTK. Characterization techniques for nanoparticles: comparison
        and complementarity upon studying nanoparticle properties. Nanoscale 2018; 10(27): 12871-934.
        [http://dx.doi.org/10.1039/C8NR02278J] [PMID: 29926865]

[48]    Yamada M, Foote M, Prow TW. Therapeutic gold, silver, and platinum nanoparticles. Wiley
        Interdiscip Rev Nanomed Nanobiotechnol 2015; 7(3): 428-45.
        [http://dx.doi.org/10.1002/wnan.1322] [PMID: 25521618]

[49]    Nath D, Banerjee P. Green nanotechnology – A new hope for medical biology. Env Tox Pharm 36:
        997-1014.

[50]    Adeola HA, Sabiu S, Adekiya TA, *et al.* Prospects of nanodentistry for the diagnosis and treatment of
        maxillofacial pathologies and cancers. Heliyon 2020; 6: 9.
        [http://dx.doi.org/10.1016/j.heliyon.2020.e04890]

[51]    Barabadi H, Ovais M, Shinwari ZK, Saravanan M. Anti-cancer green bionanomaterials: present status
        and future prospects. Green Chem Lett Rev 2017; 10: 285-314.
        [http://dx.doi.org/10.1080/17518253.2017.1385856]

[52]    Goel A, Bhatia AK. Phytosynthesized Nanoparticles for effective cancer treatment: A review. Nanosci
        Nanotech-Asia 2019; 9: 001-9.
        [http://dx.doi.org/10.2174/2210681208666180724100646]

[53]    Dadashpour M, Firouzi-Amandi A, Pourhassan-Moghaddam M, *et al.* Biomimetic synthesis of silver
        nanoparticles using *Matricaria chamomilla* extract and their potential anticancer activity against
        human lung cancer cells. Mater Sci Eng C 2018; 92: 902-12.
        [http://dx.doi.org/10.1016/j.msec.2018.07.053] [PMID: 30184820]

[54]    Lakshmanan G, Sathiyaseelan A, Kalaichelvan P, Murugesan K. Plant-mediated synthesis of silver
        nanoparticles using fruit extract of *Cleome viscosa* L.: assessment of their antibacterial and anticancer
        activity. Karbala Int J Mod Sci 2018; 1: 61-8.

[55]    Anandan M, Poorani G, Boomi P, *et al.* Green synthesis of anisotropic silver nanoparticles from the
        aqueous leaf extract of *Dodonaea viscosa* with their antibacterial and anticancer activities. Process
        Biochem 2019; 80: 80-8.
        [http://dx.doi.org/10.1016/j.procbio.2019.02.014]

[56]    Fard SE, Tafvizi F, Torbati MB. Silver nanoparticles biosynthesised using *Centella asiatica* leaf
        extract: apoptosis induction in MCF-7 breast cancer cell line. IET Nanobiotechnol 2018; 12(7): 994-
        1002.
        [http://dx.doi.org/10.1049/iet-nbt.2018.5069] [PMID: 30247143]

[57]    Oves M, Aslam M, Rauf MA, *et al.* Antimicrobial and anticancer activities of silver nanoparticles
        synthesized from the root hair extract of *Phoenix dactylifera.* Mater Sci Eng C 2018; 89: 429-43.
        [http://dx.doi.org/10.1016/j.msec.2018.03.035] [PMID: 29752116]

[58]    Umar H, Kavaz D, Rizaner N. Biosynthesis of zinc oxide nanoparticles using *Albizia lebbeck* stem
        bark, and evaluation of its antimicrobial, antioxidant, and cytotoxic activities on human breast cancer
        cell lines. Int J Nanomedicine 2018; 14: 87-100.
        [http://dx.doi.org/10.2147/IJN.S186888] [PMID: 30587987]

[59]    Vemuri SK, Banala RR, Mukherjee S, *et al.* Novel biosynthesized gold nanoparticles as anti-cancer

agents against breast cancer: Synthesis, biological evaluation, molecular modelling studies. Mater Sci Eng C 2019; 99: 417-29.
[http://dx.doi.org/10.1016/j.msec.2019.01.123] [PMID: 30889716]

[60]    Sunderam V, Thiyagarajan D, Lawrence AV, Mohammed SSS, Selvaraj A. *In-vitro* antimicrobial and anticancer properties of green synthesized gold nanoparticles using *Anacardium occidentale* leaves extract. Saudi J Biol Sci 2019; 26(3): 455-9.
[http://dx.doi.org/10.1016/j.sjbs.2018.12.001] [PMID: 30899157]

[61]    Mousavi B, Tafvizi F, Zaker Bostanabad S. Green synthesis of silver nanoparticles using *Artemisia turcomanica* leaf extract and the study of anti-cancer effect and apoptosis induction on gastric cancer cell line (AGS). Artif Cells Nanomed Biotechnol 2018; 46(sup1): 499-510.
[http://dx.doi.org/10.1080/21691401.2018.1430697] [PMID: 29361855]

[62]    Yadav P, Bandyopadhyay A, Chakraborty A, Sarkar K. Enhancement of anticancer activity and drug delivery of chitosan-curcumin nanoparticle *via* molecular docking and simulation analysis. Carb Poly 2018; 182: 188-98.
[http://dx.doi.org/10.1016/j.carbpol.2017.10.102] [PMID: 29279114]

[63]    Sanaeimehr Z, Javadi I, Namvar F. Antiangiogenic and antiapoptotic effects of green-synthesized zinc oxide nanoparticles using Sargassum muticum algae extraction Cancer Nanotech 2018; 9: 3-19.

[64]    Saratale RG, Benelli G, Kumar G, Kim DS, Saratale GD. Bio-fabrication of silver nanoparticles using the leaf extract of an ancient herbal medicine, dandelion (Taraxacum officinale), evaluation of their antioxidant, anticancer potential, and antimicrobial activity against phytopathogens. Environ Sci Pollut Res Int 2018; 25(11): 10392-406.
[http://dx.doi.org/10.1007/s11356-017-9581-5] [PMID: 28699009]

[65]    Vijayan R, Joseph S, Mathew B. Indigofera tinctoria leaf extract mediated green synthesis of silver and gold nanoparticles and assessment of their anticancer, antimicrobial, antioxidant and catalytic properties. Artif Cells Nanomed Biotechnol 2018; 46(4): 861-71.
[http://dx.doi.org/10.1080/21691401.2017.1345930] [PMID: 28681622]

[66]    Bin-Jumah M, Al-Abdan M, Albasher G, Alarifi S. Al-Abdan M, Albasher G, Alarifi S. Effects of green silver nanoparticles on apoptosis and oxidative stress in normal and cancerous human hepatic cells *in vitro*. Int J Nanomedicine 2020; 15: 1537-48.
[http://dx.doi.org/10.2147/IJN.S239861] [PMID: 32210550]

[67]    Yakop F, Abd Ghafar SA, Yong YK. Silver nanoparticles Clinacanthus Nutans leaves extract induced apoptosis towards oral squamous cell carcinoma cell lines. Art Cells Nanomed Biotech 2018; 1-9.

[68]    Chugh H, Sood D, Chandra I, Tomar V, Dhawan G, Chandra R. Role of gold and silver nanoparticles in cancer nano-medicine. Artif Cells Nanomed Biotechnol 2018; 46(sup1): 1210-20.
[http://dx.doi.org/10.1080/21691401.2018.1449118] [PMID: 29533101]

[69]    Chellapandian C, Ramkumar B, Puja P, *et al.* Shanmuganathan, R. Gold nanoparticles using red seaweed *Gracilaria verrucosa*: Green synthesis, characterization, and biocompatibility studies. Process Biochem 2019; 80: 58-63.
[http://dx.doi.org/10.1016/j.procbio.2019.02.009]

[70]    Wang L, Xu J, Yan Y, Liu H, Karunakaran T, Li F. Green synthesis of gold nanoparticles from *Scutellaria barbata* and its anticancer activity in pancreatic cancer cell (PANC-1). Artif Cells Nanomed Biotechnol 2019; 47(1): 1617-27.
[http://dx.doi.org/10.1080/21691401.2019.1594862] [PMID: 31014134]

[71]    Navya PN, Kaphle A, Srinivas SP, Bhargava SK, Rotello VM, Daima HK. Current trends and challenges in cancer management and therapy using designer nanomaterials. Nano Converg 2019; 6(1): 23-9.
[http://dx.doi.org/10.1186/s40580-019-0193-2] [PMID: 31304563]

**CHAPTER 12**

# Oxidative Stress Involvement in Antibacterial Therapy

**Christiana E. Aruwa[1]** and **Saheed Sabiu[1,\*]**

[1] *Department of Biotechnology and Food Science, Faculty of Applied Sciences, Durban University of Technology, P.O. Box 1334, Durban 4000, South Africa*

**Abstract:** Antimicrobial therapy is necessary to reduce the global burden of disease and infection. Oxidative stress (OS) may play a key function in determining the extent of efficacy of antimicrobial treatment regimens. However, whether the agent has a 'static' (inhibitory) or 'cidal' (killing) effect or the ability to induce an oxidative state, achieving therapy is a complex one. Bactericidal agents are known to induce a downstream cascade of responses in bacteria beyond their direct target(s). These responses correspond with the generation of reactive oxygen species (ROS) and the development of OS that eventually results in the disruption/destruction of integral components and/or processes within bacteria cells. In contrast, bacteriostatic antibiotics may not always induce cell death. Both classes of antimicrobials are useful in antibacterial therapy. The actualization of an oxidatively stressed microbial cell is key to optimizing the available antibiotic therapy options for efficient treatment and reducing the acquisition of microbial resistance. Studies are still required to expatiate on the role played by OS in antimicrobial therapy. This chapter, therefore, focuses on discussing available research data and knowledge on this complex role by OS, while highlighting potential future application and development prospects. In addition, the chapter touched OS and their sources, antimicrobial lethality-OS association, factors affecting OS-mediating therapy and efficacy, bacterial adaptations to OS in response to antimicrobial treatment and prospects for combination therapy with bactericidal agents and adjuvants.

**Keywords:** Oxidative stress, Reactive species, Antibiotics, Antimicrobial therapy, Bacteria, Adaptations.

## 1. INTRODUCTION

Antimicrobials-induced cell apoptosis is a multifaceted and complex process [1, 2]. While more effort has been directed towards the derivation or discovery of

---

\* **Corresponding author Saheed Sabiu:** Department of Biotechnology and Food Science, Faculty of Applied Sciences, Durban University of Technology, P.O. Box 1334, Durban, 4000, South Africa; Tel: +2731 373 5330; E-mail: sabius@dut.ac.za

new antimicrobials and their specific target(s) in microbial cells, this approach is simplistic. This approach points to the view that antimicrobials evince their effects through the inhibition of specified targets only. However, the upgrades in high-throughput techniques have empowered scientific analysis into microbial responses to stress or toxic conditions [3]. In other words, microbial cell death or inhibition could be a function of more than the antibiotic-target specific theory. It may also be a consequence of affected cell processes, for example, physiological and metabolic processes, as well as interactions that transcend cell target(s), and may be associated with the development of oxidative stress (OS) in cells under treatment conditions [3]. The accumulation and excessive presence of reactive oxygen species (ROS) in a living system could culminate in oxidative stress (OS). Oxidative stress has also been defined as a state of antioxidant deficiency [4]. ROS usually target lipids, proteins, RNA and DNA [5], and their occurrence beyond optimal level is harmful to cells [6].

Generally, antimicrobial therapy faces pertinent challenges on a global scale, given the increase in antimicrobial resistance (AMR) of microbial species to available antibiotics or antimicrobial agents [7]. In a bid to tackle AMR, research should not be limited to the discovery or synthesis of novel antimicrobials and new modes of action but also extended to investigations on integral factors that contribute to the development of AMR and antimicrobial tolerance [7]. Under certain conditions, exposure of bacterial cells to some classes of antimicrobials could enhance increased production of ROS, that may cause death and disruption of the target with which the drug or agent interacts within the cells [3]. In contrast, antioxidants and OS defences could contribute to reducing susceptibility to antibiotics and be involved in bacterial responses to antibacterial or antimicrobial agents [7].

Antibacterial agents, especially bactericidal antibiotics, disrupt the bacterial cells they permeate and may cause irreversible damage or death to the cells through breakage in deoxyribonucleic acid (DNA), and induction of oxidative stress biomarkers. These effects are, however more pronounced in bactericidal agents [8, 9]. In the Fenton pathway, DNA is damaged by hydrogen peroxide ($H_2O_2$), a ROS [10]. It has also been reported that aerobic microbial species such as *Escherichia coli* produce significant quantities of intracellular peroxide to induce OS and cause damage to their own DNA [11].

Again, in the study of the *E. coli* metabolome, some changes were profiled in response to three antibacterial agents, that is, quinolones, aminoglycosides, and β-lactams antibiotics. *Escherichia coli* cells showed a decrease in lipid quantities, breaks in the nucleotide chain, an increase in the redox condition within cells, and upregulated levels of central carbon metabolites [12, 13]. The loss of homeostasis in the cell's metabolic state led to toxic shifts which was an evidence of OS in treated cells. Following the establishment of an oxidatively stressed state, breakage in DNA, increase in nucleotide oxidation, malondialdehyde adducts, and carbonylation of protein were also reported [8]. Hence, shifts in cell metabolism may function in the regulation of bacterial susceptibility responses [14, 15]. The disturbance of metabolic processes has been reported to stall the uptake of antibiotics [16] and induce bacterial protection by decreasing cell growth [13]. It may also downregulate the generation of by-products which are toxic to the cells [3]. Thus, microbial reactions to antibiotics used in antimicrobial treatment can be a function of several interactions that induce a stressed oxidative state in affected cells.

Considering the foregoing, increasing research insights into how antimicrobial agents impact microbial physiological and metabolic responses, as well as the OS-bacterial cell disruption link in antimicrobial therapy, could also be key to solving the nagging global challenge of AMR. This would further aid the evolution of therapeutic techniques to improve the efficacy of treatment regimens in the future. This chapter, therefore, aims to synergize a range of relevant and available information in the literature on the OS function in antibacterial therapy. Information for the chapter was derived from research and review articles and an array of online databases.

## 2. DISCUSSION

### 2.1. Sources of Oxidative Stress

Some of the known sources of oxidative stress include, but are not limited to obesity or metabolic syndrome, leukocytospermia, alcohol and tobacco usage, bacterial prostatitis; sexually transmitted disease (STDs), for example, those caused by *Chlamydia trachomatis*, *Neisseria gonorrhoeae* (Gonorrhoea), and *Treponema pallidum* (Syphilis); viral infections like hepatitis, human immunodeficiency virus (HIV), mutations that occur in microorganisms which increase OS stress levels [4], and antimicrobial agents used in antimicrobial therapy. However, the effects of ROS generation leading to oxidative stress as a mechanism of antibacterial action, the OS-antibacterial lethality link in antimicrobial chemotherapy, and bacterial mutations in response to OS and antibacterial agents are the subjects of focus.

### 2.2. Mechanism of Action of Antibacterial Agents

Some antibacterial agents that have shown ROS-generating capacity as a mode of action include the fluoroquinolones known to cease the fragmentation and replication of the bacterial cell chromosome. Examples are norfloxacin and moxifloxacin [17]. Quinones antibiotics produce thiol-depletion in prokaryotic cells though a one-electron reduction pathway. Quinone examples include methyl benzoquinone, mitomycin and nitrofurantoin [18]. β-lactams inhibit cell wall synthesis and facilitate ROS production in cells. Ampicillin, ceftriaxone and meropenem are examples β-lactam antibiotics [12]. Aminoglycosides disrupt protein synthesis, trigger ROS generation and bind ribosomes. Gentamicin is an aminoglycoside antibiotic [3, 19].

The establishment of OS may participate actively in the mechanism of action of antibacterial agents. Antibiotics such as the aminoglycosides can cause membrane protein changes upon ROS induction [20]. A similar action pathway occurs with quinolone and β-lactam antibacterial agents when respiratory metabolism is disturbed by pathogen presence. Both agents trigger hydroxyl radical (OH•) production, followed by ferrous iron release and superoxide anion upregulation [20]. Besides these antibiotic classes, antimicrobial action has also been shown in other chemotherapeutic agents such as antidepressant, antipsychotic, anti-inflammatory, anxiolytic and antineoplastic agents. The antimicrobial action of these agents was also linked to their disturbance of the redox metabolism in microorganisms [21]. OS or ROS-mediated cell killing is a pharmacological effect and strategy that may shape new drugs development through repurposing approach for antibacterial therapy [21, 22].

At high concentrations of free radicals and reactive oxygen species, lipids can be directly damaged. OH• enhance lipid peroxidation and induces an oxidative chain reaction in the cell membrane polyunsaturated phospholipids (PUPL) leading to inhibited or reduced functions [23]. The bacterial cell damage triggered by ROS varies from that evinced in eukaryotic organisms since most prokaryotes lack the PUPL in their cell membrane [24]. ROS antibacterial effects are initiated upon their interaction with protein, membrane, and DNA thiol groups, but depending on the dosage [25]. In peroxide cell toxicity, DNA is the primary target such that the DNA double strand structure is broken, or bases are affected. Also, DNA breakage may occur as a by-product of lipid peroxidation [26, 27]. ROS disruption of the lipid bilayer may also deactivate membrane proteins and receptors, thus causing loss of membrane functions, efflux and loss of cell constituents, and cell fluidity [24, 28]. When ROS target proteins, damages such as peptide breakup, protein-protein cross-lining, the generation of amino acid oxidation adducts that are close to metal-binding positions *via* metal-dependent oxidation, disulphides reduction, changes in metal clusters and prosthetic groups, sulfhydryl groups oxidation, and interference with aldehydes can occur [29]. Peroxide species also cause oxidative changes in proteins like the F0F1-ATPase of *Escherichia coli*, enolase, alcohol dehydrogenase E, and elongation factor G [30, 31]. Proteins also experience oxidative changes at the phenylalanine, tyrosine, cysteine, tryptophan, and methionine residues. ROS damage caused by the presence of protein carbonyls produced through oxidative reactions involving proline, arginine, or lysine amino acids have also been observed [30, 31]. Table **1** shows the mode of action of a range of ROS-producing antibacterial agents and test bacteria cell(s) studied.

Table 1. ROS-generating antimicrobial agents, the mechanism of action and bacteria tested on.

| Test Bacteria | Antibacterial (Antibiotic) Agent | Primary Mechanism of Action | Reference |
|---|---|---|---|
| *Enterococcus sp.* *Streptococcus sp.* *Staphylococcus sp.* *Moraxela catarrhalis* | Quinones | Varied cell targets | [32] |
| *Rhodococcus equi* | Erythromycin | Inhibition of protein synthesis | [17] |
| *R. equi* | Rifampicin | RNA synthesis inhibition | [17] |
| *Mycobacterium tuberculosis* *R. equi* *S. aureus* | Vancomycin | Cell wall synthesis inhibition | [33] [17] [20] |
| *M. tuberculosis* | Clofazimine | DNA replication inhibition | [33] |
| *M. tuberculosis* | Isoniazid | Cell wall synthesis inhibition | [33] |
| *M. tuberculosis* | Ethambutol | Cell wall synthesis inhibition | [33] |
| *R. equi* *S. aureus* *Escherichia coli* | Norfloxacin | DNA gyrase inhibition | [17] [20] [34] |
| *E. coli* | Ampicillin | Cell membrane disruption, DNA damage | [12] [13] |
| *E. coli MG1655* | Gentamycin Ampicillin Norfloxacin | Cell membrane disruption, DNA damage, Alteration of redox state | [3] |
| *S. aureus* *E. coli* *Pseudomonas aeruginosa* | Ceftazidima Piperacillin, Chloramphenicol Ciprofloxacin | Cell wall inhibition, Macromolecule oxidation (DNA, lipid) | [35 - 37] |

Adapted with permission from Mourenza *et al.* [38].

## 2.3. The Antimicrobial Lethality-Oxidative Stress Link

Bactericidal antibiotics are believed to cause lethal damage to cells by interacting with target-specific processes [3]. Microbial and bacterial cell death could occur beyond cell membrane permeabilization and disruption and may involve OS generation [39]. The roles played by OS in antimicrobial therapy have been referred to as reactive oxygen therapy (ROT) [40]. Although, ROS are regarded as non-specific, reactive, and promiscuous molecules due to their instability, they are integral determinants of the cross between resistance and susceptibility to infectious agents [41, 42]. ROT was suggested as a new antimicrobial approach for the management of AMR or multi-drug resistance (MDR) and infection treatment. ROT is an alternative mode of bactericidal action of conventional antimicrobials [40]. The generation of ROS is also the mechanism of action behind therapeutic strategies like medical honey and nanoparticle use, as well as photodynamic [9, 38, 40], and hyperbaric oxygen [43] treatments. The generation of ROS and OS are linked with antimicrobial lethality and efficacy. Besides their specific cell targets, 'cidal' agents also trigger oxidative destruction in microorganisms [44].

Cytotoxic reactive species interfere with the electron transport chain and tricarboxylic acid (TCA) cycle [44, 45]. The hydroxyl radical (OH•) production process involves the TCA pathway, transiently depleting NADH, disruption of iron regulations and iron-sulphur cluster instability [46]. A high-level generation of OH• could also be a common mode of action in antibacterial-mediated lethality in antimicrobial treatment [47]. In strict anaerobic conditions, lethality is greatly reduced. Nonetheless, bacterial kill rate could be improved by introducing another electron acceptor such as nitrate, sulphate, or oxygen [40]. A basic representation of the ROS-lethality link is shown in Fig. (**1**). Basically, bactericidal agents interact with specific cell targets and induce cell damage. Likewise, they also trigger a stressed state by initiating redox-related pathways like the Fenton and Haber-Weiss reactions and the oxidative phosphorylation pathway, for cytotoxic ROS generation, causing damage and killing cells [40].

In contrast to bactericidal agents' lethality, noteworthy is the fact that little or no research data exists to understand the OS-lethality link due to the use of bacteriostatic chemotherapeutic agents. To bridge the gap, a study recently tested for the first time, the effect of bacteriostatic linezolid antibiotic on three bacterial strains of *Staphylococcus aureus*. The species did not experience severe damage and oxidation of protein macromolecules since OS levels were insignificant. The generated ROS were also insufficient to counter antioxidant responses, but reactive species produced were more detectable in clinical microbial isolates, compared to reference strains [48]. Bacteriostatic agents, therefore, can trigger increased formation of ROS, but at negligible levels which do not result in substantial OS and damage to cells. Hence, the contribution of ROS and OS in linezolid's inhibitory activity may not be significant when compared with a bactericidal agent. So, lethality in respect to use of bacteriostatic agents is negligible [48].

# Bactericidal antibiotics

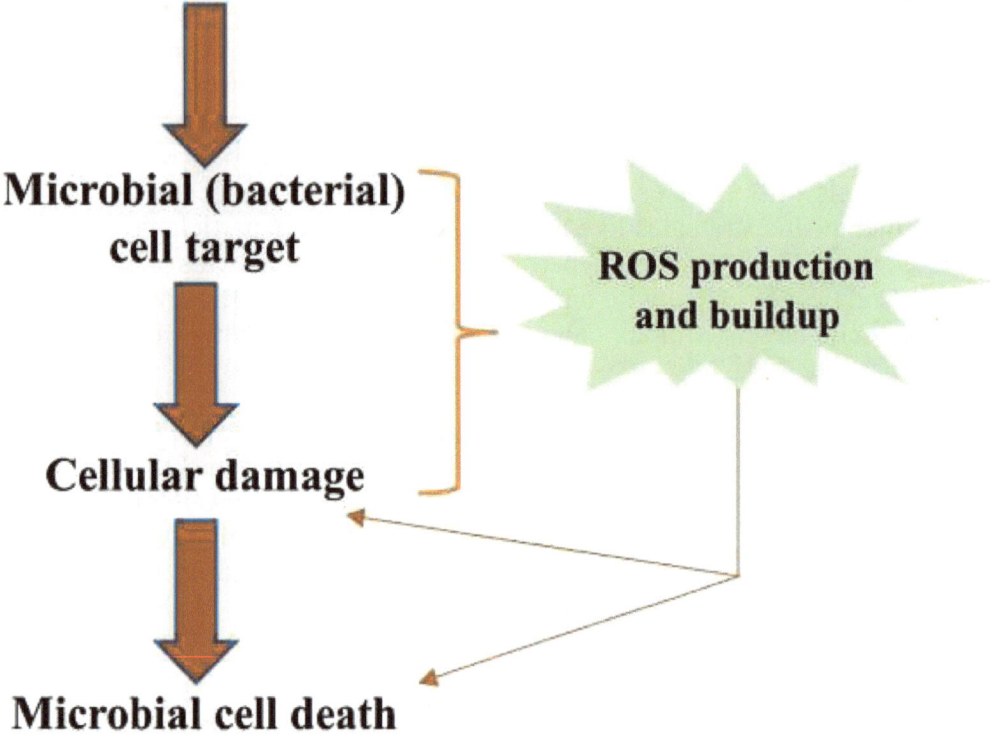

**Fig. (1).** Lethality-ROS link in response to antibiotics (antibacterial agents). Adapted with permission from Memar *et al*. [40].

In further discussions, there are some well-known traditional antimicrobials that evince their antimicrobial action by generating ROS within the target microbial cells. There are those that cycle redox reactions by shuttling electrons from the cell's reducing powers directly to oxygen for conversion to reactive oxygen species. Examples of this first group include mitomycin, nitrofurantoin (in treatment of urinary tract infections - UTIs) [49] and artemisinin [50]. Another category is the antimicrobial peptides (AMPs) that impact membrane integrity by disruption of the cell membrane. An example of AMP includes polymyxin B used in drug resistance therapy of Gram-negative bacteria such as Enterobacteriaceae bacteria that produce carbapenemase, *Pseudomonas aeruginosa* and *Acinetobacter baumanii* [51]. These are said to be membrane active and thought to significantly affect the respiratory chain structure leading to the leakage of electrons. The last group are bactericidal antimicrobials that generate ROS below inhibitory concentrations as their mechanism of action [52]. Examples of this third class include the quinolone, norfloxacin; the β-lactam, ampicillin and the aminoglycoside, kanamycin. Bactericidal antibiotics can also cause microbial cell death even in conditions that are anaerobic if electron acceptors such as sulphates and nitrates are introduced [53, 54].

In environments totally lacking oxygen bactericidal agents' lethality is diminished. Even at high antibiotic concentrations, lethality was not significant. This led to the hypothesis that ROS is not the only cause, but a contributor to antibiotic-induced lethality [3]. The same observations were made in use of moxifloxacin, a fluoroquinolone, and ceftriaxone and meropenem β-lactam antibiotics. Hence, the presence of electron acceptors such as oxygen, sulphate and nitrate are relevant in determining the rate and level of lethality of bactericidal antibiotics [3]. Metabolism and antibiotics may fuel ROS formation as a mechanism for acquisition of beneficial mutations when small and insufficient stresses are generated [55]. In the reverse case, lethality ensues if the stress created is significant [56]. ROS production by quinone-based antimicrobial agents like benzoquinone and mitomycin have been reported. Mitomycin undergoes flavoprotein-mediated one-electron reduction to a semiquinone radical which spontaneously reacts with oxygen to turn back to quinone and produce $O_2^-$ [52].

While the techniques for ROT delivery which enhance for pathogen selectivity are welcome, reducing adverse effects to the host could also have great prospects for disease therapy. In the same vein, ROS can adversely impact the host microflora, cells, tissues, and organs after production from activated leukocytes in response to pathogen presence [57 - 59]. Hence, this should also constitute the subject of future research to ensure the safe channelling of ROS in future antimicrobial therapies [40]. In addition, novel ROS-producing antimicrobials such as ebselen [60], allicin [61] and silver [62] have been reported. Ebselen, an antioxidant molecule known as SPI-1005, is a synthetic organoselenium-based compound with cytoprotective and anti-inflammatory properties [60, 63]. There is the potential application for use of ebselen in atherosclerosis, cancer, stroke, arthritis, and cardiovascular disease therapy, when the drug acts by mimicking glutathione peroxidase (GluP) in mammalian cells [64]. The compound also actively inhibits thioredoxin/thioredoxin reductases (TrxR) in bacteria like *M. tuberculosis* and *S. aureus* that lack glutathione [65, 66], and induces oxidative stress [60, 67]. Ebselen can also be combined with other ROS inducing molecules such as silver nanoparticles which have the capability to block antioxidant fortifications in bacteria [67].

Another possibility is the utilization of an antimicrobial coating called AGXX® (Largetec GmbH, Berlin), which is a novel broad-spectrum antimicrobial. AGXX® is an ROS-inspired preventive approach against AMR bacteria. The coating is made up of ruthenium and silver metals that cause loss of iron homeostasis and produce OS in methicillin-resistant *S. aureus*. AGXX® is also known to prevent bacterial attachment to their target cells and surface and kill all kinds of bacteria and other microbial classes such as viruses, yeasts, and fungi [68]. Allicin is a plant metabolite derived from garlic (*Allium sativum*). It is a reactive sulphur specie that acts by oxidizing protein thiol groups in a dose-dependent manner. Its antimicrobial activity and ability to generate and induce OS has been shown in *Bacillus subtilis* and *S. aureus* where allicin creates a significant disulphide stress that greatly reduces viability in bacteria [61, 69]. The near future may yet see the discovery and evolution of new antimicrobials. In line with this, it has been suggested that new treatment regimens should include the combination of two or more ROS-generating antibacterial agents. A combination therapy using bactericidal agents with other bioactive molecules, adjuvants, or enhancers, could also prove to be efficient [17, 38, 62, 70]. This would contribute to decreasing the development of microbial resistance.

Lastly, the modulation of redox metabolism in different microbial strains could be a more rational route to take in infections treatment compared to modulating same in vertebrate, or eukaryotic hosts [59, 71]. Since many antioxidant molecules in pathogenic microorganisms are not produced in eukaryotes, the molecules or enzymes could serve as possible targets in the design of new medications and antimicrobials for use in antibacterial chemotherapy [72, 73]. Since antimicrobial resistance may not be phased out soon, strengthening our insight into antimicrobial mechanisms and how they impact on bacterial lethality through relevant research cannot be overemphasized.

### 2.3.1. Additional Notes and Considerations

The mechanism of action of antimicrobials are targeted towards achieving the death or inhibition of the target microorganism or pathogen [47]. Microbial killing or inhibition need to be reached to treat or manage an infection or disease. Bactericidal antimicrobials that bring about their cidal effects rapidly could also better reduce the emergence of AMR compared to bacteriostatic antimicrobial agents. Microbial cell death or apoptosis is believed to be elicited through the active interaction of antimicrobials with specific targets in the target microbial cells. Such interaction may then result in the disruption or break-down of cellular processes within the cell [74]. Some authors have however put forward that, bactericidal agents may have common mechanism of action that involves the production and elevation of hydroxyl radicals [20, 34]. This hypothesis remains the subject of many studies.

During microbial aerobic respiration, ROS such as hydrogen peroxide ($H_2O_2$), hydroxyl radicals (OH•) and superoxide ($O_2^{\cdot-}$) are usually produced [75]. These species are toxic to microbial cells, but to varying degrees and through varied pathways. The peroxide and superoxide radicals have a reduced effect compared to the OH• radical [76]. Their reduced toxicity is closely linked to the ease with which they are detoxified by scavenging enzymes such as flavoenzymes, peroxidases, superoxide dismutase (SOD) and catalases produced within the organism. On the other hand, OH• cannot be detoxified by induced scavenging enzymes. This enhances the lethality and toxicity of OH•. Again, in the Fenton reaction, the OH• is generated from hydrogen peroxide within cells. Thus, in the intracellular control of peroxide levels, scientists may begin to find answers to the pathways that impact on OH•-mediated 'cidal' action [76, 77]. The dismutation of superoxide species to produce peroxide occurs through the catalytic action of SOD [78, 79]. The inhibition of this pathway could reduce peroxide accumulation and production of OH• [80, 81]. The break-down of peroxide to water is achieved through the action of catalases or peroxidases. When these enzyme genes are disrupted, level of peroxide is raised followed by OH•, thus reducing the cell's ability to survive antimicrobial therapy [34]. Hence, many bactericidal antimicrobial agents are cell stressors that upregulate superoxide production, which is converted to peroxide and the highly toxic hydroxyl radical. The generated radical then enhances the killing effect of the agents in antimicrobial treatment [47].

The bactericidal action of antibacterial agents may involve the 'creation' of an 'oxidatively stressed' microenvironment in target cells. This has been demonstrated in studies involving antimicrobial groups which brought about cell death by accumulating superoxide anions within the bacterial cells [45, 82, 83]. The generation of ROS in association with susceptibility to ciprofloxacin has also been reported [84]. Also, antimicrobial lethality in the presence or absence of single and/or multiple mutations in enzyme genes and pathways was shown by Wang and Zhao [47]. The authors successfully showed that mutations can have varied effects on antimicrobial agents' lethality, and lethality could also be dependent on other factors such as length of therapy and agent concentrations. They submitted that OS pathways are closely linked to the level of killing of an antimicrobial agent, as was the case in β-lactam, fluoroquinolone, and aminoglycoside lethality. A closer investigation of these pathways could point to novel targets for molecules (known and new) that can evince a static or 'cidal' antimicrobial action [47].

Toxic reactive species contribute to the killing efficiency of antibacterial gents used in therapy. Interestingly, it has been demonstrated that cell death and accumulation of ROS continued in *E. coli* even after the antibacterial stressor or antibiotic was removed. The post-stress killing effect was only slowed when mitigating agents were added. Authors surmised that the killing efficacy of an antimicrobial is a partial derivative of the stimulation of a self-boosting build-up of ROS that inundates initial damage repairs, and this effect varies for different antimicrobial stressors [85]. In other words, under post-treatment and post-stress conditions, microbial cells may still be alive but can be killed eventually due to increase of ROS. It also provides scientific backing into the search for broad-spectrum ROS-linked optimizers of antimicrobial action [85].

## 2.3.2. Factors Impacting OS-mediated Antibacterial Therapy and Efficacy

The effect of antibiotic use cannot be overemphasized in global health systems. Antibiotics have paved the way for developments in the society, and pharmaceutical and medical industries [86]. The development of resistance by microorganisms is a subject closely linked to antimicrobial therapy such that one cannot be discussed without mention of the other. This is a major concern to stakeholders in the health sectors. Likewise, the issues of correct/appropriate dosage, treatment regimen and duration of therapy to stem the tide of AMR development are also relevant [87]. In a section of the medical sector such as dentistry, research continues to emerge on the inefficiency of the adjuvant systemic antibiotic administration procedures for patient therapy [88, 89].

In the use of the antibiotic regimen, metronidazole, and amoxicillin, to treat chronic periodontitis, the reactive oxygen metabolites derived during treatment were examined as a measure of the level of OS generated. Antimicrobial resistance response of associated bacteria was also investigated [90]. Prior to treatment, amoxicillin resistance was not detected, but after patient treatment, two microbial strains developed resistance. Surprisingly, thirteen microbial species showed resistance to metronidazole prior to patient therapy. The numbers reduced to two strains following the course of treatment. In a patient, one strain that showed susceptibility prior to therapy, expressed resistance to both metronidazole and amoxicillin after patient treatment [90]. The patient group that received both antibiotics over the longest period of 7 days showed fewer developments of resistance in the periodontal pathogens identified. The same group demonstrated an upregulation of OS, as well as the most reduced presence of pathogens. This result contrasted with that reported for the patient groups that received a 3-day treatment regimen of the antibiotics [90]. From the study, one may also point out an often-forgotten factor in therapy, that is, that individual pharmacokinetics or drug response vary from one person to another. This is similar in the case of pathogens, as pathogens often show varied susceptibility response to specific antibiotics [91]. ROS also contribute to inflaming the respiratory tract [92]. In certain cases, such as those involving respiratory diseases, OS can give rise to inflammations which need to be appropriately managed to efficiently treat the infection [93].

Another issue worthy of discussion is the persistence of bacterial infections. Persistent infections can boomerang into a higher risk of spreading the disease and invariably higher mortality and morbidity rates [94]. Attempts at nipping such infections in the bud often involve the administration of repeated or long-term doses of antibiotics [94]. Most persistent infections are chronic and asymptomatic, for example, infections associated with *Salmonella typhi* or *Mycobacterium tuberculosis* [95, 96]. In contrast, symptomatic chronic and acute infections can be caused by certain pathogens like *E. coli* and *Pseudomonas aeruginosa*. Factors which contribute to the development of persistent infections include both bacteria-related and host-related factors. Bacterial factors involve those that increase the adaptability and evasive capabilities of bacterial species and ensure the infectious state continues within the host. Host-related factors may include innate host response to drugs, genetics, history of drug abuse and alcoholism [97]. The highlighted factors must be appropriately resolved to ensure improved antibacterial lethality and efficacy during disease therapy.

## 2.4. Adaptations in OS and Antimicrobial Therapy

**i. *Adaptations in response to polyamines*** - The contribution of *in vivo* natural molecules to the efficiency of antimicrobial agents used in therapy cannot be overlooked. These molecules are used as adaptive mechanisms by bacteria and other prokaryotic species to protect themselves against the deleterious effects of antibiotics. One of such molecules produced by microorganisms include polyamines. A study has demonstrated that the accumulation of polyamines in *E. coli* bacteria resulted in a lowered antibiotic induced oxidative damage to cell macromolecules, thus aiding cell survival. Antibacterial agents used were the β-lactam and fluoroquinolone class of antibiotics. Polyamines reduced superoxide species production, and significantly inhibited peroxide species [7]. The supplementation of the reaction mixture with exogenous polyamines under laboratory conditions also impacted bacterial susceptibility to antibiotics [19, 98].

A class of polyamines known as biogenic polyamines are considered as aliphatic hydrocarbons that possess 2 or more imino- or amino groups. The major polyamines produced within prokaryotic cells include putrescine or 1,4-diaminobutane, cadaverine or 1,5-diaminopentane, and spermidine or N-(-aminopropyl)-1,4-diaminobutane. These, alongside spermine are also expressed in eukaryotes, and through the active transport system they are accumulated in microbial pathogens, as well as commensal microbes [99]. Polyamine particles are capable of electrostatic interactions. As positively charged ions they bind to negatively charged cell components such as proteins, nucleic acids, phospholipids and ribosomes. This interaction enhances their ability to regulate the cell's adaptation to stress, as well as basic metabolic processes [100].

Putrescine and spermidine polyamines are known to contribute to adaptive cell responses to high temperatures, osmotic shock and OS, and the protection and stabilization of cell DNA, osmotic shock, and heat [100, 101]. Polyamines may be said to have antioxidant roles. They provide bacterial defence in response to OS *via* one or more of the following means.

  i. by downregulating ROS [102];
 ii. by protecting and binding negatively charged macromolecules [103];
iii. by regulating adaptive genes expression [104], and
iv. by preventing the ROS formation, for example, through chelation and scavenging effects [105].

The antioxidant efficacy of polyamines against hydroxyl radical species have only been demonstrated in spermidine and spermine [102, 106]. Also, it is important to state that the urogenital and intestinal tracts in humans also produce polyamines, and this may affect bacterial susceptibility and efficacy of antimicrobial therapy [107]. It has been recently opined that reduction in antibiotic susceptibility in the presence of polyamines could be due to their competitive binding to target cell sites and macromolecules such as the DNA or ribosome. So, ROS neutralization and the antibacterial availability within the cell are lowered [7].

**ii. *Bacterial mutations* -** The presence of a stressed cellular microenvironment can induce mutational changes in microorganisms. For bacteria to rapidly adapt to changing environmental conditions mutations may occur. The rate of mutation may also be increased depending on the stressor(s) to ensure optimal adaptation or alterations, and survival. Even inhibitory concentrations of bactericides have been demonstrated to upregulate mutations in *E. coli* [55]. In another study, ampicillin at below bacteriostatic levels was believed to involve the uptake of nucleotides that had been oxidized into nascent DNA followed by a mismatch repair that was temporarily suppressed to prevent their removal [108]. Bacteria are often exposed to antimicrobials at dosages that do not achieve killing under natural conditions. Therefore, a pathway that involves the upregulation of ROS-dependent mutations under stress of low antibiotic doses evolved and could have had some benefits. Hence, microbial death that is dependent on the generation of ROS at antimicrobial concentrations used clinically and that results in DNA damage could be an adverse effect of a means that usually benefits adaptation in a condition that experiences less or reduced stress [1].

**iii. *Physiological adaptations* -** The adaptive measures used by bacteria in response to host-imposed stressors like antibiotics make cells transform to a different physiological state. Such physiological changes could impact on bacterial replication or reduce their rate of replication. This may constitute an added advantage of strengthening a pathogen's defence against exposure to antimicrobials as actively growing and replicating cells facilitate antibiotic uptake and increase antimicrobial efficacy [109]. In the new physiological state, bacteria metabolism impacts on the efficiency of the antibiotic such that cells become 'numb' or 'unaffected' by the antimicrobial agent [94, 97]. In nature, bacterial biofilms can create an environment low in oxygen supply, and physiological changes can also be studied within bacterial biofilm populations [110]. Nevertheless, since oxygen levels are directly proportional to ROS production, the generation of reactive molecules within cells that make up the biofilm is minimal [109].

**iv. *Other adaptive bacterial mechanisms and structures* -** The presence of the enzyme, superoxide dismutase (SOD), in the *Bacillus anthracis* exosporium is suspected to regulate levels of ROS in the host [111, 112]. The excision of this outer layer from the sporulated microorganism resulted in higher levels of ROS. It was then suspected that the exosporium plays a critical role in protecting the microbe from the harmful effect of antibiotics used in antibacterial therapy. It achieves this by regulating the production of free radicals [113]. The same mechanism may be applicable to bacterial respiratory diseases. Various bacteria also possess the cytochrome bd oxidase enzyme that helps them resist OS and bypass defences of the immune system [114]. Bacteria may also induce the production of antioxidant moieties like an oxygen regulator (OxyR) and catalase [52]. The regulatory action of OxyR was recorded in oral pathogens, *Porphyromonas gingivalis* [115] and *Tannerella forsythia* [116] exposed to ROS in the dental cavity. OxyR also increased *Klebsiella pneumoniae* defences by enhancing its ability to colonize mucosal surfaces, inducing the expression of fimbriae, and helping to form biofilms, in response to OS [117].

Antimicrobial reactive species produced by macrophages have also been reported in infections linked to *M. tuberculosis* [118, 119]. Low quantities of peroxide and superoxide anion reactive species were not efficient in killing cultures of *M. tuberculosis* [120], but nitric oxide species at the same levels were toxic to the cells. The observation was, however, acknowledged to be dependent on strain [121].

Superoxide regulating species (SoxRS) are also used in *Salmonella* species and *E. coli* as a defence against OS [122]. Molecules that act by the redox-cycling mechanism to produce superoxide anions activate SoxR [123]. Upon SoxR activation, the generation of superoxide species is stimulated. This gives rise to the induction of OS defence genes [5, 124]. In another adaption, bacterial efflux pump (EP) systems are well known. The EP is a transport protein that actively contributes to the removal of cytotoxic substances from cells into the external environment [125]. EPs can pump out a specific substrate, compound, or specie. They may also transport an array of compounds that are structurally different.

Having highlighted some adaptive mechanisms utilized by microbial species to evade OS and agents used in antimicrobial therapy, microbial MDR remains an ever-present threat which calls for outside-the-box thinking by members of the scientific community. This is essential to prevent a deluge of infections that defy therapy and the emergence of totally resistant strains. An option that has come to the limelight and is under scientific investigation is the application of non-antimicrobial methods. It has been opined that this strategy may act faster and be more efficient compared to antibiotics currently used. An example is the application of antimicrobial photodynamic inactivation (APDI) (Fig. **2**). In the non-antibiotic APDI approach, ROS are also produced when light and certain dyes are combined [126]. However, pertinent aspects which require further clarification, such as the practical evaluation of APDI efficacy and the extent of damage that APDI can have on a host of microbial biomolecules, need to be addressed. Likewise, much research data is required to ensure and ascertain its safe use as a potential alternative [5].

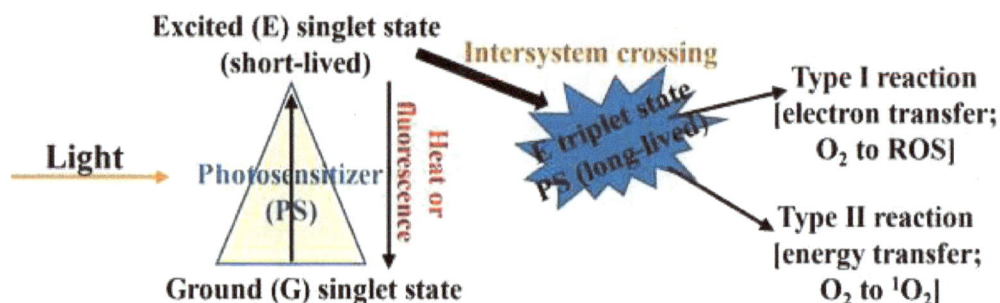

**Fig. (2).** Principle of the Antimicrobial Photodynamic Inactivation (APDI) demonstrated in a Jablonski diagram. Adapted from Kashef and Hamblin [5].

## 2.5. Oxidative Stress Assessment

The generation of OS is a significant organic or metabolic stressor which is indicative of an oxidant-antioxidant imbalance, and this has implications in the development of diseases [93]. The mitochondria and microsomes are cell organelles that produce reactive organic moieties that usually play beneficial roles in the cell. ROS participates in several cellular processes such as enzyme activation, the expression of genes, vascular tone, signal transduction, and oxygen tension monitoring [6, 127].

In an infection state, the host generates reactive species as a defence line against disease-causing agents [42, 128], but certain microbes can circumvent these fortifications. Nonetheless, OS has merits and demerits which are best exemplified in respiratory infections. Since most reactive species are radicals and unstable in nature, their direct measurement is difficult, but indirect techniques are available for OS measurement, especially in respiratory infections [93]. Samples of blood, sputum, condensates of exhaled air have been used to determine and manage infectious respiratory ailments [129]. In the laboratory, immunoassays, chemical and chromatographic methods can be used to assess OS in respiratory and other disease conditions [93]. A technique that monitors OS biomarkers like advanced oxidation protein products (AOPP), activity of SOD, and base amounts of glutathione in microbial species have also proved to be effective to assess OS effect [48].

In a recent report, an assessment method was devised to achieve separation of the effects due to the initial antibiotic stressor from that linked to ROS build-up within the microbial cell. The *E. coli* cells were treated with a bactericidal agent, the agent was then removed, and the cells were plated on agar media free of the primary stressor antibiotic. The media, however, contained an agent known to suppress cytotoxic ROS accumulation. The ROS suppressor interfered with *E. coli* cell killing induced by the bactericidal agent. This interference continued after the bactericide was removed, showing that ROS are a cause of stress-induced cell death [85].

Studies have also demonstrated the semiquantitative means that utilize fluorescein derivatives for ROS assessment. The reduced forms of fluorescein penetrate microbial cells, become oxidized, and are transformed into molecules whose fluorescence can be detected by cell sorting or microscopy [20, 109]. Generally, an assortment of assay techniques for the qualitative and quantitative measurement of ROS involved in OS and bacterial cell damage continue to be devised and modified in many studies and have led to interesting findings. Still, novel, more specific and sensitive assays may be essential to unify research reports on antibiotic induced-OS lethality. This would aid the clarification of inconsistencies on the link between antibiotic induced-OS lethality [122, 130].

## CONCLUDING REMARKS AND PERSPECTIVES

Antibiotic efficacy in therapy against bacteria involves varying aspects, which should be considered for good comprehension of the mechanism(s) of action and resistance evolution [36, 37]. Not much is known of the extent of contribution of OS relative to other organic stressors in microbial cells and disease therapy. However, microbes continue to evolve means to evade antimicrobials and treatment regimens. This is the foundation of persistent infections and resistance development in certain microorganisms. The role of OS, which is mostly induced by bactericidal antibiotics in antibacterial therapy, is a complex one that involves several physiological and metabolic interactions that cause damage to macromolecules and cell death.

Also, the contribution of combination therapies with bactericidal agents and/or adjuvants cannot be overemphasised in enhancing antibiotic efficacy and reducing antimicrobial resistance. Hence, it may suffice to say that targeting and studying cellular processes through unified assessment methods could aid our current understanding of the OS-antibiotic treatment link. In addition, in order to significantly decrease the burden of persistent, emerging, and re-emerging infections, targeting microbial metabolic processes beyond the primary antibiotic cell target could improve the antibacterial action of many antibiotics [131]. Also, increasing knowledge and investigations into the roles played by antimicrobial agents, strain-specificity, the presence or absence of electron acceptors, and bacterial adaptation mechanisms are important. In addition, the effect of host and microenvironment inducing factors in bacterial inhibition and death in the course of infection treatment can help tailor future research for the development of new therapies and antimicrobials. Such enhanced therapies could circumvent the current global challenge of AMR and stem the upsurge in emerging and re-emerging infections. Lastly, the use and availability of OS biomarkers in measurement platforms could also assist in the effective diagnosis, management, and treatment of persistent, emerging, and re-emerging diseases.

## CONSENT FOR PUBLICATION

Not applicable.

## CONFLICT OF INTEREST

The authors declare no conflict of interest, financial or otherwise.

## ACKNOWLEDGEMENTS

Declared none.

## REFERENCES

[1]    Dwyer DJ, Collins JJ, Walker GC. Unraveling the physiological complexities of antibiotic lethality. Annu Rev Pharmacol Toxicol 2015; 55: 313-32.
       [http://dx.doi.org/10.1146/annurev-pharmtox-010814-124712] [PMID: 25251995]

[2]    Zhao X, Hong Y, Drlica K. Moving forward with reactive oxygen species involvement in antimicrobial lethality. J Antimicrob Chemother 2015; 70(3): 639-42.
       [http://dx.doi.org/10.1093/jac/dku463] [PMID: 25422287]

[3]    Dwyer DJ, Belenky PA, Yang JH, *et al.* Antibiotics induce redox-related physiological alterations as

part of their lethality. Proc Natl Acad Sci USA 2014; 111(20): E2100-9.
[http://dx.doi.org/10.1073/pnas.1401876111] [PMID: 24803433]

[4]     Agarwal A, Rana M, Qiu E, AlBunni H, Bui AD, Henkel R. Role of oxidative stress, infection and inflammation in male infertility. Andrologia 2018; 50(11): e13126.
[http://dx.doi.org/10.1111/and.13126] [PMID: 30569652]

[5]     Kashef N, Hamblin MR. Can microbial cells develop resistance to oxidative stress in antimicrobial photodynamic inactivation? Drug Resist Updat 2017; 31: 31-42.
[http://dx.doi.org/10.1016/j.drup.2017.07.003] [PMID: 28867242]

[6]     Valavanidis A, Vlachogianni T, Fiotakis K, Loridas S. Pulmonary oxidative stress, inflammation and cancer: respirable particulate matter, fibrous dusts and ozone as major causes of lung carcinogenesis through reactive oxygen species mechanisms. Int J Environ Res Public Health 2013; 10(9): 3886-907.
[http://dx.doi.org/10.3390/ijerph10093886] [PMID: 23985773]

[7]     Akhova AV, Tkachenko AG. Multifaceted role of polyamines in bacterial adaptation to antibiotic-mediated oxidative stress. Korea J Microbiol 2020; 56: 103-10.

[8]     Belenky P, Ye JD, Porter CB, *et al.* Bactericidal antibiotics induce toxic metabolic perturbations that lead to cellular damage. Cell Rep 2015; 13(5): 968-80.
[http://dx.doi.org/10.1016/j.celrep.2015.09.059] [PMID: 26565910]

[9]     Vatansever F, de Melo WCMA, Avci P, *et al.* Antimicrobial strategies centered around reactive oxygen species--bactericidal antibiotics, photodynamic therapy, and beyond. FEMS Microbiol Rev 2013; 37(6): 955-89.
[http://dx.doi.org/10.1111/1574-6976.12026] [PMID: 23802986]

[10]    Imlay JA, Chin SM, Linn S. Toxic DNA damage by hydrogen peroxide through the Fenton reaction *in vivo* and *in vitro.* Science 1988; 240(4852): 640-2.
[http://dx.doi.org/10.1126/science.2834821] [PMID: 2834821]

[11]    Park S, You X, Imlay JA. Substantial DNA damage from submicromolar intracellular hydrogen peroxide detected in Hpx- mutants of *Escherichia coli.* Proc Natl Acad Sci USA 2005; 102(26): 9317-22.
[http://dx.doi.org/10.1073/pnas.0502051102] [PMID: 15967999]

[12]    Thomas VC, Kinkead LC, Janssen A, *et al.* A dysfunctional tricarboxylic acid cycle enhances fitness of *Staphylococcus epidermidis* during β-lactam stress. MBio 2013; 4(4): 4.
[PMID: 23963176]

[13]    Baek S-H, Li AH, Sassetti CM. Metabolic regulation of mycobacterial growth and antibiotic sensitivity. PLoS Biol 2011; 9(5): e1001065.
[http://dx.doi.org/10.1371/journal.pbio.1001065] [PMID: 21629732]

[14]    Van Acker H, Van Dijck P, Coenye T. Molecular mechanisms of antimicrobial tolerance and resistance in bacterial and fungal biofilms. Trends Microbiol 2014; 22(6): 326-33.
[http://dx.doi.org/10.1016/j.tim.2014.02.001] [PMID: 24598086]

[15]    Cohen NR, Lobritz MA, Collins JJ. Microbial persistence and the road to drug resistance. Cell Host Microbe 2013; 13(6): 632-42.
[http://dx.doi.org/10.1016/j.chom.2013.05.009] [PMID: 23768488]

[16]    Allison KR, Brynildsen MP, Collins JJ. Metabolite-enabled eradication of bacterial persisters by aminoglycosides. Nature 2011; 473(7346): 216-20.
[http://dx.doi.org/10.1038/nature10069] [PMID: 21562562]

[17]    Mourenza Á, Gil JA, Mateos LM, Letek M. A novel screening strategy reveals ROS-Generating antimicrobials that act synergistically against the intracellular veterinary pathogen *Rhodococcus equi.* Antioxidants 2020; 9(2): 114.
[http://dx.doi.org/10.3390/antiox9020114] [PMID: 32012850]

[18]    Liebeke M, Pöther DC, van Duy N, *et al.* Depletion of thiol-containing proteins in response to

quinones in *Bacillus subtilis*. Mol Microbiol 2008; 69(6): 1513-29.
[http://dx.doi.org/10.1111/j.1365-2958.2008.06382.x] [PMID: 18673455]

[19]　Tkachenko AG, Akhova AV, Shumkov MS, Nesterova LY. Polyamines reduce oxidative stress in *Escherichia coli* cells exposed to bactericidal antibiotics. Res Microbiol 2012; 163(2): 83-91.
[http://dx.doi.org/10.1016/j.resmic.2011.10.009] [PMID: 22138596]

[20]　Kohanski MA, Dwyer DJ, Hayete B, Lawrence CA, Collins JJ. A common mechanism of cellular death induced by bactericidal antibiotics. Cell 2007; 130(5): 797-810.
[http://dx.doi.org/10.1016/j.cell.2007.06.049] [PMID: 17803904]

[21]　Beltran-Hortelano I, Perez-Silanes S, Galiano S. Trypanothione reductase and superoxide dismutase as current drug targets for *Trypanosoma cruzi*: an overview of compounds with activity against Chagas disease. Curr Med Chem 2017; 24(11): 1066-138.
[http://dx.doi.org/10.2174/0929867323666161227094049] [PMID: 28025938]

[22]　May HC, Yu JJ, Guentzel MN, Chambers JP, Cap AP, Arulanandam BP. Repurposing auranofin, ebselen, and PX-12 as antimicrobial agents targeting the thioredoxin system. Front Microbiol 2018; 9: 336.
[http://dx.doi.org/10.3389/fmicb.2018.00336] [PMID: 29556223]

[23]　Ayala A, Muñoz MF, Argüelles S. Lipid peroxidation: production, metabolism, and signaling mechanisms of malondialdehyde and 4-hydroxy-2-nonenal. Oxid Med Cell Longev 2014; 2014: 360438.
[http://dx.doi.org/10.1155/2014/360438] [PMID: 24999379]

[24]　Avery SV. Molecular targets of oxidative stress. Biochem J 2011; 434(2): 201-10.
[http://dx.doi.org/10.1042/BJ20101695] [PMID: 21309749]

[25]　Dryden M, Cooke J, Salib R, Holding R, Pender SLF, Brooks J. Hot topics in reactive oxygen therapy: Antimicrobial and immunological mechanisms, safety and clinical applications. J Glob Antimicrob Resist 2017; 8: 194-8.
[http://dx.doi.org/10.1016/j.jgar.2016.12.012] [PMID: 28219826]

[26]　Cadet J, Douki T, Gasparutto D, Ravanat J-L. Oxidative damage to DNA: formation, measurement and biochemical features. Mutat Res 2003; 531(1-2): 5-23.
[http://dx.doi.org/10.1016/j.mrfmmm.2003.09.001] [PMID: 14637244]

[27]　Beckman KB, Ames BN. Oxidative decay of DNA. J Biol Chem 1997; 272(32): 19633-6.
[http://dx.doi.org/10.1074/jbc.272.32.19633] [PMID: 9289489]

[28]　Birben E, Sahiner UM, Sackesen C, Erzurum S, Kalayci O. Oxidative stress and antioxidant defense. World Allergy Organ J 2012; 5(1): 9-19.
[http://dx.doi.org/10.1097/WOX.0b013e3182439613] [PMID: 23268465]

[29]　Cabiscol E, Tamarit J, Ros J. Oxidative stress in bacteria and protein damage by reactive oxygen species. Int Microbiol 2000; 3(1): 3-8.
[PMID: 10963327]

[30]　Fang FC. Antimicrobial reactive oxygen and nitrogen species: concepts and controversies. Nat Rev Microbiol 2004; 2(10): 820-32.
[http://dx.doi.org/10.1038/nrmicro1004] [PMID: 15378046]

[31]　Tamarit J, Cabiscol E, Ros J. Identification of the major oxidatively damaged proteins in *Escherichia coli* cells exposed to oxidative stress. J Biol Chem 1998; 273(5): 3027-32.
[http://dx.doi.org/10.1074/jbc.273.5.3027] [PMID: 9446617]

[32]　Iorio M, Cruz J, Simone M, *et al.* Antibacterial paramagnetic quinones from Actinoallomurus. J Nat Prod 2017; 80(4): 819-27.
[http://dx.doi.org/10.1021/acs.jnatprod.6b00654] [PMID: 28218529]

[33]　Bhaskar A, Chawla M, Mehta M, *et al.* Reengineering redox sensitive GFP to measure mycothiol redox potential of *Mycobacterium tuberculosis* during infection. PLoS Pathog 2014; 10(1): e1003902.

[http://dx.doi.org/10.1371/journal.ppat.1003902] [PMID: 24497832]

[34]   Dwyer DJ, Kohanski MA, Hayete B, Collins JJ. Gyrase inhibitors induce an oxidative damage cellular death pathway in *Escherichia coli*. Mol Syst Biol 2007; 3: 91.
[http://dx.doi.org/10.1038/msb4100135] [PMID: 17353933]

[35]   Páez PL, Becerra MC, Albesa I. Comparison of macromolecular oxidation by reactive oxygen species in three bacterial genera exposed to different antibiotics. Cell Biochem Biophys 2011; 61(3): 467-72.
[http://dx.doi.org/10.1007/s12013-011-9227-z] [PMID: 21739263]

[36]   Becerra MC, Páez PL, Laróvere LE, Albesa I. Lipids and DNA oxidation in *Staphylococcus aureus* as a consequence of oxidative stress generated by ciprofloxacin. Mol Cell Biochem 2006; 285(1-2): 29-34.
[http://dx.doi.org/10.1007/s11010-005-9051-0] [PMID: 16541200]

[37]   Guerzoni ME, Lanciotti R, Cocconcelli PS. Alteration in cellular fatty acid composition as a response to salt, acid, oxidative and thermal stresses in *Lactobacillus helveticus*. Microbiology 2001; 147(Pt 8): 2255-64.
[http://dx.doi.org/10.1099/00221287-147-8-2255] [PMID: 11496002]

[38]   Mourenza Á, Gil JA, Mateos LM, Letek M. Oxidative stress-generating antimicrobials, a novel strategy to overcome antibacterial resistance. Antioxidants 2020; 9(5): 361. b
[http://dx.doi.org/10.3390/antiox9050361] [PMID: 32357394]

[39]   Sato H, Feix JB. Peptide-membrane interactions and mechanisms of membrane destruction by amphipathic α-helical antimicrobial peptides. Biochim Biophys Acta 2006; 1758(9): 1245-56.
[http://dx.doi.org/10.1016/j.bbamem.2006.02.021] [PMID: 16697975]

[40]   Memar MY, Ghotaslou R, Samiei M, Adibkia K. Antimicrobial use of reactive oxygen therapy: current insights. Infect Drug Resist 2018; 11: 567-76.
[http://dx.doi.org/10.2147/IDR.S142397] [PMID: 29731645]

[41]   Pohanka M. Role of oxidative stress in infectious diseases. A review. Folia Microbiol (Praha) 2013; 58(6): 503-13.
[http://dx.doi.org/10.1007/s12223-013-0239-5] [PMID: 23504625]

[42]   Ivanov AV, Bartosch B, Isaguliants MG. Oxidative stress in infection and consequent disease. Oxid Med Cell Longev 2017; 2017: 3496043.
[http://dx.doi.org/10.1155/2017/3496043] [PMID: 28255425]

[43]   Thom SR. Oxidative stress is fundamental to hyperbaric oxygen therapy. J Appl Physiol 2009; 106(3): 988-95.
[http://dx.doi.org/10.1152/japplphysiol.91004.2008] [PMID: 18845776]

[44]   Dridi B, Lupien A, Bergeron MG, Leprohon P, Ouellette M. Differences in antibiotic-induced oxidative stress responses between laboratory and clinical isolates of *Streptococcus pneumoniae*. Antimicrob Agents Chemother 2015; 59(9): 5420-6.
[http://dx.doi.org/10.1128/AAC.00316-15] [PMID: 26100702]

[45]   Becerra MC, Albesa I. Oxidative stress induced by ciprofloxacin in *Staphylococcus aureus*. Biochem Biophys Res Commun 2002; 297(4): 1003-7.
[http://dx.doi.org/10.1016/S0006-291X(02)02331-8] [PMID: 12359254]

[46]   Dwyer DJ, Kohanski MA, Collins JJ. Role of reactive oxygen species in antibiotic action and resistance. Curr Opin Microbiol 2009; 12(5): 482-9.
[http://dx.doi.org/10.1016/j.mib.2009.06.018] [PMID: 19647477]

[47]   Wang X, Zhao X. Contribution of oxidative damage to antimicrobial lethality. Antimicrob Agents Chemother 2009; 53(4): 1395-402.
[http://dx.doi.org/10.1128/AAC.01087-08] [PMID: 19223646]

[48]   Martínez SR, Aiassa V, Sola C, Becerra MC. Oxidative stress response in reference and clinical *Staphylococcus aureus* strains under Linezolid exposure. J Glob Antimicrob Resist 2020; 22: 257-62.

[http://dx.doi.org/10.1016/j.jgar.2020.02.032] [PMID: 32169679]

[49]   Barber AE, Norton JP, Spivak AM, Mulvey MA. Urinary tract infections: current and emerging management strategies. Clin Infect Dis 2013; 57(5): 719-24.
[http://dx.doi.org/10.1093/cid/cit284] [PMID: 23645845]

[50]   Yan ZQ, Wang DD, Ding L, *et al.* Mechanism of artemisinin phytotoxicity action: induction of reactive oxygen species and cell death in lettuce seedlings. Plant Physiol Biochem 2015; 88: 53-9.
[http://dx.doi.org/10.1016/j.plaphy.2015.01.010] [PMID: 25658194]

[51]   Chua NG, Zhou YP, Tan TT, *et al.* Polymyxin B with dual carbapenem combination therapy against carbapenemase-producing *Klebsiella pneumoniae.* J Infect 2015; 70(3): 309-11.
[http://dx.doi.org/10.1016/j.jinf.2014.10.001] [PMID: 25305144]

[52]   Kim SY, Park C, Jang H-J, *et al.* Antibacterial strategies inspired by the oxidative stress and response networks. J Microbiol 2019; 57(3): 203-12.
[http://dx.doi.org/10.1007/s12275-019-8711-9] [PMID: 30806977]

[53]   Keren I, Wu Y, Inocencio J, Mulcahy LR, Lewis K. Killing by bactericidal antibiotics does not depend on reactive oxygen species. Science 2013; 339(6124): 1213-6.
[http://dx.doi.org/10.1126/science.1232688] [PMID: 23471410]

[54]   Liu Y, Imlay JA. Cell death from antibiotics without the involvement of reactive oxygen species. Science 2013; 339(6124): 1210-3.
[http://dx.doi.org/10.1126/science.1232751] [PMID: 23471409]

[55]   Kohanski MA, DePristo MA, Collins JJ. Sublethal antibiotic treatment leads to multidrug resistance *via* radical-induced mutagenesis. Mol Cell 2010; 37(3): 311-20.
[http://dx.doi.org/10.1016/j.molcel.2010.01.003] [PMID: 20159551]

[56]   Foti JJ, Devadoss B, Winkler JA, Collins JJ, Walker GC. Oxidation of the guanine nucleotide pool underlies cell death by bactericidal antibiotics. Science 2012; 336(6079): 315-9.
[http://dx.doi.org/10.1126/science.1219192] [PMID: 22517853]

[57]   Sorci G, Faivre B. Inflammation and oxidative stress in vertebrate host-parasite systems. Philos Trans R Soc Lond B Biol Sci 2009; 364(1513): 71-83.
[http://dx.doi.org/10.1098/rstb.2008.0151] [PMID: 18930878]

[58]   Kalghatgi S, Spina CS, Costello JC, *et al.* Bactericidal antibiotics induce mitochondrial dysfunction and oxidative damage in Mammalian cells. Sci Transl Med 2013; 5(192): 192ra85.
[http://dx.doi.org/10.1126/scitranslmed.3006055] [PMID: 23825301]

[59]   Novaes RD, Santos EC, Fialho MDCQ, *et al.* Nonsteroidal anti-inflammatory is more effective than anti-oxidant therapy in counteracting oxidative/nitrosative stress and heart disease in *T. cruzi*-infected mice. Parasitology 2017; 144(7): 904-16.
[http://dx.doi.org/10.1017/S0031182016002675] [PMID: 28134069]

[60]   Dong C, Zhou J, Wang P, *et al.* Topical therapeutic efficacy of ebselen against multidrug-resistant *Staphylococcus aureus* LT-1. Front Microbiol 2020; 10: 3016.
[http://dx.doi.org/10.3389/fmicb.2019.03016] [PMID: 32010088]

[61]   Chi BK, Huyen NTT, Loi VV, *et al.* The disulfide stress response and protein s-thioallylation caused by allicin and diallyl polysulfanes in *Bacillus subtilis* as revealed by transcriptomics and proteomics. Antioxidants 2019; 8(12): 605.
[http://dx.doi.org/10.3390/antiox8120605] [PMID: 31795512]

[62]   Zou L, Wang J, Gao Y, *et al.* Synergistic antibacterial activity of silver with antibiotics correlating with the upregulation of the ROS production. Sci Rep 2018; 8(1): 11131.
[http://dx.doi.org/10.1038/s41598-018-29313-w] [PMID: 30042429]

[63]   Zhao R, Masayasu H, Holmgren A. Ebselen: a substrate for human thioredoxin reductase strongly stimulating its hydroperoxide reductase activity and a superfast thioredoxin oxidant. Proc Natl Acad Sci USA 2002; 99(13): 8579-84.

[http://dx.doi.org/10.1073/pnas.122061399] [PMID: 12070343]

[64] Nakamura Y, Feng Q, Kumagai T, *et al.* Ebselen, a glutathione peroxidase mimetic seleno-organic compound, as a multifunctional antioxidant. Implication for inflammation-associated carcinogenesis. J Biol Chem 2002; 277(4): 2687-94.
[http://dx.doi.org/10.1074/jbc.M109641200] [PMID: 11714717]

[65] Lu J, Vlamis-Gardikas A, Kandasamy K, *et al.* Inhibition of bacterial thioredoxin reductase: an antibiotic mechanism targeting bacteria lacking glutathione. FASEB J 2013; 27(4): 1394-403.
[http://dx.doi.org/10.1096/fj.12-223305] [PMID: 23248236]

[66] Thangamani S, Younis W, Seleem MN. Repurposing clinical molecule ebselen to combat drug resistant pathogens. PLoS One 2015; 10(7): e0133877.
[http://dx.doi.org/10.1371/journal.pone.0133877] [PMID: 26222252]

[67] Zou L, Lu J, Wang J, *et al.* Synergistic antibacterial effect of silver and ebselen against multidrug-resistant Gram-negative bacterial infections. EMBO Mol Med 2017; 9(8): 1165-78.
[http://dx.doi.org/10.15252/emmm.201707661] [PMID: 28606995]

[68] Loi VV, Busche T, Preuß T, Kalinowski J, Bernhardt J, Antelmann H. The AGXX® antimicrobial coating causes a thiol-specific oxidative stress response and protein s-bacillithiolation in *Staphylococcus aureus*. Front Microbiol 2018; 9: 3037.
[http://dx.doi.org/10.3389/fmicb.2018.03037] [PMID: 30619128]

[69] Loi VV, Huyen NTT, Busche T, *et al. Staphylococcus aureus* responds to allicin by global S-thioallylation - Role of the Brx/BSH/YpdA pathway and the disulfide reductase MerA to overcome allicin stress. Free Radic Biol Med 2019; 139: 55-69.
[http://dx.doi.org/10.1016/j.freeradbiomed.2019.05.018] [PMID: 31121222]

[70] Ibitoye OB, Ajiboye TO. Ferulic acid potentiates the antibacterial activity of quinolone-based antibiotics against *Acinetobacter baumannii*. Microb Pathog 2019; 126: 393-8.
[http://dx.doi.org/10.1016/j.micpath.2018.11.033] [PMID: 30476577]

[71] Sigler K, Chaloupka J, Brozmanová J, Stadler N, Höfer M. Oxidative stress in microorganisms--I. Microbial *vs.* higher cells--damage and defenses in relation to cell aging and death. Folia Microbiol (Praha) 1999; 44(6): 587-624.
[http://dx.doi.org/10.1007/BF02825650] [PMID: 11097021]

[72] Becker K, Gromer S, Schirmer RH, Müller S. Thioredoxin reductase as a pathophysiological factor and drug target. Eur J Biochem 2000; 267(20): 6118-25.
[http://dx.doi.org/10.1046/j.1432-1327.2000.01703.x] [PMID: 11012663]

[73] Turrens JF. Oxidative stress and antioxidant defenses: a target for the treatment of diseases caused by parasitic protozoa. Mol Aspects Med 2004; 25(1-2): 211-20.
[http://dx.doi.org/10.1016/j.mam.2004.02.021] [PMID: 15051329]

[74] Keren I, Shah D, Spoering A, Kaldalu N, Lewis K. Specialized persister cells and the mechanism of multidrug tolerance in *Escherichia coli*. J Bacteriol 2004; 186(24): 8172-80.
[http://dx.doi.org/10.1128/JB.186.24.8172-8180.2004] [PMID: 15576765]

[75] Hassan HM, Fridovich I. Intracellular production of superoxide radical and of hydrogen peroxide by redox active compounds. Arch Biochem Biophys 1979; 196(2): 385-95.
[http://dx.doi.org/10.1016/0003-9861(79)90289-3] [PMID: 225995]

[76] Fridovich I. Superoxide dismutases: regularities and irregularities. Harvey Lect 1983-1984; 79: 51-75.
[PMID: 6100676]

[77] Fenton HJH. Oxidation of tartaric acid in presence of iron. J Chem Soc Trans 1894; 65: 899-11.
[http://dx.doi.org/10.1039/CT8946500899]

[78] Liochev SI, Fridovich I. The effects of superoxide dismutase on $H_2O_2$ formation. Free Radic Biol Med 2007; 42(10): 1465-9.
[http://dx.doi.org/10.1016/j.freeradbiomed.2007.02.015] [PMID: 17448892]

[79]    Fridovich I. Superoxide dismutases. An adaptation to a paramagnetic gas. J Biol Chem 1989; 264(14): 7761-4.
[http://dx.doi.org/10.1016/S0021-9258(18)83102-7] [PMID: 2542241]

[80]    Moore RL, Powell LJ, Goodwin DC. The kinetic properties producing the perfunctory pH profiles of catalase-peroxidases. Biochim Biophys Acta 2008; 1784(6): 900-7.
[http://dx.doi.org/10.1016/j.bbapap.2008.03.008] [PMID: 18413236]

[81]    Claiborne A, Fridovich I. Purification of the o-dianisidine peroxidase from *Escherichia coli* B. Physicochemical characterization and analysis of its dual catalatic and peroxidatic activities. J Biol Chem 1979; 254(10): 4245-52.
[http://dx.doi.org/10.1016/S0021-9258(18)50722-5] [PMID: 374409]

[82]    Baba T, Ara T, Hasegawa M, *et al.* Construction of *Escherichia coli* K-12 in-frame, single-gene knockout mutants: the Keio collection. Mol Syst Biol 2006; 2: 2006-8.

[83]    Albesa I, Becerra MC, Battán PC, Páez PL. Oxidative stress involved in the antibacterial action of different antibiotics. Biochem Biophys Res Commun 2004; 317(2): 605-9.
[http://dx.doi.org/10.1016/j.bbrc.2004.03.085] [PMID: 15063800]

[84]    Goswami M, Mangoli SH, Jawali N. Involvement of reactive oxygen species in the action of ciprofloxacin against *Escherichia coli.* Antimicrob Agents Chemother 2006; 50(3): 949-54.
[http://dx.doi.org/10.1128/AAC.50.3.949-954.2006] [PMID: 16495256]

[85]    Hong Y, Zeng J, Wang X, Drlica K, Zhao X. Post-stress bacterial cell death mediated by reactive oxygen species. Proc Natl Acad Sci USA 2019; 116(20): 10064-71.
[http://dx.doi.org/10.1073/pnas.1901730116] [PMID: 30948634]

[86]    Laxminarayan R, Duse A, Wattal C, *et al.* Antibiotic resistance-the need for global solutions. Lancet Infect Dis 2013; 13(12): 1057-98.
[http://dx.doi.org/10.1016/S1473-3099(13)70318-9] [PMID: 24252483]

[87]    Mah MW, Memish ZA. Antibiotic resistance. An impending crisis. Saudi Med J 2000; 21(12): 1125-9.
[PMID: 11360084]

[88]    Cosgarea R, Heumann C, Juncar R, *et al.* One year results of a randomized controlled clinical study evaluating the effects of non-surgical periodontal therapy of chronic periodontitis in conjunction with three or seven days systemic administration of amoxicillin/metronidazole. PLoS One 2017; 12(6): e0179592.
[http://dx.doi.org/10.1371/journal.pone.0179592] [PMID: 28662049]

[89]    Cosgarea R, Juncar R, Heumann C, *et al.* Non-surgical periodontal treatment in conjunction with 3 or 7 days systemic administration of amoxicillin and metronidazole in severe chronic periodontitis patients. A placebo-controlled randomized clinical study. J Clin Periodontol 2016; 43(9): 767-77.
[http://dx.doi.org/10.1111/jcpe.12559] [PMID: 27027501]

[90]    Boia S, Boariu M, Baderca F, *et al.* Clinical, microbiological and oxidative stress evaluation of periodontitis patients treated with two regimens of systemic antibiotics, adjunctive to non-surgical therapy: A placebo-controlled randomized clinical trial. Exp Ther Med 2019; 18(6): 5001-15.
[http://dx.doi.org/10.3892/etm.2019.7856] [PMID: 31819766]

[91]    Lakhssassi N, Elhajoui N, Lodter JP, Pineill JL, Sixou M. Antimicrobial susceptibility variation of 50 anaerobic periopathogens in aggressive periodontitis: an interindividual variability study. Oral Microbiol Immunol 2005; 20(4): 244-52.
[http://dx.doi.org/10.1111/j.1399-302X.2005.00225.x] [PMID: 15943770]

[92]    Andreadis AA, Hazen SL, Comhair SA, Erzurum SC. Oxidative and nitrosative events in asthma. Free Radic Biol Med 2003; 35(3): 213-25.
[http://dx.doi.org/10.1016/S0891-5849(03)00278-8] [PMID: 12885584]

[93]    Bwititi PT, Chinkwo K. Oxidative stress markers in infectious respiratory diseases: current clinical practice. Int J Res Med Sci 2016; 4: 1802-13.

[http://dx.doi.org/10.18203/2320-6012.ijrms20161727]

[94] Grant SS, Hung DT. Persistent bacterial infections, antibiotic tolerance, and the oxidative stress response. Virulence 2013; 4(4): 273-83.
[http://dx.doi.org/10.4161/viru.23987] [PMID: 23563389]

[95] Gomez JE, McKinney JD. *M. tuberculosis* persistence, latency, and drug tolerance. Tuberculosis (Edinb) 2004; 84(1-2): 29-44.
[http://dx.doi.org/10.1016/j.tube.2003.08.003] [PMID: 14670344]

[96] Monack DM, Mueller A, Falkow S. Persistent bacterial infections: the interface of the pathogen and the host immune system. Nat Rev Microbiol 2004; 2(9): 747-65.
[http://dx.doi.org/10.1038/nrmicro955] [PMID: 15372085]

[97] McDERMOTT W. Microbial persistence. Yale J Biol Med 1958; 30(4): 257-91.
[PMID: 13531168]

[98] Kwon DH, Lu CD. Polyamines induce resistance to cationic peptide, aminoglycoside, and quinolone antibiotics in *Pseudomonas aeruginosa* PAO1. Antimicrob Agents Chemother 2006; 50(5): 1615-22.
[http://dx.doi.org/10.1128/AAC.50.5.1615-1622.2006] [PMID: 16641426]

[99] Igarashi K, Kashiwagi K. Modulation of cellular function by polyamines. Int J Biochem Cell Biol 2010; 42(1): 39-51.
[http://dx.doi.org/10.1016/j.biocel.2009.07.009] [PMID: 19643201]

[100] Rhee HJ, Kim EJ, Lee JK. Physiological polyamines: simple primordial stress molecules. J Cell Mol Med 2007; 11(4): 685-703.
[http://dx.doi.org/10.1111/j.1582-4934.2007.00077.x] [PMID: 17760833]

[101] Yoshida M, Kashiwagi K, Shigemasa A, *et al.* A unifying model for the role of polyamines in bacterial cell growth, the polyamine modulon. J Biol Chem 2004; 279(44): 46008-13.
[http://dx.doi.org/10.1074/jbc.M404393200] [PMID: 15326188]

[102] Gaboriau F, Vaultier M, Moulinoux JP, Delcros JG. Antioxidative properties of natural polyamines and dimethylsilane analogues. Redox Rep 2005; 10(1): 9-18.
[http://dx.doi.org/10.1179/135100005X21561] [PMID: 15829106]

[103] Muscari C, Guarnieri C, Stefanelli C, Giaccari A, Caldarera CM. Protective effect of spermine on DNA exposed to oxidative stress. Mol Cell Biochem 1995; 144(2): 125-9.
[http://dx.doi.org/10.1007/BF00944391] [PMID: 7623783]

[104] Tkachenko A, Nesterova L, Pshenichnov M. The role of the natural polyamine putrescine in defense against oxidative stress in *Escherichia coli*. Arch Microbiol 2001; 176(1-2): 155-7.
[http://dx.doi.org/10.1007/s002030100301] [PMID: 11479716]

[105] Løvaas E. Antioxidative and metal-chelating effects of polyamines. Adv Pharmacol 1997; 38: 119-49.
[http://dx.doi.org/10.1016/S1054-3589(08)60982-5] [PMID: 8895807]

[106] Ha HC, Sirisoma NS, Kuppusamy P, Zweier JL, Woster PM, Casero RA Jr. The natural polyamine spermine functions directly as a free radical scavenger. Proc Natl Acad Sci USA 1998; 95(19): 11140-5.
[http://dx.doi.org/10.1073/pnas.95.19.11140] [PMID: 9736703]

[107] Ramani D, De Bandt JP, Cynober L. Aliphatic polyamines in physiology and diseases. Clin Nutr 2014; 33(1): 14-22.
[http://dx.doi.org/10.1016/j.clnu.2013.09.019] [PMID: 24144912]

[108] Gutierrez A, Laureti L, Crussard S, *et al.* β-Lactam antibiotics promote bacterial mutagenesis *via* an RpoS-mediated reduction in replication fidelity. Nat Commun 2013; 4: 1610.
[http://dx.doi.org/10.1038/ncomms2607] [PMID: 23511474]

[109] Hassett DJ, Imlay JA. Bactericidal antibiotics and oxidative stress: a radical proposal. ACS Chem Biol 2007; 2(11): 708-10.

[http://dx.doi.org/10.1021/cb700232k] [PMID: 18030985]

[110]  Parsek MR, Singh PK. Bacterial biofilms: an emerging link to disease pathogenesis. Annu Rev Microbiol 2003; 57: 677-701.
[http://dx.doi.org/10.1146/annurev.micro.57.030502.090720] [PMID: 14527295]

[111]  Peranzoni E, Marigo I, Dolcetti L, *et al.* Role of arginine metabolism in immunity and immunopathology. Immunobiology 2007; 212(9-10): 795-812.
[http://dx.doi.org/10.1016/j.imbio.2007.09.008] [PMID: 18086380]

[112]  Steichen C, Chen P, Kearney JF, Turnbough CL Jr. Identification of the immunodominant protein and other proteins of the *Bacillus anthracis* exosporium. J Bacteriol 2003; 185(6): 1903-10.
[http://dx.doi.org/10.1128/JB.185.6.1903-1910.2003] [PMID: 12618454]

[113]  Raines KW, Kang TJ, Hibbs S, *et al.* Importance of nitric oxide synthase in the control of infection by *Bacillus anthracis.* Infect Immun 2006; 74(4): 2268-76.
[http://dx.doi.org/10.1128/IAI.74.4.2268-2276.2006] [PMID: 16552057]

[114]  Borisov VB, Forte E, Siletsky SA, *et al.* Cytochrome bd protects bacteria against oxidative and nitrosative stress: a potential target for next-generation antimicrobial agents. Biochemistry (Mosc) 2015; 80(5): 565-75.
[http://dx.doi.org/10.1134/S0006297915050077] [PMID: 26071774]

[115]  Meuric V, Gracieux P, Tamanai-Shacoori Z, Perez-Chaparro J, Bonnaure-Mallet M. Expression patterns of genes induced by oxidative stress in *Porphyromonas gingivalis.* Oral Microbiol Immunol 2008; 23(4): 308-14.
[http://dx.doi.org/10.1111/j.1399-302X.2007.00429.x] [PMID: 18582330]

[116]  Honma K, Mishima E, Inagaki S, Sharma A. The OxyR homologue in *Tannerella forsythia* regulates expression of oxidative stress responses and biofilm formation. Microbiology 2009; 155(Pt 6): 1912-22.
[http://dx.doi.org/10.1099/mic.0.027920-0] [PMID: 19389765]

[117]  Hennequin C, Forestier C. oxyR, a LysR-type regulator involved in Klebsiella pneumoniae mucosal and abiotic colonization. Infect Immun 2009; 77(12): 5449-57.
[http://dx.doi.org/10.1128/IAI.00837-09] [PMID: 19786563]

[118]  Ehrt S, Schnappinger D. Mycobacterial survival strategies in the phagosome: defence against host stresses. Cell Microbiol 2009; 11(8): 1170-8.
[http://dx.doi.org/10.1111/j.1462-5822.2009.01335.x] [PMID: 19438516]

[119]  Voskuil MI, Bartek IL, Visconti K, *et al.* The response of Mycobacterium tuberculosis to reactive oxygen and nitrogen species. Front Microbiol Cell Infect Micro 2011; p. 2.

[120]  Jones GS, Amirault HJ, Andersen BR. Killing of *Mycobacterium tuberculosis* by neutrophils: a nonoxidative process. J Infect Dis 1990; 162(3): 700-4.
[http://dx.doi.org/10.1093/infdis/162.3.700] [PMID: 2167338]

[121]  Long R, Light B, Talbot JA. Mycobacteriocidal action of exogenous nitric oxide. Antimicrob Agents Chemother 1999; 43(2): 403-5.
[http://dx.doi.org/10.1128/AAC.43.2.403] [PMID: 9925545]

[122]  Imlay JA. Cellular defenses against superoxide and hydrogen peroxide. Annu Rev Biochem 2008; 77: 755-76.
[http://dx.doi.org/10.1146/annurev.biochem.77.061606.161055] [PMID: 18173371]

[123]  Gu M, Imlay JA. The SoxRS response of *Escherichia coli* is directly activated by redox-cycling drugs rather than by superoxide. Mol Microbiol 2011; 79(5): 1136-50.
[http://dx.doi.org/10.1111/j.1365-2958.2010.07520.x] [PMID: 21226770]

[124]  Pomposiello PJ, Bennik MH, Demple B. Genome-wide transcriptional profiling of the *Escherichia coli* responses to superoxide stress and sodium salicylate. J Bacteriol 2001; 183(13): 3890-902.
[http://dx.doi.org/10.1128/JB.183.13.3890-3902.2001] [PMID: 11395452]

[125]  Van Bambeke F, Glupczynski Y, Plésiat P, Pechère JC, Tulkens PM. Antibiotic efflux pumps in prokaryotic cells: occurrence, impact on resistance and strategies for the future of antimicrobial therapy. J Antimicrob Chemother 2003; 51(5): 1055-65.
[http://dx.doi.org/10.1093/jac/dkg224] [PMID: 12697642]

[126]  Kharkwal GB, Sharma SK, Huang YY, Dai T, Hamblin MR. Photodynamic therapy for infections: clinical applications. Lasers Surg Med 2011; 43(7): 755-67.
[http://dx.doi.org/10.1002/lsm.21080] [PMID: 22057503]

[127]  Mak JC. Pathogenesis of COPD. Part II. Oxidative-antioxidative imbalance. Int J Tuberc Lung Dis 2008; 12(4): 368-74.
[PMID: 18371260]

[128]  Novaes RD, Teixeira AL, de Miranda AS. Oxidative stress in microbial diseases: pathogen, host, and therapeutics. Oxid Med Cell Longev 2019; 2019: 8159562.
[http://dx.doi.org/10.1155/2019/8159562] [PMID: 30774746]

[129]  Domej W, Oettl K, Renner W. Oxidative stress and free radicals in COPD--implications and relevance for treatment. Int J Chron Obstruct Pulmon Dis 2014; 9: 1207-24.
[http://dx.doi.org/10.2147/COPD.S51226] [PMID: 25378921]

[130]  Imlay JA. Diagnosing oxidative stress in bacteria: not as easy as you might think. Curr Opin Microbiol 2015; 24: 124-31.
[http://dx.doi.org/10.1016/j.mib.2015.01.004] [PMID: 25666086]

[131]  Brynildsen MP, Winkler JA, Spina CS, MacDonald IC, Collins JJ. Potentiating antibacterial activity by predictably enhancing endogenous microbial ROS production. Nat Biotechnol 2013; 31(2): 160-5.
[http://dx.doi.org/10.1038/nbt.2458] [PMID: 23292609]

**CHAPTER 13**

# Phytotherapy and the 'Omics Concept

**Ismaila O. Nurain[1,*]**

[1] *Department of Pharmacology, the University of Minnesota Medical School, Minneapolis, USA*

**Abstract:** Medicinal plants are particularly important biobanks for chemical and structural diversity and the identification and characterization of druggable agents in the pharmaceutical developmental processes. Many researchers are now striving to upgrade traditional medicine to match modern medicine. One of the greatest means to do this is by omics sciences. This chapter focuses on the description of 'omics technologies as a pivotal tool in the standardization and modernization of phytotherapy. Some of the 'omics approaches discussed are genomics, proteomics, chemoproteomics, glycoproteomics, immunoproteomics, interactomics, transcriptomics, metabolomics, toxicogenomics, pharcogenomics, pharmacometabolomics, phytochemomics, toxicometabolomics, phenomics, cytomics, and metallomics. These fields of sciences are very important for the understanding of components and mechanisms of actions of cells, tissues, organs, and systems with disease mechanisms. Thus, 'omics sciences have been gaining ground and acceptance in the drug development processes of modern medicine and as a precision medicine for disease management. Overall, utilizing 'omics technologies as tools for the standardization and modernization of phytotherapy is a promising way to improve traditional medicine in tackling several life-threatening and deadly diseases.

**Keywords:** Phytotherapy, Medicinal plant, Omics technology, Genomics, Transcriptomics, Proteomics, Metabolomics.

## 1. INTRODUCTION

The study of the use of plant extracts or extracts from another natural origin as therapeutic agents that promote the healthy living of organisms is referred to as phytotherapy or herbal therapy. It involves the use of the whole plant or parts of the plant as foods, teas, powdered herbs, liquid extracts, incense, smudges, and skin preparations to manage organisms' conditions. Examples are adaptogens, adjuvants, analgesic, antiemetics, aperients, astringents, *etc*. Adaptogens are herbs

---

[*] **Corresponding author Ismaila O. Nurain:** Department of Pharmacology, the University of Minnesota Medical School, Minneapolis, USA; Tel: +2348068088828; E-mail: isnurain@gmail.com

**Saheed Sabiu (Ed)**

that are used for the improvement of the adaptability of the body to stress. Adjuvants enhance the body's response to a remedy. Also, analgesic and anodynes plants are used for pain relief in the same manners and antiemetics are used for lessening nausea and preventing vomiting. Aperients are mostly used as moderate laxative and digestion or appetite modifiers. Astringents could be used in tissue contraction and regulation of body secretion. They are also used to tighten or change the tone of the body. To mitigate or soothe inflammation, Balsamic herbs are extremely useful. Other uses of plants and plant extracts are as an expectorant, emmenagogue, hypnotics, and demulcent to mention a few. Currently, it has been reported that 38% of United States adults depend on some kind of herbal medicine as part of their alternative medicine. Being that as it is, there are a lot of concerns on their effects in the general biological system, toxicological effects, efficacy, and reproducible method of preparations, *etc*.

Historically, phytotherapy as a way of disease management is as old as the age of man on earth. The first man to use the term "phytotherapy" as a concept in 1913 was Henri Leclerc, who was a French physician. Since the beginning of the world, there was always quest to search for the rescue for human discomfort or disease. The act of using medicinal plants for different human conditions (disease states or discomfort of any form) is natural [1]. Moreover every knowledge about herbs was gained by experience. The reason for using a particular plant or plant product would be as a result of other user experiences and that was how thousands of plants become known for their roles and functions in biological system. One of the written evidence of the use of herbal terapy was found in Nagpur with a Sumerian Clay Slab about 5000 years old. It has more than 250 different plant components made up of 12 different recipes [2]. "Pen T'Sao" was written by Emperor Shen Nung circa 2500 BC. In the book, about 365 drugs were proposed from dried plants' parts. Some of these prescriptions are still in use today e.g., *podophyllum*, *Rhei rhizoma*, camphor, *Theae folium*, cinnamon bark, ginseng, jimson weed, gentian *etc* [3, 4]. In India, a book, "Vedas" described the most abundant plants for disease treatment. It is established that most numerous spice plants used until today originated from India e.g., pepper, nutmeg, clove. *etc* [5]. Also, in 1550 BC, about 700 different plant species such as willow, fig, juniper, onion, common centaury, aloe, castor oil pomegranate to mention, but few were gathered and enumerated for the bioactivity potentials [6, 7]. Other historical information about the use of herbal medicine can be found in the literature [8 - 13].

As mention above, the use of phytotherapy in the management of different diseases has been existent for centuries. Many researchers have worked on the cytotoxicity effects of several medicinal plants in the efforts to provide a cure for cancer disease. Wargovich and co-workers have reported the effect of herbs in the prevention of cancer and other diseases [14]. For prostate cancer, *Pygeum africanum*, which is commonly used in Europe and the USA for benign prostatic hypertrophy (BPH, has been proven to be very efficacious against cancer and safe for consumption at the described dosage [15]. Thus, this plant could be a good supplement for the prevention of prostate cancer. In another research *Boophone disticha*, a South African ethnomedicinal plant, was investigated phytochemically and phytotherapeutically for its usage in the management of diseases such as inflammatory disease, mental illness, and wounds healing [16]. Also, phytochemical analysis of *Genus uncaria* was carried out on nineteen species of the plant, which revealed some important pharmacological properties, including usage for rheumatism, hyperpyrexia, asthma, hypertension, *etc.*, in South America, Malaysia, Africa, Philippines, and China [17]. Other applications of phytotherapy in diseases' management have been enumerated, such as liver disease [18, 19], skin disease [20], Alzheimer's disease [21], urologic disease [22], nonsurgical treatment of periodontal disease [23], Parkinson's disease [24], cardiovascular disease [25] coronavirus [26, 27], urinary stone disease [28], and cancer [29].

The different kinds of phytomedicines used in the management of various conditions are also referred to as phytotherapy. The combined approach to bridge phytotherapy and modern medicine and between available genomic information and several biological processes involve the use of the different strategies from many analytical strata in combination with sophisticated computational studies [30, 31]. Although the genomic study is very significant and impactful, it is imperative to fill the gap between the series of information for the identification and characterization of probable biomarkers with the physiological and pathological processes in the living system coupled with potential therapeutic agents [32]. The field of science responsible for this is omics science. It is relevant in the standardization and characterization of phytomedicine with correlation to genomic information. An omics concept is a vital technique in the modernization of phytotherapy. It involves technologies that measure some characteristic of a large family of cellular molecules, such as genes, proteins, or small metabolites. It is a branch of science comprised of many disciplines in biological sciences with their names ending in omics such as genomics, proteomics, transcriptomics, metabolomics, glycomics, lipidomics. It involves the characterization and quantification of structure, function, and dynamism which make up the organism. As a concept, omics science is commonly used by research and medical professionals like bioinformaticians and molecular biologists. The importance of the application of omics in phytotherapy cannot be overemphasized since it has penetrated almost all aspects of medicine.

Omics can be considered as a basis for precision medicine. The results of the data analysis from the omics studies usually lead to disease management [33]. The fundamental basics for the genome project were to match the vast knowledge of the abnormalities in cancers and several other diseases [34, 35] with accurate disease management strategy by the identification of molecular abnormalities which can lead to the disease detection and diagnosis. The relevance of omics sciences in research and development has also been reported [30]. Through the development of omics-based analysis of clinical data and tests, omics has been proven essential in the prognosis and therapy selection in the management of diseases including cancer [36, 37]. Omics science is particularly important in the biobank which serves as a repository tool where biological samples (especially human samples) and data are stored for further use in research studies. The biobank is a very important resource in biomedical research such as genomics and personalized medicine [34].

Due to the fast technology development, many research tools have also been innovated to aid the understanding of the study of biological systems. In traditional medicine where the use of herbal products is dominant, several researchers have put forward the most recent current advancement in technologies to overcome the problems in research. The first and best scientific achievement and breakthrough in the past century is the completion of the human genome project [38]. The identification of drugs, drug targets, validation of drug targets, and explanation of etiology of several diseases has been made easier since the genomic revolution in the human genome project [32, 39]. These advancements in technology including but are not limited to genetic markers through DNA, miniaturization and automation technologies cloning procedures, Sanger DNA sequencing, genotyping, polymerase chain reaction (PCR), and nanotechnology [40]. These techniques have bridged many gaps in deciphering procedures in biological processes [39]. However, it is imperative to fill the gap between the therapeutic targets and the organism's physiological and pathological processes. This is where omics comes in to play. Omics involves the combination of sophisticated analytical technologies and computational strategies from various analytical strata. To understand the molecular mechanisms, there is a need to integrate scientific technology, bioinformatics, and molecular biology, which is the work of omics sciences [30, 31, 40]. The post-genomic era represents the beginning of system biology for the evolution of the sciences of omics and the result of any omics analysis can be considered as the wholeness of organismal systems gathered from bioinformatic analyses [41]. Thus, the omics science in traditional medicine approaches to therapy in the management of diseases is a powerful tool in the development of high quality and standardized herbal products. The following next headings explain the concept of omics sciences in the field of phytotherapy as shown in Table **1**.

**Table 1. List of omics sciences in system biology.**

| S/N | Areas of System Biology | Omics Sciences |
|:---:|:---:|:---:|
| 1 | DNA | Genomics<br>Epigenomics<br>Metagenomics<br>Toxicogenomics<br>Pharmacogenomics<br>herbogenomics |
| 2 | RNA | Transcriptome |
| 3 | Proteins | Proteomics<br>Phosphoproteomics<br>Glycoproteomics<br>Toxicoproteomics<br>Chemoproteomics<br>Immunoproteomics<br>Interactomics |
| 4 | Metabolites | metabolomics<br>Pharmacometabolomics<br>Phytochemomics<br>Lipidomics<br>Toxicometabolomics |
| 5 | Ions | Metallomics<br>Ionomics |
| 6 | Cell | Phenomics<br>Cytomics |

## 2. THE 'OMICS CONCEPT IN PHYTOTHERAPY

### 2.1. 'OMICS Concept in Phytotherapy at DNA Level

Both the genes and the gene products (RNA or protein resulting from gene expression) are related and not independent in various molecular pathways in the system. The analysis of the levels of gene products could be used to determine the activity or inactivity of a gene. A good target or biomarker could be identified at each level of any gene product. Therefore, omics technologies (also DNA or RNA sequencing approaches as well as network pharmacology) can be applied for diverse treatment approaches as in chemotherapy as well as phytochemicals and phytotherapy [42]. Epigenomics deals with the heritable and reversible DNA changes but which do not affect DNA sequence. So, as omics science, epigenomics deals with the identification of alteration in gene and gene activities through the epigenetic changes that take place in the genome [41, 43]. Metagenomics is also an omics science at the DNA level. It is concerned with the analysis of a group of genes from the environment which have a relationship with the host biological system. An example of this is the study of the relationship between the host's pathophysiology and drug metabolism during microflora infection in the gut [40, 44]. Toxicogenomics is also part of the omics concept in phytotherapy at the DNA level. It is the study of the changes in gene expression due to the exposure to some chemicals which lead to the identification of probable genetic toxicants such as environmental stress in the history of the disease [45, 46]. At the DNA level also, pharmacogenomics is an omics concept in phytotherapy. This aims at the identification and explanation of genes that participate in the response to a drug by the system to recognize the individual differences among genes and their reaction to the changes [47]. This kind of analysis, coupled with the data from other multidisciplinary omics approaches, leads to important information on safe and effective doses of therapeutic agents. Botanogenomics is an omics science that involves the combined information from genomics and proteomics for the study of effect of herbs on several biological systems. This is the omics concept where a specialized herbal remedy is introduced. Example is the treatment of immunoinflammatory disease with plant products [48, 49]. The difference in the changes that occur between the treated and the control group provides understanding of the effects of herbal products.

On quality control and sample variability of medicinal plant materials, omics approaches have been essential and inevitable. Several procedures on polymerase chain reaction have been designed and considered essential and inevitable in the omics sciences to determine and identify the herbal products. The DNA after amplified, cDNA would then be sequenced to identify species of medicinal plants, an example is the determination and identification of Fritillaria species [50]. This is possible because DNA sequences of DNA chips are unique for a given species of medicinal plant [51]. Omics is a very important tool in the analysis of herbal mixtures [52] since the approach provides a fast, high-throughput, and highly informative ways to decipher medicinal plant materials and their bioactive contents [53, 54]. In the same way, the DNA barcoding method is a very vital tool and the approach to analyze medicinal plant materials. DNA barcode is a small and short sequence fragment present in all plant species, which have identical nucleotide sequence in all members of the same species, but with sufficient variation to discriminate it from species. This is done by comparing sequences of standard DNA fragments (called DNA barcode) of an unknown specimen with the ones in the library of reference sequences from the known species [55, 56]. DNA barcoding is a powerful tool when compared with old techniques like DNA fingerprint [57], microchip electrophoresis coupled with PCR-short tandem repeats, and fluorescence detection [58]. Other new DNA assays and tools, which are very innovative include mini sequencing, nanoscale DNA sequencing. These together with DNA barcoding contribute greatly to the next-generation genomic technologies [59]. Although DNA-based techniques represent an unbeatable way for medicinal plant component identification, the limitation lies in the quantity and quality of DNA samples from plant materials, i.e dried, fresh, processed, or raw material. the presence of particular metabolites may also hinder the DNA extraction and other analysis such as non-water-soluble components.

## 2.2. 'OMICS Concept in Phytotherapy at the RNA Level

The omics science at the level of RNA is transcriptomics. It is concerned with the study of the complete set of messenger RNA levels. The measure of the number of transcripts could be determined to know the expression level of the genes. Transcriptomics analysis has been used in the analysis of the biological activities of several medicinal plants. Some good example is the study of the wound-healing activity of *Moros alba* root extract through the up-regulating keratin filament and the CXCL 12/CXCR4 signaling [60, 61], the use of phytochemicals in phytotherapy for the treatment of cancer [42, 62], and the integration of transcriptomics and metabolomics in the study of *Astragalus membranaceus Bae. var. mongolicus (Bge.) Hsiao* which reveals the phytochemicals profile and their biological roles in the plant [63]. The correlation among the gene expression profile under certain treatment, herbal formulae (or any known drug or therapeutics agent), and the disease state profile could be determined by making use of databases for the gene association. And the results from this correlation can be used to predict the unknown physiological and toxicological effects of the formulae [64]. Thus, transcriptomics in combination with multi-omic technologies is a very pivotal tool in the standardization of phytotherapy.

Gene expression studies through microarray analysis are one of the important DNA chip technology through which a rapid and extensive study of several RNA transcripts could be studied. This transcriptomic approach can identify concurrently the difference in expression level of multiple genes. This denotes one of the great tools for deciphering the molecular mechanisms and networks underlying the complex pharmacological function of an ethnomedicinal plant used in phytotherapy. Coupling microarray gene expression analysis with sophisticated bioinformatics tools and other statistical software, the pharmacokinetics, pharmacodynamics, and toxicological characteristics of medicinal plants can be elucidated and standardized. When a transcriptomic database profile of a plant is compared with herbal induced transcriptional effects, the mechanism of action, target specificity, and downstream effects of that plant material could be ascertained. It could also provide insight into the toxicological impact by comparing the transcriptomic profile and the toxicological profile in the databases [53]. Moreover, this is a good approach to explain the molecular mechanism and targeted pathways of the pharmacological agent.

For instance, a report by Zhuang and co-workers [65] indicated that cDNA microarray studies have shown pro-apoptotic effects on *Tripterygium hypoglaucum*-induced apoptosis in HL-60 cells. Another work by Kang et al., *Coptidis rhizoma* (the rhizome of *Coptis* chinensis) on breast cancer indicated that the plant upregulated IFN-mRNA in the DNA microarray study as its cell growth arrest and apoptotic effects [66] just as cytokines were induced in a treatment *with a combined formulation of Radix Ginseng, Cornu Cervi Pantotrichum,* and *Fructus Cnidii.* This means that they have biological roles on innate and acquired immune system [67]. Synergistic effect of root extracts of *Scutellaria baicalensis, Coptis chinensis and rhubarb* species (Rheum sp.) was also investigated on human hepatoma cell line (HepG2 cells) using microarrays. The results implied a cytotoxic effect on p53 signaling pathway [68, 69]. Several other research reports have shown the significance and relevance of transcriptomics in phytotherapy [69 - 74].

## 2.3. 'OMICS Concept in Phytotherapy at Protein Level

The omics science at the protein level is called proteomics. This is one of the important omics sciences which bridges the information from genomics and the biological system. It is a powerful scientific tool used for the assessment of several physiological processes in biological systems. And it has been integrated into many analytical levels, pharmaceutical research, and development [75]. Proteomics involves the study of the whole population of proteins in the cell, tissue, organ, or system at a particular time [76]. Not always that the number of genes plays roles in the complex mechanism of reaction in the system, but some gene expression mechanisms do. Such gene expression processes include alternative splicing and posttranslational modifications. These play a vital role in protein variability. Thirty-five percent of human genes undergo alternative splicing, resulting in one gene translated in to many protein, which means it is one gene-many protein and not one gene-one protein as traditionally agreed [31, 77]. Proteomics is very important in the discovery of drug targets and their validation [75]. Phosphorylation is the most common posttranslational modification process to proteins. The science of protein phosphorylation is phosphoproteomics. About 17,500 genes and gene products have been reported to be modified by phosphorylation [78] which indicates its important roles in cell processes and mechanisms. Some of the undeniably important roles of phosphorylation are in cell signaling, gene expression, metabolism, and cell growth and differentiation. In the same manner, glycoproteomics is the study of posttranslational modification in which proteins are glycosylated, *i.e* addition of sugar to the proteins. About 25% of the human proteins have been discovered to be glycosylated [78]. Glycosylation helps in processes such as cell adhesion, cell immunity, protein translation, protein degradation to mention but a few cellular functions [41]. It is, however, unfortunate that despite the importance and viability of this glycoproteomics science, little efforts have been put by researchers to explore the technique for the characterization and standardization of traditional medicine.

Moreover, toxicoproteomics is a science concerning the quantitative and qualitative study of the effects of exposure to toxic agents on cells, tissue, organ, or even the whole system. This study avail researcher and pharmacologists the prediction of possible toxic response to herbal agents [79]. In the same realm, chemoproteomics deals with the interactions of chemicals with proteins due to their structures. It requires the use of bioinformatics tools to characterize the resulting protein functions and structures [41]. During the study, care must be taken with optimized study conditions to prevent alteration to the protein structure, any interaction with regulatory proteins, and all the posttranslational modifications. Chemoproteomics could be a general study that deals with a cellular response such as protein expression, or a targeted (specific) study which deals with a specific posttranslational modification that occurs due to the treatment with a particular compound [80]. Another proteomics concept in phytotherapy is immunomics. It involves the study of how pathogens regulate the immune system due to the recognition by the antigen and immune response of the host [81]. As the final note on the omics concept in phytotherapy at the protein level (proteomics), interactomics is the amalgamation of all data from different omics studies to formulate networks of reactions and interactions among drugs and drug targets. This is called integrome. Integrome is the result of the integration of numerous amounts of data from different multi-omics data analysis for the vast understanding of biological processes at various analytical levels. Using some sophisticated bioinformatics tools, interaction networks could be constructed to monitor the characteristics of the networks, the major focus of which is drug discovery and development [40].

Proteomics is a scientific field that shed light on the transformation of the biological system and machine/technology since mRNA expression always comparable with protein expression and protein function depends on posttranslational modifications, which in turn depends on protein localization. Therefore, proteomics study deals with a fundamental understanding of the expression and function of proteins, which is needed to be integrated with other biological information like mRNA, secondary and primary metabolites, and gene profiles. The knowledge of the vast usage of this technique will provide full understanding of the functional architecture of the biological system. The two current approaches used in protein profiling are two-dimensional electrophoresis and isotopic label protein in liquid chromatography-mass spectrometry [82, 83].

The most important application of proteomics science in phytotherapy is its ability to identify different plant species [84] which is a very vital tool in standardization, quality control, and toxicity investigation.

## 2.4. 'OMICS Concept in Phytotherapy at Metabolites Level

Metabolomics is the quantitative and qualitative study of all metabolites (including secondary and primary metabolites) and their characteristics in the biological system [85]. It focuses on the determination of the effects of specific internal or external stimuli on the biological pathways. Stimuli such as genetic modifications are considered as internal factors while environmental pharmaceutical agents are termed external factors [30]. Alterations to the metabolic content of any biological system will lead to changes in the metabolomics of the system and ultimately ulter the biological roles. So, factors that can influence the metabolic content of an individual are genetic, environmental, and some gut microbiomes. By profiling the metabolites, the information about their pharmacokinetics, pharmacodynamics, and pathophysiology can be determined and made available for development into therapeutic agents for disease management [41, 64]. The effectiveness or ineffectiveness of a treatment outcome can be determined by comparing the metabolic profiles of an individual and this provides information about the metabolic effects of the drug on the system metabolism. Pharmacometabolomics is a branch of metabolomics [86]. Is also called pharmacometabonomics. It is a field that is concerned with the determination of metabolic contents in an individual to predict and understand the pharmacokinetics of the pharmaceutical compounds. This avails the general effect of the drug on the metabolism. At the moment, Pharmacometabolomics is widely being used in drug discovery and development as well as in general pharmacological procedures [87]. In omics sciences, when metabolomics is combined with toxicology study in comparative studies of metabolites, it is called toxicometabolomics. Toxicometabolomics is the omics science which deals with the comparison of the metabolic analysis of system before and after treatment [88]. To ensure the safety of herbs and herbal components, the use of metabolomics and toxicometabolomics are important tools in the toxicological studies [64, 89].

Several reports have been put forward to buttress the importance of metabolomics and toxicometabolomics in drug discovery and development. Metabolomics approach was utilized to authenticate the effect of *Schisandra sinensis* (common name: magnolia-vine, Chinese magnolia-vine, schisandra). The results of this method were not different from that of NMR [90, 91]. And in the study of herbal therapy pharmacovigilant, metabolomics has been a proven exalted tool. Despite the constant growth of herbal therapy in the world, the quality and safety of these products remain questionable because most of the products are either adulterated, contaminated, or even processed in a fraudulent way without any medical regulations or quality control. Thus, the emergence of the metabolomics approach to research therefore serves as a biochemical profiling tool, which provides solutions for the various problems [92]. Another instance of the importance of metabolomics and toxicometabolomics is in the investigation of the mechanism of action of aristolochic acid in the nephrotoxicity study using a techniques that combined LC-MS, 1H-NMR spectroscopy, and GC-MS to elucidate and characterize the plant metabolites. The results of the study indicated that aristolochic acid-treated rats developed nephrotoxicity which might have been caused by the decreasing concentrations of prostaglandins leading to reversible vasoconstrictive conditions and kidney problems [93 - 96]. Ricin-based preparation was also investigated for its nephrotoxic effects in a long term used. Ricin, which a water-soluble glycoprotein is known to cause toxin in castor oil plant (*Ricinus communis*). Long term treatment with ricin induced perturbations in many metabolic pathways. Examples of the pathways are amino acid metabolism pathway and oxidative stress. These partially explained the observed nephrotoxicity [97]. In another investigation using GC-MS techniques, an active anti-inflammatory component in *Tripterygium wilfordii*, triptolide, was reported to cause changes in the beta-oxidation pathway [98].

Besides, lipids are essential biological components that also play pivotal roles in several biological processes ranging from being energy reservoir, structural and cellular components to units in the signaling pathways [99]. Lipidome is the lipid profile in the biological systems and disturbances in these metabolites have been shown to cause several deadly and life-threatening diseases like diabetes [100], obesity, Alzheimer's disease, and some dangerous infectious diseases [41, 101]. The widely diverse chemical structures of lipids in biological complexity have made it difficult to carry out lipidomics studies on the metabolites. For this, it is imperative for researchers to constantly improve the technologies in this omics science to achieve accurate results in the lipid profiling analysis in experimental samples. Phytochemome includes alkaloids, flavonoids, polyphenols, terpenes, sulfides, plant peptides, thiols, and their metabolites. Phytochemomics is the study of the intracellular and extracellular chemical structure and mechanism of actions of phytochemicals at the different molecular levels [102]. Phytochemomics is the same as metabolomics but only different in that phytochemomics focuses on the studies of plant chemicals. Unfortunately, phytochemomic concept has not be utilized in the phytotherapy, the reason the term phytochemomics is not common in the literature as does metabolomics when studying phytochemicals.

Applications of metabolomics in pharmaceutical research and development have been published [103]. It has been employed in the investigation composition of *Panax ginseng* from different origins using NMR-based spectroscopy [104, 105]. It has also been used in another research where Panax herbs were characterized using ultra-performance liquid chromatography–quadrupole TOF MS (UPLC–QTOFMS) [105]. Ultra-performance liquid chromatography is capable of generating different distinct chromatographic peaks within a very short period, making it a great tool that facilitates the concurrent analysis of complex samples with different chemical characteristics, coupled with high precision of the mass information generated with TOF MS analysis [105]. Gas chromatographic-mass spectrometry has also been used in metabolomics profiling of herbal preparations [106]. This method, apart from diverse statistical analysis of the results, was able to differentiate the quality of the herbal samples from different species. It is a very efficient and accurate method in metabolomics profiling.

## 2.5. 'OMICS Concept in Phytotherapy at the Electrolytes Level

Metallomics focuses on the study of the functions of proteins since many proteins require metal as cofactors, such as zinc, copper, molybdenum, and ion, to function. It deals with the quantitative and qualitative analysis of the entire sum of metals and metalloids species in a cell, tissue, organ, systems, and whole organisms [107].

## 2.6. 'OMICS Concept in the Phytotherapy at the Cellular Level

The omics concept can be applied to everything that happens to organisms at cellular levels. Phenome is the total expressed traits in an organism in a population in relation to the organism's genetic composition [108]. Phenotype is the totality of physical and biochemical characteristics in a living organism due to its interactions with genetic and environmental factors. So, in the disease condition, the disease manifestation, its progression, severity, whether it is improving with treatment or not, are all closely inter-related to the genetic composition of the organism and are referred to as the disease phenotype [109]. Therefore, phenomics is the study of the changes in phenome due to environmental and genetic factors [41]. Although it is exceedingly difficult in phytotherapy to study the component(s) of a plant that is responsible for its biological activities, the use of phenomics is a very important tool that should be utilized in the standardization of traditional medicine. Cytomics is also an omics science that deals with the understanding of the disease networks. The human cytometry project was put forward to explain the molecular processes at the cellular level [110]. Unfortunately, not many researchers make use of this tool in the phytotherapy to standardize the phytomedicines.

## CONCLUSION

Overall, the importance of the concept of omics in modern phytotherapy cannot be overemphasized. It was a technique invented to fill the knowledge gap on correct and accurate information on the genetic and physiological levels of ethnomedicinal plants. Several omics techniques are now being used every day for the purposes of standardization, characterization, and methodological and analytical quality control of herbs used in phytotherapy. Omics also aids the identification of the molecular mechanism of actions of plant materials for the prediction of its bioactivities and toxicological effects. Considering the usability of all the omics sciences in phytotherapy research, metabolomics is the most important in phytotherapy because its experimental design and methodology seem noncomplicated, which give the opportunity for direct and accurate analysis of an enormous amount of biological samples

## CONSENT FOR PUBLICATION

Not applicable.

## CONFLICT OF INTEREST

The authors declare no conflict of interest, financial or otherwise.

## ACKNOWLEDGEMENTS

Declared none.

## REFERENCES

[1]     Stojanoski N. Development of health culture in Veles and its region from the past to the end of the 20th century. Veles: Society of Science and Art 1999; 13

[2]     Kelly K. History of medicinethe middle ages 500-1450. Facts on File 2009.

[3]     Bottcher H. Miracle drugs. Zagreb: Zora 1965; pp. 23-139.

[4]     Wiart C. Ethnopharmacology of medicinal plants: Asia and the Pacific. Springer Science & Business Media 2007.

[5]     Tucakov J. *Healing with plants–phytotherapy*. Beograd. Culture (Que) 1971; 180-90.

[6]     Glesinger L. Medicine through centuries. Zagreb: Zora 1954; pp. 21-38.

[7]     Tucakov J. Pharmacognosy. Beograd: Academic books 1948; 8-21.

[8]     Dimitrova Z. The history of pharmacy. Sofija: St Clement of Ohrid 1999; 13-26.

[9]     Toplak Galle K. Domestic medicinal plants. Zagreb: Mozaic book 2005; 60-1.

[10]    Bojadzievski P. The health services in Bitola through the centuries. Bitola: Society of science and art 1992; 1992: 15-27.

[11]    Nikolovski B. Essays on the history of health culture in Macedonia. Skopje: Macedonian

Pharmaceutical Association 1995; 17-27.

[12]   Revision USPCCo. US pharmacopeia & national formulary. United States Pharmacopeial Convention, Inc 2008.

[13]   Monograph T. European Pharmacopoeia. European Directorate for the Quality of Medicine & Health Care of the Council of Europe (EDQM), edn 2017; 9: 3104-5.

[14]   Wargovich MJ, Woods C, Hollis DM, Zander ME. Herbals, cancer prevention and health. J Nutr 2001; 131(11) (Suppl.): 3034S-6S.
       [http://dx.doi.org/10.1093/jn/131.11.3034S] [PMID: 11694643]

[15]   Shenouda NS, Sakla MS, Newton LG, *et al.* Phytosterol Pygeum africanum regulates prostate cancer *in vitro* and *in vivo*. Endocrine 2007; 31(1): 72-81.
       [http://dx.doi.org/10.1007/s12020-007-0014-y] [PMID: 17709901]

[16]   Nair JJ, Van Staden J. Traditional usage, phytochemistry and pharmacology of the South African medicinal plant *Boophone disticha* (L.f.) Herb. (Amaryllidaceae). J Ethnopharmacol 2014; 151(1): 12-26.
       [http://dx.doi.org/10.1016/j.jep.2013.10.053] [PMID: 24211396]

[17]   Zhang Q, Zhao JJ, Xu J, Feng F, Qu W. Medicinal uses, phytochemistry and pharmacology of the genus Uncaria. J Ethnopharmacol 2015; 173: 48-80.
       [http://dx.doi.org/10.1016/j.jep.2015.06.011] [PMID: 26091967]

[18]   Parturier G. Phytotherapy of liver disease. Rev Med-Chir Mal Foie 1950; 25(8-9): 5-32.
       [PMID: 14786976]

[19]   Li Z, Zhang H, Li Y, *et al.* Phytotherapy using blueberry leaf polyphenols to alleviate non-alcoholic fatty liver disease through improving mitochondrial function and oxidative defense. Phytomedicine 2020; 69: 153209.
       [http://dx.doi.org/10.1016/j.phymed.2020.153209] [PMID: 32240928]

[20]   Rai MK, Upadhyay SK. Phytotherapy of skin disease by plants of patalkot and tamiya. Anc Sci Life 1997; 16(4): 337-46.
       [PMID: 22556809]

[21]   Perry EK, Pickering AT, Wang WW, Houghton PJ, Perry NS. Medicinal plants and Alzheimer's disease: from ethnobotany to phytotherapy. J Pharm Pharmacol 1999; 51(5): 527-34.
       [http://dx.doi.org/10.1211/0022357991772808] [PMID: 10411211]

[22]   Kim SW. Phytotherapy: emerging therapeutic option in urologic disease. Transl Androl Urol 2012; 1(3): 181-91.
       [PMID: 26816707]

[23]   Moro MG, Silveira Souto ML, Franco GCN, Holzhausen M, Pannuti CM. Efficacy of local phytotherapy in the nonsurgical treatment of periodontal disease: A systematic review. J Periodontal Res 2018; 53(3): 288-97.
       [http://dx.doi.org/10.1111/jre.12525] [PMID: 29352465]

[24]   Rabiei Z, Solati K, Amini-Khoei H. Phytotherapy in treatment of Parkinson's disease: a review. Pharm Biol 2019; 57(1): 355-62.
       [http://dx.doi.org/10.1080/13880209.2019.1618344] [PMID: 31141426]

[25]   Chávez-Castillo M, Ortega Á, Duran P, *et al.* Phytotherapy for Cardiovascular Disease: A Bench-t--Bedside Approach. Curr Pharm Des 2020; 26(35): 4410-29.
       [http://dx.doi.org/10.2174/1381612826666200420160422] [PMID: 32310044]

[26]   Koshak DAE, Koshak PEA. *Nigella sativa* L as a potential phytotherapy for coronavirus disease 2019: A mini review of *in silico* studies. Curr Ther Res Clin Exp 2020; 93: 100602.
       [http://dx.doi.org/10.1016/j.curtheres.2020.100602] [PMID: 32863400]

[27]   Levy E, Delvin E, Marcil V, Spahis S. Can phytotherapy with polyphenols serve as a powerful

approach for the prevention and therapy tool of novel coronavirus disease 2019 (COVID-19)? Am J Physiol Endocrinol Metab 2020; 319(4): E689-708.
[http://dx.doi.org/10.1152/ajpendo.00298.2020] [PMID: 32755302]

[28]    Saenko VS, Lachinov EL, Zhantlisov DA, Gorbachev MI, Soltanov AA. Adjustment of urine PH as effective tool for successful metaphylaxis of urinary stone disease phytotherapy. Urologiia 2020; (3): 104-10.
[http://dx.doi.org/10.18565/urology.2020.3.104-110] [PMID: 32597596]

[29]    Xu M, Deng PX, Qi C, *et al.* Adjuvant phytotherapy in the treatment of cervical cancer: a systematic review and meta-analysis. J Altern Complement Med 2009; 15(12): 1347-53.
[http://dx.doi.org/10.1089/acm.2009.0202] [PMID: 19954338]

[30]    Pelkonen O, Pasanen M, Lindon JC, *et al.* Omics and its potential impact on R&D and regulation of complex herbal products. J Ethnopharmacol 2012; 140(3): 587-93.
[http://dx.doi.org/10.1016/j.jep.2012.01.035] [PMID: 22313626]

[31]    Reiss T. Drug discovery of the future: the implications of the human genome project. Trends Biotechnol 2001; 19(12): 496-9.
[http://dx.doi.org/10.1016/S0167-7799(01)01811-X] [PMID: 11711192]

[32]    Chanda SK, Caldwell JS. Fulfilling the promise: drug discovery in the post-genomic era. Drug Discov Today 2003; 8(4): 168-74.
[http://dx.doi.org/10.1016/S1359-6446(02)02595-3] [PMID: 12581711]

[33]    Garay JP, Gray JW. Omics and therapy - a basis for precision medicine. Mol Oncol 2012; 6(2): 128-39.
[http://dx.doi.org/10.1016/j.molonc.2012.02.009] [PMID: 22445068]

[34]    Luo J, Guo XR, Tang XJ, *et al.* Intravital biobank and personalized cancer therapy: the correlation with omics. Int J Cancer 2014; 135(7): 1511-6.
[http://dx.doi.org/10.1002/ijc.28632] [PMID: 24285244]

[35]    Ternès N, Arnedos M, Koscielny S, Michiels S, Lanoy E. Statistical methods applied to omics data: predicting response to neoadjuvant therapy in breast cancer. Curr Opin Oncol 2014; 26(6): 576-83.
[http://dx.doi.org/10.1097/CCO.0000000000000134] [PMID: 25210869]

[36]    McShane LM, Polley MY. Development of omics-based clinical tests for prognosis and therapy selection: the challenge of achieving statistical robustness and clinical utility. Clin Trials 2013; 10(5): 653-65.
[http://dx.doi.org/10.1177/1740774513499458] [PMID: 24000377]

[37]    Oehr P. 'Omics'-based imaging in cancer detection and therapy. Per Med 2006; 3(1): 19-32.
[http://dx.doi.org/10.2217/17410541.3.1.19] [PMID: 29783424]

[38]    Olson MV. The Human Genome Project: a player's perspective. J Mol Biol 2002; 319(4): 931-42.
[http://dx.doi.org/10.1016/S0022-2836(02)00333-9] [PMID: 12079320]

[39]    Collins FS, *et al.* A vision for the future of genomics research. Nature 2003; 422(6934): 835-47.
[http://dx.doi.org/10.1038/nature01626]

[40]    Sánchez-Vidaña DI, Rajwani R, Wong M-S. The use of omic technologies applied to traditional chinese medicine research. Evidence-Based Complementary and Alternative Medicine 2017; 2017
[http://dx.doi.org/10.1155/2017/6359730]

[41]    Yan S-K, Liu RH, Jin HZ, *et al.* "Omics" in pharmaceutical research: overview, applications, challenges, and future perspectives. Chin J Nat Med 2015; 13(1): 3-21.
[http://dx.doi.org/10.1016/S1875-5364(15)60002-4] [PMID: 25660284]

[42]    Efferth T, Saeed MEM, Mirghani E, *et al.* Integration of phytochemicals and phytotherapy into cancer precision medicine. Oncotarget 2017; 8(30): 50284-304.
[http://dx.doi.org/10.18632/oncotarget.17466] [PMID: 28514737]

[43]   Zheng-Yuan S, *et al.* Perspective on Nrf2, epigenomics and cancer stem cells in cancer chemoprevention using dietary phytochemicals and traditional Chinese medicines. Huaxue Jinzhan 2013; 25(09): 1526.

[44]   Li H, Zhou M, Zhao A, Jia W. Traditional Chinese medicine: balancing the gut ecosystem. Phytother Res 2009; 23(9): 1332-5.
[http://dx.doi.org/10.1002/ptr.2590] [PMID: 19253310]

[45]   Waters MD, Fostel JM. Toxicogenomics and systems toxicology: aims and prospects. Nat Rev Genet 2004; 5(12): 936-48.
[http://dx.doi.org/10.1038/nrg1493] [PMID: 15573125]

[46]   Gao C, Weisman D, Lan J, Gou N, Gu AZ. Toxicity mechanisms identification *via* gene set enrichment analysis of time-series toxicogenomics data: impact of time and concentration. Environ Sci Technol 2015; 49(7): 4618-26.
[http://dx.doi.org/10.1021/es505199f] [PMID: 25785649]

[47]   Daly AK. Pharmacogenomics of adverse drug reactions. Genome Med 2013; 5(1): 5.
[http://dx.doi.org/10.1186/gm409] [PMID: 23360680]

[48]   Kang YJ. Herbogenomics: from traditional Chinese medicine to novel therapeutics. Exp Biol Med (Maywood) 2008; 233(9): 1059-65.
[http://dx.doi.org/10.3181/0802-MR-47] [PMID: 18535158]

[49]   Denzler KL, Waters R, Jacobs BL, Rochon Y, Langland JO. Regulation of inflammatory gene expression in PBMCs by immunostimulatory botanicals. PLoS One 2010; 5(9): e12561.
[http://dx.doi.org/10.1371/journal.pone.0012561] [PMID: 20838436]

[50]   Cai ZH, Li P, Dong TT, Tsim KW. Molecular diversity of 5S-rRNA spacer domain in Fritillaria species revealed by PCR analysis. Planta Med 1999; 65(4): 360-4.
[http://dx.doi.org/10.1055/s-1999-14003] [PMID: 10364844]

[51]   Carles M, Lee T, Moganti S, *et al.* Chips and Qi: microcomponent-based analysis in traditional Chinese medicine. Fresenius J Anal Chem 2001; 371(2): 190-4.
[http://dx.doi.org/10.1007/s002160100964] [PMID: 11678190]

[52]   Zhang Y-B, Wang J, Wang ZT, But PP, Shaw PC. DNA microarray for identification of the herb of dendrobium species from Chinese medicinal formulations. Planta Med 2003; 69(12): 1172-4.
[http://dx.doi.org/10.1055/s-2003-818015] [PMID: 14750041]

[53]   Chavan P, Joshi K, Patwardhan B. DNA microarrays in herbal drug research. Evid Based Complement Alternat Med 2006; 3(4): 447-57.
[http://dx.doi.org/10.1093/ecam/nel075] [PMID: 17173108]

[54]   Tsoi P-Y, Woo HS, Wong MS, *et al.* Genotyping and species identification of Fritillaria by DNA chips. Yao Xue Xue Bao 2003; 38(3): 185-90.
[PMID: 12830713]

[55]   Hollingsworth PM, Graham SW, Little DP. Choosing and using a plant DNA barcode. PLoS One 2011; 6(5): e19254.
[http://dx.doi.org/10.1371/journal.pone.0019254] [PMID: 21637336]

[56]   Zuo Y, Chen Z, Kondo K, Funamoto T, Wen J, Zhou S. DNA barcoding of Panax species. Planta Med 2011; 77(2): 182-7.
[http://dx.doi.org/10.1055/s-0030-1250166] [PMID: 20803416]

[57]   Mihalov JJ, Marderosian AD, Pierce JC. DNA identification of commercial ginseng samples. J Agric Food Chem 2000; 48(8): 3744-52.
[http://dx.doi.org/10.1021/jf000011b] [PMID: 10956181]

[58]   Qin J, Leung FC, Fung Y, Zhu D, Lin B. Rapid authentication of ginseng species using microchip electrophoresis with laser-induced fluorescence detection. Anal Bioanal Chem 2005; 381(4): 812-9.

[http://dx.doi.org/10.1007/s00216-004-2889-2] [PMID: 15750870]

[59]    Heubl G. New aspects of DNA-based authentication of Chinese medicinal plants by molecular
        biological techniques. Planta Med 2010; 76(17): 1963-74.
        [http://dx.doi.org/10.1055/s-0030-1250519] [PMID: 21058240]

[60]    Kim KH, Chung WS, Kim Y, et al. Transcriptomic analysis reveals wound healing of Morus alba root
        extract by up-regulating keratin filament and CXCL12/CXCR4 signaling. Phytother Res 2015; 29(8):
        1251-8.
        [http://dx.doi.org/10.1002/ptr.5375] [PMID: 26014513]

[61]    Lo H-Y, Li CC, Huang HC, Lin LJ, Hsiang CY, Ho TY. Application of transcriptomics in Chinese
        herbal medicine studies. J Tradit Complement Med 2012; 2(2): 105-14.
        [http://dx.doi.org/10.1016/S2225-4110(16)30083-9] [PMID: 24716122]

[62]    Wagschal I, Eggenschwiler J, Viviani A. Phytotherapy against cancer: analysis down to the
        transcriptomic level. Bioforum Eur 2007; 10(11): 34-6.

[63]    Wu X, Li X, Wang W, et al. Integrated metabolomics and transcriptomics study of traditional herb
        Astragalus membranaceus Bge. var. mongolicus (Bge.) Hsiao reveals global metabolic profile and
        novel phytochemical ingredients. BMC Genomics 2020; 21(10) (Suppl. 10): 697.
        [http://dx.doi.org/10.1186/s12864-020-07005-y] [PMID: 33208098]

[64]    Buriani A, Garcia-Bermejo ML, Bosisio E, et al. Omic techniques in systems biology approaches to
        traditional Chinese medicine research: present and future. J Ethnopharmacol 2012; 140(3): 535-44.
        [http://dx.doi.org/10.1016/j.jep.2012.01.055] [PMID: 22342380]

[65]    Zhuang W-J, Fong CC, Cao J, et al. Involvement of NF-kappaB and c-myc signaling pathways in the
        apoptosis of HL-60 cells induced by alkaloids of Tripterygium hypoglaucum (levl.) Hutch.
        Phytomedicine 2004; 11(4): 295-302.
        [http://dx.doi.org/10.1078/0944711041495128] [PMID: 15185841]

[66]    Kang JX, Liu J, Wang J, He C, Li FP. The extract of huanglian, a medicinal herb, induces cell growth
        arrest and apoptosis by upregulation of interferon-β and TNF-α in human breast cancer cells.
        Carcinogenesis 2005; 26(11): 1934-9.
        [http://dx.doi.org/10.1093/carcin/bgi154] [PMID: 15958519]

[67]    Pan-Hammarström Q, Wen S, Hammarström L. Cytokine gene expression profiles in human
        lymphocytes induced by a formula of traditional Chinese medicine, vigconic VI-28. J Interferon
        Cytokine Res 2006; 26(9): 628-36.
        [http://dx.doi.org/10.1089/jir.2006.26.628] [PMID: 16978066]

[68]    Cheng W-Y, Wu SL, Hsiang CY, et al. Relationship Between San-Huang-Xie-Xin-Tang and its herbal
        components on the gene expression profiles in HepG2 cells. Am J Chin Med 2008; 36(4): 783-97.
        [http://dx.doi.org/10.1142/S0192415X08006235] [PMID: 18711774]

[69]    Sakai R, Irie Y, Murata T, Ishige A, Anjiki N, Watanabe K. Toki-to protects dopaminergic neurons in
        the substantia nigra from neurotoxicity of MPTP in mice. Phytother Res 2007; 21(9): 868-73.
        [http://dx.doi.org/10.1002/ptr.2172] [PMID: 17486689]

[70]    Watanabe-Fukuda Y, Yamamoto M, Miura N, et al. Orengedokuto and berberine improve
        indomethacin-induced small intestinal injury via adenosine. J Gastroenterol 2009; 44(5): 380-9.
        [http://dx.doi.org/10.1007/s00535-009-0005-2] [PMID: 19319464]

[71]    Liu S-H, Cheng Y-C. Old formula, new Rx: the journey of PHY906 as cancer adjuvant therapy. J
        Ethnopharmacol 2012; 140(3): 614-23.
        [http://dx.doi.org/10.1016/j.jep.2012.01.047] [PMID: 22326673]

[72]    Wang E, Bussom S, Chen J, et al. Interaction of a traditional Chinese Medicine (PHY906) and CPT-11
        on the inflammatory process in the tumor microenvironment. BMC Med Genomics 2011; 4(1): 38.
        [http://dx.doi.org/10.1186/1755-8794-4-38] [PMID: 21569348]

[73]    Youns M, Hoheisel JD, Efferth T. Toxicogenomics for the prediction of toxicity related to herbs from

traditional Chinese medicine. Planta Med 2010; 76(17): 2019-25.
[http://dx.doi.org/10.1055/s-0030-1250432] [PMID: 20957595]

[74]   Cheng H-M, Li CC, Chen CY, *et al.* Application of bioactivity database of Chinese herbal medicine on the therapeutic prediction, drug development, and safety evaluation. J Ethnopharmacol 2010; 132(2): 429-37.
[http://dx.doi.org/10.1016/j.jep.2010.08.022] [PMID: 20713146]

[75]   Cutler P, Voshol H. Proteomics in pharmaceutical research and development. Proteomics Clin Appl 2015; 9(7-8): 643-50.
[http://dx.doi.org/10.1002/prca.201400181] [PMID: 25763573]

[76]   Cristea IM, Gaskell SJ, Whetton AD. Proteomics techniques and their application to hematology. Blood 2004; 103(10): 3624-34.
[http://dx.doi.org/10.1182/blood-2003-09-3295] [PMID: 14726377]

[77]   Twyman R, George A. Principles of proteomics. Garland Science 2013.
[http://dx.doi.org/10.1201/9780429258527]

[78]   Pagel O, Loroch S, Sickmann A, Zahedi RP. Current strategies and findings in clinically relevant post-translational modification-specific proteomics. Expert Rev Proteomics 2015; 12(3): 235-53.
[http://dx.doi.org/10.1586/14789450.2015.1042867] [PMID: 25955281]

[79]   van Breemen RB, Fong HH, Farnsworth NR. Ensuring the safety of botanical dietary supplements. Am J Clin Nutr 2008; 87(2): 509S-13S.
[http://dx.doi.org/10.1093/ajcn/87.2.509S] [PMID: 18258648]

[80]   Bantscheff M, Drewes G. Chemoproteomic approaches to drug target identification and drug profiling. Bioorg Med Chem 2012; 20(6): 1973-8.
[http://dx.doi.org/10.1016/j.bmc.2011.11.003] [PMID: 22130419]

[81]   Bulman A, Neagu M, Constantin C. Immunomics in skin cancer-improvement in diagnosis, prognosis and therapy monitoring. Curr Proteomics 2013; 10(3): 202-17.
[http://dx.doi.org/10.2174/1570164611310030003] [PMID: 24228023]

[82]   Kandpal R, Saviola B, Felton J. The era of 'omics unlimited. Biotechniques 2009; 46(5): 351-352, 354-355.
[http://dx.doi.org/10.2144/000113137] [PMID: 19480630]

[83]   Weston AD, Hood L. Systems biology, proteomics, and the future of health care: toward predictive, preventative, and personalized medicine. J Proteome Res 2004; 3(2): 179-96.
[http://dx.doi.org/10.1021/pr0499693] [PMID: 15113093]

[84]   Lum JHK, *et al.* Proteome of Oriental ginseng Panax ginseng CA Meyer and the potential to use it as an identification tool. 2002.

[85]   Ulrich-Merzenich G, Zeitler H, Jobst D, Panek D, Vetter H, Wagner H. Application of the "-Omic-" technologies in phytomedicine. Phytomedicine 2007; 14(1): 70-82.
[http://dx.doi.org/10.1016/j.phymed.2006.11.011] [PMID: 17188482]

[86]   Kaddurah-Daouk R, Kristal BS, Weinshilboum RM. Metabolomics: a global biochemical approach to drug response and disease. Annu Rev Pharmacol Toxicol 2008; 48(1): 653-83.
[http://dx.doi.org/10.1146/annurev.pharmtox.48.113006.094715] [PMID: 18184107]

[87]   Kaddurah-Daouk R, Weinshilboum RM, Network PR. Pharmacometabolomics: implications for clinical pharmacology and systems pharmacology. Clin Pharmacol Ther 2014; 95(2): 154-67.
[http://dx.doi.org/10.1038/clpt.2013.217] [PMID: 24193171]

[88]   Bouhifd M, Hartung T, Hogberg HT, Kleensang A, Zhao L. Review: toxicometabolomics. J Appl Toxicol 2013; 33(12): 1365-83.
[http://dx.doi.org/10.1002/jat.2874] [PMID: 23722930]

[89]   Araújo AM, Carvalho F, Guedes de Pinho P, Carvalho M. Toxicometabolomics: Small Molecules to

Answer Big Toxicological Questions. Metabolites 2021; 11(10): 692.
[http://dx.doi.org/10.3390/metabo11100692] [PMID: 34677407]

[90]   Kamsu-Foguem B, Foguem C. Adverse drug reactions in some African herbal medicine: literature review and stakeholders' interview. Integr Med Res 2014; 3(3): 126-32.
[http://dx.doi.org/10.1016/j.imr.2014.05.001] [PMID: 28664088]

[91]   Tian JS, Zhao L, Shen XL, Liu H, Qin XM. $^1$H NMR-based metabolomics approach to investigating the renal protective effects of Genipin in diabetic rats. Chin J Nat Med 2018; 16(4): 261-70.
[http://dx.doi.org/10.1016/S1875-5364(18)30056-6] [PMID: 29703326]

[92]   Crighton E, Mullaney I, Trengove R, Bunce M, Maker G. The application of metabolomics for herbal medicine pharmacovigilance: a case study on ginseng. Essays Biochem 2016; 60(5): 429-35.
[http://dx.doi.org/10.1042/EBC20160030] [PMID: 27980093]

[93]   Zhang X, Wu H, Liao P, Li X, Ni J, Pei F. NMR-based metabonomic study on the subacute toxicity of aristolochic acid in rats. Food Chem Toxicol 2006; 44(7): 1006-14.
[http://dx.doi.org/10.1016/j.fct.2005.12.004] [PMID: 16457928]

[94]   Ni Y, Su M, Qiu Y, *et al.* Metabolic profiling using combined GC-MS and LC-MS provides a systems understanding of aristolochic acid-induced nephrotoxicity in rat. FEBS Lett 2007; 581(4): 707-11.
[http://dx.doi.org/10.1016/j.febslet.2007.01.036] [PMID: 17274990]

[95]   Chan W, Lee KC, Liu N, Wong RN, Liu H, Cai Z. Liquid chromatography/mass spectrometry for metabonomics investigation of the biochemical effects induced by aristolochic acid in rats: the use of information-dependent acquisition for biomarker identification. Rapid Commun Mass Spectrom 2008; 22(6): 873-80.
[http://dx.doi.org/10.1002/rcm.3438] [PMID: 18288688]

[96]   Liu X, *et al. Metabonomic study of aristolochic acid I-induced acute renal toxicity urine at female and male C57BL/6J Mice based on H-1 NMR.* Gaodeng Xuexiao Huaxue Xuebao. Chem J Chin Univ 2010; 31(5): 927-32.

[97]   Guo P, Wang J, Dong G, *et al.* NMR-based metabolomics approach to study the chronic toxicity of crude ricin from castor bean kernels on rats. Mol Biosyst 2014; 10(9): 2426-40.
[http://dx.doi.org/10.1039/C4MB00251B] [PMID: 24992468]

[98]   Aa J, *et al.* Gas chromatography time-of-flight mass spectrometry based metabolomic approach to evaluating toxicity of triptolide. Metabolomics 2011; 7(2): 217-25.
[http://dx.doi.org/10.1007/s11306-010-0241-8]

[99]   Teo CC, *et al.* Advances in sample preparation and analytical techniques for lipidomics study of clinical samples. Trends Analyt Chem 2015; 66: 1-18.
[http://dx.doi.org/10.1016/j.trac.2014.10.010]

[100]  Sabiu S, *et al.* Bioactive Food as Dietary Interventions for Diabetes. 2013.

[101]  Astarita G, Ollero M. Lipidomics: an evolving discipline in molecular sciences. Multidisciplinary Digital Publishing Institute 2015.

[102]  del Castillo MD, *et al.* Phytochemomics and other omics for permitting health claims made on foods. Food Res Int 2013; 54(1): 1237-49.
[http://dx.doi.org/10.1016/j.foodres.2013.05.014]

[103]  Lindon JC, Holmes E, Nicholson JK. Metabonomics techniques and applications to pharmaceutical research & development. Pharm Res 2006; 23(6): 1075-88.
[http://dx.doi.org/10.1007/s11095-006-0025-z] [PMID: 16715371]

[104]  Kang J, Lee S, Kang S, *et al.* NMR-based metabolomics approach for the differentiation of ginseng (Panax ginseng) roots from different origins. Arch Pharm Res 2008; 31(3): 330-6.
[http://dx.doi.org/10.1007/s12272-001-1160-2] [PMID: 18409046]

[105]  Xie G, Plumb R, Su M, *et al.* Ultra-performance LC/TOF MS analysis of medicinal Panax herbs for

metabolomic research. J Sep Sci 2008; 31(6-7): 1015-26.
[http://dx.doi.org/10.1002/jssc.200700650] [PMID: 18338405]

[106]   Xiang Z, Wang XQ, Cai XJ, Zeng S. Metabolomics study on quality control and discrimination of three curcuma species based on gas chromatograph-mass spectrometry. Phytochem Anal 2011; 22(5): 411-8.
[http://dx.doi.org/10.1002/pca.1296] [PMID: 21433157]

[107]   Ogra Y. [Development of metallomics research on environmental toxicology]. Journal of the Pharmaceutical Society of Japan 2015; 135(2): 307-14.
[http://dx.doi.org/10.1248/yakushi.14-00233] [PMID: 25747230]

[108]   Monte AA, Brocker C, Nebert DW, Gonzalez FJ, Thompson DC, Vasiliou V. Improved drug therapy: triangulating phenomics with genomics and metabolomics. Hum Genomics 2014; 8(1): 16.
[http://dx.doi.org/10.1186/s40246-014-0016-9] [PMID: 25181945]

[109]   Hoehndorf R, Schofield PN, Gkoutos GV. Analysis of the human diseasome using phenotype similarity between common, genetic, and infectious diseases. Sci Rep 2015; 5(1): 10888.
[http://dx.doi.org/10.1038/srep10888] [PMID: 26051359]

[110]   Valet G. Cytomics: an entry to biomedical cell systems biology. Cytometry A 2005; 63(2): 67-8.
[http://dx.doi.org/10.1002/cyto.a.20110] [PMID: 15657925]

# CHAPTER 14

# Phytoinformatics in Disease Management

**Ismaila O. Nurain**[1,*]

[1] *Department of Pharmacology, the University of Minnesota Medical School, Minneapolis, USA*

**Abstract:** The profound importance of medicinal plants as therapeutic agents as well as their economic values has captured the attention of researchers around the world. However, it has been recognized that standardization of medicinal plant research is required for its incorporation into modern medicine and to maintain the healthy development of the traditional medicine industry. Due to this fact, several extensive research efforts have been added to the existing approaches to upgrade the sector through standardization and authentication of medicinal plant and plant products as well as bioengineering of metabolic pathways. This chapter has divulged information about the application of computational omics approaches to medicinal plant research and its relevance in disease management. Omics studies such as genomics, transcriptomics, proteomics, metabolomics as well as multi-omics data integration were accounted for their application in a medicinal plant. Some bioinformatics programs, tools, and web databases were explained and their application in the phytoinformatics analysis of medicinal plant was discussed. This chapter concluded with the importance of storing, integrating, and management of biological and medicinal plant data to make them available as information used in disease management. It is, therefore, hoped that this chapter will enlighten medicinal plant researchers more on the availability of computational tools to use in standardizing traditional medicine and authenticate the methodologies by making them reproducible and applicable to disease management.

**Keywords:** Omics studies, Medicinal plants, Bioinformatics tools, Databases, Standardization, Plant metabolites, Disease management.

## 1. INTRODUCTION

Every living organism is bound to pass through both healthy and disease states at certain times in its life span. The change in the biological system from healthy to disease state quest for remedy, and this gingers the search for various sources of traditional medicines. The use of plants and plant products as remedies for human diseases dates back to time immemorial. The recognition of medicinal plants as a vital source of remedies for several human diseases came into play when modern

---

\* **Corresponding author Ismaila O. Nurain:** Department of Pharmacology, the University of Minnesota Medical School, Minneapolis, USA; Tel: +2348068088828; E-mail: isnurain@gmail.com

**Saheed Sabiu (Ed)**

medicine practitioners started questioning the safety, standardization, reproducibility of methods, and authenticity of traditionally based remedies [1]. Even though it cannot be disproved that medicinal plants are efficacious, some questions could not be answered. However, with time, the introduction of sciences into traditional medicine enlighten the dark spot in the use of ethnomedicinal plants to treat human diseases. Tradition medicine is common in Africa, India, China, Arab and other countries with western countries accepting it later after some facts have been established regarding the potency and safety of plants [2, 3]. Thus, the world depends on medicinal plants for the management of disease and other unhealthy states. The allopathic, which is widely accepted nowadays, is also based on medicines from the animal source, plants origin, and mineral resources. Medicinal plants are renewables reservoirs, safe for consumption, readily available, and cheap [4, 5]. Medicinal plants are good sources of useful chemicals with bioactive properties and so they are the most acceptable sources of drug and therapeutic agents in traditional medicines, complementary and alternative medicine, and also in the allopathic system of medicines [6]. Several ethnomedicinal plants have been proved efficacious in the management of many diseases such as neurodegenerative diseases [7], inflammatory and cardiovascular diseases [8], HIV/AIDS [9], plants' diseases [10 - 12], sickle cell disease [13, 14], cancer [15], and infectious diseases [16 - 18].

Even though medicinal plants are particularly important sources of therapeutic agents used by humans for ages, the knowledge of the vital information about the molecular, chemical, and cellular systems is just gaining ground with the invention of modern technologies and molecular biology techniques, jointly referred to as omics sciences. The advent of omics sciences enables scientists and researchers to explain complex information in genes and genomes coupled with metabolic proteins involved in biological systems [19]. Currently, in all the continents, medicinal plants have provided substantial advantages to the pharmaceutical industry in the same ways as they have provided stability to the biomedicine industry. This was possible through the establishment of pressing and urgently standardized and advanced research activities on the medicinal plants. So, in disease management, there is a need for phytochemical informatics to decipher and understand the biomarkers and bioactivities of phytochemicals. Two tasks in the applications of phytoinformatics to medicinal plant research in disease management are to provide standardization and characterization of the plant materials as well as to decipher the mechanistic annotations of the metabolic pathways of the plants' bioactivities. These applications of phytoinformatics would be accomplished through medicinal plant research using multi-omics data integration and technologies such as genomics, proteomics, transcriptomics, *etc* [20, 21]. On the other hand, phytoinformatics is combined with system biology to bridge the gap between the phytochemical information, their bioactivities, and disease management. The system biology approach is a multidisciplinary way to understand the complex processes in the human biological system. It is the combined efforts of chemists, biologists, physicists, mathematicians, and bioengineers to integrate an enormous amount of data from omics studies to arrive at a precise medicine for a disease. Reports have indicated the importance of system biology in the understanding of the regulatory and metabolic pathways networks in plants [22 - 24]. But what is disease management? The concept of cost reduction and improved life quality of individuals living with disease through total prevention, cure, and integrated care from professionals is referred to as disease management. Disease management is the way of a regulated and coordinated intervention program for the health sector. So, to be able to outline proper and accurate disease management, there is a need for integrated information from genomics, proteomics, transcriptomics, metabolomics, and other omics science to identify, characterize, and validate the targeted disease biomarkers as well bioactive ingredients from medicinal plants.

This chapter is aimed at deciphering and elucidating the phytoinformatics concept in disease management. It will include the relevance of medicinal plants in disease management, informatics from omics sciences and their relevance in disease management, phyto-bioactive chemical data integration from different databases, tools, and some computational and bioinformatics analyses to integrate Phyto-bioactive chemical data for disease management. The chapter will be concluded with further and prospective areas to be explored by the traditional medicine researchers in the phytoinformatics for increasing the standardization of the medicinal plant plant-based diseases management.

## 2. RELEVANCE OF MEDICINAL PLANTS IN DISEASE MANAGEMENT

In the quest for the efficacious, safe, cheap, and readily available cure and treatment for various human diseases, the human being has explored several other organismal species including plant and plant-related species. The ethnomedicinal plant has been the most important and reliable source compared to other sources of human cure and treatment; they possess various secondary and primary metabolites required by the living organisms and metabolic pathways that make up the organism [25, 26]. The metabolites modulate the pathways or cause biochemical changes that could help in the treatment of diseases. Moreover, for every plant identified for its bioactive chemicals, all parts of the plant are particularly useful. These include the fruits, seed, leaf, bark, stem, roots, flowers, all prepared in different forms depending on the diseases and method of development [27].

The use of the plant as a remedy dated back to the prehistoric era. Not only that plants are used for the cure and treatment of diseases alone they are also used as an integral part of rituals substances [28, 29]. Nowadays, pharmaceuticals and biomedical systems are relying on plant phytochemicals and plants' parts for synthetic or plant derivatives for disease treatment. The economic and non-readily available medical care have made it important to utilize traditional medicines as an alternative healing approach [3]. In fact, it has been estimated that above 80% of the world population relies on traditional herbal medicine for the treatment of various diseases [2, 30]. Medicinal plants contain several vital phytochemicals such as alkaloids, flavonoids, glycoside, phenols, polyphenols, terpenes, *etc* [31, 32]. Not only do medicinal plants use for diseases, but they are also a great source of food for human consumption. The pharmacological actions of the phytochemicals make them pivotal components of the drugs. Research has shown how relevant and important medicinal plants are in modern-day disease management. Ranging from inflammatory and cardio vascular disease management [33], Parkinson's [34, 35], and gastroesophageal reflux disease [36] to cancer [37 - 40], medicinal plants have been proven to be inevitable in disease management. The availability and ease of access of these plants, coupled with their reduced negative effects, lead to their increased usage, especially in the form of extracts, concoction, pastes, powders, balm, raw, and prepared. *Aloe vera* and its other species are used in various forms throughout the world [41] the same way black pepper, ginger, clover arc used for wound healing, sores, and boils treatment [42], and *Hydrocotyl bonariensis* Comm. Ex Lam (Apiaceae) leaves extract for cataracts [43].

Several researchers are now tailoring their research towards understanding the molecular mechanism involves in the production of plant metabolites. They use omics sciences to achieve this objective. By carry out genomics, proteomics, transcriptomics, and other omics studies on many plant species, it is possible to identify and develop an appropriate medicinal product for disease management. The ultimate goals of many traditional/herbal medicine researchers are to standardize the approach and incorporate the medicinal plant and plant product in modern medicine.

## 3. MEDICINAL PLANT INFORMATICS AND APPLICATION IN DISEASE MANAGEMENT

To be able to standardize medicinal plants as an agent in disease management and make them incorporated into modern medicine, current advanced technology and improved curated research techniques must be applied. An interdisciplinary field of science that combines many subject fields of science including biology, computer science, information engineering and technology, mathematics, and statistics in analyzing and interpreting biological data, bioinformatics, is essential and required [21]. In the case of medicinal plant research for disease management, phytoinformatics is a pivotal tool in the correlation of the human genome and its metabolic processes information with phytochemical ingredients in plant materials. This has upgraded the medicinal plant and its products to the standardized and regulated mode of disease management. Phytoinformatics involves the use of bioinformatics tools to divulge information embedded in the genome and characterize and elucidate its metabolic processes for the purpose of matching it with the appropriate therapeutic agent from plants. It also involves the application of the bioinformatics approach in the plant system analysis to decipher the plant components with their bioactive properties through the metabolomics concept. Therefore, phytoinformatics is the bioinformatics-assisted computational application of different integrated omics fields to the medicinal plants for its standardized use in disease management. Some omics sciences considered in this chapter include genomics, proteomics, transcriptomics, metabolomics, and functional applications.

Large and nano-scale scale data storage, management, and analysis have been made easy through the advancement in technology and instrumentation. The current era technologies enable accurate probing of biological samples and deposit data in the databases. The vast enormous amount of available data is beyond human brain capacity and so there is a need for a supercomputing system to manage the sea of data. Bioinformatics is defined as an interdisciplinary bioscience field that includes biological sciences, computer and information science, engineering, mathematics, and statistics, and other related fields of study to manage biological data [44, 45]. It is the study of biological information through computational analysis coupled with statistical modeling and engineering. So, it is divided into the management of biological information and computation of the biological data and information. By managing the biological information, it means to research or apply computational tools through acquiring, describing, representing, storing, analyzing, and visualizing the biological data in the medical, health, or behavioral sectors [46]. On the other hand, the computation of biological data is the development and application of theoretical and analytical, mathematical modeling, computational simulations approach to the acquisition, storage, analysis, and visualization of biological data, behavioral and social systems. There is no clear boundary between the management and computation of biological data since as both of them increased in advancement, they become interwoven. so, in medicinal plant science, phytoinformatics play the same role as bioinformatics. This section aims at elucidating the application of phytoinformatics in biological data management and integration to help in cost and time effective disease management [21, 22]. The major concept, methods, and tools in the phytoinformatics pertinent in medicinal plant research as applied to disease management will be discussed.

Several plants have been sequenced through the next-generation sequencing (NGS) approach and their full sequence lengths are available in different online databases. For the easy management of the sequences, several expressed sequence tags (ESTs) have also been identified [47, 48]. This process is very cost and time-efficient and aids accurate analysis of medicinal plants. Later new techniques were invented including various advanced bioinformatics techniques, polymorphism ratio sequencing, comparative hybridization of probes [42]. Also, bioinformatics is important in the identification and analysis of introns, exons, and other regions of the sequenced gene. Analysis of coding and noncoding regions of the gene enables characterization of the gene, which could be important in the growth and development of the plant. Then, follows the identification of metabolites in the plant. The secondary and primary metabolites and genetic factors responsible for the metabolites in the plants could be identified using bioinformatics tools. Functional annotation and phylogenetic studies help in the identification and comparison of genes and genomes [49]. Moreover, sequence alignment is use for comparison and identification of differences in genes due to evolution. Sequence alignment is divided into two, local, and global sequence alignment [50, 51].

## COMPUTATIONAL GENOMICS ANALYSIS

The most fundamental sequences in the biological system at the molecular level are DNA, RNA, and protein sequences. Thousands of plant genomes have been sequenced *e.g.* rice [52, 53], *Arabidopsis thaliana,* and many more are still in the process [54]. Examples of genome sequence databases are listed in Table **1**. Through the sequence analysis, research has generated several expressed sequence tags (ESTs) from several plant sequences including lotus, beet, soybean, cotton, wheat, and sorghum (Table **1**). Many bioinformatics tools and software are available for the sequence of these analyses. This advancement in informatics studies including shotgun sequencing in medicinal plants has availed researchers the opportunity for accurate managing processing, analyzing, and storing curated biological data. The shotgun is a powerful approach in DNA sequencing, in which DNA pieces are scattered randomly, then cloned and re-sequenced in a parallel manner, and then paired all the randomly overlapping short sequences together in a coherent and accurate contiguous sequence [46]. For assembly of sequences sea of software has been developed (Table **2**) [55, 56]. Some methods in use now reduce the time and cost of sequencing analysis including differential hybridization of oligonucleotide probes, polymorphism ratio sequencing, four-color DNA sequencing by synthesis on a chip [46]. To identify a functional gene or regulatory gene sequence, there is a need for analysis of introns, exons, coding, noncoding, *etc.* sequences in the gene. Large numbers of computer programs are available online for gene and protein-coding identification [57 - 59]. Table **2** shows the non-exhaustive list of programs and bioinformatics tools for medicinal plant research. Most of these tools are specifically for plant gene and bioactivity identification analysis [60 - 62].

**Table 1. Non-exhaustive List of Databases for Phyto-Bio-Informatics Studies.**

| S/NO | Classification of Study | Name of Database | URL |
|---|---|---|---|
| 1 | Genomics | **MGHa** | **http://maca.eplant.org** |
| | | MMDBD | http://www.cuhk.edu.hk/icm/mmdbd.htm |
| | | HopBase | http://hopbase.org/ |
| | | CmMDB | http://bigd.big.ac.cn/databasecommons/database/id/1052 |
| 2 | Transcriptomics | miRBase | http://www.mirbase.org/ |
| | | MepmiRDB | http://mepmirdb.cn/mepmirdb/index.html |
| | | ArrayExpress | https://www.ebi.ac.uk/arrayexpress/ |
| | | GEO | https://www.ncbi.nlm.nih.gov/geo/ |
| | | SRA | https://www.ncbi.nlm.nih.gov/sra/ |
| | | croFGD | http://bioinformatics.cau.edu.cn/croFGD/ |
| 3 | Proteomics | UniProt | https://www.uniprot.org/ |
| | | Pfam | http://pfam.xfam.org/ |
| | | BioGRID | https://thebiogrid.org/ |
| | | STRING | http://string-db.org |
| | | IntAct | https://www.ebi.ac.uk/intact/ |
| | | PRIN | http://bis.zju.edu.cn/prin/ |
| | | Others | http://au.expasy.org/melanie/ <br> http://open2dprot.sourceforge.net/Flicker/ <br> http://www.proteomeworks.bio-rad.com <br> https://www.expasy.org/resources/swiss-2dpage. |
| 4 | Metabolomics | CathaCyc | http://www.cathacyc.org |
| | | KEGG | https://www.kegg.jp/kegg/pathway.html |
| | | ArMet | https://users.aber.ac.uk/nwh/Research/armet.html |
| 5 | General Omics | MPGR | http://medicinalplantgenomics.msu.edu/ |
| | | HMOD | http://herbalplant.ynau.edu.cn/ |

*(Table 1) cont.....*

| S/NO | Classification of Study | Name of Database | URL |
|---|---|---|---|
| | | **MGHa** | **http://maca.eplant.org** |
| 1 | **Genomics** | AromaDb | http://bioinfo.cimap.res.in/aromadb/ |
| | | Phytochemica | http://faculty.iiitd.ac.in/~bagler/webservers/Phytochemica/ |
| | | SerpentinaDB | http://faculty.iiitd.ac.in/~bagler/webservers/SerpentinaDB/ |
| 6 | Databases Specific for Medicinal Plant | TCM Database@Taiwan | http://tcm.cmu.edu.tw/ |
| | | IPPAT | https://cb.imsc.res.in/imppat |
| | | InDiaMed | http://www.iibt.in/IndiaMed/Home.aspx |
| | | NeMedPlantb | http://bif.uohyd.ac.in/nemedplant/ |
| | | NPASS | http://bidd2.nus.edu.sg/NPASS/ |
| | | CMAUP | http://bidd2.nus.edu.sg/CMAUP/ |
| | | DIACAN | http://bic.kau.in/diacan/ |
| | | SACPD | https://teeqrani1.wixsite.com/sapd |
| | | KNApSAcK | http://kanaya.naist.jp/MetaboliteActivity/top.jsp |
| | | TCMGeneDIT | http://tcm.lifescience.ntu.edu.tw/ |
| | | HIT | https://openebench.bsc.es/tool/hit |
| 7 | Taxonomics and Phenomics | MPDB | http://www.medicinalplantbd.net |
| | | MPID | https://library.hkbu.edu.hk/electronic/libdbs/mpd/ |
| | | ebDB | https://www.quantumimagery.com/software-ebDB.html |
| | | lantCLEF 2019 | https://www.imageclef.org/PlantCLEF2019 |
| 8 | Sequence Alignment and Analysis | - | https://zhanglab.ccmb.med.umich.edu/TM-align/<br>http://www.ncbi.nlm.nih.gov/dbEST/)<br>https://zhanglab.ccmb.med.umich.edu/MM-align/<br>https://zhanglab.ccmb.med.umich.edu/RNA-align/<br>http://genome.jgi-psf.org/Poptr1/<br>http://www.kazusa.or.jp/lotus/<br>http://genes.mit.edu/GENSCAN.html<br>http://opal.biology.gatech.edu/GeneMark/<br>http://compbio.ornl.gov/Grail-1.3/<br>http://www.fruitfly.org/seqtools/genie.html<br>http://www.tigr.org/softlab/glimmer |

Sequence comparison allows structural, functional, and evolutionary inference from genomes and genes. It provides the basis for the modeling of genes [46] such as a homology study [63, 64], though homology results may not mean conservation of function. Sequence comparison is based on the sequence similarity between two strings of text in a sequence (amino acids), especially when the confident level of comparison is low, which do not or may not correspond to the exact evolutionary or common ancestor. Several other websites and tools for genomics analysis of medicinal plants are listed in Tables 1 and 2.

The most important aspect of genome study is functional genomics. The genome-wide study has generated enough data for the functional genomic study. A good way to apply genomic functional study is in the production of plant secondary metabolite in metabolic pathway influenced by the production of bioactive molecules in the medicinal plant. Benzylisoquinoline alkaloids such as sanguinarine and chelerythrine possess antimicrobial properties and are produced from *Mocleaya cordata*. It has been reported that about 22000 predicted protein-coding genes are contained in the *M. cordata* [65]. Sixteen of them were functionally identified as metabolic genes involved in the biosynthesis of sanguinarine and chelerythrine. This provided insight into the application of bioengineering on the metabolic pathway of the alkaloids. Another one with anti-viral and anti-inflammatory properties is Neoandrographolide.

**Table 2. Non-exhaustive list of software for Phytoinformatics Research.**

| S/NO | Classification of Study | Name of Tools | URL |
|---|---|---|---|
| 1 | Functional Annotation | PlantTFcat | http://plantgrn.noble.org/PlantTFcat/ |
| | | Cytoscape | http://www.cytoscape.org/ |
| | | agriGO v2.0 | http://systemsbiology.cau.edu.cn/agriGOv2/ |
| | | WGCNA | https://horvath.genetics.ucla.edu/html/CoexpressionNetwork/Rpackages/WGCNA/index.html |
| | | INfORM | https://github.com/Greco-Lab/INfORM |
| | | PathPred | https://www.genome.jp/tools/pathpred/ |
| 2 | Phenomics and Taxonomics | TNRS | http://tnrs.iplantcollaborative.org/ |
| | | ImageJ | https://imagej.nih.gov/ij/ |
| | | HTPheno | http://htpheno.ipk-gatersleben.de/ |
| | | PlantCV | https://plantcv.danforthcenter.org/ |

(Table 2) cont.....

| S/NO | Classification of Study | Name of Tools | URL |
|------|------------------------|---------------|-----|
|      |                        | **PlantTFcat** | **http://plantgrn.noble.org/PlantTFcat/** |
| 1 | **Functional Annotation** | PLACE | https://www.dna.affrc.go.jp/PLACE/?action=newplace |
|   |   | WebLogo | http://weblogo.berkeley.edu/logo.cgi |
|   |   | PlantCARE | http://bioinformatics.psb.ugent.be/webtools/plantcare/html/ |
|   |   | Vienna RNA server | http://rna.tbi.univie.ac.at/ |
|   |   | RNAshapes | https://bibiserv.cebitec.unibielefeld.de/rnashapes |
| 3 | Genomics, transcriptomics | Bowtie | (1) http://bowtie-bio.sourceforge.net/index.shtml (2) http://bowtie-bio.sourceforge.net/bowtie2/index.shtml |
|   |   | Trinity | https://github.com/trinityrnaseq/trinityrnaseq/wiki |
|   |   | SOAPdenovo-Trans | https://sourceforge.net/projects/soapdenovotrans/ |
|   |   | TopHat +Cufflinks | http://ccb.jhu.edu/software.shtml |
|   |   | StringTie | https://ccb.jhu.edu/software/stringtie/ |
|   |   | PEA | https://hub.docker.com/r/malab/pea |
|   |   | SAM | http://www.biostat.umn.edu/&#x007E;baolin/research/ |
|   |   | miRPlant | http://sourceforge.net/projects/mirplant/ |
|   |   | miRDeep-P | https://sourceforge.net/projects/mirdp/ |
|   |   | PmiRDiscVali | https://github.com/unincrna/pmirdv |
|   |   | P-SAMS | http://p-sams.carringtonlab.org/ |
|   |   | NATpipe | www.bioinfolab.cn/NATpipe/NATpipe.zip |
|   |   | PLncPRO | http://ccbb.jnu.ac.in/plncpro/ |
|   |   | PcircRNA_finder | http://ibi.zju.edu.cn/bioinplant/tools/manual.htm |
|   |   | psRNATarget | http://plantgrn.noble.org/psRNATarget/ |
|   |   | TAPIR | http://bioinformatics.psb.ugent.be/webtools/tapir/ |
|   |   | CleaveLand | http://sites.psu.edu/axtell/software/cleaveland4/ |
|   |   | IIKmTA | http://www.bioinformatics.org/iikmta/ |
| 4 | Array and Omics Analysis | mixOmics | http://mixomics.org/ |
|   |   | BRB-ArrayTools | https://brb.nci.nih.gov/BRBArrayTools/index.html |
| 5 | Assembly of Sequences | - | (http://www.phrap.org (http://www.broad.mit.edu/wga/ (http://staden.sourceforge.net/overview.html (http://www.tigr.org/software/AMOS/ |
| 6 | Regulatory Analysis | - | http://rsat.sb-roscoff.fr/ |

It's a depterpenoids family. It contains a high content of *Andrographis aniculata.* Besides, *A. paniculate* was investigated and found to contain about 25000 protein-coding genes in a research method involving coupling illumine short-read sequencing, PacBio long-read sequencing, and High-confidence platforms [66]. Moreover, the integration of many analytical techniques has made it possible to integrate genome and transcriptome sequencing data and results indicated the presence of some important biological pathways modulator including diterpenoid synthases, 2-oxoglutarate-dependent dioxygenases, cytochrome P450 (CytP450), and UDP-dependent glycosyltransferases in the biosynthesis pathway of diterpenoid lactone. Moreover, transgenic experiment such as over expression and targeted mutagenesis has also been carried out on *Salvia. miltiorrhiza*, a medicinal plant that is highly potent in the treatment of cardiovascular and cerebrovascular diseases in East Asia including Korea as well as inflammation, fibrosis, oxidative stress, and apoptosis [67 - 69]. Regulatory genes are very important in the metabolic processes. Sea of tools is available for this purpose to identify and characterize regulatory mechanisms in medicinal plants in the genome-based analysis. Several other tools used in functional genomics are listed in Table **2**. Proper utilization of listed tools in medicinal plant research could be a breakthrough in traditional medicine.

## COMPUTATIONAL TRANSCRIPTOMICS ANALYSIS

Transcriptomics analysis is aimed at deciphering the transcript level of a gene in relation to the metabolic processes in the biological system. The major reason being to understand the level of mRNA that contributes to the growth and development in an organism or due to environmental response. DNA microarray is a powerful tool for this purpose [70]. Microarray analysis involves the simultaneous determination of transcript level for many genes. The data from microarray coupled with ones from regulatory sequence studies, gene ontology study, regulatory pathway analysis, could be sum together in inferring the regulatory or co-regulatory processes in an organism or a system. Chromatin immunoprecipitation (ChIP)-chip and DNA tiling are the methods which are used in detecting unbiased transcription level. Regulatory Sequence Analysis is based on the understanding of how some segments of genes behave in the way they do in the modification of gene functions. Several websites and tools are available for the regulatory analysis (Table **2**), which offers analyses like motif discovery (support genome-wide data sets like ChIP-seq), transcription factor binding motif analysis (quality assessment, comparisons, and clustering), comparative genomics analysis of regulatory variations. Transcriptomics is the study of the complete set of transcripts of RNA (transcriptome) in the genome in a certain condition and a certain cell with high-throughput techniques like microarray analysis. Through transcriptomics, the role of the genetic transcript in the growth and development can be elucidated. This study has helped in the determination of plants' structural and functional proteins which are responsible for plants' various bioactivities. By carrying out studies such as regulatory sequences analysis, metabolic pathways analysis, gene ontology, specific plant components could be identified and characterized [71]. Since transcriptomics study generates an enormous amount of data, there is a need for data mining and the tools for the mining. Various computational tools are available for this purpose.

## COMPUTATIONAL PROTEOMICS ANALYSIS

One of the leading advanced technologies in quantitative and qualitative analysis of proteins and their interactions in the genomes is proteomics. Through the omics, vast numbers of proteins are identified in the cells, tissues, or system, including posttranslational modification. It also includes the characterization of protein activity-functions and structures [72]. This approach is not popular with the medicinal plant researcher because of many limitations, especially the availability of phytoinformatics tools and knowledge of advanced technology. What is currently common in proteomics of plants is the identification of proteins in the plants [73]. Other areas of proteomics that are not widely utilized in medicinal plant research include proteomics applications in protein-protein interactions, protein structure/activity profiling, protein subcellular localization, and so on [74]. One of the qualitative and quantitative protein analyses is electrophoresis. It is a laboratory technique of separating DNA, RNA, and protein molecule based on their size and charges. Bioinformatics tools are developed for the analysis of gel images through analysis, comparison, and interpreting the results [75]. One more advanced and sophisticated tool in proteomics for qualitative study on proteins is mass spectrometry. It gives room for a high-throughput method for large-scale protein characterization [76]. Data generated from spectrometry analysis need to be analyzed. This is done through the computational tool to identify and interpret the results [77]. Other available programs for studying plant protein are tandem mass spectrometry (MS-MS) for comparison of the masses generated from proteins [78] and peptide mass fingerprinting (PMF), which performs its works by breaking the digested peptide into the smaller fragment of detailed amino acid content [79]. There are many websites for the analysis of protein, examples are listed in Table **1**. Some of them are used for two-dimensional electrophoresis analysis of proteins, while others like mass spectrometry are used for the identification of proteins using a high-throughput approach.

## COMPUTATIONAL METABOLOMICS ANALYSIS

The most important application of the omics concept in medicinal plants is metabolomics, which is the study and analysis of the complete reservoir of metabolites in a cell. The fact that it is extremely useful in deciphering the secondary metabolites in the plant, which are principally responsible for the plant activity, metabolomics is proved to be particularly important in medicinal plant studies. Thousands of metabolites have been identified in the plant with millions of such yet to be explored [46, 80]. metabolomics is used for metabolites profiling by extracting the metabolite from the tissues, separate them, and analyze with a high-throughput approach [81]. Metabolite fingerprinting study entails differentiation of samples based on the phenotype or biological relevance to identify various metabolic components in the sample, manually [82] or automated [83]. Available repository metabolomics includes an architecture for metabolomics (ArMet) [84], which provides annotation of plant metabolites experimental analysis. Similarly, minimum information about a metabolomics experiment (MIAMET) describes the requirements for reporting experiment methodologies standardize experimental methodologies [85]. Moreover, there is a working group on the standardized metabolic reporting structures (SMRS), which developed basic standards for explaining and reporting techniques, methods and the origin of biological sample under the experiment for metabolic profiling [86]. The data gather from metabolic profiling have been used for network of metabolic correlation which will reveal the net carbon-nitrogen partitioning resulting from transcriptional and biochemical processes as a result of direct or indirect enzymatic regulations [87]. Meanwhile, it is not possible to make an inference in a metabolic profiling correlation reaction network that a change in one metabolite level causes the change in another one [88]. In the metabolic flux studies, the flow of the steady-state of metabolites is determined, although, this is rather more difficult to measure than measuring the metabolic level due to intracellular transport complication coupled with the lack of understanding of the *in-vivo* pathway processes [89]. The metabolic flux measures the stoichiometric of the metabolites, which calculate the number of reactants and products of a reaction to know the metabolite fluxes, even though it numerically hard to do so for a large reaction volume or in a reversible reaction [90, 91]. A package called flux analyzer is available from MATLAB [92]. It integrates the pathway and the flux analysis for metabolic networks study [93]. A more accurate study of metabolic flux analysis could be done using E-cell (http://www.e-cell.org/), a cellular modelling environment that integrates all the simulation and information in the metabolic analysis. Another better metabolic flux analyzer is the Cell Designer (http://www.systems-biology.org).

## 4. NON-EXHAUSTIVE LIST OF DATABASES AND TOOLS FOR PHYTOINFORMATICS

For ages, biologists have been dependent on textbooks and journal publications for information, but the advent of the internet, web browsers, and databases has drastically changed the system. Now, the internet is the first place of contact for any meaningful information especially when one needs to compare sources. Databases are an indispensable tool for biological research, that almost every research groups tend to create a database for their research. There are three types of biological databases. These are largescale public repositories or databases, community-specific databases, and project-specific databases. A good example of a large-scale database is GenBank for sequence, which is developed and maintained by government agencies of international consortia [90]. Another example of a large-scale repository database is UniProt for resources about protein information [94], Protein Data Bank is for information about protein structure [95], while ArrayExpress [96, 97] and Gene Expression Omnibus (GEO) (38) for microarray data [98]. For the community-specific, there are several databases available, which are curated and standardized for information for a particular community or groups of researchers [99 - 102]. The small-scale databases are created purposely for data concerning project data management for a short period. They are usually for funding projects to allow members to have access to information about the ongoing research and fund management. Tables **1** and **2** show the non-exhaustive list of databases and tools or software for phytoinformatics studies. Some of these databases and tools are free for access online while some are not. It is imperative that medicinal plant researchers improve and widen their scope of studies by explore research areas in phytoinformatics.

## 5. FROM DATA ACQUISITION TO DISEASE MANAGEMENT

The results of phytoinformatics studies on medicinal plants do not end in the databases or journal publications. Effective utilization of data gathered from phytoinformatics should include their availability to the experimental and medical researchers for administration into the disease management program. The size of data acquired determines their storage, retrieval, curation, and administration [103, 104] and also their availability to the research and caregiver. So, the factors that enable us to translate the vast and enormous amount of data information into a clearer and better understanding of various disease mechanisms that are applied to personalized medicine range from the knowledge of how to manage complex biological information, how to integrate data from heterogeneity sources to what types and kinds of principles should be followed for analysis of large biomedical data. To properly make use of these data extensively, three things needed to be put in place. It is imperative to develop a bioinformatics tool, interdependent databases, and state-of-the-art high-performance supercomputing system [105]. In essence, the main aim and objective of the modern data acquisition and management system should include gathering all data from all experimental levels. To achieve this, a bioinformatics data mining tool is necessary, which enables a better understanding of the information in the data [106]. Thus, the availability of data to the medical personnel will enable proper disease management. Knowing the properties and potential functions of a particular plant will lead to matching the plant with disease and biomarkers and thereby solve the disease problem. For example, the identification of a particular metabolite in an antimalaria plant will shed light on its antiparasitic properties and biomedical personnel will be able to recommend this for treatment. Another instance is in the identification of a transcriptional factor in a plant that modulates growth and development. An accurate characterization of the gene could lead to the development of a good metabolic modulator for use in disease treatment.

## CONCLUSION

The application of high-throughput and advanced technologies and the related analytical tools have profoundly improved the omics and system biology research progression. The omics sciences, including genomics, transcriptomics, proteomics, and metabolomics, and their relevance in medicinal plant study have been deciphered. Functional omics studies confirmed the relevance of computational omics studies in medicinal plant research. This chapter has also enumerated the application of bioinformatics (phytoinformatics) and the achievement of omics science in medicinal plant research. To be able to incorporate medicinal plants in modern medicine, the chapter has recommended that accurate data storage and management should be followed. It was suggested that researchers should improve and widen the scope of their research to include a vast number of bioinformatics tools and databases in medicinal plant research to standardize the results from reproducible research methodologies. The chapter also pointed out that omics and phytoinformatics research is just at their very beginning stages in medicinal pant research and needs improvement. Moreover, the relevance of medicinal plants in disease management was accounted for in this chapter, where data management was related to the cost and time effective disease management. A non-exhaustive list of bioinformatics tool and databases has been provided for medicinal plant researchers to move the area of the research to the next higher level.

## CONSENT FOR PUBLICATION

Not applicable.

## CONFLICT OF INTEREST

The authors declare no conflict of interest, financial or otherwise.

## ACKNOWLEDGEMENTS

Declared none.

## REFERENCES

[1]     Choudhary N, Sekhon BS. An overview of advances in the standardization of herbal drugs. Journal of Pharmaceutical Education and Research 2011; 2(2): 55.

[2]     Ahn K. The worldwide trend of using botanical drugs and strategies for developing global drugs. BMB Rep 2017; 50(3): 111-6.
[http://dx.doi.org/10.5483/BMBRep.2017.50.3.221] [PMID: 27998396]

[3]     Leonti M, Casu L. Traditional medicines and globalization: current and future perspectives in ethnopharmacology. Front Pharmacol 2013; 4: 92.
[http://dx.doi.org/10.3389/fphar.2013.00092] [PMID: 23898296]

[4]     Saxena M, *et al.* Phytochemistry of medicinal plants. J Pharmacogn Phytochem 2013; 1: 6.

[5]     Arnason JT, Mata R, Romeo JT. Phytochemistry of medicinal plants. Springer Science & Business Media 2013; Vol. 29.

[6]     Karunamoorthi K, *et al.* Traditional medicinal plants: a source of phytotherapeutic modality in resource-constrained health care settings. J Evid Based Complementary Altern Med 2013; 18(1): 67-74.
[http://dx.doi.org/10.1177/2156587212460241]

[7]     Auddy B, Ferreira M, Blasina F, *et al.* Screening of antioxidant activity of three Indian medicinal plants, traditionally used for the management of neurodegenerative diseases. J Ethnopharmacol 2003; 84(2-3): 131-8.
[http://dx.doi.org/10.1016/S0378-8741(02)00322-7] [PMID: 12648805]

[8]     Shayganni E, Bahmani M, Asgary S, Rafieian-Kopaei M. Inflammaging and cardiovascular disease: Management by medicinal plants. Phytomedicine 2016; 23(11): 1119-26.
[http://dx.doi.org/10.1016/j.phymed.2015.11.004] [PMID: 26776956]

[9]     Chinsembu KC. Ethnobotanical study of plants used in the management of HIV/AIDS-related diseases in Livingstone, Southern Province, Zambia. Evidence-based complementary and alternative medicine 2016.

[10]    Johal G, Huber D. Glyphosate effects on diseases of plants. Eur J Agron 2009; 31(3): 144-52.
[http://dx.doi.org/10.1016/j.eja.2009.04.004]

[11]    Divya Rani V, Sudini H. *Management of soilborne diseases in crop plants: an overview.* International Journal of Plant. Animal and Environmental Sciences 2013; 3(4): 156-64.

[12]    Gahukar RT. Management of pests and diseases of important tropical/subtropical medicinal and aromatic plants: A review. J Appl Res Med Aromat Plants 2018; 9: 1-18.
[http://dx.doi.org/10.1016/j.jarmap.2018.03.002]

[13]    Okpuzor J, *et al.* The potential of medicinal plants in sickle cell disease control: A review. Int J

Biomed Health Sci 2008; 4(2): 47-55.

[14]    Nurain IO, Bewaji CO, Johnson JS, Davenport RD, Zhang Y. Potential of Three Ethnomedicinal Plants as Antisickling Agents. Mol Pharm 2017; 14(1): 172-82.
[http://dx.doi.org/10.1021/acs.molpharmaceut.6b00767] [PMID: 28043127]

[15]    Ochwang'i DO, Kimwele CN, Oduma JA, Gathumbi PK, Mbaria JM, Kiama SG. Medicinal plants used in treatment and management of cancer in Kakamega County, Kenya. J Ethnopharmacol 2014; 151(3): 1040-55.
[http://dx.doi.org/10.1016/j.jep.2013.11.051] [PMID: 24362078]

[16]    Runyoro DK, Ngassapa OD, Matee MI, Joseph CC, Moshi MJ. Medicinal plants used by Tanzanian traditional healers in the management of Candida infections. J Ethnopharmacol 2006; 106(2): 158-65.
[http://dx.doi.org/10.1016/j.jep.2005.12.010] [PMID: 16458463]

[17]    Shaheen G, Akram M, Jabeen F, *et al.* Therapeutic potential of medicinal plants for the management of urinary tract infection: A systematic review. Clin Exp Pharmacol Physiol 2019; 46(7): 613-24.
[http://dx.doi.org/10.1111/1440-1681.13092] [PMID: 30932202]

[18]    Otang WM, Grierson DS, Ndip RN. Phytochemical studies and antioxidant activity of two South African medicinal plants traditionally used for the management of opportunistic fungal infections in HIV/AIDS patients. BMC Complement Altern Med 2012; 12(1): 43.
[http://dx.doi.org/10.1186/1472-6882-12-43] [PMID: 22502778]

[19]    Van Emon JM. The omics revolution in agricultural research. J Agric Food Chem 2016; 64(1): 36-44.
[http://dx.doi.org/10.1021/acs.jafc.5b04515] [PMID: 26468989]

[20]    Buriani A, Garcia-Bermejo ML, Bosisio E, *et al.* Omic techniques in systems biology approaches to traditional Chinese medicine research: present and future. J Ethnopharmacol 2012; 140(3): 535-44.
[http://dx.doi.org/10.1016/j.jep.2012.01.055] [PMID: 22342380]

[21]    Ma X, Meng Y, Wang P, Tang Z, Wang H, Xie T. Bioinformatics-assisted, integrated omics studies on medicinal plants. Brief Bioinform 2020; 21(6): 1857-74.
[http://dx.doi.org/10.1093/bib/bbz132] [PMID: 32706024]

[22]    Pinu FR, Beale DJ, Paten AM, *et al.* Systems biology and multi-omics integration: Viewpoints from the metabolomics research community. Metabolites 2019; 9(4): 76.
[http://dx.doi.org/10.3390/metabo9040076] [PMID: 31003499]

[23]    Bassel GW, Gaudinier A, Brady SM, Hennig L, Rhee SY, De Smet I. Systems analysis of plant functional, transcriptional, physical interaction, and metabolic networks. Plant Cell 2012; 24(10): 3859-75.
[http://dx.doi.org/10.1105/tpc.112.100776] [PMID: 23110892]

[24]    Fukushima A, Kusano M, Redestig H, Arita M, Saito K. Integrated omics approaches in plant systems biology. Curr Opin Chem Biol 2009; 13(5-6): 532-8.
[http://dx.doi.org/10.1016/j.cbpa.2009.09.022] [PMID: 19837627]

[25]    Incarbone M, Dunoyer P. RNA silencing and its suppression: novel insights from in planta analyses. Trends Plant Sci 2013; 18(7): 382-92.
[http://dx.doi.org/10.1016/j.tplants.2013.04.001] [PMID: 23684690]

[26]    Agyare C, *et al.* Anti-inflammatory and analgesic activities of African medicinal plants.Medicinal Plant Research in Africa. Elsevier 2013; pp. 725-52.
[http://dx.doi.org/10.1016/B978-0-12-405927-6.00019-9]

[27]    Chanda S. Importance of pharmacognostic study of medicinal plants: An overview. J Pharmacogn Phytochem 2014; 2: 5.

[28]    Petrovska BB. Historical review of medicinal plants' usage. Pharmacogn Rev 2012; 6(11): 1-5.
[http://dx.doi.org/10.4103/0973-7847.95849] [PMID: 22654398]

[29]    Wilkins J. Galen's simple medicines: problems in ancient herbal medicine. Critical approaches to the

history of Western herbal medicine: from classical antiquity to the early modern period. USA: A&C Black 2014; pp. 173-90.
[http://dx.doi.org/10.5040/9781474210577-ch-009]

[30]     Chattopadhyay N, Maurya R. Herbal Medicine 2015.
[http://dx.doi.org/10.1016/B978-0-12-801238-3.05061-3]

[31]     Yadav R, Agarwala M. Phytochemical analysis of some medicinal plants. J Phytol 2011.

[32]     Kamal A, Khan MMR. Phytochemical evaluation of some medicinal plants. Int J Plant Sci 2014; 3(4): 5-8.

[33]     Geetha RG, Ramachandran S. Recent Advances in the Anti-Inflammatory Activity of Plant-Derived Alkaloid Rhynchophylline in Neurological and Cardiovascular Diseases. Pharmaceutics 2021; 13(8): 1170.
[http://dx.doi.org/10.3390/pharmaceutics13081170] [PMID: 34452133]

[34]     Pathak-Gandhi N, Vaidya AD. Management of Parkinson's disease in Ayurveda: Medicinal plants and adjuvant measures. J Ethnopharmacol 2017; 197: 46-51.
[http://dx.doi.org/10.1016/j.jep.2016.08.020] [PMID: 27544001]

[35]     Moraes LS, Rohor BZ, Areal LB, *et al.* Medicinal plant Combretum leprosum mart ameliorates motor, biochemical and molecular alterations in a Parkinson's disease model induced by MPTP. J Ethnopharmacol 2016; 185: 68-76.
[http://dx.doi.org/10.1016/j.jep.2016.03.041] [PMID: 26994817]

[36]     Salehi M, Karegar-Borzi H, Karimi M, Rahimi R. Medicinal Plants for Management of Gastroesophageal Reflux Disease: A Review of Animal and Human Studies. J Altern Complement Med 2017; 23(2): 82-95.
[http://dx.doi.org/10.1089/acm.2016.0233] [PMID: 27996295]

[37]     Malami I, Jagaba NM, Abubakar IB, *et al.* Integration of medicinal plants into the traditional system of medicine for the treatment of cancer in Sokoto State, Nigeria. Heliyon 2020; 6(9): e04830.
[http://dx.doi.org/10.1016/j.heliyon.2020.e04830] [PMID: 32939417]

[38]     Tesfaye S, Asres K, Lulekal E, *et al.* Ethiopian Medicinal Plants Traditionally Used for the Treatment of Cancer, Part 2: A Review on Cytotoxic, Antiproliferative, and Antitumor Phytochemicals, and Future Perspective. Molecules 2020; 25(17): E4032.
[http://dx.doi.org/10.3390/molecules25174032] [PMID: 32899373]

[39]     Aiello P, Sharghi M, Mansourkhani SM, *et al.* Medicinal Plants in the Prevention and Treatment of Colon Cancer. Oxid Med Cell Longev 2019; 2019: 2075614.
[http://dx.doi.org/10.1155/2019/2075614] [PMID: 32377288]

[40]     Yedjou CG, Mbemi AT, Noubissi F, *et al.* Prostate Cancer Disparity, Chemoprevention, and Treatment by Specific Medicinal Plants. Nutrients 2019; 11(2): E336.
[http://dx.doi.org/10.3390/nu11020336] [PMID: 30720759]

[41]     Witkin JM, Li X. Curcumin, an active constiuent of the ancient medicinal herb Curcuma longa L.: some uses and the establishment and biological basis of medical efficacy. CNS & Neurological Disorders-Drug Targets (Formerly Current Drug Targets-CNS & Neurological Disorders) 2013; 12(4): 487-97.

[42]     Babar MM, *et al.* Application of bioinformatics and system biology in medicinal plant studies.Plant Bioinformatics. Springer 2017; pp. 375-93.
[http://dx.doi.org/10.1007/978-3-319-67156-7_15]

[43]     Ajani EO, Salako AA, Sharlie PD, *et al.* Chemopreventive and remediation effect of Hydrocotyl bonariensis Comm. Ex Lam (Apiaceae) leave extract in galactose-induced cataract. J Ethnopharmacol 2009; 123(1): 134-42.
[http://dx.doi.org/10.1016/j.jep.2009.02.006] [PMID: 19429352]

[44]     Lesk A. Introduction to bioinformatics. Oxford university press 2019.

[45]    Baxevanis AD, Bader GD, Wishart DS. Wishart, Bioinformatics 2020.

[46]    Rhee SY, Dickerson J, Xu D. Bioinformatics and its applications in plant biology. Annu Rev Plant Biol 2006; 57: 335-60.
[http://dx.doi.org/10.1146/annurev.arplant.56.032604.144103] [PMID: 16669765]

[47]    Benson DA, Cavanaugh M, Clark K, *et al.* GenBank. Nucleic Acids Res 2013; 41(Database issue): D36-42.
[PMID: 23193287]

[48]    Ueno S, Moriguchi Y, Uchiyama K, *et al.* A second generation framework for the analysis of microsatellites in expressed sequence tags and the development of EST-SSR markers for a conifer, Cryptomeria japonica. BMC Genomics 2012; 13(1): 136.
[http://dx.doi.org/10.1186/1471-2164-13-136] [PMID: 22507374]

[49]    Shinwari ZK, *et al.* Identification and phylogenetic analysis of selected medicinal plant species from pakistan: dna barcoding approach. Pak J Bot 2018; 50(2): 553-60.

[50]    Bhargava M, Sharma A. DNA barcoding in plants: evolution and applications of *in silico* approaches and resources. Mol Phylogenet Evol 2013; 67(3): 631-41.
[http://dx.doi.org/10.1016/j.ympev.2013.03.002] [PMID: 23500333]

[51]    Rivas E, Eddy SR. Parameterizing sequence alignment with an explicit evolutionary model. BMC Bioinformatics 2015; 16(1): 406.
[http://dx.doi.org/10.1186/s12859-015-0832-5] [PMID: 26652060]

[52]    Sang J, Zou D, Wang Z, *et al.* IC4R-2.0: rice genome reannotation using massive RNA-seq data. Genomics Proteomics Bioinformatics 2020; 18(2): 161-72.
[http://dx.doi.org/10.1016/j.gpb.2018.12.011] [PMID: 32683045]

[53]    Paul A. Sequencing the Rice Genome: Gateway to Agricultural Development 2020.
[http://dx.doi.org/10.1007/978-981-15-4120-9_6]

[54]    Steenwyk JL, Buida TJ III, Li Y, Shen XX, Rokas A. ClipKIT: A multiple sequence alignment trimming software for accurate phylogenomic inference. PLoS Biol 2020; 18(12): e3001007.
[http://dx.doi.org/10.1371/journal.pbio.3001007] [PMID: 33264284]

[55]    Pereira R, Oliveira J, Sousa M. Bioinformatics and Computational Tools for Next-Generation Sequencing Analysis in Clinical Genetics. J Clin Med 2020; 9(1): 132.
[http://dx.doi.org/10.3390/jcm9010132] [PMID: 31947757]

[56]    Singh H, *et al.* Computational Metagenomics: State-of-the-Art, Facts and Artifacts 2020.
[http://dx.doi.org/10.1007/978-981-15-6529-8_13]

[57]    Kelley DR. Cross-species regulatory sequence activity prediction. PLOS Comput Biol 2020; 16(7): e1008050.
[http://dx.doi.org/10.1371/journal.pcbi.1008050] [PMID: 32687525]

[58]    Kulkarni SR, Vandepoele K. Inference of plant gene regulatory networks using data-driven methods: A practical overview. Gene Regulatory Mechanisms 2020; 1863(6): 194447.
[http://dx.doi.org/10.1016/j.bbagrm.2019.194447] [PMID: 31678628]

[59]    Singh S, Geeta R, Das S. Comparative sequence analysis across Brassicaceae, regulatory diversity in KCS5 and KCS6 homologs from Arabidopsis thaliana and Brassica juncea, and intronic fragment as a negative transcriptional regulator. Gene Expr Patterns 2020; 38: 119146.
[http://dx.doi.org/10.1016/j.gep.2020.119146] [PMID: 32947048]

[60]    Mahood EH, Kruse LH, Moghe GD. Machine learning: A powerful tool for gene function prediction in plants. Appl Plant Sci 2020; 8(7): e11376.
[http://dx.doi.org/10.1002/aps3.11376] [PMID: 32765975]

[61]    Michael TP, VanBuren R. Building near-complete plant genomes. Curr Opin Plant Biol 2020; 54: 26-33.

[http://dx.doi.org/10.1016/j.pbi.2019.12.009] [PMID: 31981929]

[62]    Hasan MM, *et al.* Meta-i6mA: an interspecies predictor for identifying DNA N6-methyladenine sites of plant genomes by exploiting informative features in an integrative machine-learning framework. Brief Bioinform 2020.
[PMID: 32910169]

[63]    Chikhale RV, Gupta VK, Eldesoky GE, Wabaidur SM, Patil SA, Islam MA. Identification of potential anti-TMPRSS2 natural products through homology modelling, virtual screening and molecular dynamics simulation studies. J Biomol Struct Dyn 2020; 1-16.
[PMID: 32741259]

[64]    Stitou M, *et al.* Quantitative structure–activity relationships analysis, homology modeling, docking and molecular dynamics studies of triterpenoid saponins as Kirsten rat sarcoma inhibitors. J Biomol Struct Dyn 2020; 1-19.
[PMID: 31870215]

[65]    Liu X, Liu Y, Huang P, *et al.* The genome of medicinal plant Macleaya cordata provides new insights into benzylisoquinoline alkaloids metabolism. Mol Plant 2017; 10(7): 975-89.
[http://dx.doi.org/10.1016/j.molp.2017.05.007] [PMID: 28552780]

[66]    Zhang D, Jiang C, Huang C, *et al.* The light-induced transcription factor FtMYB116 promotes accumulation of rutin in Fagopyrum tataricum. Plant Cell Environ 2019; 42(4): 1340-51.
[http://dx.doi.org/10.1111/pce.13470] [PMID: 30375656]

[67]    Jung I, Kim H, Moon S, Lee H, Kim B. Overview of *Salvia miltiorrhiza* as a Potential Therapeutic Agent for Various Diseases: An Update on Efficacy and Mechanisms of Action. Antioxidants 2020; 9(9): 857.
[http://dx.doi.org/10.3390/antiox9090857] [PMID: 32933217]

[68]    Sun W, Wang B, Yang J, *et al.* Weighted gene co-expression network analysis of the dioscin rich medicinal plant Dioscorea nipponica. Front Plant Sci 2017; 8: 789.
[http://dx.doi.org/10.3389/fpls.2017.00789] [PMID: 28638386]

[69]    Li B, Cui G, Shen G, *et al.* Targeted mutagenesis in the medicinal plant Salvia miltiorrhiza. Sci Rep 2017; 7: 43320.
[http://dx.doi.org/10.1038/srep43320] [PMID: 28256553]

[70]    Sarfraz I, Asif M, Hijazi K. MiCA: An extended tool for microarray gene expression analysis. Comput Biol Med 2020; 116: 103561.
[http://dx.doi.org/10.1016/j.compbiomed.2019.103561] [PMID: 31785415]

[71]    Singh A, Kumar N. A review on DNA microarray technology. Int J Curr Res Rev 2013; 5(22): 1.

[72]    Sánchez-Vidaña DI, Rajwani R, Wong M-S. The use of omic technologies applied to traditional chinese medicine research. Evidence-Based Complementary and Alternative Medicine 2017.
[http://dx.doi.org/10.1155/2017/6359730]

[73]    Huang X, Zhou H-w. Evaluation of six different protocols for protein extraction from rice young panicles by two-dimensional electrophoresis 2020.
[http://dx.doi.org/10.21203/rs.3.rs-16995/v1]

[74]    Wright EP, Partridge MA, Padula MP, Gauci VJ, Malladi CS, Coorssen JR. Top-down proteomics: enhancing 2D gel electrophoresis from tissue processing to high-sensitivity protein detection. Proteomics 2014; 14(7-8): 872-89.
[http://dx.doi.org/10.1002/pmic.201300424] [PMID: 24452924]

[75]    Caccia D, *et al.* Bioinformatics tools for secretome analysis. Biochimica et Biophysica Acta (BBA)-. Proteins and Proteomics 2013; 1834(11): 2442-53.
[http://dx.doi.org/10.1016/j.bbapap.2013.01.039]

[76]    Chambers MC, Maclean B, Burke R, *et al.* A cross-platform toolkit for mass spectrometry and proteomics. Nat Biotechnol 2012; 30(10): 918-20.

[http://dx.doi.org/10.1038/nbt.2377] [PMID: 23051804]

[77]     Bensimon A, Heck AJ, Aebersold R. Mass spectrometry-based proteomics and network biology. Annu Rev Biochem 2012; 81: 379-405.
[http://dx.doi.org/10.1146/annurev-biochem-072909-100424] [PMID: 22439968]

[78]     Zhang G, *et al.* Overview of peptide and protein analysis by mass spectrometry. Current protocols in protein science 2010; 62(1): 16.1. 1-16.1. 30.
[http://dx.doi.org/10.1002/0471140864.ps1601s62]

[79]     Su Y, Wang H, Liu J, Wei P, Cooks RG, Ouyang Z. Quantitative paper spray mass spectrometry analysis of drugs of abuse. Analyst (Lond) 2013; 138(16): 4443-7.
[http://dx.doi.org/10.1039/c3an00934c] [PMID: 23774310]

[80]     Rameshkumar K, *et al.* Threatened Medicinal Plants in the Western Ghats–Phytochemical Perspective 2020.
[http://dx.doi.org/10.1007/978-3-030-39793-7_10]

[81]     Sharanya C, Sabu A, Haridas M. Plant Metabolomics: Current Status and Prospects 2020.
[http://dx.doi.org/10.1007/978-981-15-5136-9_1]

[82]     Bizzarri M, Minini M, Monti N. Revisiting the Concept of Human Disease 2020.
[http://dx.doi.org/10.1007/978-3-030-32857-3_1]

[83]     Lénárt J, *et al.* LC–MS based metabolic fingerprinting of apricot pistils after self-compatible and self-incompatible pollinations. Plant Mol Biol 2020; 1-13.
[PMID: 33296063]

[84]     Mayneris-Perxachs J, Fernández-Real JM. Exploration of the microbiota and metabolites within body fluids could pinpoint novel disease mechanisms. FEBS J 2020; 287(5): 856-65.
[http://dx.doi.org/10.1111/febs.15130] [PMID: 31709683]

[85]     Bino RJ, Hall RD, Fiehn O, *et al.* Potential of metabolomics as a functional genomics tool. Trends Plant Sci 2004; 9(9): 418-25.
[http://dx.doi.org/10.1016/j.tplants.2004.07.004] [PMID: 15337491]

[86]     Lindon JC, Nicholson JK, Holmes E, *et al.* Summary recommendations for standardization and reporting of metabolic analyses. Nat Biotechnol 2005; 23(7): 833-8.
[http://dx.doi.org/10.1038/nbt0705-833] [PMID: 16003371]

[87]     Steuer R, *et al.* Interpreting correlations in metabolomic networks. Portland Press Ltd. 2003.
[http://dx.doi.org/10.1042/bst0311476]

[88]     Steuer R, Kurths J, Fiehn O, Weckwerth W. Observing and interpreting correlations in metabolomic networks. Bioinformatics 2003; 19(8): 1019-26.
[http://dx.doi.org/10.1093/bioinformatics/btg120] [PMID: 12761066]

[89]     Shanks JV. Phytochemical engineering: combining chemical reaction engineering with plant science. AIChE J 2005; 51(1): 2-7.
[http://dx.doi.org/10.1002/aic.10418]

[90]     Wheeler DL, Smith-White B, Chetvernin V, *et al.* Plant genome resources at the national center for biotechnology information. Plant Physiol 2005; 138(3): 1280-8.
[http://dx.doi.org/10.1104/pp.104.058842] [PMID: 16010002]

[91]     Wiechert W, Möllney M, Petersen S, de Graaf AA. A universal framework for 13C metabolic flux analysis. Metab Eng 2001; 3(3): 265-83.
[http://dx.doi.org/10.1006/mben.2001.0188] [PMID: 11461148]

[92]     Morales Y, Bosque G, Vehí J, Picó J, Llaneras F. PFA toolbox: a MATLAB tool for Metabolic Flux Analysis. BMC Syst Biol 2016; 10(1): 46.
[http://dx.doi.org/10.1186/s12918-016-0284-1] [PMID: 27401090]

[93]     Klamt S, Stelling J, Ginkel M, Gilles ED. FluxAnalyzer: exploring structure, pathways, and flux

distributions in metabolic networks on interactive flux maps. Bioinformatics 2003; 19(2): 261-9.
[http://dx.doi.org/10.1093/bioinformatics/19.2.261] [PMID: 12538248]

[94] Schneider M, Bairoch A, Wu CH, Apweiler R. Plant protein annotation in the UniProt Knowledgebase. Plant Physiol 2005; 138(1): 59-66.
[http://dx.doi.org/10.1104/pp.104.058933] [PMID: 15888679]

[95] Deshpande N, Addess KJ, Bluhm WF, *et al.* The RCSB Protein Data Bank: a redesigned query system and relational database based on the mmCIF schema. Nucleic Acids Res 2005; 33(Database issue) (Suppl. 1): D233-7.
[http://dx.doi.org/10.1093/nar/gki057] [PMID: 15608185]

[96] Parkinson H, Sarkans U, Shojatalab M, *et al.* ArrayExpress--a public repository for microarray gene expression data at the EBI. Nucleic Acids Res 2005; 33(Database issue) (Suppl. 1): D553-5.
[http://dx.doi.org/10.1093/nar/gki056] [PMID: 15608260]

[97] Brazma A, Parkinson H, Sarkans U, *et al.* ArrayExpress--a public repository for microarray gene expression data at the EBI. Nucleic Acids Res 2003; 31(1): 68-71.
[http://dx.doi.org/10.1093/nar/gkg091] [PMID: 12519949]

[98] Edgar R, Domrachev M, Lash AE. Gene Expression Omnibus: NCBI gene expression and hybridization array data repository. Nucleic Acids Res 2002; 30(1): 207-10.
[http://dx.doi.org/10.1093/nar/30.1.207] [PMID: 11752295]

[99] Lawrence CJ, Seigfried TE, Brendel V. The maize genetics and genomics database. The community resource for access to diverse maize data. Plant Physiol 2005; 138(1): 55-8.
[http://dx.doi.org/10.1104/pp.104.059196] [PMID: 15888678]

[100] Matthews DE, Carollo VL, Lazo GR, Anderson OD. GrainGenes, the genome database for small-grain crops. Nucleic Acids Res 2003; 31(1): 183-6.
[http://dx.doi.org/10.1093/nar/gkg058] [PMID: 12519977]

[101] Zhang P, Foerster H, Tissier CP, *et al.* MetaCyc and AraCyc. Metabolic pathway databases for plant research. Plant Physiol 2005; 138(1): 27-37.
[http://dx.doi.org/10.1104/pp.105.060376] [PMID: 15888675]

[102] Tchieu JH, Fana F, Fink JL, *et al.* The PlantsP and PlantsT functional genomics databases. Nucleic Acids Res 2003; 31(1): 342-4.
[http://dx.doi.org/10.1093/nar/gkg025] [PMID: 12520018]

[103] Luo J, *et al.* Big data application in biomedical research and health care: a literature review. 2016.

[104] Schadt EE, Linderman MD, Sorenson J, Lee L, Nolan GP. Computational solutions to large-scale data management and analysis. Nat Rev Genet 2010; 11(9): 647-57.
[http://dx.doi.org/10.1038/nrg2857] [PMID: 20717155]

[105] Li Y, Chen L. Big biological data: challenges and opportunities. Genomics Proteomics Bioinformatics 2014; 12(5): 187-9.
[http://dx.doi.org/10.1016/j.gpb.2014.10.001] [PMID: 25462151]

[106] Musa A, Ghoraie LS, Zhang SD, *et al.* A review of connectivity map and computational approaches in pharmacogenomics. Brief Bioinform 2018; 19(3): 506-23.
[PMID: 28069634]

**CHAPTER 15**

# Computational Applications in the Drug Discovery and Development Processes

**M.O. Kaka[1], J.O. Aribisala[2], S. Karishma[2], A.K. Oyebamiji[3], T.A. Ajayeoba[1], N.J. Ohanaka[4] and S. Sabiu[2,*]**

[1] *Department of Microbiology, Adeleke University, Ede, Osun State, Nigeria*

[2] *Department of Biotechnology and Food Science, Faculty of Applied Sciences, Durban University of Technology, South Africa*

[3] *Computational Chemistry Research Laboratory, Department of Pure and Applied Chemistry, Ladoke Akintola University of Technology, Ogbomoso, Oyo State, Nigeria*

[4] *Department of Biochemistry, Nile University of Nigeria, Abuja, Nigeria*

**Abstract:** The traditional drug discovery and development process has been shown to be not only time-consuming and risky, but also expensive. The identification of disease-related targets, the identification and optimization of novel leads, and drug development are the three critical steps in modern drug discovery. Approaches such as genomics, proteomics, molecular biology, cell biology, structure biology, computational biology, and bioinformatics are commonly used to identify disease-related targets. Here, we appraised the significance of computational applications in modern drug discovery and development. It was revealed that the adoption of novel computational technologies has proven to be efficient in identifying drug targets and drug candidates against degenerative diseases such as diabetes, cancer and bacterial infections, and the concept holds significant promise for a future breakthrough in drugs discovery, design and development. The challenges involved with computational applications in drug discovery are basically those of precision and accuracy in handler and software limitations. However, future breakthroughs and effective outcomes depend on the combination of advanced models with vast experience in the field of drug discovery and an understanding of the limitations of the existing computational tools.

**Keywords:** Bioinformatics, Computational Science, Drug Discovery, Drug Development, Life Sciences, Therapeutic Target.

* **Corresponding author S. Sabiu:** Department of Biotechnology and Food Science, Faculty of Applied Sciences, Durban University of Technology, South Africa; Tel: +2731 373 5330; E-mail: sabius@dut.ac.za

Saheed Sabiu (Ed)

# 1. INTRODUCTION

Historically, medicines have often been derived from fungi, herbs, plants and other natural sources known to man [1]; the naturally derived drugs constituted those of plant, animal, and microbiological sources. Many important drugs were derived from plants, both directly and indirectly- hence, plants were deemed to be vital sources of novel pharmacologically active compounds [2]. Until the mid 19th century, there was little to no scientific understanding of why certain substances (mostly natural products) produced medicinal effects. There was also a non-existent use of man-made/synthetic drugs for disease cure. Basically, pharmaceutical drug discovery trended through a different era and commenced with the discovery of the first synthetic compound (chloral hydrate) in 1832, which was not used medically until 1969. Drug discovery from synthetic compounds of organic molecules such as citric, gallic, malic, lactic, oxalic and uric acids was rampant [3]. In the 20th century, fusion of knowledge from biochemistry, microbiology and synthetic organic chemistry yielded the production of natural, semi-synthetic, and synthetic drugs, whereas the discovery of antibiotics by Alexander Fleming aided the development of more antibiotics in order to treat infectious diseases [4]. Further advances in drugs discovery, design and development took place with the discovery of vaccines, active modified purines as anticancer drugs, and antiviral drugs [5, 6], which were greatly helped by the discovery and the knowledge of DNA Recombinant Technology. In the 21st century, multidisciplinary approaches, bioinformatics, combination chemistry and molecular modeling have aided pharmaceutical advances in drugs design and development [7].

In modern day trends, drugs discovery occurs through gaining new insights into a disease process, allowing the design of an agent(s) that stops or reverses the effects of the disease [8]. Drugs are also discovered when many tests of molecular compounds are carried out in order to observe their effects against certain diseases (Fig. **1**). The discovery of new drugs also stems from the knowledge of existing treatments that have unanticipated effects and furthermore, new technologies, these include technologies which work in the manipulation of genetic material and those that function in the specific targeting of drugs/medical products to body sites [9].

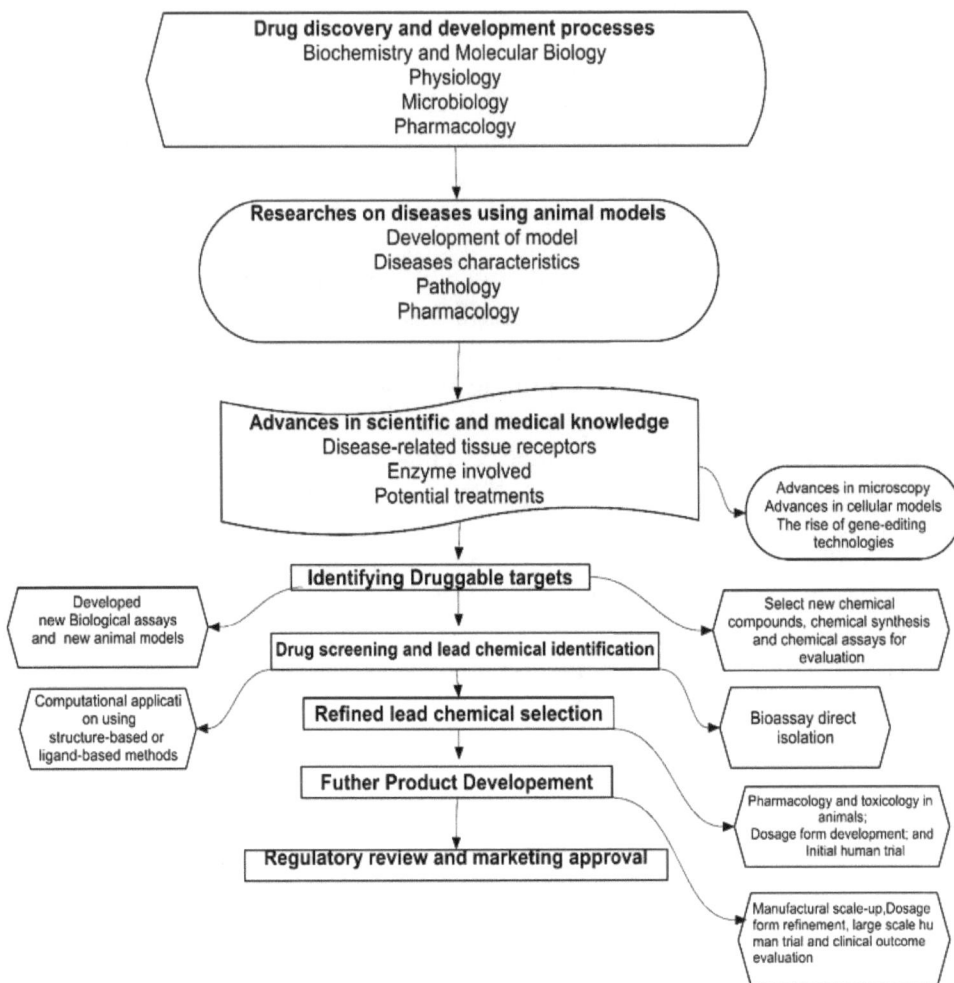

**Fig. (1).** Flow Chart of Drug Discovery and Development.

After identifying promising/lead compounds, experiments are carried out in the development of new drugs (Fig. **1**) to gather information on the drug's absorption, distribution, metabolism, and excretion [10]. The potential benefits of the new drug in addition to its mechanisms of action and the best dosage for effective use, are also examined. Furthermore, the method of ingestion, adverse effects, toxicity, and the drugs' interaction and effectiveness in comparison with other drugs are observed and studied [7, 10] to gather information on the absorption, distribution, metabolism and excretion of the drug [10]. They also examine its potential benefits and mechanisms of action in addition to the best dosage for effective use.

## 2. HISTORY OF DRUGS DISCOVERY, DESIGN AND DEVELOPMENT

Drug discovery spans three major timelines. The first timeline is the nineteenth century, and era where drugs were derived from natural sources (plants) with limited to no knowledge of their toxicity [5]. Preceding this period, plants, animals, minerals that were believed to be capable of exerting therapeutic activities were manipulated by men in a futile attempt to disease cure [5, 6]. The initial stages of drugs design in the early 19th century ranged from natural to semi-synthetic; however, from the mid-19th century [5 - 7, 10], synthetic methods were developed, allowing the structural modification that yielded active semisynthetic analogues. In the late 19th century, organic synthesis provided a way to produce purely synthetic structures that reduced the dependence of pharmaceutical medicines on the natural world. These then became important in the course of the twentieth century for the discovery of novel agents for drugs design.

Pharmaceutical companies in the twentieth century focused on synthesizing as many compounds as possible by discovering active compounds in a rather disorganized and irrational format. With the development of agents such as the antiulcer drug cimetidine in the 1960s, rational drug design began to have an impact. Because of advances in genomics and proteomics based on the discovery of computational drug design method [11], significantly huge amounts of breakthrough in organized and rational drug design have occurred, beginning in the 1980s. This was due to the fact that the 'omics' help in identifying an increased number of potential drug targets [12].

Rapid advancements in molecular modeling tools have occurred since the 1990s [13], as has the application of combinatorial chemistry and automated high-throughput screening, which has resulted in enormous benefits in transitioning from "lead discovery" to "lead optimization" [12, 13]. Rationally designed libraries of compounds based on known drug scaffolds were created in a relatively short period of time, and by the end of the twentieth century, advances in molecular and cell biology, such as recombinant DNA techniques, had helped to revolutionize the pharmaceutical industry [13]. The conventional methods of carrying out research especially the ones involved in drug development and design are mostly time consuming and involve trial and error which constitutes exertion of resources which might have otherwise been converted to better use. These also sometimes cause environmental pollution. Hence, this work is aimed at projecting the significance of computational applications in drug development for the purpose of faster and efficient research.

Scientific journals are well-indexed in prominent databases; and ranging from the last five to ten years were gathered and used for the purpose of this research.

## 3. CHALLENGES INVOLVED WITH CONVENTIONAL METHODS OF DRUG DEVELOPMENT

Drugs were primarily derived from natural sources in the early days of drug discovery, with no prior knowledge of their toxicity. Traditional techniques of drug discovery until the late 1980s were, therefore excessively time consuming and inefficient, and several treatments were not applied as a beneficial therapy. Thus, relying on automated and computer-assisted rational drug design, the industry began to evaluate purified biological targets by performing campaigns of high-throughput screening of large combichem libraries [14]. From the ancient Egypt Pharmacopeia described in the Ebers Papyrus to the early 1990s emergence of high throughput screening, drug discoveries were mostly the result of serendipity, intuition, and trial-and-error efforts (forward pharmacology) or first-generation rational drug design (reverse pharmacology) (HTS) [15]. It is reasonable to conclude that Fleming discovered penicillin from mold secretions by chance and intuition.

Scientists working on drug discovery face challenges that are associated with disease complexity and the inherent need to bring patients in contact with safer drugs at a faster and lower rate [16]. The workflow of drug discovery which was developed for HTS a few decades ago [17] is seen to be evolving under the guidance of multidisciplinary scientists. Computational Associated Drug Design (CADD) has reemerged in the last decade as a method to effectively reduce the number of compounds for screening while maintaining the same level for lead compound discovery [18]. As a result, many previously classified and predicted inactive compounds can be avoided, while those that are active can be prioritized as useful. As a result, the cost and workload of a full HTS screen for lead discovery could be reduced while maintaining accuracy [17, 18]. Furthermore, before they can be used, traditional HTS assays frequently require extensive development and validation. [18, 16]. Since CADD requires less time to prepare, experimenters can conduct CADD studies concurrently; this is in the sense that comparative cases in the use of CADD and HTS for the examination of inhibitory activities of pharmacophores against important receptor enzymes has effectively demonstrated the power of CADD [19].

Researchers gain from advanced technologies that enable new disease targets to better be identified and validated. These advances also enable scientists in the design of more biologically-relevant disease models and in the development of unbiased assays for the purpose of finding relatively safer and efficient therapies based on small or large molecules [20].

In the previous half century, the history of drug development in the pharmaceutical business and academic laboratories evolved, starting soon after the Penicillins, known as "miracles" which was later made available to the public. In the same decade synthetic organic chemistry developed into the commercially practical manufacture of "non-natural" therapeutic possibilities. This advancement was deemed significant at the time because bacteria developed resistance to natural penicillin. Synthetic chemistry offers a solution: the capacity to generate analogs that demonstrate their action under resistant stresses (with the natural lactam core but with a non-normal side chain) [20, 21]. There remained, however, a number of disorders for which therapy was not effective and synthetic chemistry promised it could be developed, provided a medicine were imaginable [21]. On the other hand, biology took some further years to catch up by supplying more detailed knowledge, which would be necessary at the molecular level. Drug creation became more erudite over time, eventually taking the lead in the development of novel drugs, particularly in the pharmaceutical industry. especially in the optimization of the drugs activity. There was a strong empirical nature of analog models resulting from the drug discovery (methyl, ethyl, isopropyl). However, for many decades, especially the 1970s, they were highly popular. Initially isolating, identified and screened in panels of tests for various kinds of desired activity, for example, toxicity in cancer cells [20, 21], the commercial availability of powerful spectrometers (particularly NMR and MS and separation techniques (HPLCs) for the determination of minute quantities of biologically active natural products led to a new revolution.

In the following decade the emphasis switched toward a more rational approach to computer-assisted drug design in the searches for active natural compounds. This paradigm shift was triggered not just by progress in computer power at the beginning of the 1980s, but also by significant and parallel advancements in structural biology that provided a continual flow of protein structures based on computer drug design research [22]. The discovery paradigm in general was poorly carried out and a return to largely empirical approaches – small molecule library synthesis and high-performance screening – was superseded in the early 1990s [18, 22].

In this situation, sophisticated robotics and biological procedures were technological developments (used in simultaneously assaying thousands of compounds), and enhanced methodology in synthetic chemistry which led to this change [17, 18, 20]. However, the output of the large pharmaceutical medication pipeline seems to have reached another low, which shows a growing consensus that these high-performance screening programs, too, have not been implemented. This could be because the incredibly huge industrial libraries, which have been produced and tested, lack real chemical diversity [23]. Thus, there is a clear need for new ideas required in opening the pipeline. This could include the same fundamental scientific facts at the heart of the pharmaceutical development for a long time, which are structural biology, which provides information about the target bio macromolecules [22]; chemical chemicals that design and synthesize drug candidates [24]. Consequently, the next stage of drug development requires an altogether new methodology, as a result of the incorporation of new disciplines and better technology in the process.

The incorporation into the process of the future phase of drug findings will be emphasis on sophisticated new computational, biomedical, pharmacogens, engineering and nanotechnology methods [26].

Finding drug candidates capable of combating the scourge of communicable and non-communicable ailments with minimal or no adverse effects is a great challenge. Many drug advances have been related with the treatment and management of diseases such as HIV/AIDS, malaria, hypertension, diabetes and cancer, yet they remain a source of considerable associated deaths in many populations around the world [27]. As a result, novel drug discovery techniques that incorporate current blockbuster Pharma R&D strategies are required [28]. Furthermore, an effective approach is to rationally return to nature for answers, as has been done in the past for drug discovery. In the treatment of these diseases, anticancer drugs such as Taxol (*Taxus brevifolia*), Vinblastine (*Catharanthus roseus*) and antimalarial drugs such as quinine (*Cinchona* spp.) and Artemisinin (*Artemisia annua*) which were all derived from natural sources have proven to be effective. As a result, natural product research & development plays a key role in new drug discovery, in the face of increasing global health challenges [26 - 28].

Nicholas *et al.* [29] report some challenges to the therapeutic usage of natural products that include difficulty accepting the fact that they are therapeutic, the lack of standardization procedures, lack of isolation for pure chemical products, the unclearing of biological mechanisms and the lack of documented clinical trials according to established standard [28]. Historical scientific data has been provided regarding the therapeutic effectiveness of natural compounds that have led to the development of key conventional drugs [30]. Due to the complexity of molecular mixtures, it is sometimes challenging to discover new drug candidates using natural products. The synergistic effect of many compounds is responsible for the medicinal effectiveness of plant extracts. Thus, given the complexity of many diseases, particularly degenerative ones such as cancer, it's not surprising that single compound-based drug discovery hasn't resulted in effective therapy. The essence of a combinatorial strategy to assessing potential compounds is the plant-driven medicines discovery. Scientists can take a combinatorial approach in order to harness the therapeutic characteristic of plant-based natural products, and, in physiological conditions study their molecular effects, such as new technologies such as the quantum computing, profiling, computational biology techniques, big data, microfluidics and artificial intelligence [30, 31].

# 4. ADVANCES IN DRUGS DISCOVERY AND DEVELOPMENT PROCESSES

There has been a reduction in the overall efficiency of pharmaceutical research and development, [which is also known as the ratio of New Molecular Entities (NMEs) and Biologic License Applications (BLAs)] launched over the last decade as a function of their associated R&D investments [32]. Numerous advances in the drug discovery process have been made to improve the situation [32 - 34]. Predictive toxicology, for example, was introduced during absorption, distribution, metabolism, elimination, and toxicity (ADMET) to fail drug candidates more quickly and reduce drug attrition rate related to safety [35]. Traditional toxicity assessment was done using animal models, and predictive toxicology necessitated the development of *in silico* and *in vitro* methods that could be used on a large scale, as well as in the drug discovery workflow [36].

Quantitative structure activity relationships (QSAR) are used in *in silico* methods to filter potentially toxic compounds from libraries based on their structure. They used specialized cell lines, microscale physiological systems, and small animal models for the *in vitro* tests [37].

The primary technological arsenal available to scientists in the early days of modern drug discovery consisted of microscopes, pipettes, test tubes, and primitive immunoassays such as radioimmunoassay's (RIAs) [37, 38]. Microscopes were demoted to a secondary role as target-based drug discovery became more industrialized, while pipettes, test tubes, and immunoassays improved significantly, leading to automated liquid handlers, microplates, ultrasensitive non-radiometric immunoassays, and associated multi-level detectors [38].

## 4.1. Advances in Microscopy

The need to change the drug discovery workflow, as well as the subsequent resurgence of phenotypic assays, necessitated the advancement of time-tested/relegated technologies like microscopy [39]. One example is the development of electron microscopy (EM), which has proven to be a valuable structural technique; in fact, recent technological advances now allow for the analysis of high-resolution structures. As a result, potential applications of EM have been transformed, particularly in the field of drug discovery. Cryo-EM is now used extensively in drug discovery programs, particularly for difficult targets that were previously difficult to characterize structurally, such as membrane proteins [40]. The advent of new technologies, including enhancements to existing techniques, are currently addressing technical issues that previously have limited the usefulness of microscopic imaging; together, these developments augment the existing assays. It also enables new disease models [41].

High-content image analysis (HCIA) and high-content screening (HCS) which are new microscopy-based technologies have proven to be extremely useful in drug discovery efforts [39]. The generation of high-quality images not only allows for the detection of a specific target signal but also allows for the detection of multiple target signals, they also enable the recording of holistic whole cell phenotypic changes as well as the analysis of organoid or small organism [38, 39].

However, a literature survey indicated that the majority of high content data previously published relied solely on a few measured image-based traits from all tested samples, limiting the use of additional significant phenotypic data [42].

Initially, a lack of modern technology that permits multi parametrical analysis of all collectible data was a key constraint that limited HCS and HCIA potential [39, 42]. Surprisingly, these limitations are overcome by artificial intelligence, particularly machine learning.

HCS and HCIA are both based on traditional optical microscopy, with a diffraction-limited resolution of about 200 nm [43, 44]. The invention of the Stimulated Emission Depletion (STED) microscopy technique aids in overcoming the diffraction-limited resolution barrier by precisely controlling the excitation state of fluorescent molecules with a precision of 50 nm or less [43, 45].

Human stem cell–derived cultures can now be used thanks to three (3) significant technological advances. The first step was to identify actively dividing intestinal stem cells molecularly [46], and the second step was to use previously developed methods to differentiate inducible pluripotent stem cells (iPSCs) into a multicellular culture model of the fetal intestine that included epithelial cells and human intestinal organoids [47]. The third step was the creation of platforms, which included simple culture dishes, Trans well filters, and micro physiological systems. All of these contribute to the growth and differentiation of human stem cells [48]. These advancements are aided by the creation of improved cellular models that mimic *in vivo* systems [49]. For example, *in vitro* cell-based assays aid in replicating the complexities of the biological environment are generally predictive of how a compound will behave *in vivo*.

Immortalized cell lines, primary cell cultures, and human pluripotent stem cells have recently been shown to be useful in basic research models (hPSCs). They are also helpful in efforts to develop drugs [49]. Several laboratories still use immortalized cell lines like HEK-293 and CHO-K1. However, these cell lines have very little biological significance, particularly when used to overexpress exogenous proteins [49, 50].

Introduction to both basic and implemented research was achieved by stem cells, specifically inducible pluripotent stem cells (iPSCs). They can be used in every phase of the drug discovery, all from ADMET research to target identification [34, 36]. Due to the fact that stem cells are able to renew themselves unlimitedly, when differentially controlled, they are regarded as reliable physiologically significant cell sources. Stem cells are an excellent alternative to recombinant/immortalized cell lines and primary cells because of these two characteristics. However, greater use of stem cells is hampered by challenges with directed differentiation and the associated maintenance costs [39]. Furthermore, scientists must pay close attention to cell culture conditions because they have the potential to significantly alter cellular phenotype and biological functions. Moreover, as cells are normally cultivated and employed (as suspensions or monocultures adhering to them), co-culture with different types of cells occurring in the natural surroundings may be needed to better adapt and respond to them. In addition, numerous studies have found that cells have different structures and functions when used in suspension *versus* adherent forms. The results were comparable when cells grown on 2D surface-coated support were compared to cells grown on 3D scaffolds [51].

Growing cells in 3D has piqued the interest of many researchers because it is said to be more similar to *in vivo* natural systems and provide more biologically relevant information than single cell populations [49]. The ability to generate patient-specific tissues using human-induced pluripotent stem cells (hiPSCs) and obtain any cell type composed in the human body using hPSCs enables significant advances in personalized medicine. Recently disclosed 3D matrix and cell printing capabilities should aid in the latter efforts in the near future [49, 51].

## 4.2. The Rise of Gene-editing Technologies

The technology of gene editing has been shown to be one of the most significant scientific breakthroughs of the twentieth century. Scientists can use these technologies to add, delete, or modify genetic material at specific locations in the genome. The CRISPR-Cas9 method is widely used in science because it has been demonstrated to be more accurate and efficient than other gene editing systems while also being quick and cheap to implement [52].

This technology (gene editing) is used at all stages of drug discovery, from target identification to the development of new models and therapies. Identifying and validating new disease targets (oncology) is made possible by high resolution CRISPR screens of gRNA libraries [52]. CRISPR technology has also been used in drug absorption studies, distribution, metabolism and excretion (ADME) and for ADME model generation [53].

CRISPR-Cas9 is also being used in immuno-oncology research to engineer T-cells to treat hematological and solid tumors. T-cells that have been engineered can thus be (re)injected into cancer patients during autologous or allogenic grafting. As a result of collaborative translational oncology efforts, a growing number of clinical trials involving CRISPR-Cas9 engineered T-cells have been established. Meanwhile, specialized organizations began offering T-cell engineering and grafting services to cancer patients [52, 53].

## 4.3. Other Advances

High-performance liquid chromatography technologies, nuclear magnetic resonance spectroscopy, mass spectrometry, microfluidics, and computational algorithms advanced medicinal chemistry significantly during the twentieth century [54]. This has made it possible to identify plant chemical components and use them in drug discovery. The utilization of bioreactors and microfluidic technologies in high-performance tests led to the discovery of various drugs based on natural plant products [55].

Innovative medicine design based on natural ingredients, thanks to technology advancement, are necessary to address global health concerns. Above all, new and creative computer and analytical methods for identifying chemical components in crude plant extracts are necessary for the determination and optimization of the extraction of compounds causing the desired therapeutic effect, to prevent interference in components [56]. Further investigations should also focus on the combinatory effects and not only single compounds of chemicals from plant extracts. The mechanisms of how these combinations influence genes and proteins in several biological processes must be examined by existing "omics" platforms [57] Microfluidic and computer analyses developments have permitted plant extract chemical design and testing in drug discovery. plant extract chemical [58]. New analytical and bioinformatics techniques, for example, will aid in the design, synthesis, and biological testing of new compounds.

## 5. ROLE AND SIGNIFICANCE OF COMPUTATIONAL APPLICATIONS IN TRANSLATIONAL SCIENCE/PERSONALIZED MEDICINE

The pharmaceutical sector is already reducing the time scale for all areas of drug detection [59, 60]. Though computational progress, structural chemistry and molecular modeling have helped to rationalize design, empirical screening still remains vital in the identification of lead compounds [60]. In many businesses, HTS has become a valuable tool. due to the fact that testing large numbers of compounds in an efficient form allows a competitive advantage [59] As a result, in order to achieve the required productivity, compound supply integration, testing and data management is essential. For this purpose, HTS has fully taken advantage of recent progress in biology, biotechnology, engineering and the information science [61, 62].

## 5.1. Computer-aided Drug Discovery

Over three decades These processes have been fundamental for the discovery of small compounds of therapeutic importance [63, 64]. Computer-aided methods are often characterized as structural or ligand-based (Fig. **2**). Structure-based methods need knowledge on targets and ligands, and procedures like as ligand docking, pharmacophores and ligand design are used [64].

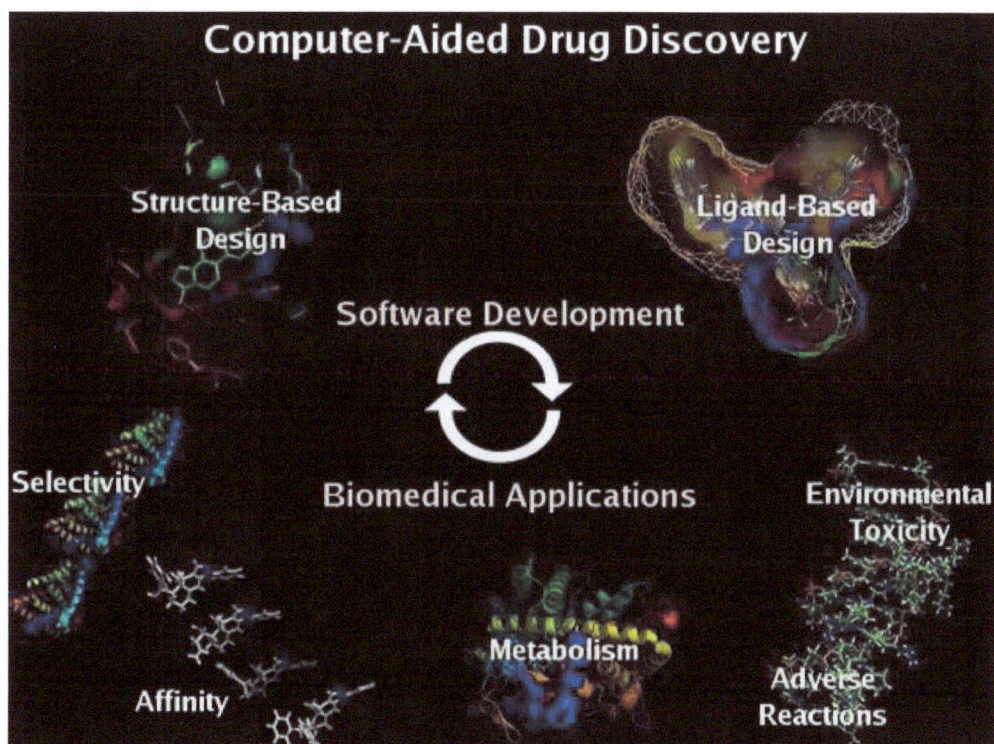

**Fig. (2).** Classification of CADD and their Biomedical Applications [75].

CADD could boost the hits of new medicinal compounds as they have a much more specific search than conventional HTS and combination chemistry [65]. It aims not only at explaining the molecular foundation of therapeutic activities, but also at predicting the prospective derivatives that improve activities. CADD is primarily used in three ways: (1) the filtering of large compound libraries into small sets of predictable, experimentally testable active compounds; (2) the supervision of lead optimization to determine whether its association increases and optimizes drug metabolism and pharmacokinetics, such as absorption, distribution and optimization; and (3) the optimization of drug metabolism and pharmacokinetics (DMPK) properties [64, 66, 67]. CADD is separated into two different categories: ligand-based and structural. In order to compute the energy interaction of all tested compounds, structural CADD relies on an understanding of the target protein structure, whereas ligand CADD utilizes known active and inactive molecules by searches with chemical similitudes or the development of predicted QSAR models [67]. Another difference is, while structural CADD is preferred when structural high resolution target protein structure data are available (soluble protéins that can easily be crystallized) [68], ligand based CADD is preferred when structural data are scarce or not available, common to membrane protein targets [69].

Through the targeting of its ATP binding site, structure-based high-throughput screening (SBHTS) has been useful in the identification of protein kinase CK2 inhibitors (an important target in the development of antitumor drugs) [70]. Out of the 400,000 compounds which have been screened, twelve (12) hits were selected, out of these emanated a novel drug with the ability to inhibit CK2 enzymatic activity with an $IC_{50}$ of 80 nM. On discovery, this novel drug was thought to be one of the most potent drugs for a protein kinase. In addition, SBHTS has been used in examining proliferator-activated target agonistic behavior with Sulfonylureas and Glinides binding [71]. This discovery has been linked to the treatment of type 2 diabetes and has been validated by experimental assays. SBHTS has also recently been used in the discovery of antiviral inhibitors that target the Ebola virus [72].

When the receptor 3D information is not available, Ligand-based drug design depends on the knowledge of the molecules involved to link to the biological objective of interest [73]. Three dimensional quantitative structure activity relationship (3D QSAR) and pharmacophore models are one of the most important technologies used to create ligand-based medicinal products as at today. 3D QSAR can provide prediction models ideal to identify and optimize leads. QSAR is the name given to approaches that connect the chemical structure with qualities as biological activity *in vitro* or *in vivo*. Ligand-based drug design has also been widely applied in the quantitative exploration of shared chemical properties among a large number of known 5-LOX inhibitors of varying diversity [74]. 5-LOX is an enzyme that is essential for the biosynthesis of leukotrienes, which are the mediators of allergies, asthma, GERD, Crohn's disease, and other inflammatory disorders. It is also linked to a variety of cancers, and many pharmaceutical companies and academic research groups are focusing on the development of effective 5-LOX inhibitors [73].

## 5.2. Therapeutic Targets in Degenerative and Microbial Diseases

The basic physical, functional and molecular heritage unit is the gene [76]. Genes are a set of guidelines governing the appearance, survival and behavior of the organism. The genes vital to the survival of an organism are called essential genes. These are the least necessary genes for a living cell's survival and are considered a crucial source of life. Modern drug finding is founded on the identification and evaluation of drug candidates who act on predetermined therapeutic targets. Advances in the areas of genetics, protein structure, proteomics and causes for disease have reawaken interest in discovering and exploring new and existing objectives effectively [76].

Identification of genes in bacterial organisms is crucial for the identity of genes and new targets for bacterial disease and the development of antibacterial agents. Because they avoid costly and difficult experimental checks, computational methods are more appealing for avoiding experimental constraints. Furthermore, these methods could help guide the prediction of new organisms for accurately predicting essential genes [77]. Knowledge about existing targets can help you find clues to identify new targets. It is also important that drug operations be molecularly dissected, that characteristics that drive the new design of drug be predicted, and that instruments be developed for these tasks [78]. The examination of these objectives also provides helpful information about trends, current research areas, and success and challenges in exploring therapeutic objectives for the creation of medicines against certain diseases [79].

Various computer methods have been created for the prediction of basic genes as a result of a variety of factors: sequenced data collections for a large number of organisms and virtually validated gene collections for certain similar organizations. Different methods have been used to determine the essentiality of genes in genome-based organisms [69, 76, 77]. The combination of the intrinsic characteristics of the investigated organisms with features from the experimental data has been shown to greatly increase prediction accuracy. Comprehensive study of many important genes can help to develop a training package that will improve basic genetic prediction for different bacteria.

The technological basis of the present approach of drug finding is the search for drug leads against preset therapeutic aims followed by the tests of the candidates for derived drugs [69]. Numerous efforts have been made to investigate the targets of highly effective and potent drugs, and there is a growing interest in identifying new targets. Rapid advances in genomics, protein structures, proteomics, and disease molecular mechanisms [78, 80] not only allow for the discovery of new targets, but also allow for the investigation of existing targets. These advancements also allow for the discovery of new targets and the investigation of the molecular mechanisms of drug action. In addition, these advances help in studying adverse drug reactions, pharmacogenetic implications of gene sequence variations, expression profiles, and post-transcriptional processing [80]. The discovery of an increasing number of new and novel targets has resulted from advancements in target identification and validation technologies. The following are some druggable targets for degenerative diseases, as shown in Table **1**.

**Table 1. Selected druggable targets of some degenerative diseases.**

| Disease | Molecular/Therapeutic Targets | References |
|---|---|---|
| **Cancers** | | |
| Prostate cancer | Glucose transporter, HK2, Proteasome | [81] |
| Metastatic RCC, melanoma | PKM2, DNA alkylating agent | [82] |
| Multiple cancers | LDHA, Folate cycle (DHFR), Thymidine synthesis (TYMS), Deoxynucleotide synthesis (Ribonucleotide reductase: RNR), Nucleotide incorporation (DNA polymerase/RNR) | [81, 83] |
| Brain cancer | Pyruvate dehydrogenase kinase (PDK) | [84, 85] |
| Head and neck cancer | Pyruvate dehydrogenase kinase (PDK) | [84, 86] |
| Non-small cell lung cancer (NSCLC) | Pyruvate dehydrogenase kinase (PDK), Tyrosine kinases; KIT, BCR-Abl, PDGFR, | [87] |
| Advanced solid tumors | MCT1 | [82] |
| Leukemia | Tyrosine kinases; KIT, BCR-Abl, PDGFR, mTORC1, EGFR, Bcl2 | [88] |
| Cutaneous T cell lymphoma (CTCL) | Nicotinamide phosphoribosyl-transferase (NAMPT), HDAC | [83] |
| B-Cell Chronic Lymphocytic Leukemia (CLL) | Nicotinamide phosphoribosyl-transferase (NAMPT) | [87, 89] |
| Lymphomas | Nicotinamide phosphoribosyl-transferase (NAMPT), HDAC | [90] |
| Colorectal cancer | Class III PI3 kinase | [91] |
| Cervical cancer | Lysosomal protease (Cathepsin) | [85] |
| Renal cancer | mTORC1 | [92] |
| Glioma | Tyrosine kinases; KIT, BCR-Abl, PDGFR | [84, 86, 93] |
| Pancreatic carcinoma | Bcl2 | [88] |
| Brest Cancer | Vacuolar-ATPase | [94] |

| Disease | Molecular/Therapeutic Targets | References |
|---|---|---|
| **Diabetes** | | |
| Type-2 Diabetes | Glucose transporter type 4 (GLUT4); G-protein coupled receptor (GPR); Protein tyrosine phosphatase 1B (PTP1B); Glutamine fructose-6-phosphate amidotransferase (GFAT); 17β-Hydroxysteroid dehydrogenase type 1 (17β-HSD1); 11β -Hydroxysteroid dehydrogenase (11β HSD); Peroxisome proliferator-activated receptor-gamma (PPAR-γ); Dipeptidylpepdidase 4 (DPP-4); Sodium glucose transporter (SGLT2); alpha-glucosidase; alpha-amylase | [95 - 101] |
| **Bacterial Infections** | | |
| Pneumonia | Penicillin binding protein; Folic acid synthesis enzyme; DNA Gyrase; Topo IV isomerase; 50S ribosomal subunit | [102] |
| Bacterial meningitis | 30S ribosomal subunit; Penicillin binding protein | [102, 103] |
| Salmonellosis | DNA Gyrase; Topo IV isomerase; Penicillin binding protein, Penicillin binding protein | [102, 103] |
| Cholera | Topo IV isomerase, DNA Gyrase, | [104, 105] |
| Syphilis | 30S ribosomal subunit; Penicillin binding protein | [106; - 108] |
| Gonorrhea | Penicillin binding protein; 50S ribosomal subunit | [107, 109] |
| Dysentery | DNA Gyrase; Topo IV isomerase, Penicillin binding protein | [103] |
| Urinary tract infection | Penicillin binding protein; Folic acid synthesis enzyme; DNA Gyrase; Topo IV isomerase; 50S ribosomal subunit | [103] |
| Chlamydia | Topo IV isomerase, DNA Gyrase, 50S ribosomal subunit | [107, 108] |

## 5.3. Application of Molecular Dynamics Simulation in the Drug Discovery and Development Processes for Degenerative and Microbial Diseases

Over the last few years, computational chemistry methods have become ingrained in the drug discovery process, expanding significantly beyond early work on QSAR [110], computerized chemical structure representation [110, 111], and computerized databases on structure–activity [111]. Computational methods have been established to being an intrinsic part of the drugs discovery process. Nonetheless, there have been questions regarding their continued role in drug discovery since the pharmaceutical industry tends to face looming scientific and economic challenges in its application. Molecular dynamics simulations (MDS) not only offer various structural dynamic information on bio macromolecules, but also a vast of knowledge regarding protein-ligand interactions [112]. This type of information is ultimately important in understanding the structural and functional relationship of the target, as well as the essence of protein-ligand interactions, which guides the drug discovery and design process. As a result, MD simulations are now widely used in modern drug discovery procedures [113].

There are numerous cases where MD simulation has been applied to decipher the nature of molecular interactions between bioactive compounds and the targets for lead compound identification [88, 90]. This concept has been used with promising outcomes in understanding the nature of molecular interactions between drug candidates and therapeutic targets in several degenerative human ailments such as diabetes, cancer, and microbial diseases such as bacterial and viral infections [110, 111, 114].

## 5.4. Diabetes

Several efforts have been made to find effective treatments for Type 2 diabetes. Scientists have been working hard over many years to utilize pharmacological and non-pharmacological techniques; however, none of them have been able to meet all medication safety requirements. In a study by Nguyen Vo *et al.* [115], molecular interactions that exist between different bioactive compounds in *Euphorbia thymifolia* and targeted proteins (11-β HSD1, GFAT, PTP1B, and SIRT6) related to Type 2 Diabetes Mellitus (T2DM) were evaluated. The chemical composition analyzed by GC–MS from arial part of *E. thymifolia* comprises three (3) main families: tannin, flavonoid and terpenoid. They were able to achieve their main goal of displaying a variety of bioactive compounds from all three families and determining how they interact with proteins that are important in T2DM by using computational approaches. The methodology used included molecular docking using Autodock Vina, a tool which allows for binding affinity measurement [115, 116]. The results of the analysis revealed that seven compounds were chosen from a list of 20 compounds based on their high binding energy to all four receptors (>8 kcal/mol) [115]. They included β-amyrine, taraxerol, 1-O-galloyl-β-d-glucose, corilagin, cosmosiin, quercetin-3-galactoside and quercitrin. Furthermore, the polyphenol and flavonoid family was discovered to have high binding affinity to the four receptors. They also discovered that the binding affinity of two of the terpenoid compounds indicated that they would be promising candidates for diabetes treatment [116].

In a study by Thakral *et al.* [117], a series of compounds including **5o** (2-chlor--5-[(4-chlorophenyl) sulfamoyl]-*N*-(2-methyl-5-nitrophenyl)-4-nitrobenzamide) was synthesized which compared to the drug standard acarbose, was discovered to be highly active, with a four-fold inhibitory effect against -glucosidase and a six-fold inhibition potential against -amylase. The anti-diabetic results of the molecular docking studies revealed the synthesized molecules had reasonable docking scores and binding interactions with their respective targets. Molecular dynamic simulations of the ligand protein complex revealed the stability of the most active compounds 5o in the binding sites of the respective target proteins, namely the -glucosidase and -amylase enzymes.

Furthermore, a study by Jeyabeskar *et al.* [118], reported on the docking analysis of compound nerolidol from *Momordica charantia* and further revealed that the compound exhibited good binding interaction with diabetic protein [118]. Also, an *in silico* approach by Thkral *et al.* [119] was used to study the major phytochemical properties and interactions of *P. longum* constituents. Using a molecular docking technique, they observed the interaction of four bioactive compounds from *P. longum* (piperine, piperlongumine, piperlonguminine, and retrofractamide A) with diabetic proteins. The compounds' strong binding to the proteins receptors confirmed that they act as inhibitors for dipeptidyl peptidase-4, GKRP, 11-hydroxysteroid dehydrogenase type 1, glutamine-fructose-6-phosphate transaminase 1, and protein tyrosine phosphatase 1B, which promote glucose digestion and increase insulin affectability.

In addition, Kaushik *et al.* [120] investigated the selection of four different receptors in order to identify the major pathway by which *Pinus roxburghii* exhibits its antidiabetic potential. The active constituents of *Pinus roxburghii* were found to be most active on aldose reductase, as previously confirmed by other researchers, according to their docking results.

## 5.5. Cancer

The primary goal of anti-cancer drug development is to re-induce "programmed cell death" in cancer cells [121]. Many of our efficient chemotherapy medications, such as vincristine, vinblastine, doxorubicin, etoposide and paclitaxel, stem from natural products that demonstrate the relevance as a lynchpin of cancer therapy [121]. Most bioactive compounds can concurrently target several signaling routes that are critical for the survival of cancer cells while they spare healthy cells, making them potential cancer-controlled silver bullets [121, 122]. A number of bioactive compounds have been identified that support this concept, with recognized anticancer potentials, the underlying processes by which cell death is induced and preclinical/clinical development [123]. Bioactive compounds have been studied and are reported to be multifunctional; they may limit cancer cell proliferation, cause apoptosis, trigger several tumor suppressors, inhibit angiogenesis, inhibit invasion and probable migration of cancer cells, and lower or inhibit inflammation [124]. Together, these study projects give significant assistance in the clinical development of various bioactive compounds, including Withaferin A, Honokiol, Benzyl Isothiocyanate, Resveratrol, Turmeric, Genistein, Epigallocatechin-3-Gallate [125, 126].

Breast cancer is another example of a multi-stage, multifactoral, and heterogeneous disease. The systemic management of breast cancer in the recent decade has undergone substantial alterations [125, 126]. As a result of a better understanding of pathogenesis, several studies have identified signaling pathways and therapeutic targets in breast cancer, including hormone receptor, human epidermal growth factor receptor 2 (HER2), epidermal growth factor receptor (EGFR), vascular endothelial growth factor (VEGF), phosphoinositide-3-kinase (PI3K), v-akt murine thymoma viral oncogene homolog (AKT), mechanistic target of rapamycin (mTOR), cyclin-dependent kinase 4/6 (CDK4/6), poly (adenosine diphosphate-ribose) polymerase (PARP), and programmed death-1 (PD-1) [98, 101].

Hinkson *et al.* [127] conducted research to predict the interaction between selected anticancer compounds and cancer target proteins from various types of cancer. Breast cancer associated protein, BRCA1-1JNX, gastric cancer-1BJ7, brain cancer (brain-type creatine kinase)- 1QH4, lung cancer (EGFR kinase)- 2ITO and skin cancer (Hsp90 molecular chaperone)- 2VCJ were the target proteins downloaded from the Protein Data Bank (PDB) database to study their susceptibility to selected anticancer compounds. Using *in silico* studies, the extent of interaction of the selected anticancer compound with the target proteins was predicted [128, 129]. According to their findings, the anticancer drug cabazitaxel had the highest binding energy against the skin cancer protein (2VCJ) and the brain cancer protein (2VCJ) (1QH4). Among the drugs tested, cabazitaxel was found to be effective and interacted strongly with all cancer target proteins tested. The analysis therefore showed that the interaction and binding between selected ligands, and targets for cancer are crucial for *in silico* investigations [129, 130].

In a study by Oyebamiji *et al.* [131], five selected compounds from *Annona muricata* were evaluated against type 3 of 3α-hydroxysteroid dehydrogenase (3α-HSD) [131]. Their action against cancer was examined with a quantum chemistry technique, molecular docking and molecular dynamics modeling approaches. A large number of descriptors have been derived, which describe the anti-cancer action of the chemicals examined (EHOMO, ELUMO, dipole moment, energy gaps, area, volume, polarization, polar surface area, log P, donor of hydrogen bonds or acceptor of hydrogen binding), The docking analysis also shows that the chemical studied has a larger inhibitory capacity than other compounds studied and the standard (compound C) has a greater ability to inhibit (5FU).

Shikder *et al.* [132] also examined the anti-cancer activity of the bioactive substances of *Withinia Somnifera* and predicted the relationship between phytochemicals (Withanolide, Withaferin-A) and cancer cell proliferation macromolecules. In a computational approach, Reddy *et al.* [133] explored the potential of Withaferin-A in attenuating Indoleamine 2,3-dioxygenase (IDO) for immunotherapeutic tumor arresting activity and elucidated its underlying mode of action.

In addition to letrozole(LTZ), the most powerful inhibitor of aromatase in human enzymes, which has been utilized as an antestrogen in breast cancer, research from MebarkA *et al.* [134] investigated the inhibitory effect of 1.2.3 triazole on human aroma enzyme (a major enzyme involved in breast cancer). The usage of MOLEGRO software was used for the analysis of the triazol inhibition energy (IE) of the aromatase enzyme p450 (3EQM.PDB).

Researchers have recently established an increased desire to create a mechanism for prediction before synthesis of biological activity. The invention of the QSAR model enables quantitative structure-activity relationship in the quest of data that connects chemical structures/ molecular properties to biological and other activities (QSAR). This approach can be used before synthesis to anticipate new chemical activity. Recent advances in QSAR studies have broadened the scope of drug design and examination of drug activity processes [135]. A study by Oyebami *et al.* [136] evaluated the bioactivity of thirty-two (32) sets of 1, 2, 3-triazolo [4, 5-d] pyrimidine derivatives by observing the calculated electronic descriptors using density functional theory (DFT) method. The molecular descriptors chosen were used to create QSAR models for anti-gastric cancer activity. The molecular docking study revealed the binding interactions between the compounds studied and the receptor. The results revealed that 2-(1-(2-(3-benzyl-5-(benzylthio)-3H- [1 - 3] was a 2-(1-(2-(3-benzyl-5-(benzylthio)-3H-[1 - 3] was a 2-(1-(2-(3-benzyl-5-(benzylthio)-3H- [1 - 3] -triazolo[4,5-d] When compared to the other compounds, the compound -pyrimidin-7-yl)-hydraz-no)-ethyl)-phenol (A22) had the lowest affinity and the highest inhibitory activity, making it the most promising drug-like compound for gastric cancer inhibition.

In another study, Iheagwam *et al.* [137] used *in silico* methods to discover potential inhibitors of VEGF, TK, and MMP (from *Caesalpinia bonduc*) as a potential cancer therapy. When compared to existing anti-cancer drugs, the binding energy and interactions with proteins were highly comparable.

## 5.6. Malaria

The protein-ligand interaction is critical in the design and development of structurally based drugs. A docking investigation of proguanil and its analog with the Human Dihydrofolate Reductase Receptor was conducted by Prakash *et al.* [138] with computer docking software. For analysis in this study, biological databases such as PubChem, Drug Bank, PDB and programs such as Hex, Arguslab, Molinspiration, FROG and ADME Tox were used. Findings of their results concluded that some of the modified drugs (Proguanil Analog 2 which was synthesized computationally due to the fact that side effects of the original drugs had been reported) are superior to commercially available drugs on the market.

They also suggested that these compounds' ADMET (Absorption, Distribution, Metabolism, Excretion/Toxicity) properties be tested in a wet lab before proceeding with clinical trials [139, 140].

A study by Collins [141] investigated the activities of *Ajuga remota* and *Azadirachta indica* against *Plasmodium falciparum*. They evaluated the molecular docking analysis of the herbal compounds against *Plasmodium falciparum's* protein targets, empirically comparing them with FDA-approved drugs known to inhibit the protein targets. The bioactivity prediction revealed that majority of the ligands have a good biological activity as an enzyme inhibitor. Finally, pharmacokinetic properties showed that all ligands possess the ability to permeate biological systems while portraying no carcinogenicity.

Temitope *et al.* [142] used molecular docking to screen *Cannabis sativa* compounds for antimalarial activity against *Plasmodium falciparum* drug target dihydrofolate reductase. Their findings revealed that phytochemicals from *Cannabis sativa* bind to isovitexin and vitexin with greater affinity and lower free energy than the standard ligand, shedding new light on *Cannabis sativa's* potential as an antimicrobial agent.

Furthermore, Kurniawan *et al.* [143] used a comparison of molecular field analysis (CoMFA), molecular docking, and molecular dynamics simulations to investigate cycloguanil analogues as a potent antimalarial agent. A CoMFA model with five partial least square regressions (PLSR) was developed to predict the $pIC_{50}$ value of 42 cycloguanil analogues. Docking analysis revealed that the attached substituent on the cycloguanil backbone structure was critical for antimalarial activity, and MD simulation confirmed the stability of the docking-derived binding pose.

Given the possible anti malaria-related activities, host non-toxicity, excellent pharmacokinetic and medicinal qualities, the leading compound for further comprehensive *in-silico*, pharmacological, and biological research has been identified as 18β Glycyrrhetinic Acid of *Glycyrrhiza glabra* (GA). Kalani *et al.* [144] studied the antimalarial activity of GA *in vitro*, *in silico*, and *in vivo*. *In vitro* anti-malarial activity of GA against *P. falciparum* was demonstrated ($IC_{50}$ 1.69g/ml). Similarly, molecular docking studies revealed that GA had a LibDock score of 71.18, while chloroquine had a score of 131.15. GA also has drug-like properties, according to *in silico* pharmacokinetic and drug-likeness studies. Finally, on day eight, *in vivo* testing revealed dose-dependent antimalarial activity ranging from 62.5–100% at doses ranging from 62.5–250mg/kg.

Furthermore, Rivo *et al.* [145] investigated the antimalarial activity of *S. hygroscopicus* derivative compounds by examining the binding affinity, pharmacokinetic profile, and bond interaction. The reverse molecular docking method was used to screen protein targets for the derivative compound. The isoquinoline derivative was able to bind to all of the protein targets, and its pharmacokinetic profile demonstrated that it met the drug-likeness criteria. Based on reverse molecular docking studies and pharmacokinetic profiles, they discovered that 6,7-Dinitro-2- [1, 2, 4]triazole-4-yl-benzo[de]isoquinoline-1,3-dione has antimalarial activity. Furthermore, based on bond affinity, adenylosuccinate synthetase was discovered to have the best inhibitory ability of all compounds.

## 5.7. Bacterial, Fungal and Viral Infections

The high rate of reports on complications encountered in diagnosing and treating multiple drug resistant (MDR) infections poses a threat to global health care [146]. For several years, docking as a way of determining the relationship between the drug-like molecules and the receptor has been widely acknowledged. This is a function of its capacity to basically select vast set of molecules and scoring, in addition to revealing the steps involved in drug-like molecule inhibition of a targeted binding site [147].

Oyebamiji *et al.* [148] used the quantum chemical method to investigate the biological activities of a set of seven hydrazone derivatives. Many molecular descriptors were obtained. In addition, docking studies on the investigated compounds were performed against the *Candida albicans* cell line (receptor) 1q42 in order to obtain the binding affinity and observe the intermolecular interactions between the ligand and the receptor. Clotrimazole, the standard drug, was used to compare the compounds studied. Each molecule's binding energy with the receptors AB7 AB1 AB5 AB6= AB4 AB3 AB2 inhibited better than the standard Clotrimazole.

The anti-Bacillus subtilis activity was reported by Oyebamiji *et al.* [147] by applying the descriptors generated using the density functional theory approach of QSAR studies using the 2-[5-(aryloxymethyl)-1,3,4-oxadiazol-2-ylsulfanyl] acetic acids derivative. The QSAR model created reproduced the observed bioactivities and the results of the docking research expected stable ligand configuration in the active region of the enzyme. They also investigated the inhibitory activity of 2-[-(aryloxymethyl)-1, 3, 4-oxadiazol-2-ylsulfanyl] acetic acid derivatives against *Staphylococcus aureus* cell line using density functional theory (DFT), quantitative structure activity relationship (QSAR), and docking methods [150]. In addition, the cytotoxicity of fifteen molecular compounds was studied using the quantum chemical method, QSAR, and docking studies [151]. The descriptors obtained were used to assess the anti-Sclerotinia sclerotiorum activity of 3,5-

dimethoxy-N-vinylbenzenamine derivatives, and a QSAR model was developed. The docking studies revealed the molecular interaction between the ligands and protein studied and hence the results demonstrate that all the compounds studied were more efficient than the standard drug in inhibiting *Sclerotinia sclerotiorum.*

In another study, Iheagwam *et al.* [152] researched Africa medicinal plant compounds as prospective candidates against multiple SARS-CoV-2 therapeutic targets. Possessing some therapeutics, these compounds were virtually screened against six SARS-CoV-2 and two human drug targets. The best hits were further simulated using molecular docking and ADMET. Three major compounds found in almond (*Terminalia catappa*), grape (*Vitis vinifera*), and common verbena (*Verbena officinalis*) were able to bind to all eight targets better than conventional drugs: 3-galloylcatechin, proanthocyanidin B1, and luteolin 7-galactoside. As a result of their multi-target activity, these molecules were concluded to be capable of serving as therapeutic leads in the fight against SARS-CoV-2. Similarly, Shode *et al.* [153] used *in silico* methods to report the potential of geraniin, 6-hydroxylcyanidin-3-rutinoside, epigallocatechin gallate, and cyanindin--glucoside as SARS-CoV-2 spike glycoprotein and main protease enzyme inhibitors. Further MDS revealed the compounds to be promising SARS-CoV-2 Mpro inhibitors, with significantly higher binding energies than the reference standards used in the study.

## 6. CHALLENGES WITH COMPUTATIONAL APPLICATIONS IN THE DRUG DISCOVERY PROCESS

The molecular docking method is widely used in computational science. Molecular docking is a technique that can be used in structure-based drug design, virtual screening, and lead compound optimization. It aids in the understanding of compound activity at the molecular level or in the selection of compounds for further investigation [153]. In general, current docking programs can predict correct binding modes. Most docking protocols, on the other hand, have a significant limitation in calculating accurate binding energies. During a docking process, many approaches such as solvent processing, macro-molecular flexibility, and protein-ligand complex, contributes to these constraints [154]. Covalent docking and accurate and quick modeling of metal interactions throughout the docking process represent major hurdles [155].

However, other methods for improving binding energies predictions include molecular dynamics, free energy disturbing methods and quantum mechanics/molecular mechanics (QM/MM) calculations [156]. While there are certain parts of simulation and computation that demand refinement, current drug design and optimization methodologies could provide valuable information

Presently, the presence of water molecules may be detected during the measurements in most docking algorithms. However, there are still certain problems, such as parameter scoring, comparison with interacting waters and correct discrimination of displaceable/non-displaceable waters [157]. Docking very large data sets has become a common task due to tremendous progress throughout the previous quarter of a century. Despite these developments, it is evident that a lot still has to be done, especially in the field of score-and-binding relationships. The increasing application of physical measurement processes may be associated with regression or machine learning methods that utilize structure-activity data for the receptor family or ligand chemical type [158], may be the most promising path forward. The second most important area to address is the routine incorporation of receptor flexibility. Secondly, the routine inclusion of receptor flexibility is the most significant region. Although combination docking and flexible receptor docking offer substantial progress towards a more realistic paradigm, they raise worry regarding the accuracy of conformal flexibility inside the receptor and its contribution to ligand binding affinity [159].

## 7. RECENT AND EMERGING ROLES OF COMPUTATION APPLICATIONS IN DRUG DISCOVERY

Bringing engineering to biology was one of the paradigm shifts that influenced the development of predictive, preventive, personalized, and participatory medicine, also known as P4 Medicine [160]. Several large international projects, including The Human Genome Project, the National Center for Biotechnology Information, the European Biotechnology Institute, and the Cancer Genome Atlas have all laid the groundwork for P4 medicine.

### Progress in Molecular Targeted Therapies

In recent years, molecular targeted therapy for breast cancer has made significant progress [161, 162]. Trastuzumab is widely regarded as the cornerstone of HER2-positive breast cancer targeted therapy, with significant efficacy in both neoadjuvant and adjuvant settings. Targeted therapy based on trastuzumab and pertuzumab ushers in a new era of cancer treatment [161]. T-DM1 is important in heavily pretreated HER2-positive advanced breast cancer patients and contributes to blood-brain barrier breakdown [161, 162]. With a better understanding of the pathogenesis of breast cancer, increasingly effective targeted drugs can be taken to lessen symptoms in the clinical setting, and further look towards developing a cure for breast cancer in the near future.

In addition, Alzheimer's (AD) disease is a complex multifactorial condition with unknown mechanisms [163]. The failure of the A-centered single goal strategy is convincing proof that the AD drug design paradigm has to be changed. The development of new biomarkers and imaging technologies for Alzheimer's disease has made substantial progress in the past decade. However, these instruments have not yet been thoroughly perfected in clinical trial practice. As such, effective and safe preventative treatments can be obtained by adopting personalized multi-target and biomarker-oriented techniques depending on the illness features of each individual patient [164].

Recent neurobiological progress has provided a more comprehensive view into neurodegenerative disease pathogenesis, paving the way for molecular targeted therapeutics to evolve. Integrated approaches should be employed to increase the effectiveness of both basic and clinical trials to examine the efficacy of putative illness modifications with limited financial and patient resources [165]. As it becomes obvious now that the creation of molecular targeted medicines is not always suitable for traditional methodologies, conceptual innovation is necessary both in basic and in clinical research.

## CONCLUSION AND PERSPECTIVES

Bioinformatics is seen as a technology that can greatly increase drug discovery, testing and commercialization in clinical trials. In addition to the possibility of accelerating drug discovery and hence reducing costs, computer biology and biological informatics have the ability to alter medicine design [166]. Rational Drug Design (RDD) supports the process of drug design, which incorporates a number of methodologies for determining new compounds, facilitates and speeds up [167, 168]. Docking is a molecular modeling process that predicts the preferred molecule orientation when bonded to create a stable complex. Then, the best orientation can be used to predict the interactions or the binding affinity of two molecules. Docking is often used to anticipate how small molecular therapeutic candidates have a binding orientation to their protein goals, which predicts the affinity and activity of the small molecule [168]. Molecular dynamics simulations can be used to produce a set of ligand-protein interactions or to refine the docking results. The latter is a non-exhaustive computer-intensive strategy (the results are biased by the starting docking position and the setting of the dynamic run parameters). Therefore, it is only beneficial at the lead optimization stage and well beyond the existing virtual screening resources/functions [169].

We examined the role of computational science in drug discovery and development processes in this review. Finally, this review comprehensively summarizes the applications of computational applications throughout the process of novel drug discovery, design, and development, further deepening our understanding of Molecular Dynamics simulations, Bioinformatics, and all other applications mentioned above and providing useful drug discovery ideas. Despite the obstacles associated with drug discovery computational applications, increased access to high-performance computing (including grid and cloud resources) can be a time for additional effort to improve protein-ligand docking accuracy and dependability.

## CONSENT FOR PUBLICATION

Not applicable.

## CONFLICT OF INTEREST

The authors declare no conflict of interest, financial or otherwise.

## ACKNOWLEDGEMENTS

Declared none.

## REFERENCES

[1]     Harvey AL, Edrada-Ebel R, Quinn RJ. The re-emergence of natural products for drug discovery in the genomics era. Nat Rev Drug Discov 2015; 14(2): 111-29.
        [http://dx.doi.org/10.1038/nrd4510] [PMID: 25614221]

[2]     Veeresham C. Natural products derived from plants as a source of drugs. J Adv Pharm Technol Res 2012; 3(4): 200-1.
        [http://dx.doi.org/10.4103/2231-4040.104709] [PMID: 23378939]

[3]     Yuan H, Ma Q, Ye L, Piao G. The traditional medicine and modern medicine from natural products. Molecules 2016; 21(5): 559.
        [http://dx.doi.org/10.3390/molecules21050559] [PMID: 27136524]

[4]     Newman DJ, Cragg GM, Snader KM. The influence of natural products upon drug discovery. Nat Prod Rep 2000; 17(3): 215-34.
        [http://dx.doi.org/10.1039/a902202c] [PMID: 10888010]

[5]     Sneader W. Drug Discovery: The Evolution of Modern Medicines. Chichester, UK: Wiley 1985.

[6]     History of Drug Discovery. eLS. Chichester, UK: John Wiley & Sons 2013.
        [http://dx.doi.org/10.1002/9780470015902.a0003090.pub2]

[7]     Balaram P. Drug discovery: myth and reality. Curr Sci 2004; 87: 847-8.

[8]     Xiang M, Cao Y, Fan W, Chen L, Mo Y. Computer-aided drug design: lead discovery and optimization. Comb Chem High Throughput Screen 2012; 15(4): 328-37.
        [http://dx.doi.org/10.2174/138620712799361825] [PMID: 22221065]

[9]     Zhang S. Computer-aided drug discovery and development. Methods Mol Biol 2011; 716: 23-38.
        [http://dx.doi.org/10.1007/978-1-61779-012-6_2] [PMID: 21318898]

[10]    Triggle DJ. Drug discovery and delivery in the 21st century. Med Princ Pract 2007; 16(1): 1-14.
        [http://dx.doi.org/10.1159/000096133] [PMID: 17159357]

[11]    Leelananda SP, Lindert S. Computational methods in drug discovery. Beilstein J Org Chem 2016; 12: 2694-718. [Internet].
        [http://dx.doi.org/10.3762/bjoc.12.267] [PMID: 28144341]

[12]    Chang J, Kim Y, Kwon HJ. Advances in identification and validation of protein targets of natural products without chemical modification. Nat Prod Rep 2016; 33(5): 719-30.
[http://dx.doi.org/10.1039/C5NP00107B] [PMID: 26964663]

[13]    Özdemir V, Hekim N. Birth of industry 5.0: Making sense of big data with artificial intelligence, "the internet of things" and next-generation technology policy. OMICS 2018; 22(1): 65-76.
[http://dx.doi.org/10.1089/omi.2017.0194] [PMID: 29293405]

[14]    Reitz AB, Czupich KM. The challenge of drug discovery in the 21$^{st}$ century. Open Conf Proc J 2010; 45-53.

[15]    Hassan HM. A short history of the use of plants as medicines from ancient times. Chimia (Aarau) 2015; 69(10): 622-3.
[http://dx.doi.org/10.2533/chimia.2015.622] [PMID: 26598407]

[16]    DiMasi JA. Assessing pharmaceutical research and development costs. JAMA Intern Med 2018; 178(4): 587.
[http://dx.doi.org/10.1001/jamainternmed.2017.8703] [PMID: 29610869]

[17]    Annang F, Pérez-Moreno G, García-Hernández R, *et al.* High-throughput screening platform for natural product-based drug discovery against 3 neglected tropical diseases: human African trypanosomiasis, leishmaniasis, and Chagas disease. J Biomol Screen 2015; 20(1): 82-91.
[http://dx.doi.org/10.1177/1087057114555846] [PMID: 25332350]

[18]    Soleilhac E, Nadon R, Lafanechere L. High-content screening for the discovery of pharmacological compounds: advantages, challenges and potential benefits of recent technological developments. Expert Opin Drug Discov 2010; 5(2): 135-44.
[http://dx.doi.org/10.1517/17460440903544456] [PMID: 22822913]

[19]    Doman TN, McGovern SL, Witherbee BJ, *et al.* Molecular docking and high-throughput screening for novel inhibitors of protein tyrosine phosphatase-1B. J Med Chem 2002; 45(11): 2213-21.
[http://dx.doi.org/10.1021/jm010548w] [PMID: 12014959]

[20]    De Vivo M, Masetti M, Bottegoni G, Cavalli A. Role of molecular dynamics and related methods in drug discovery. J Med Chem 2016; 59(9): 4035-61.
[http://dx.doi.org/10.1021/acs.jmedchem.5b01684] [PMID: 26807648]

[21]    Santos R, Ursu O, Gaulton A, *et al.* A comprehensive map of molecular drug targets. Nat Rev Drug Discov 2017; 16(1): 19-34.
[http://dx.doi.org/10.1038/nrd.2016.230] [PMID: 27910877]

[22]    Atangcho L, Navaratna T, Thurber GM. Hitting undruggable targets: viewing stabilized peptide development through the lens of quantitative systems pharmacology. Trends Biochem Sci 2019; 44(3): 241-57.
[http://dx.doi.org/10.1016/j.tibs.2018.11.008] [PMID: 30563724]

[23]    Bjerrum EJ. Machine learning optimization of cross docking accuracy. Comput Biol Chem 2016; 62: 133-44.
[http://dx.doi.org/10.1016/j.compbiolchem.2016.04.005] [PMID: 27179709]

[24]    Brás NF, Cerqueira NMFSA, Sousa SF, Fernandes PA, Ramos MJ. Protein ligand docking in drug discovery. Protein Modelling 2014.
[http://dx.doi.org/10.1007/978-3-319-09976-7_11]

[25]    Ashtawy HM, Mahapatra NR. Molecular Docking for Drug Discovery: Machine-Learning Approaches for Native Pose Prediction of Protein-Ligand Complexes. International Meeting on Computational Intelligence Methods for Bioinformatics and Biostatistics 2014; 8452: 15-32.
[http://dx.doi.org/10.1007/978-3-319-09042-9_2]

[26]    Pushpakom S, Iorio F, Eyers PA, *et al.* Drug repurposing: progress, challenges and recommendations. Nat Rev Drug Discov 2019; 18(1): 41-58.
[http://dx.doi.org/10.1038/nrd.2018.168] [PMID: 30310233]

[27]   Nar H, Fiegen D, Hörer S, Pautsch As, Reinert D. High Throughput Crystallography and its Applications Drug Discovery, Comprehensive Medicinal Chemistry. 3rd ed. Elsevier 2017; pp. 153-79.

[28]   Renaud J-P, Chung CW, Danielson UH, *et al.* Biophysics in drug discovery: impact, challenges and opportunities. Nat Rev Drug Discov 2016; 15(10): 679-98.
[http://dx.doi.org/10.1038/nrd.2016.123] [PMID: 27516170]

[29]   Thomford NE, Senthebane DA, Rowe A, *et al.* Natural Products for Drug Discovery in the 21st Century: Innovations for Novel Drug Discovery. Int J Mol Sci 2018; 19(6): 1578.
[http://dx.doi.org/10.3390/ijms19061578] [PMID: 29799486]

[30]   David B, Wolfender J-L, Dias DA. The pharmaceutical industry and natural products: historical status and new trends. Phytochem Rev 2015; 14: 299-315.
[http://dx.doi.org/10.1007/s11101-014-9367-z]

[31]   Alemayehu C, Mitchell G, Nikles J. Barriers for conducting clinical trials in developing countries- a systematic review. Int J Equity Health 2018; 17(1): 37.
[http://dx.doi.org/10.1186/s12939-018-0748-6] [PMID: 29566721]

[32]   Eder J, Sedrani R, Wiesmann C. The discovery of first-in-class drugs: origins and evolution. Nat Rev Drug Discov 2014; 13(8): 577-87.
[http://dx.doi.org/10.1038/nrd4336] [PMID: 25033734]

[33]   Song , *et al.* Recent advances in computer-aided drug design. Brief Bioinform 2009; 10(5): 579-91.
[http://dx.doi.org/10.1093/bib/bbp023]

[34]   Baldi A, *et al.* Computational Approaches for Drug Design and Discovery: An Over View. IP: 11720464189 2010.

[35]   Alonso H, Bliznyuk AA, Gready JE. Combining docking and molecular dynamic simulations in drug design. Med Res Rev 2006; 26(5): 531-68.
[http://dx.doi.org/10.1002/med.20067] [PMID: 16758486]

[36]   Paul SM, Mytelka DS, Dunwiddie CT, *et al.* How to improve R&D productivity: the pharmaceutical industry's grand challenge. Nat Rev Drug Discov 2010; 9(3): 203-14.
[http://dx.doi.org/10.1038/nrd3078] [PMID: 20168317]

[37]   Bohacek RS, McMartin C, Guida WC. The art and practice of structure-based drug design: a molecular modeling perspective. Med Res Rev 1996; 16(1): 3-50.
[http://dx.doi.org/10.1002/(SICI)1098-1128(199601)16:1<3::AID-MED1>3.0.CO;2-6]   [PMID: 8788213]

[38]   Genovesio A, Kwon Y-J, Windisch MP, *et al.* Automated genome-wide visual profiling of cellular proteins involved in HIV infection. J Biomol Screen 2011; 16(9): 945-58.
[http://dx.doi.org/10.1177/1087057111415521] [PMID: 21841144]

[39]   Scannell JW, Blanckley A, Boldon H, Warrington B. Diagnosing the decline in pharmaceutical R&D efficiency. Nat Rev Drug Discov 2012; 11(3): 191-200.
[http://dx.doi.org/10.1038/nrd3681] [PMID: 22378269]

[40]   Ceska T, Chung CW, Cooke R, Phillips C, Williams PA. Cryo-EM in drug discovery. Biochem Soc Trans 2019; 47(1): 281-93.
[http://dx.doi.org/10.1042/BST20180267] [PMID: 30647139]

[41]   Drulyte I, *et al.* Approaches to altering particle distributions in cryo-electron microscopy sample preparation. Acta Crystallogr. Sect. D Struct. Biol 2018; 74: 1-12.

[42]   Zhang J-H, Chung TD, Oldenburg KR. A Simple Statistical Parameter for Use in Evaluation and Validation of High Throughput Screening Assays. J Biomol Screen 1999; 4(2): 67-73.
[http://dx.doi.org/10.1177/108705719900400206] [PMID: 10838414]

[43]   Kümmel A, Selzer P, Siebert D, *et al.* Differentiation and visualization of diverse cellular phenotypic

responses in primary high-content screening. J Biomol Screen 2012; 17(6): 843-9.
[http://dx.doi.org/10.1177/1087057112439324] [PMID: 22396475]

[44]    Walter CT, Barr JN. Recent advances in the molecular and cellular biology of bunyaviruses. J Gen Virol 2011; 92(Pt 11): 2467-84.
[http://dx.doi.org/10.1099/vir.0.035105-0] [PMID: 21865443]

[45]    Deshpande Dhruva, Grieshober Mark, Wondany Fanny, *et al.* Super-Resolution Microscopy Reveals a Direct Interaction of Intracellular Mycobacterium tuberculosis with the Antimicrobial Peptide LL-37. Int J Mol Sci 21, 18(6741)2020;
[http://dx.doi.org/10.3390/ijms21186741]

[46]    Vernetti L, Gough A, Baetz N, *et al.* Corrigendum: Functional coupling of human microphysiology systems: intestine, liver, kidney proximal tubule, blood-brain barrier and skeletal muscle. Sci Rep 2017; 7: 44517.
[http://dx.doi.org/10.1038/srep44517] [PMID: 28300206]

[47]    Jang KJ, Otieno MA, Ronxhi J, *et al.* Reproducing human and cross-species drug toxicities using a Liver-Chip. Sci Transl Med 2019; 11(517): eaax5516.
[http://dx.doi.org/10.1126/scitranslmed.aax5516] [PMID: 31694927]

[48]    Marx U, Akabane T, Andersson TB, *et al.* Biology-inspired microphysiological systems to advance patient benefit and animal welfare in drug development. Altern Anim Exp 2020; 37(3): 365-94. [published online February 28, 2020].
[http://dx.doi.org/10.14573/altex.2001241] [PMID: 32113184]

[49]    Ravi M, Paramesh V, Kaviya SR, Anuradha E, Solomon FDP. 3D cell culture systems: advantages and applications. J Cell Physiol 2015; 230(1): 16-26.
[http://dx.doi.org/10.1002/jcp.24683] [PMID: 24912145]

[50]    Kinch MS, Haynesworth A, Kinch SL, Hoyer D. An overview of FDA-approved new molecular entities: 1827-2013. DDT 2014; 19(8): 1033-9.
[http://dx.doi.org/10.1016/j.drudis.2014.03.018] [PMID: 24680947]

[51]    Yuan H, Xing K, Hsu H-Y. Trinity of Three-Dimensional (3D) Scaffold, Vibration, and 3D Printing on Cell Culture Application: A Systematic Review and Indicating Future Direction. Bioengineering (Basel) 2018; 5(3): 57.
[http://dx.doi.org/10.3390/bioengineering5030057] [PMID: 30041431]

[52]    Hart T, Chandrashekhar M, Aregger M, *et al.* High-Resolution CRISPR Screens Reveal Fitness Genes and Genotype-Specific Cancer Liabilities. Cell 2015; 163(6): 1515-26.
[http://dx.doi.org/10.1016/j.cell.2015.11.015] [PMID: 26627737]

[53]    Karlgren , *et al.* Drug Metab Dispos 2018.

[54]    Agarwal S, Mehrotra R. An overview of Molecular Docking. JSM Chem 2016; 4(2): 1024.

[55]    Cole J, Davis E, Jones G, Sage CR. Molecular Docking—A Solved Problem? In Comprehensive Medicinal Chemistry III. Elsevier 2017; pp. 297-318.
[http://dx.doi.org/10.1016/B978-0-12-409547-2.12352-2]

[56]    Allen WJ, Balius TE, Mukherjee S, *et al.* DOCK 6: Impact of new features and current docking performance. J Comput Chem 2015; 36(15): 1132-56.
[http://dx.doi.org/10.1002/jcc.23905] [PMID: 25914306]

[57]    Legut M, Dolton G, Mian AA, Ottmann OG, Sewell AK. CRISPR-mediated TCR replacement generates superior anticancer transgenic T cells. Blood 2018; 131(3): 311-22.
[http://dx.doi.org/10.1182/blood-2017-05-787598] [PMID: 29122757]

[58]    Chaput L, Mouawad L. Efficient conformational sampling and weak scoring in docking programs? Strategy of the wisdom of crowds. J Cheminform 2017; 9(1): 37.
[http://dx.doi.org/10.1186/s13321-017-0227-x] [PMID: 29086077]

[59]    Agyeman AA, Ofori-Asenso R. Perspective: Does personalized medicine hold the future for medicine? J Pharm Bioallied Sci 2015; 7(3): 239-44.http://www.ncbi.nlm.nih.gov/pubmed/26229361 [Internet]. [http://dx.doi.org/10.4103/0975-7406.160040] [PMID: 26229361]

[60]    Pasipoularides A. Genomic translational research: Paving the way to individualized cardiac functional analyses and personalized cardiology. Int J Cardiol 2017; 230: 384-401. [Internet]. [http://dx.doi.org/10.1016/j.ijcard.2016.12.097] [PMID: 28057368]

[61]    Fröhlich H, Balling R, Beerenwinkel N, *et al.* From hype to reality: data science enabling personalized medicine. BMC Med 2018; 16(1): 150. [Internet]. [http://dx.doi.org/10.1186/s12916-018-1122-7] [PMID: 30145981]

[62]    Mathur S, Sutton J. Personalized medicine could transform healthcare. Biomed Rep 2017; 7(1): 3-5. [http://dx.doi.org/10.3892/br.2017.922] [PMID: 28685051]

[63]    Forli S, Huey R, Pique ME, Sanner MF, Goodsell DS, Olson AJ. Computational protein-ligand docking and virtual drug screening with the AutoDock suite. Nat Protoc 2016; 11(5): 905-19. [http://dx.doi.org/10.1038/nprot.2016.051] [PMID: 27077332]

[64]    Schneider G, Clark DE. Automated de novo drug design: Are we nearly there yet? Angew Chem Int Ed Engl 2019; 58(32): 10792-803. [http://dx.doi.org/10.1002/anie.201814681] [PMID: 30730601]

[65]    Chen X, Ji ZL, Chen YZ. TTD: Therapeutic target database. Nucleic Acids Res 2002; 30(1): 412-5. [http://dx.doi.org/10.1093/nar/30.1.412] [PMID: 11752352]

[66]    Jorgensen WL. The many roles of computation in drug discovery. Science 2004; 303(5665): 1813-8. [http://dx.doi.org/10.1126/science.1096361] [PMID: 15031495]

[67]    Lin X, Li X, Lin X. A Review on Applications of Computational Methods in Drug Screening and Design. Molecules 2020; 25(6): 1375. [http://dx.doi.org/10.3390/molecules25061375] [PMID: 32197324]

[68]    Schneider G, Fechner U. Computer-based de novo design of drug-like molecules. Nat Rev Drug Discov 2005; 4(8): 649-63. [http://dx.doi.org/10.1038/nrd1799] [PMID: 16056391]

[69]    Bosse R. The future of drug discovery – cutting-edge technologies meet traditional paradigms in assay development. In: Drug Discovery World (DDW). Nuvomondo Ltd., Manchester, UK (2018).

[70]    Vangrevelinghe E, Zimmermann K, Schoepfer J, Portmann R, Fabbro D, Furet P. Discovery of a potent and selective protein kinase CK2 inhibitor by high-throughput docking. J Med Chem 2003; 46(13): 2656-62. [http://dx.doi.org/10.1021/jm030827e] [PMID: 12801229]

[71]    Scarsi M, Podvinec M, Roth A, *et al.* Sulfonylureas and glinides exhibit peroxisome proliferator-activated receptor gamma activity: a combined virtual screening and biological assay approach. Mol Pharmacol 2007; 71(2): 398-406. [http://dx.doi.org/10.1124/mol.106.024596] [PMID: 17082235]

[72]    Lu Y, Nikolovska-Coleska Z, Fang X, *et al.* Discovery of a nanomolar inhibitor of the human murine double minute 2 (MDM2)-p53 interaction through an integrated, virtual database screening strategy. J Med Chem 2006; 49(13): 3759-62. [http://dx.doi.org/10.1021/jm060023+] [PMID: 16789731]

[73]    Zhu J, Mishra RK, Schiltz GE, *et al.* Virtual High-Throughput Screening To Identify Novel Activin Antagonists. J Med Chem 2015; 58(14): 5637-48. [http://dx.doi.org/10.1021/acs.jmedchem.5b00753] [PMID: 26098096]

[74]    Gilbert NC, Bartlett SG, Waight MT, *et al.* The structure of human 5-lipoxygenase. Science 2011; 331(6014): 217-9. [http://dx.doi.org/10.1126/science.1197203] [PMID: 21233389]

[75]    Morshed MN, Cho YS, Seo SH, Han K-C, Yang EG, Pae AN. Computational approach to the identification of novel Aurora-A inhibitors. Bioorg Med Chem 2011; 19(2): 907-16.
[http://dx.doi.org/10.1016/j.bmc.2010.11.064] [PMID: 21194953]

[76]    Zhang X, Acencio ML, Lemke N. Predicting essential genes and proteins based on machine learning and network topological features: a comprehensive review. Front Physiol 2016; 7: 75.
[PMID: 27014079]

[77]    Hua H-L, Zhang F-Z, Labena AA, Dong C, Jin Y-T, Guo F-B. An approach for predicting essential genes using multiple homology mapping and machine learning algorithms. BioMed Res Int 2016; 2016: 7639397.
[http://dx.doi.org/10.1155/2016/7639397] [PMID: 27660763]

[78]    Cardoso F, van't Veer LJ, Bogaerts J, *et al.* 70-Gene Signature as an Aid to Treatment Decisions in Early-Stage Breast Cancer. N Engl J Med 2016; 375(8): 717-29.
[http://dx.doi.org/10.1056/NEJMoa1602253] [PMID: 27557300]

[79]    Chiesi M, Huppertz C, Hofbauer KG. Pharmacotherapy of obesity: targets and perspectives. Trends Pharmacol Sci 2001; 22(5): 247-54.
[http://dx.doi.org/10.1016/S0165-6147(00)01664-3] [PMID: 11339976]

[80]    Miotto R, Li L, Kidd BA, Dudley JT. Deep Patient: An Unsupervised Representation to Predict the Future of Patients from the Electronic Health Records. Sci Rep 2016; 6: 26094.
[http://dx.doi.org/10.1038/srep26094] [PMID: 27185194]

[81]    Zhu K, Dunner K Jr, McConkey DJ. Proteasome inhibitors activate autophagy as a cytoprotective response in human prostate cancer cells. Oncogene 2010; 29(3): 451-62.
[http://dx.doi.org/10.1038/onc.2009.343] [PMID: 19881538]

[82]    Kanzawa T, Germano IM, Komata T, Ito H, Kondo Y, Kondo S. Role of autophagy in temozolomide-induced cytotoxicity for malignant glioma cells. Cell Death Differ 2004; 11(4): 448-57.
[http://dx.doi.org/10.1038/sj.cdd.4401359] [PMID: 14713959]

[83]    Ellis L, Bots M, Lindemann RK, *et al.* The histone deacetylase inhibitors LAQ824 and LBH589 do not require death receptor signaling or a functional apoptosome to mediate tumor cell death or therapeutic efficacy. Blood 2009; 114(2): 380-93.
[http://dx.doi.org/10.1182/blood-2008-10-182758] [PMID: 19383971]

[84]    Boya P, González-Polo R-A, Casares N, *et al.* Inhibition of macroautophagy triggers apoptosis. Mol Cell Biol 2005; 25(3): 1025-40.
[http://dx.doi.org/10.1128/MCB.25.3.1025-1040.2005] [PMID: 15657430]

[85]    Hsu K-F, Wu C-L, Huang S-C, *et al.* Cathepsin L mediates resveratrol-induced autophagy and apoptotic cell death in cervical cancer cells. Autophagy 2009; 5(4): 451-60.
[http://dx.doi.org/10.4161/auto.5.4.7666] [PMID: 19164894]

[86]    Yamamoto A, Tagawa Y, Yoshimori T, Moriyama Y, Masaki R, Tashiro Y. Bafilomycin A1 prevents maturation of autophagic vacuoles by inhibiting fusion between autophagosomes and lysosomes in rat hepatoma cell line, H-4-II-E cells. Cell Struct Funct 1998; 23(1): 33-42.
[http://dx.doi.org/10.1247/csf.23.33] [PMID: 9639028]

[87]    Milano V, Piao Y, LaFortune T, de Groot J. Dasatinib-induced autophagy is enhanced in combination with temozolomide in glioma. Mol Cancer Ther 2009; 8(2): 394-406.
[http://dx.doi.org/10.1158/1535-7163.MCT-08-0669] [PMID: 19190119]

[88]    Kayser S, Levis MJ. FLT3 tyrosine kinase inhibitors in acute myeloid leukemia: clinical implications and limitations. Leuk Lymphoma 2014; 55(2): 243-55.
[http://dx.doi.org/10.3109/10428194.2013.800198] [PMID: 23631653]

[89]    Qian W, Liu J, Jin J, Ni W, Xu W. Arsenic trioxide induces not only apoptosis but also autophagic cell death in leukemia cell lines *via* up-regulation of Beclin-1. Leuk Res 2007; 31(3): 329-39.
[http://dx.doi.org/10.1016/j.leukres.2006.06.021] [PMID: 16882451]

[90] Maclean KH, Dorsey FC, Cleveland JL, Kastan MB. Targeting lysosomal degradation induces p53-dependent cell death and prevents cancer in mouse models of lymphomagenesis. J Clin Invest 2008; 118(1): 79-88.
[http://dx.doi.org/10.1172/JCI33700] [PMID: 18097482]

[91] Petiot A, Ogier-Denis E, Blommaart EF, Meijer AJ, Codogno P. Distinct classes of phosphatidylinositol 3'-kinases are involved in signaling pathways that control macroautophagy in HT-29 cells. J Biol Chem 2000; 275(2): 992-8.
[http://dx.doi.org/10.1074/jbc.275.2.992] [PMID: 10625637]

[92] Yazbeck VY, Buglio D, Georgakis GV, et al. Temsirolimus downregulates p21 without altering cyclin D1 expression and induces autophagy and synergizes with vorinostat in mantle cell lymphoma. Exp Hematol 2008; 36(4): 443-50.
[http://dx.doi.org/10.1016/j.exphem.2007.12.008] [PMID: 18343280]

[93] Aliberti S, Cook GS, Babu BL, et al. International prevalence and risk factors evaluation for drug-resistant Streptococcus pneumoniae pneumonia. J Infect 2019; 79(4): 300-11.
[http://dx.doi.org/10.1016/j.jinf.2019.07.004] [PMID: 31299410]

[94] Rahim R, Strobl JS. Hydroxychloroquine, chloroquine, and all-trans retinoic acid regulate growth, survival, and histone acetylation in breast cancer cells. Anticancer Drugs 2009; 20(8): 736-45.
[http://dx.doi.org/10.1097/CAD.0b013e32832f4e50] [PMID: 19584707]

[95] Ahmad JB, Ajani EO, Sabiu S. Chemical group profiling, *in vitro* and *in silico* evaluation of *Aristolochia ringens* on α-amylase and α-glucosidase activity. Evid Based Complement Alternat Med 2021; 2021: : 6679185.
[http://dx.doi.org/10.1155/2021/6679185] [PMID: 34194523]

[96] Henquin JC. Pathways in beta-cell stimulus-secretion coupling as targets for therapeutic insulin secretagogues. Diabetes 2004; 53 (Suppl. 3): S48-58.
[http://dx.doi.org/10.2337/diabetes.53.suppl_3.S48] [PMID: 15561921]

[97] Shravanti K, Kumar PK, Raju MB, Madhusudhanareddy I, Atyam G. A Review on structure based drug design of Protein Tyrosine Phosphatase 1B Inhibitors for Target for obesity and Type 2 Diabetes Mellitus. J Pharma Res 2010; 3: 2939-40.

[98] Trinh KY, O'Doherty RM, Anderson P, Lange AJ, Newgard CB. Perturbation of fuel homeostasis caused by overexpression of the glucose-6-phosphatase catalytic subunit in liver of normal rats. J Biol Chem 1998; 273(47): 31615-20.
[http://dx.doi.org/10.1074/jbc.273.47.31615] [PMID: 9813078]

[99] Odermatt A, Atanasov AG, Balazs Z, et al. Why is 11beta-hydroxysteroid dehydrogenase type 1 facing the endoplasmic reticulum lumen? Physiological relevance of the membrane topology of 11beta-HSD1. Mol Cell Endocrinol 2006; 248(1-2): 15-23.
[http://dx.doi.org/10.1016/j.mce.2005.11.040] [PMID: 16412558]

[100] Neumiller JJ, White JR Jr, Campbell RK. Sodium-glucose co-transport inhibitors: progress and therapeutic potential in type 2 diabetes mellitus. Drugs 2010; 70(4): 377-85.
[http://dx.doi.org/10.2165/11318680-000000000-00000] [PMID: 20205482]

[101] Gerich JE, Bastien A. Development of the sodium-glucose co-transporter 2 inhibitor dapagliflozin for the treatment of patients with type 2 diabetes mellitus. Expert Rev Clin Pharmacol 2011; 4(6): 669-83.
[http://dx.doi.org/10.1586/ecp.11.54] [PMID: 22111852]

[102] Nguyen F, Starosta AL, Arenz S, Sohmen D, Dönhöfer A, Wilson DN. Tetracycline antibiotics and resistance mechanisms. Biol Chem 2014; 395(5): 559-75.
[http://dx.doi.org/10.1515/hsz-2013-0292] [PMID: 24497223]

[103] Amieva MR. Important bacterial gastrointestinal pathogens in children: a pathogenesis perspective. Pediatr Clin North Am 2005; 52(3): 749-777, vi.
[http://dx.doi.org/10.1016/j.pcl.2005.03.002] [PMID: 15925661]

[104]    Saha D, Karim MM, Khan WA, Ahmed S, Salam MA, Bennish ML. Single-dose azithromycin for the treatment of cholera in adults. N Engl J Med 2006; 354(23): 2452-62.
[http://dx.doi.org/10.1056/NEJMoa054493] [PMID: 16760445]

[105]    Weil AA, Khan AI, Chowdhury F, *et al.* Clinical outcomes in household contacts of patients with cholera in Bangladesh. Clin Infect Dis 2009; 49(10): 1473-9.
[http://dx.doi.org/10.1086/644779] [PMID: 19842974]

[106]    Shields M, Guy RJ, Jeoffreys NJ, Finlayson RJ, Donovan B. A longitudinal evaluation of Treponema pallidum PCR testing in early syphilis. BMC Infect Dis 2012; 12: 353.
[http://dx.doi.org/10.1186/1471-2334-12-353] [PMID: 23241398]

[107]    Al-Younes HM. High prevalence of Chlamydia pneumoniae infection in an asymptomatic Jordanian population. J Microbiol Immunol Infect 2014; 47(5): 412-7.
[http://dx.doi.org/10.1016/j.jmii.2013.04.004] [PMID: 23751768]

[108]    Owusu-Edusei K Jr, Chesson HW, Gift TL, *et al.* The estimated direct medical cost of selected sexually transmitted infections in the United States, 2008. Sex Transm Dis 2013; 40(3): 197-201.
[http://dx.doi.org/10.1097/OLQ.0b013e318285c6d2] [PMID: 23403600]

[109]    Suay-García B, Pérez-Gracia MT. Drug-resistant *Neisseria gonorrhoeae*: latest developments. Eur J Clin Microbiol Infect Dis 2017; 36(7): 1065-71.
[http://dx.doi.org/10.1007/s10096-017-2931-x] [PMID: 28210887]

[110]    Bichsel VE, Liotta LA, Petricoin EF III. Cancer proteomics: from biomarker discovery to signal pathway profiling. Cancer J 2001; 7(1): 69-78.
[PMID: 11269650]

[111]    Chang RL, Xie L, Xie L, Bourne PE, Palsson BØ. Drug off-target effects predicted using structural analysis in the context of a metabolic network model. PLOS Comput Biol 2010; 6(9): e1000938.
[http://dx.doi.org/10.1371/journal.pcbi.1000938] [PMID: 20957118]

[112]    Karplus M, Kuriyan J. Molecular dynamics and protein function. Proc Natl Acad Sci USA 2005; 102(19): 6679-85.
[http://dx.doi.org/10.1073/pnas.0408930102] [PMID: 15870208]

[113]    Khalil HS, Langdon SP, Goltsov A, *et al.* A novel mechanism of action of HER2 targeted immunotherapy is explained by inhibition of NRF2 function in ovarian cancer cells. Oncotarget 2016; 7(46): 75874-901.
[http://dx.doi.org/10.18632/oncotarget.12425] [PMID: 27713148]

[114]    Durrant JD, McCammon JA. Molecular dynamics simulations and drug discovery. BMC Biol 2011; 9: 71.
[http://dx.doi.org/10.1186/1741-7007-9-71] [PMID: 22035460]

[115]    Nguyen NDT, Le LT. Targeted proteins for diabetes drug design. Adv Nat Sci Nanosci Nanotechnol 2012; 3: : 013001.
[http://dx.doi.org/10.1088/2043-6262/3/1/013001]

[116]    Nguyen Vo TH, Tran N, Nguyen D, Le L. An in silico study on antidiabetic activity of bioactive compounds in Euphorbia thymifolia Linn. Springerplus 2016; 5(1): 1359.
[http://dx.doi.org/10.1186/s40064-016-2631-5] [PMID: 27588252]

[117]    Thakral S, Narang R, Kumar M, Singh V. Synthesis, molecular docking and molecular dynamic simulation studies of 2-chloro-5-[(4-chlorophenyl)sulfamoyl]-*N*-(alkyl/aryl)-4-nitrobenzamide derivatives as antidiabetic agents. BMC Chem 2020; 14(1): 49.
[http://dx.doi.org/10.1186/s13065-020-00703-4] [PMID: 32789301]

[118]    Jeyabaskar Suganya Radha Mahendran, Sharanya Manoharan. Virtual Screening and Analysis of Bioactive Compounds of Momordica charantia against Diabetes using Computational Approaches. Research Journal of Pharmacy and Technology 2017; 10(10): 3353-60.
[http://dx.doi.org/10.5958/0974-360X.2017.00596.0]

[119] Thakuria B, Laskar S, Adhikari S. A bioinformatics-based investigation to screen and analyze the bioactivity of *Piper longum* Linn. compounds as a ground-breaking hostile to antidiabetic activity. Pharmacogn Mag 2020; 16 (Suppl. S1): 199-205.
[http://dx.doi.org/10.4103/pm.pm_400_19]

[120] Kaushik PSLK. A. C. Rana, and Dhirender Kaushik A bioinformatics-based investigation to screen and analyze the bioactivity of *Piper longum* Linn. compounds as a ground-breaking hostile to antidiabetic activity. Pharmacogn Mag 2020; 16 (Suppl. S1): 199-205.
[http://dx.doi.org/10.4103/pm.pm_400_19]

[121] Ernst M, Grace OM, Saslis-Lagoudakis CH, Nilsson N, Simonsen HT, Rønsted N. Global medicinal uses of Euphorbia L. (Euphorbiaceae). J Ethnopharmacol 2015; 176: 90-101.
[http://dx.doi.org/10.1016/j.jep.2015.10.025] [PMID: 26485050]

[122] Ji S, Fattahi A, Raffel N, *et al.* Antioxidant effect of aqueous extract of four plants with therapeutic potential on gynecological diseases; Semen persicae, Leonurus cardiaca, Hedyotis diffusa, and Curcuma zedoaria. Eur J Med Res 2017; 22(1): 50.
[http://dx.doi.org/10.1186/s40001-017-0293-6] [PMID: 29178942]

[123] Becker AS, Marcon M, Ghafoor S, Wurnig MC, Frauenfelder T, Boss A. Deep learning in mammography diagnostic accuracy of a multipurpose image analysis software in the detection of breast cancer. Invest Radiol 2017; 52(7): 434-40.
[http://dx.doi.org/10.1097/RLI.0000000000000358] [PMID: 28212138]

[124] Zhao B, Wang L, Qiu H, *et al.* Mechanisms of resistance to anti-EGFR therapy in colorectal cancer. Oncotarget 2017; 8(3): 3980-4000.
[http://dx.doi.org/10.18632/oncotarget.14012] [PMID: 28002810]

[125] Noguchi T, Toiyama Y, Kitajima T, *et al.* MiRNA-503 promotes tumor progression and is associated with early recurrence and poor prognosis in human colorectal cancer. Oncology 2016; 90(4): 221-31.
[http://dx.doi.org/10.1159/000444493] [PMID: 26999740]

[126] Ramanto KN, Parikesit AA. The usage of deep learning algorithm in medical diagnostic of breast cancer. Malaysian J Fundam Appl Sci [Internet] 2019; 15(2): 274-81.
[http://dx.doi.org/10.11113/mjfas.v15n2.1231]

[127] Hinkson IV, Davidsen TM, Klemm JD, Kerlavage AR, Kibbe WA, Chandramouliswaran I. A comprehensive infrastructure for big data in cancer research: accelerating cancer research and precision medicine. Front Cell Dev Biol 2017; 5: 83.
[http://dx.doi.org/10.3389/fcell.2017.00083] [PMID: 28983483]

[128] Muthumani D, Hedina A, Kausar J, Anand V. Phytopharmacological activities of Euphorbia thymifolia Linn. Syst Rev Pharmacy 2016; 7(1): 30-4.
[http://dx.doi.org/10.5530/srp.2016.7.4]

[129] Alakwaa FM, Chaudhary K, Garmire LX. Deep learning accurately predicts estrogen receptor status in breast cancer metabolomics data. J Proteome Res 2018; 17(1): 337-47.
[http://dx.doi.org/10.1021/acs.jproteome.7b00595] [PMID: 29110491]

[130] Kahn B, Collazo J, Kyprianou N. Androgen receptor as a driver of therapeutic resistance in advanced prostate cancer. Int J Biol Sci 2014; 10(6): 588-95.
[http://dx.doi.org/10.7150/ijbs.8671] [PMID: 24948871]

[131] Oyebamiji Abel Kolawole, Tolufashe Gideon Femi, Oyawoye Olubukola Monisola, Oyedepo Temitope A, Semire Banjo. Biological Activity of Selected Compounds from Annona muricata Seed as Antibreast Cancer Agents: Theoretical Study. Journal of Chemistry 2020; 10.
[http://dx.doi.org/10.1155/2020/6735232]

[132] Shikder M, Al Hasib T, Kabir M. Anticancer Mechanism of Withania Somnifera and Its Bioactive Compounds : A Short Review Along with Computational Molecular Docking Study. ChemRxiv Preprint 2020.

[http://dx.doi.org/10.26434/chemrxiv.13038236.v1]

[133] Reddy SVG, Reddy KT, Kumari VV, Basha SH. Molecular docking and dynamic simulation studies evidenced plausible immunotherapeutic anticancer property by Withaferin A targeting indoleamine 2,3-dioxygenase. J Biomol Struct Dyn 2015; 33(12): 2695-709.
[http://dx.doi.org/10.1080/07391102.2015.1004834] [PMID: 25671592]

[134] Mebarka O, Salah B, Khaled L, Ismail D, Houmam B. Molecular docking studies and ADMET properties of new 1.2.3 triazole derivatives for anti-breast cancer activity. Journal of Bionanoscience 2018; 12: 26-36.
[http://dx.doi.org/10.1166/jbns.2018.1505]

[135] Abolghasem B, Eslam P, Mehdi N, Saadat V. QSAR modelling of antimalarial activity of urea derivatives using genetic algorithm–multiple linear regressions. J Saudi Chem Soc 2012; 20(3): 282-90.

[136] Kolawole OA, Olatomide A F, Banjo S. Anti-gastric cancer activity of 1,2,3-triazolo[4,5-d]pyrimidine hybrids (1,2,3-TPH): QSAR and molecular docking approaches. Heliyon 2020; 6(3): : e03561.
[http://dx.doi.org/10.1016/j.heliyon.2020.e03561] [PMID: 32215327]

[137] Iheagwam FN, Ogunlana OO, Ogunlana OE, Isewon I, Oyelade J. Potential Anti-Cancer Flavonoids Isolated From *Caesalpinia bonduc* Young Twigs and Leaves: Molecular Docking and In Silico Studies. Bioinform Biol Insights 2019; 13: : 1177932218821371.
[http://dx.doi.org/10.1177/1177932218821371] [PMID: 30670919]

[138] Muegge I. Selection criteria for drug-like compounds. Med Res Rev 2003; 23(3): 302-21.
[http://dx.doi.org/10.1002/med.10041] [PMID: 12647312]

[139] Bnouham M, Ziyyat A, Mekhfi H, Tahri A, Legssyer A. Medicinal plants with potential antidiabetic activity—a review of ten years of herbal medicine research (1990–2000). Int J Diabetes Metab 2006; 14(1): 1-25.
[http://dx.doi.org/10.1159/000497588]

[140] Chou K-C. Molecular therapeutic target for type-2 diabetes. J Proteome Res 2004; 3(6): 1284-8.
[http://dx.doi.org/10.1021/pr049849v] [PMID: 15595739]

[141] Kugen Collins. *In silico* prediction of anti-malarial activity and pharmacokinetic properties of herbal derivatives of ajuga remota and azadirachta indica. International Centre of Insect Physiology and Ecology 2019.

[142] David TI, Adelakun NS, Omotuyi OI, *et al.* Molecular docking analysis of phyto-constituents from Cannabis sativa with pfDHFR. Bioinformation 2018; 14(9): 574-9.
[http://dx.doi.org/10.6026/97320630014574] [PMID: 31223216]

[143] Kurniawan, Isman; Fareza, Muhammad Salman; Iswanto, Ponco. COMFA, Molecular Docking and Molecular Dynamics Studies on Cycloguanil Analogues as Potent Antimalarial Agents. Indonesian Journal of Chemistry 2020; 21(1): 66-76.

[144] Kalani K, Agarwal J, Alam S, Khan F, Pal A, Srivastava SK. *In silico* and *in vivo* anti-malarial studies of 18β glycyrrhetinic acid from Glycyrrhiza glabra. PLoS One 2013; 8(9): e74761.
[http://dx.doi.org/10.1371/journal.pone.0074761] [PMID: 24086367]

[145] Rivo YB. Antimalarial Properties of Isoquinoline Derivative from Streptomyces hygroscopicus subsp. Hygroscopicus: An In Silico Approach. BioMed Research International 2020; Article ID 6135696: 15.
[http://dx.doi.org/10.1155/2020/6135696]

[146] Subhedar DD, Shaikh MH, Shingate BB, *et al.* Quinolidene-rhodanine conjugates: Facile synthesis and biological evaluation. Eur J Med Chem 2017; 125: 385-99.
[http://dx.doi.org/10.1016/j.ejmech.2016.09.059] [PMID: 27688192]

[147] Oyebamiji AK, Semire B. Studies of 2-[5- (aryloxymethyl)-1, 3, 4-oxadiazol-2-ylsulfanyl] acetic acid derivatives for antibacterial activities *via* dft, qsar and docking approaches. Bulletin of Pharmaceutical Research 2017; 7(3): 148.

[148] Oyebamiji, Abel Kolawole Folashade O. Oyedeji, Isaiah A. Adejoro And Babatunde Benjamin Adeleke. AntiFungal Activities Of 2,4-Dintrophenyl Hydrazones Derivatives: Dft And Docking Approaches. Academ Arena 2018; 10(6): 12-6.

[149] Abel K. Oyebamiji and Semire Banjo. DFT-QSAR and Docking Studies of 2-[5-(aryloxymethyl)-1,3,4-oxadiazol-2-ylsulfanyl] acetic acids Derivatives against *Bacillus subtilis*. Pharma Chemica 2018; 10(3): 135-9.

[150] Abel Kolawole Oyebamiji and Banjo Semire. Studies of 2-[5-(Aryloxymethyl)-1, 3, 4-oxadiazol2-Ylsulfanyl] acetic acid derivative for antibacterial activities *via* DFT. QSAR and docking approaches Bulletin of Pharmaceutical Research 2017; 7(3): 148.

[151] Oyebamiji, A.K., Kaka, M.O., Akintelu S.A., Semire B., Adelowo J.M. (2020) Theoretical Bio-evaluation of 3,5-dimethoxy-N-vinylbenzenamine Analogues as Potential anti-Sclerotinia sclerotiorum. Pharmacology Online; Vol. 3. Pp 427-439.

[152] Iheagwam FNSOR. Computer-Aided Analysis of Multiple SARS-CoV-2 Therapeutic Targets: Identification of Potent Molecules from African Medicinal Plants. 2020. [http://dx.doi.org/10.1155/2020/1878410]

[153] Shode FO, Idowu ASK, Uhomoibhi OJ, Sabiu S. Repurposing drugs and identification of inhibitors of integral proteins (spike protein and main protease) of SARS-CoV-2. J Biomol Struct Dyn 2021; 1-16. [http://dx.doi.org/10.1080/07391102.2021.1886993] [PMID: 33590806]

[154] Tarasov D, Tovbin D. How sophisticated should a scoring function be to ensure successful docking, scoring and virtual screening? J Mol Model 2009; 15(3): 329-41. [http://dx.doi.org/10.1007/s00894-008-0390-0] [PMID: 19066998]

[155] Pham TA, Jain AN. Customizing scoring functions for docking. J Comput Aided Mol Des 2008; 22: 269-286. 50.

[156] Seifert MHJ. Robust optimization of scoring functions for a target class. J Comput Aided Mol Des 2009; 23(9): 633-44. [http://dx.doi.org/10.1007/s10822-009-9276-1] [PMID: 19471858]

[157] O'Boyle NM, Liebeschuetz JW, Cole JC. Testing assumptions and hypotheses for rescoring success in protein-ligand docking. J Chem Inf Model 2009; 49(8): 1871-8. [http://dx.doi.org/10.1021/ci900164f] [PMID: 19645429]

[158] Waszkowycz B, Clark DE, Gancia E. Outstanding challenges in protein-ligand docking and structurebased virtual screening. Wiley Interdiscip Rev Comput Mol Sci 2011; 1(2): 229-59. [http://dx.doi.org/10.1002/wcms.18]

[159] Englebienne P, Moitessier N. Docking ligands into flexible and solvated macromolecules. 4. Are popular scoring functions accurate for this class of proteins? J Chem Inf Model 2009; 49(6): 1568-80. [http://dx.doi.org/10.1021/ci8004308] [PMID: 19445499]

[160] Klebe G. Virtual ligand screening: strategies, perspectives and limitations. Drug Discov Today 2006; 11(13-14): 580-94. [http://dx.doi.org/10.1016/j.drudis.2006.05.012] [PMID: 16793526]

[161] Sagner M, McNeil A, Puska P, *et al.* The P4 Health Spectrum - A Predictive, Preventive, Personalized and Participatory Continuum for Promoting Healthspan. Prog Cardiovasc Dis 2017; 59(5): 506-21. [http://dx.doi.org/10.1016/j.pcad.2016.08.002] [PMID: 27546358]

[162] Djuric U, Zadeh G, Aldape K. Precision histology: how deep learning is poised to revitalize histomorphology for personalized cancer care. npj Precision Onc 2017; 1: 22. [http://dx.doi.org/10.1038/s41698-017-0022-1]

[163] Ashburner M, Ball CA, Blake JA, *et al.* Gene ontology: tool for the unification of biology. Nat Genet 2000; 25(1): 25-9. [http://dx.doi.org/10.1038/75556] [PMID: 10802651]

[164]  Folch J, Petrov D, Ettcheto M, *et al.* Current research therapeutic strategies for Alzheimer's disease treatment. Neural Plast 2016; 2016: 8501693.
[http://dx.doi.org/10.1155/2016/8501693] [PMID: 26881137]

[165]  Pasquier F, Sadowsky C, Holstein A, *et al.* Two phase 2 multiple ascending-dose studies of Vanutide Cridificar (ACC-001) and QS-21 adjuvant in mild-to-moderate Alzheimer's disease. J Alzheimers Dis 2016; 51(4): 1131-43.
[http://dx.doi.org/10.3233/JAD-150376] [PMID: 26967206]

[166]  Katsuno M, Tanaka F, Sobue G. Perspectives on molecular targeted therapies and clinical trials for neurodegenerative diseases. J Neurol Neurosurg Psychiatry 2012; 83(3): 329-35.
[http://dx.doi.org/10.1136/jnnp-2011-301307] [PMID: 22323772]

[167]  Piening BD, Zhou W, Contrepois K, Röst H, Gu Urban GJ, Mishra T, *et al.* Integrative Personal Omics Profiles during Periods of Weight Gain and Loss. Cell Syst 2018; 6: 157-170.e8.
[http://dx.doi.org/10.1016/j.cels.2017.12.013]

[168]  Usha T, Shanmugarajan D, Goyal AK, Kumar CS, Middha SK. Recent updates on computer-aided drug discovery: time for a paradigm shift. Curr Top Med Chem 2017; 17(30): 3296-307.
[http://dx.doi.org/10.2174/1568026618666180101163651] [PMID: 29295698]

[169]  Varela JN, Lammoglia Cobo MF, Pawar SV, Yadav VG. Cheminformatic analysis of antimalarial chemical space illuminates therapeutic mechanisms and offers strategies for therapy development. J Chem Inf Model 2017; 57(9): 2119-31.
[http://dx.doi.org/10.1021/acs.jcim.7b00072] [PMID: 28810125]

# SUBJECT INDEX

**H**

liquid chromatography (HPLCs) 29, 370, 375
thin layer chromatography (HPTLC) 29
High resolution transmission electron microscopy 250
High throughput screening (HTS) 28, 34, 35, 36, 369, 376
HIV therapy 31
*Holarrhena* 172, 193
  *antidysenterica* 172
  *floribunda* 172, 193
Homeostasis 52, 147, 273, 298, 305
  disorder 273
Homoharringtonine 95, 96, 201
Human 39, 40, 163, 194, 195, 196, 254, 284, 299, 373, 381
  African Trypanosomiasis 40
  ailments, degenerative 381
  colon adenocarcinoma 254
  gastric adenocarcinoma 284
  immunodeficiency virus (HIV) 39, 194, 195, 196, 299
  intestinal organoids 373
  lung adenocarcinoma 254
  papillomavirus 195
  pathogens 163
Huntington's disease 215, 222, 231, 232
Hydrocortisone 71
Hydrogen 89, 167, 298, 305, 306
  bonding 167
  peroxide 89, 298, 305, 306
Hydrophobic 11, 123, 167
  aglycone 11
Hyperglycaemia 241
Hyperlipidemia 203
Hyperpyrexia 325
Hypertension 244, 325, 371
Hypodermic syringes 194
Hypoglycemia 204
Hypoglycemic activities 11

# I

Illnesses 85, 144, 215, 230, 233

cancer-related 144
multifactorial 230
neurodegenerative 233
Immune 69, 87, 93, 101, 116, 147, 174, 175, 191, 200, 201, 225, 310, 331
  reactions 225
  response 93, 101, 116, 174, 175, 200, 331
  system 69, 87, 116, 147, 174, 191, 201, 310, 331
Immunity 122, 174, 331
  effector-triggered 174
  microbial-associated molecular-patterns-triggered 174
Immunization, global 23
Immunoassays 29, 312, 372
  ultrasensitive non-radiometric 372
Immunosuppressing effects 69
Immunosuppression 113
Immunotherapeutic tumor arresting activity 383
Immunotherapy drugs 116
Inactivation 168, 169, 196, 202, 311
  antimicrobial photodynamic 311
Induced 283, 285, 329
  cell death 283
  cytotoxicity 285
  transcriptional effects 329
Induction 10, 11, 95, 101, 118, 126, 147, 201, 273, 298, 310
  tumour suppressor proteins 118
Industries 33, 35, 41, 50, 51, 53, 64, 74, 75, 307, 369
  agrochemical 35
  medical 307
  nutraceutical 51
  perfume 53
Infections 2, 6, 8, 22, 31, 32, 40, 55, 140, 143, 144, 145, 150, 167, 233, 235, 305, 307, 308, 310, 311, 312, 328
  dental 6
  invasive 144
  methicillin-resistant *Staphylococcus aureus* 150
  microbially-induced 167
  microflora 328

polymerase 170
synthesis inhibition 301
transcripts 329
ROS-lethality link 302
*Rosmarinus officinalis* 50, 51, 53, 54, 55, 69
ROS 301, 300, 304, 309, 312
   mediated cell killing 300
   neutralization 309
   producing antibacterial agents and test
      bacteria cell 301
   production by quinone-based antimicrobial
      agents 304
   production in cells 300
   suppressor 312
   target proteins 300

# S

*Saccharomyces cerevisae* 67
*Salmonella* 57, 58, 59, 60, 62, 63, 64, 276,
   308
   *enterica* 57, 58, 59, 60, 62, 63, 64
   *typhi* 276, 308
Salmonellosis DNA Gyrase 380
*Salvia cadmica* 148
*Sambucus nigra* 196, 249, 256
Saponins 1, 7, 11, 12, 141, 151, 245, 247, 248,
   249, 259
*Saraca asoca* 249, 256
*Sargassum* 249, 256, 277, 284
   *muticum* 277, 284
   *swartzii* 249, 256
SARS-CoV-2 spike glycoprotein and main
   protease enzyme inhibitors 387
Scanning electron microscopy 165, 250, 281
Scavenging enzymes 306
*Scutellaria barbata* 285
Seaweeds 121, 126, 249, 290
   edible 121
Secondary metabolites 1, 2, 3, 7, 51, 52, 103,
   141, 161, 162, 165, 169, 171, 185, 187,
   191, 195, 196, 197, 200, 204, 205
   of plant products 195
   plant-derived 103, 171

production of 2, 51
Severe 97, 194
   acute respiratory syndrome 194
   multiple organ toxicity 97
Sexually transmitted disease (STDs) 55, 299
Signal 89, 98, 311
   transducing kinases 98
   transduction 89, 311
Signaling molecules, proinflammatory 8
Signalling pathways 121, 202
   targeting numerous 121
*Silybum marianum* 249
Sinensis 205, 332
   schisandra 332
Skin 6, 112, 113, 118, 123, 127, 148, 151,
   227, 250, 282, 325
   disease 325
   healthy 227
   melanoma 123
   transitions 112
Skin cancer 112, 113, 114, 119, 121, 123, 124,
   125, 126, 127, 203, 383
   non-melanoma 112, 113, 119, 125, 126
   protein 383
   treatment of 114, 121
Software, computer docking 384
Sol gel process 240
Solvents, toxic 241
Sources 21, 24, 25, 26, 36, 37, 51, 98, 99, 100,
   121, 186, 187, 197, 215, 224, 225, 227,
   299, 343, 356, 366, 368, 369, 371
   heterogeneity 356
   marine 100
   natural 26, 37, 121, 197, 366, 368, 369, 371
   of oxidative stress 299
Spanish sage thyme 188
Spectroscopic techniques 29
Spectroscopy 37, 250, 333
   diffuse reflectance 250
   dispersive 250
   infrared 250
Squamous cell carcinomas (SCC) 112, 114
*Staphylococcus aureus* 57, 58, 59, 60, 61, 62,
   63, 144, 148, 150, 151, 152, 166, 172,
   193

Xenobiotics 9
X-ray 238, 239, 240, 245, 246, 247, 248, 249,
    250, 280, 281
  diffraction (XRD) 238, 240, 245, 246, 247,
    248, 249, 250, 280, 281
  diffractometer 250
  imaging 239
  photoelectron spectroscopy 250, 281
XRD techniques 280

# Z

Zika virus 195
Zinc oxide 26, 238, 239, 245, 246, 247, 248,
    249, 250, 259, 282, 283, 284, 285
*Zingiber officinale* 250
Zoopharmacognosy 26

www.ingramcontent.com/pod-product-compliance
Lightning Source LLC
Chambersburg PA
CBHW050758220326
41598CB00006B/58